The ESC Textbook of

Preventive Cardiology

European Society of Cardiology publications

The ESC Textbook of Cardiovascular Medicine (Second Edition)
Edited by A. John Camm, Thomas F. Lüscher, and Patrick W. Serruys

The EAE Textbook of Echocardiography
Editor-in-Chief: Leda Galiuto, with Co-editors: Luigi Badano, Kevin Fox, Rosa Sicari, and José Luis Zamorano

The ESC Textbook of Intensive and Acute Cardiovascular Care (Second Edition)
Edited by Marco Tubaro, Pascal Vranckx, Susanna Price, and Christiaan Vrints

The ESC Textbook of Cardiovascular Imaging (Second Edition)
Edited by José Luis Zamorano, Jeroen Bax, Juhani Knuuti, Patrizio Lancellotti, Luigi Badano, and Udo Sechtem

The ESC Textbook of Preventive Cardiology
Edited by Stephan Gielen, Guy De Backer, Massimo Piepoli, and David Wood

The EHRA Book of Pacemaker, ICD, and CRT Troubleshooting: Case-based learning with multiple choice questions
Edited by Haran Burri, Jean-Claude Deharo, and Carsten Israel

Forthcoming
The EACVI Echo Handbook
Edited by Patrizio Lancellotti and Bernard Cosyns

The ESC Handbook of Preventive Cardiology: Putting prevention into practice
Edited by Catriona Jennings, Ian Graham, and Stephan Gielen

The ESC Textbook of
Preventive Cardiology

Edited by

Stephan Gielen
Guy De Backer
Massimo F. Piepoli
and
David Wood

OXFORD
UNIVERSITY PRESS

EACPR
European Association for Cardiovascular Prevention and Rehabilitation
A Registered Branch of the ESC

EUROPEAN SOCIETY OF CARDIOLOGY®

OXFORD
UNIVERSITY PRESS

Great Clarendon Street, Oxford, OX2 6DP,
United Kingdom

Oxford University Press is a department of the University of Oxford. It furthers the University's objective of excellence in research, scholarship, and education by publishing worldwide. Oxford is a registered trade mark of Oxford University Press in the UK and in certain other countries

Impression: 1

Published in the United States of America by Oxford University Press
198 Madison Avenue, New York, NY 10016, United States of America

British Library Cataloguing in Publication Data

Data available

Library of Congress Control Number: 2015934880

ISBN 978–0–19–965665–3

Printed in Italy by L.E.G.O. S.p.A.—Lavis TN

Foreword

Cardiovascular diseases represent the main cause of mortality worldwide, accounting for 36% of all deaths in the European Union in 2010. A wide range of diseases related to the circulatory system is responsible for this epidemic, with ischemic heart disease (IHD) and cerebro-vascular disease (together comprising 60% of all cardiovascular deaths, and causing more than one-fifth of all deaths in EU member states), as the main ones responsible.

The enormous advances in the field of cardiovascular medicine in the last few years have proven to be important in the decrease of mortality in many clinical conditions. However, the growing prevalence of several risk factors, such as hypertension, diabetes, dyslipidemia, obesity, smoking and others, account for an increase in the prevalence and severity of cardiovascular disease. The increase of some of these risk factors occurring in some regions more than others may partially explain the differences observed between the different regions across the globe, and even within the same continent. There are underlying risk factors, such as diet, which may explain differences in IHD mortality across countries. For instance, across EU member states, IHD mortality rates in 2010 were, on average, nearly double for men.

The impact of treatment improvement should therefore be accompanied by an absolute need to promote and improve healthy lifestyles and reduce the weight of the different risk factors, particularly the ones that can be easily prevented if appropriate steps are taken (exercise, smoking, overweight/obesity, diabetes, hypertension and dyslipidemia).

The relationship of prevention strategies with cardiovascular events and death rates is clearly established through different scientific studies. Therefore, the efficacy of primary prevention programs in patients with recognized, treatable risk factors such as hypercholesterolemia, hypertension, diabetes and smoking should be a priority across the different countries. It is also important to recognize the need for a tailored approach considering the differences between different countries, which reinforces the importance of putting surveillance systems in place that may be able to properly monitor the need and implementation of preventable measures.

This is of crucial importance for a successful fight against inequality concerning access to appropriate healthcare in different countries. The role of scientific societies in the dissemination of information and the promotion of different activities (for the public as well as the decision makers) can fill an important gap in this regard. *The ESC Textbook of Preventive Cardiology* represents a major achievement of our European Association of Cardiovascular Prevention and Rehabilitation (EACPR) and, of course, results from the hard work of the editors and outstanding group of authors that have been able to put together a wonderful book that I am sure will become the key reference in the field. Whoever is involved in cardiovascular prevention (basically all health professionals should be) has, in this textbook, a reference that goes from a more detailed description through to practical advice. I am sure this will represent another important element in the road to improving and promoting healthy lifestyles and, consequently, reduce the burden of cardiovascular disease in Europe and beyond.

Prof. Fausto J. Pinto, MD, PhD, FESCC, FACC
President, European Society of Cardiology (ESC)
Cardiology Dpt, CCUL, CAML,
University of Lisbon, Portugal

Preface

What is preventive cardiology?

Preventive cardiology, as the editors see it, encompasses all aspects of knowledge related to the prevention of premature cardiovascular disease—either its manifestation or its progression—with the aim of averting life-threatening cardiovascular events and reducing cardiac mortality.

However, beyond the mere facts preventive cardiology also calls for a different approach to our patients: rather than focusing on the resolution of an acute clinical problem (such as performing a revascularization intervention in an acute myocardial infarction) preventive cardiology aims to influence the underlying systemic disease process of atherosclerosis, of which the acute events are just short manifestations. It focuses on the improvement of long-term outcome rather than acute symptomatic relief, and accepts the fact that the modification of risk factors may have a greater impact on patient longevity than sophisticated interventions.

Cardiovascular prevention faces the dilemma of multiple terminologies coming from diverse historic backgrounds: Cardiac rehabilitation, for example, was established as a combined medical and economic intervention in the 1960s with the primary aim of bringing patients after a myocardial infarction back into work. The focus here was to regain their previous exercise capacity. Secondary prevention relates to the comprehensive pharmaceutical and lifestyle interventions aimed at reducing event recurrence after a first acute coronary or vascular event. Primary prevention tries to identify and to manage individuals at high risk for developing atherosclerotic disease. Primordial prevention comes from a public health perspective to influence the prevalence of risk factors in the general population and aims to prevent people from taking up risky behaviours in the first place. Each nation has its own historical background which is also manifest in different insurance structures to pay for cardiovascular rehabilitation and prevention interventions.

The term preventive cardiology tries to bring these diverse backgrounds together in a single approach. It also accepts the fact that the line separating primary and secondary prevention is increasingly fading away. Novel imaging techniques identify subclinical atherosclerosis, and most patients with coronary artery disease are diagnosed before their first event. The Fifth Joint Task Force Guideline of the European Society of Cardiology (ESC) therefore abolished the differentiation between primary and secondary prevention entirely and looked at the continuum of cardiovascular risk instead. Because of the diversity of healthcare infrastructures, preventive cardiology separates the components of interventions (i.e. lifestyle changes, hypertension treatment, management of dyslipidaemia, etc.) from the actual setting of preventive care (i.e. acute care hospital, rehabilitation institution, community prevention centre, etc.). *The ESC Textbook of Preventive Cardiology* follows this structure because there is enormous variation in healthcare delivery between ESC member states and beyond which determines how cardiovascular prevention is implemented. Whilst the aim of prevention remains the same, the individual pathway for implementation will differ between countries. In this book we give different models from hospital-based rehabilitation to community prevention programmes. Each country can adopt the modules that fit into the context and structure of its healthcare system.

Who is the preventive cardiologist in clinical practice?

In contrast to terms like 'interventional cardiologist' a preventive cardiologist does not depend on a single methodology to define his or her work. In fact everyone who takes a genuine interest in his or her patient's well-being beyond acute care is a 'preventionist'. We address cardiovascular specialists, general physicians, general practitioners/family physicians, nurses, and allied health personnel in this textbook as they all have a role in prevention. The overriding tone of the textbook is its devotion to clinical problem solving. We have therefore introduced clinical cases at the beginning of many chapters to illustrate how difficult it sometimes is to translate guideline recommendations into clinical practice.

Why is this book needed?

In contrast to many other areas of cardiology, there is a limited choice of books on the implementation of cardiovascular prevention in clinical practice. There are academic textbooks focusing on the epidemiological and pathophysiological aspects of prevention and pocket-size checklists to optimize blood pressure or glucose control, but there is no book that unites all the specialist contributions from hypertension, dyslipidaemia, and diabetes into a single resource consistent with the respective guidelines that is accessible and well-structured. The practical hands-on approach is intended to give the reader the knowledge and tools to tackle everyday clinical challenges. This textbook finds a balance between science and practice.

A great challenge in prevention implementation is how to improve patient adherence to recommendations for lifestyle change. This book therefore contains a special chapter on behavioural tools for optimizing patient adherence.

It provides much-needed guidance in controversial areas in cardiovascular prevention such as the role of nutriceuticals, the role of thresholds and target values in lipid lowering, how to interpret novel risk factors (i.e. high-sensitivity C-reactive protein, lipoprotein(a), and how to prudently use imaging in cardiovascular risk assessment and in monitoring subclinical disease.

It answers the question 'How much pain for the cardiac gain?' with regard to the level of physical activity needed to lower mortality and disease risks.

The content of the textbook is available in both print and digital form and the online version will provide direct access to the full text of cited publications and give additional educational material on specific important but rare problems (such as training-based rehabilitation in congenital heart disease). The online version will also be updated when important new evidence is available.

How can you contribute to improving the book further?

The first edition of this textbook will not be perfect in all aspects, and while reading through the chapters you may detect errors or disagree on certain issues. The Editors would welcome your feedback on any aspects of the book that are pertinent to preventive cardiology in clinical practice. Our plan is to keep the book as up to date as possible, so should you have suggestions or ideas for improving the content in its print or online version please contact us directly, through the European Association for Cardiovascular Prevention and Rehabilitation or via the publisher, Oxford University Press. This is not a book to sit on your shelf; it should become a companion in your daily practice of preventive cardiology.

Stephan Gielen
Guy De Backer
Massimo F. Piepoli
and
David Wood

Contents

Abbreviations

2-hPG	2-hour post-load plasma glucose
AA	aldosterone antagonist
AAA	abdominal aortic aneurysm
AACVPR	American Association of Cardiovascular and Pulmonary Rehabilitation
ABI	ankle–brachial index
ACC	American College of Cardiology
ACCF	American College of Cardiology Foundation
ACE	angiotensin-converting enzyme
ACEi	angiotensin-converting enzyme inhibitor
ACS	acute coronary syndrome
ACSM	American College of Sports Medicine
ADA	American Diabetes Association
AHA	American Heart Association
AIX	augmentation index
ALA	alpha-linolenic acid
ApoB	apolipoprotein B
ARB	angiotensin II receptor blocker
ASA	acetyl salicylic acid
AUROC	area under the receiver operating curve
AV	atrioventricular [node]
AV ratio	arteriovenous ratio
BHHS	British Women's Heart and Health Study
BMI	body mass index
BNP	brain natriuretic peptide
BP	blood pressure
CABG	coronary artery bypass graft
CAC	coronary artery calcium
CAD	coronary artery disease
CBVD	cerebrovascular disease
CCB	calcium channel blocker
CCCCP	Comprehensive Cardiovascular Community Control Programme
CCS	Canadian Cardiovascular Society
cfPWV	pulse wave velocity between the carotid and femoral arteries
CFR	coronary artery flow velocity reserve
CHAP	Cardiovascular Health Awareness Program
Chr	chromosome
CHW	community health worker
CIMT	carotid intima–media thickness
CINDI	Countrywide Integrated Noncommunicable Disease Prevention Programme
CKD	chronic kidney disease
CMR	cardiac magnetic resonance imaging
CPET	cardiopulmonary exercise testing
CR	cardiac rehabilitation
CRP	C-reactive protein
CSI	calcification score index
CT	computed tomography
CTA	coronary CT angiography
CV	cardiovascular
CVD	cardiovascular disease
CX	left circumflex coronary artery
DAPT	dual antiplatelet therapy
DBP	diastolic blood pressure
DHA	docosahexanoic acid
DHEA-S	dehydroepiandrosterone sulphate
DHP	dihydropyridines
DM	diabetes mellitus
DRi	direct renin inhibitor
DSMRI	dobutamine-stress magnetic resonance imaging
EACPR	European Association for Cardiovascular Prevention and Rehabilitation
EAS	European Atherosclerosis Society
EASD	European Association for the Study of Diabetes
ECG	electrocardiogram
ECS	echocardiographic calcium score
ED	endothelial dysfunction
EELV	end-expiratory lung volume
EF	ejection fraction
EGIR	European Group for the Study of Insulin Resistance
EMA	European Medicines Agency
EMB	endomyocardial biopsy
EPA	ecosapentaenoic acid
EPIV	echo particle image velocimetry
ERI	effort–reward imbalance
ES	effect size
ESC	European Society of Cardiology

ESH	European Society of Hypertension
ESRD	end-stage renal disease
EVA	early vascular ageing
FCH	familial combined hyperlipidaemia
FDG	18F-fluorodeoxyglucose
FH	familial hypercholesterolaemia
FPG	fasting plasma glucose
FRS	Framingham risk score
GAGs	glycosaminoglycans
GFR	glomerular filtration rate
GI	glycaemic index
GWAS	genome-wide association studies
HAPA	health action process approach
Hb	haemoglobin
HbA1c	glycated haemoglobin
HDL	high-density lipoprotein
HDL-C	HDL cholesterol
HF	heart failure
HFCS	high-fructose corn syrup
HFPEF	heart failure with preserved ejection fraction
HFREF	heart failure with reduced ejection fraction
HPA	hypothalamo–pituitary–adrenocortical [axis]
HPG	hypothalamo–pituitary–gonadal [axis]
HR	hazard ratio
HRQL	health-related quality of life
HRT	hormone replacement therapy
hs-CRP	high-sensitivity CRP
ICAM-1	intercellular adhesion molecule-1
ICD	International Classification of Diseases
ICD	implantable cardioverter defibrillator
IDF	International Diabetes Federation
IDL	intermediate-density lipoprotein
IFG	impaired fasting glucose
IGT	impaired glucose tolerance
IL	interleukin
IMT	intima–media thickness
INR	international normalized ratio
ISH	International Society of Hypertension
JBS	Joint British Societies
LA	left atrial
LAD	left anterior descending coronary artery
LDL	low-density lipoprotein
LDL-C	LDL cholesterol
LGE	late gadolinium enhancement
LMCA	left main coronary artery
LMWH	low-molecular-weight heparin
LPL	lipoprotein lipase
LV	left ventricle/left ventricular
LVAD	left ventricular assist device
LVEF	left ventricular ejection fraction
LVH	left ventricular hypertrophy
MAC	mitral annular calcification
MCE	myocardial contrast echocardiography
MDCT	multidetector computed tomography
MEMS	Medication Event Monitoring System
MET	metabolic equivalent
MI	myocardial infarction
MLHF	Minnesota Living with Heart Failure Questionnaire
NCD	non-communicable disease
NCEP	National Cholesterol Education Program
NHANES	National Health and Nutrition Examination Surveys
NHLBI	National Heart Lung and Blood Institute
NICE	National Institute for Health and Care Excellence
NO	nitric oxide
NRI	net reclassification improvement
NSTEMI	non-ST-segment elevation myocardial infarction
NYHA	New York Heart Association
OCs	oral contraceptives
OGTT	oral glucose tolerance test
OR	odds ratio
PA	physical activity
PAD	peripheral arterial disease
PAR	population-attributable risk
PARs	protease-activated receptors
PARF	population attributable risk fraction
$PETCO_2$	end-tidal CO_2 pressure
Pe_{max}	maximal expiratory pressure
PTH	patient training hours
Pi_{max}	peak inspiratory muscle strength
pPCI	primary percutaneous coronary intervention
PRO	patient-reported outcome
PSC	Prospective Studies Collaboration
PUFA	polyunsaturated fatty acid
PWV	pulse wave velocity
QALY	quality-adjusted life year
RAS	renin–angiotensin system
RAAS	renin–angiotensin–aldosterone system
RCA	right coronary artery
RCT	randomized controlled trial
REACH	Reduction of Atherothrombosis for Continued Health
RPE	rating of perceived exertion
SAQ	Seattle Angina Questionnaire
SBP	systolic blood pressure
SCORE	Systematic COronary Risk Evaluation
SEE	standard error of the estimate
SF-36	Short Form 36 Survey
SFA	saturated fatty acid
SHHEC	Scottish Heart Health Extended Cohort
SHS	second-hand smoke
SIGN	Scottish Intercollegiate Guidelines Network
SPECT	single-photon emission computed tomography
STEMI	ST-segment elevation myocardial infarction
T1DM	type 1 diabetes mellitus
T2DM	type 2 diabetes mellitus
TC	total (serum) cholesterol
TG	triglycerides

THIN	The Health Improvement Network
TEE	trans-oesophageal echocardiography
TTE	transthoracic echocardiography
UA	unstable angina
UFH	unfractionated heparin
UKPDS	United Kingdom Prospective Diabetes Study
VAD	ventricular assist device
VAT	ventilatory anaerobic threshold
VBA	Very Brief Advice
VCAM-1	vascular cell adhesion molecule-1
VE	ventilation
VKA	vitamin K antagonist
WHO	World Health Organization
WMA	wall motion abnormalities

Contributors

Stephan Achenbach
Department of Cardiology, Universität Erlangen Nurnberg, Erlangen, Germany
Chapter 6

Christian Albus
Department of Psychosomatics and Psychotherapy, University of Cologne Köln, Germany
Chapter 9

Frank Bengel
Department of Nuclear Medicine, Hochschule Hannover, Germany
Chapter 6

John Betteridge
University College London Hospitals, London, UK
Chapter 15

Simone Binno
Heart Failure Unit, Cardiac Department, Guglielmo da Saliceto Polichirurgico Hospital, Piacenza, Italy
Chapter 12

Chantal Brisson
Unité de Recherche en Santé des Populations, Centre Hospitalier Universitaire de Québec, Hôpital Saint-Sacrement, Québec, Canada
Chapter 18

Simon Capewell
Department of Public Health and Policy, Institute of Psychology Health and Society, University of Liverpool, Liverpool, UK
Chapter 1

Marco Cattaneo
Ospedale San Paolo and Dipartimento di Scienze della Salute, Università degli Studi di Milano, Milan, Italy
Chapter 4

Renata Cifkova
Center for Cardiovascular Prevention, Thomayer University Hospital, Prague, Czech Republic
Chapter 14

Susan Connolly
National Heart and Lung Institute, Imperial College London, London, UK
Chapter 25

Marie Therese Cooney
Department of Cardiology, Adelaide and Meath Hospital, Dublin, Ireland
Chapter 5

Ugo Corrà
Division of Cardiology, Salvatore Maugeri Foundation, IRCCS, Veruno, Italy
Chapter 21

Margaret E. Cupples
School of Medicine, Dentistry and Biomedical Sciences, Queen's University Belfast, Belfast, UK
Chapters 24 and 25

Jean Dallongeville
Service d'Epidémiologie et Santé Publique – INSERM U1167, Institut Pasteur de Lille, Lille, France
Chapter 11

Dirk De Bacquer
Department of Public Health, University of Ghent, Ghent, Belgium
Chapter 5

Johan De Sutter
Department of Internal Medicine, University of Ghent, Ghent, Belgium
Chapter 19

Robert Fagard
Hypertension and Cardiovascular Rehabilitation Unit, Department of Cardiovascular Diseases, Faculty of Medicine, University of Leuven, Leuven, Belgium
Chapter 14

Pompilio Faggiano
Divisione di Cardiologia, Azienda Ospedaliera Santa Maria degli Angeli, Pordenone, Italy
Chapter 6

Elena M. Faioni
Ospedale San Paolo and Dipartimento di Scienze della Salute, Università degli Studi di Milano, Milan, Italy
Chapter 4

Sara Fernández
The University Hospital Ramón y Cajal, Madrid, Spain
Chapter 6

Daniel Forman
Division of Cardiovascular Medicine, Brigham and Women's Hospital, Boston, Massachusetts, USA
Chapter 12

Oscar H. Franco
Department of Epidemiology, Erasmus MC, University Medical Center, Rotterdam, The Netherlands
Chapter 19

Simona Giampaoli
Istituto Superiore di Sanità, Rome, Italy
Chapter 7

Pantaleo Giannuzzi
Fondazione Salvatore Maugeri, IRCCS, Veruno, Italy
Chapters 8 and 20

Stephan Gielen
Martin-Luther-University Halle-Wittenberg, University Hospital, Halle/Saale, Germany
Chapter 12

Mahée Gilbert-Ouimet
Unité de Recherche en Santé des Populations, Centre Hospitalier Universitaire de Québec, Hôpital Saint-Sacrement, Québec, Canada
Chapter 18

Ian Graham
Charlemont Clinic, Dublin, Ireland
Chapter 5

Christian Heiss
Cardiology Department, University Düsseldorf, Germany
Chapter 6

Christoph Herrmann-Lingen
Department of Psychosomatic Medicine and Psychotherapy, University of Göttingen Medical Centre Göttingen, Germany
Chapter 9

Lesca M. Holdt
Institute of Laboratory Medicine, Ludwig-Maximilians-University Munich, Munich, Germany
Chapter 2

Kurt Huber
Third Department of Internal Medicine, Cardiology and Emergency Medicine, Wilhelminenhospital, Vienna, Austria
Chapter 17

Christina Jarnert
Cardiology Unit, Department of Medicine, Karolinska Institutet, Stockholm, Sweden
Chapter 16

Torben Jørgensen
Research Centre for Prevention and Health, Capital Region of Denmark, Glostrup University Hospital, Copenhagen, Denmark
Chapter 1

Wolfgang Koenig
The Department of Internal Medicine II-Cardiology, University of Ulm Medical Center, Ulm, Germany
Chapter 3

Kornelia Kotseva
International Centre for Circulatory Health, National Heart and Lung Institute, Imperial College London, London, UK
Chapter 26

Ulf Landmesser
Department of Cardiology, Charité – Universitätsmedizin Berlin, Berlin, Germany
Chapter 3

Maddalena Lettino
Cardiologia I, Istituto Clinico Humanitas, Rozzano, Milano, Italy
Chapter 4

Deborah Lycett
UK Centre for Tobacco Control Studies, Primary Care Clinical Sciences, University of Birmingham, UK
Chapter 11

Giuseppe Mancia
Centro Interuniversitario di Fisiologia Clinica e Ipertensione and Istituto Auxologico Italiano IRCCS, Milano, Italy
Chapter 14

Maria Masulli
Diabetes, Nutrition and Metabolism Unit, Department of Clinical Medicine and Surgery, Federico II University, Naples, Italy
Chapter 13

Linda Mellbin
Cardiology Unit, Department of Medicine, Karolinska Institutet, Stockholm, Sweden
Chapter 16

Miguel Mendes
Instituto Do Coração, Carnaxide (Linda-a-Velha), Portugal
Chapter 19

Thomas Mengden
Kerchhoff Rehabilitationszentrum, Bad Nauheim, Germany
Chapter 6

Alessandro Mezzani
Cardiology Division, S. Maugeri Foundation, Veruno Scientific Institute, Veruno, Italy
Chapter 12

Alain Milot
Unité de Recherche en Santé des Populations, Centre Hospitalier Universitaire de Québec, Hôpital Saint-Sacrement, Québec, Canada
Chapter 18

Joao Morais
Cardiology Division, Santo Andre's Hospital, Leiria, Portugal
Chapter 17

Gian Francesco Mureddu
S. Giovanni-Addolorata Hospital, Rome, Italy
Chapter 6

Eike Nagel
Department of Cardiovascular Imaging, King's College London, London, UK
Chapter 6

Josef Niebauer
Universitätsinstitut für Präventive und Rehabilitative Sportmedizin, Universität Salzburg, Germany
Chapter 12

Uwe Nixdorff
European Prevention Center, Medical Center Düsseldorf, Düsseldorf, Germany
Chapter 6

Martin O'Flaherty
Department of Public Health and Policy, Institute of Psychology Health and Society, University of Liverpool, Liverpool, UK
Chapter 1

Neil Oldridge
College of Health Sciences, University of Wisconsin-Milwaukee, Milwaukee, Wisconsin, USA
Chapter 26

Massimo F. Piepoli
Heart Failure Unit, Cardiology, Guglielmo da Saliceto Polichirurgico Hospital, Piacenza, Italy
Chapters 8, 12, and 26

Charlotta Pisinger
Research Centre for Prevention and Health, Capital Region of Denmark, Glostrup University Hospital, Copenhagen, Denmark
Chapter 10

Paola Pontremoli
Heart Failure Unit, Cardiac Department, Guglielmo da Saliceto Polichirurgico Hospital, Piacenza, Italy
Chapter 12

Valentina Puntmann
King's College, London, UK
Chapter 6

Bernhard Rauch
Institut für Herzinfarktforschung Ludwigshafen an der Universität Heidelberg, Germany
Chapter 21

Rona Reibis
Kardiologische Gemeinschaftspraxis Am Park Sanssouci, Potsdam, Germany
Chapter 22

Željko Reiner
University Hospital Center Zagreb, School of Medicine, University of Zagreb, Zagreb, Croatia
Chapter 15

Gabriele Riccardi
Diabetes, Nutrition and Metabolism Unit, Department of Clinical Medicine and Surgery, Federico II University, Naples, Italy
Chapter 13

Lars Rydén
Cardiology Unit, Department of Medicine, Karolinska Institutet, Stockholm, Sweden
Chapter 16

Susanna Sans-Menendez
Institut d'Estudis de la Salut, Barcelona, Spain
Chapter 1

Jean-Paul Schmid
Swiss Cardiovascular Centre Bern, Cardiovascular Prevention and Rehabilitation, University Hospital (Inselspital), Bern, Switzerland
Chapters 22 and 23

Bernhard Schwaab
Curschmann Klinik der Klinikgruppe Dr Guth GmbH & Co. KG, Akademisches Lehrkrankenhaus der Medizinischen Fakultät der Universität zu Lübeck, Germany
Chapter 22

Hugo Saner
Cardiovascular Prevention and Rehabilitation Unit, Anna Seiler-Haus, University Hospitals Inselspital, Bern, Switzerland
Chapter 23

Emer Shelley
The Health Service Executive, Dublin, Ireland
Chapter 24

Daniel Teupser
Institute of Laboratory Medicine, Ludwig-Maximilians-University Munich, Munich, Germany
Chapter 2

Töres Theorell
Department of Neuroscience, Karolinska Institute, Stockholm, Sweden
Chapter 18

Serena Tonstad
School of Public Health, Loma Linda University, California, USA
Chapter 10

Jaakko Tuomilehto
Centre for Vascular Prevention, Danube-University Krems, Krems, Austria; Diabetes Prevention Unit, National Institute for Health and Welfare, Helsinki, Finland; Instituto de Investigacion Sanitaria del Hospital Universario LaPaz (IdiPAZ), Madrid, Spain; Diabetes Research Group, King Abdulaziz University, Jeddah, Saudi Arabia
Chapter 16

Diego Vanuzzo
Cardiovascular Prevention Centre, Health Unit 4 'Friuli Centrale' Udine, and General Health Directorate, Regione Autonoma Friuli Venezia Giulia, Trieste, Italy
Chapter 7

Monique Verschuren
RIVM National Institute for Public Health and the Environment, Centre for Prevention and Health Services Research, Bilthoven, The Netherlands
Chapter 11

Michel Vézina
Unité de Recherche en Santé des Populations, Centre Hospitalier Universitaire de Québec, Hôpital Saint-Sacrement, Québec, Canada
Chapter 18

Giovanni Q. Villani
Heart Failure Unit, Cardiac Department, Guglielmo da Saliceto Polichirurgico Hospital, Piacenza, Italy
Chapter 12

Heinz Völler
Center of Rehabilitation Research, University Potsdam, Potsdam, Germany
Chapter 22

Olov Wiklund
Wallenberg Laboratory for Cardiovascular Research, Sahlgrenska University Hospital, Göteborg, Sweden
Chapter 15

Jose Zamorano
University Hospital Ramón y Cajal, Madrid, Spain
Chapter 6

PART 1

Epidemiology of atherosclerotic cardiovascular disease

CHAPTER 1

Epidemiology of atherosclerotic cardiovascular disease: scope of the problem and its determinants

Martin O'Flaherty, Susanna Sans-Menendez, Simon Capewell, and Torben Jørgensen

Contents

Summary

The epidemic of cardiovascular disease (CVD) in the twentieth century prompted many population-based surveys. Now, a huge number of epidemiological studies provide a clear picture of the risk for CVD. Approximately 80% of CVD can be explained by smoking, high blood pressure, and deterioration of lipid and glucose metabolism, the two latter being mediated through an unhealthy diet (high intake of salt, saturated fat, and refined sugar) and physical inactivity. A causal web for CVD shows that the influence is seen throughout the life course, and that 'upstream' factors like socioeconomic status, health policies, and industrial influences all have a powerful impact on the more downstream parameters like lifestyle and biomarkers. This emphasizes that population-level interventions represent the most effective options for future strategies for the prevention of CVD.

Introduction

Cardiovascular disease (CVD) remains the biggest cause of death worldwide. More than 17 million people died from CVD in 2008, and 10% of the global disease burden, as measured in disability-adjusted life-years, is attributed to CVD. More than 3 millions of these deaths occurred in people below the age of 60 and could have largely been prevented [1]. The percentage of premature deaths from CVD ranges from 4% in high-income countries to 42% in low-income countries, and there are growing inequalities in the occurrence and outcome of CVD between countries and social classes. Over recent decades, CVD deaths have been declining in high-income countries, but have been increasing rapidly in low- and middle-income countries.

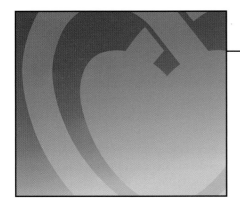

The increase in prevalence of CVD in the first half of the twentieth century prompted the need for population-based surveys. At that time the only data available on CVD were mortality statistics and clinical studies. In 1951 Dawber et al. [2] wrote: 'Of the

epidemiology of hypertensive or atherosclerotic cardiovascular disease almost nothing is known, although these two account for the great bulk of deaths from cardiovascular disease'. An initial attempt was made in St Andrews, Scotland in the 1920s, but was never completed. Instead, Dawber initiated the first population-based study of CVD in the US town of Framingham, MA. Baseline data were collected from 1948–50 on 4469 people aged 30–59 years selected at random from the population. They were followed every second year with questionnaires and clinical and biochemical examinations. Offspring of the original cohort were included and the study is now on its third generation of participants. The Framingham Study was followed by the Seven Countries Study initiated by Keys et al. [3] comprising 16 cohorts in seven countries (the United States, former Yugoslavia, Finland, the Netherlands, Greece, Italy, and Japan), thus covering various parts of the world. A total of 12 763 men aged 40–59 years were enrolled between 1958 and 1964. Parallel with and immediately after initiation of the Seven Countries Study similar studies were begun around the world in Sweden (1963), Denmark (1964), Australia (1966), and the UK (1967) [4–7].

The MONICA (multinational MONItoring of trends and determinants in CArdiovascular disease) Survey was initiated as a result of the decline in CVD mortality which started in the United States in the 1960s and continued in western Europe in the 1970s. The study involved the collection of data at 37 centres in 21 countries between 1979 and 1997. The main findings were that about one-third of the changes in mortality from coronary heart disease (CHD) could be attributed to healthcare and two-thirds to changes in risk factors [8].

Several attempts have been made to pool data from the numerous cohorts around the world, but is often a difficult task because the data were not harmonized from the outset; many of these attempts have therefore ended up with very few variables. In Oxford, Richard Peto succeeded in collecting data from nearly a million people in the Prospective Studies Collaboration (PSC). Due to the problem with data harmonization it is very valuable that the MONICA collaboration (in which many data were harmonized from the very beginning) was continued in the MORGAM study (MOnica Risk, Genetics, Archiving and Monograph), which is still on-going [9]. So that in the future data can be compared across studies and countries, new attempts to secure data harmonization from the start are being attempted in Europe by the European Health Examination Survey (EHES); the aim in this survey is to collect a nationwide, representative cohort in each country over a certain time interval to monitor the development of health indicators [10].

The causes of CVD have been very widely studied but it is still a major cause of death. Therefore, a shift in our understanding of which activities are necessary for the prevention of CVD is necessary. The paradigm says that CVD is a class of slowly developing, chronic diseases which take a long time to reach clinical manifestation; therefore it has been thought that it should also take a long time for the results of preventive measures to become apparent. This paradigm has been challenged by major structural changes in society, indicating that even small whole-society changes can lead to rapid changes in CVD mortality. This had already been seen during the Second World War, but became evident after the collapse of the Soviet Union in countries like the Czech Republic, Poland, and Cuba. This is very much in line with Rose's prevention paradox, which states that a small shift in the risk of a disease across a whole population can lead to a greater reduction in disease burden than a large shift among those people already at risk.

The huge amount of work done to unravel the causes of CVD has provided a valuable model to extend to other chronic diseases. Many epidemiological studies dealing with other chronic diseases have used data from the original CVD cohorts, but they have also initiated separate cohorts. This has led to an understanding of the many common risk factors for chronic diseases such as type 2 diabetes, chronic lung disease, and several common cancers, which have a number of the same risk factors as CVD, such as an unhealthy diet, physical inactivity, smoking, alcohol, and air pollution.

The first studies of cardiovascular epidemiology in the early 1950s together with other similar population-based observational and interventional studies made clear the need for relevant and standardized methods for analysing the data and for educating people to use these methods. The World Health Organization (WHO) published the first training manual (*Cardiovascular survey methods*) in 1968, and at the same time the International Society and Federation of Cardiology initiated annual 10-day teaching seminars, which still continue. Methods used in modern epidemiology and biostatistics were initiated in these studies. But it was not until the 1970s and 1980s that definitions of basic measures were agreed. Innovative epidemiological and biostatistical methods continue to be developed in response to the huge amount of data being collected and the research questions which are raised.

In this chapter we will discuss the scope of CVD, its causes, its burden, and the implications for prevention.

The risk factor paradigm for causation of CVD

Many factors are causally related to the development of arterial atherosclerosis. The major biological risk factors are proximal to events. However, important 'upstream' determinants of disease, including diet, environment, and socioeconomic factors are more distally related; they influence the risk of CHD indirectly through the more proximal risk factors, and also by direct links to events.

Evidence of atherosclerosis has been found in autopsies of teenagers and young adults [11], suggesting that the atheromatous process that ends in clinically apparent coronary events can start early in life [12,13]. Moreover, there is a growing body of evidence that links early life developments, childhood and adolescent trajectories, and adult levels of risk factors. This suggests that coronary disease develops over the life course, and that exposure to causative factors at early ages is also important [14].

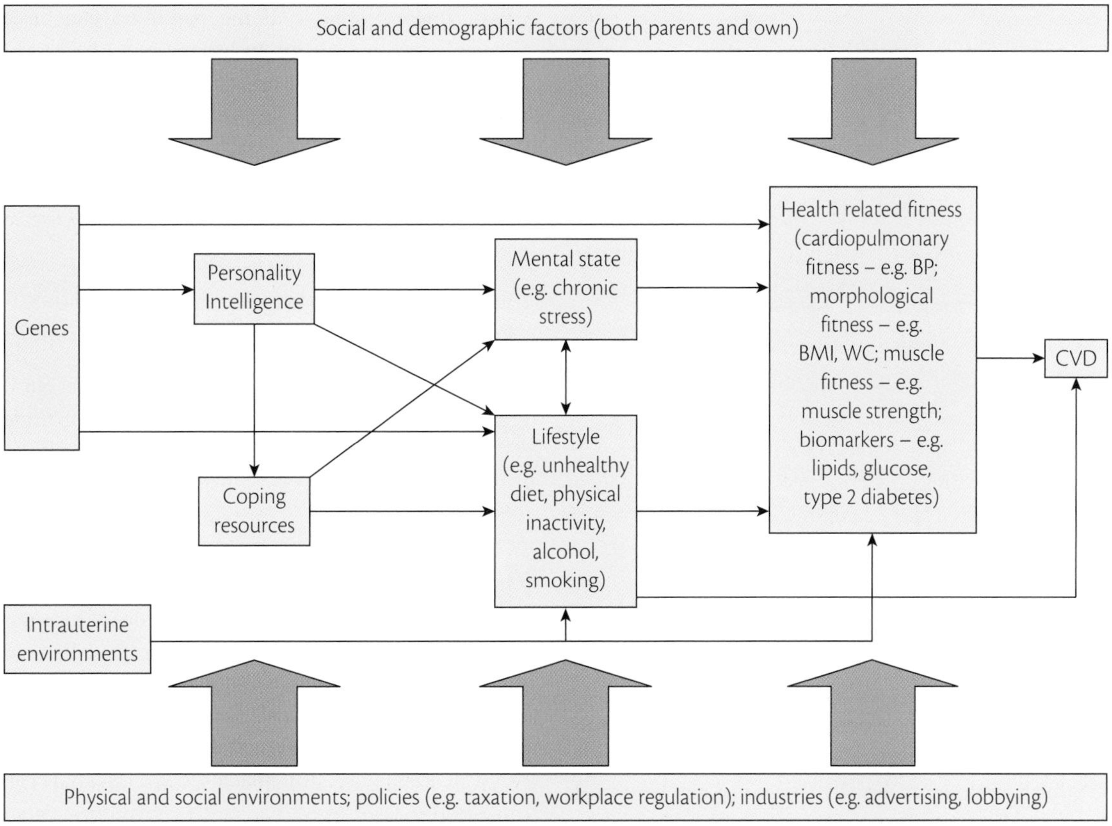

Fig. 1.1 Causal pathway in cardiovascular diseases (CVD): BMI, body mass index; BP, blood pressure; WC, waist circumference.

➲ Figure 1.1 illustrates the life course factors that are important for the development of CVD, starting with genetics and intrauterine conditions and showing the socioeconomic and environmental 'upstream' factors that influence the life course.

When we talk about the causes of CVD we do not use the word 'causes' in the everyday sense of the word. Our common sense tells us that when all causes are in place an event should happen. For example, if we press a light switch we expect the light to come on; if not we check the bulb or the power supply. If we phoned an electrician to fix the light and they said something like: 'sometimes the light is on when you press the switch, but not every time, and sometimes it will take years before it is on and other times it will be on even if you don't press the switch' we would call another electrician! But dealing with the causes of chronic diseases such as CVD is very much like that situation, so we need to explain more precisely what we are talking about when we talk about causes of diseases so we can understand this uncertainty without losing the common concept of causation.

The eighteenth-century philosopher David Hume described causes as necessary or sufficient. A necessary cause will always have been present at some time before the disease, but need not lead to the disease. A classic example of this is a virus, which is necessary to get the infection in question but will not always lead to the disease. A sufficient cause is an exposure that is always followed by the disease, but there can be other causes as well. There are few examples, but insufficient iron intake could be such a cause of anaemia, which also has other causes. We very seldom see both necessary and sufficient causes, but single-gene diseases like sickle cell anaemia are examples.

When dealing with chronic diseases like CVD we normally have a situation in which the disease sometimes follows the exposure but not always, and sometimes the disease is seen in people who have not faced the exposure. In the 1970s Mackie [15] and Rothman [16] independently introduced the INUS principle. This elegantly explains that causes may act together in concert. If we look at the causes as components of different causal fields we can still work within the common concept of causality. The INUS principle states that:

> Component causes are **I**nsufficient in themselves (as they require the presence of the other components in the causal field), but they are **N**ecessary within the causal field. Causal fields are **U**nnecessary (because there are other causal fields), but they are **S**ufficient (if they are complete).

➲ Figure 1.2 shows a very simplistic example, as there can be many causal fields and many components in each field.

The INUS principle is a theoretical model, but if it works in practice it is useful. The model can explain why not all smokers get CHD. Smoking is only one component in the causal field, and another component (or several others) needs to be present before the person will get CHD, for example certain genes. On the other hand people who have never smoked can also get CHD, which then is caused by components (e.g. high cholesterol) from other causal fields; but not all people with high cholesterol develop CHD, which means that other components need to be present too.

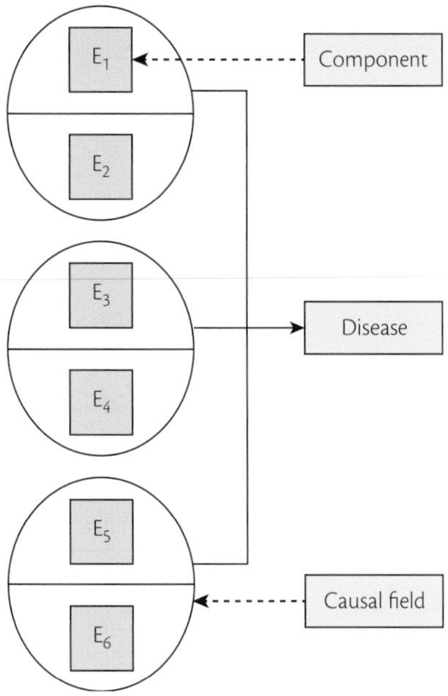

Fig. 1.2 A theoretical model for causality in chronic diseases [15,16].

The model also can be helpful in understanding the (lack of) time between exposure and disease outcome, as induction time could be one of the other components. Finally the model can be useful in prevention, as it is theoretically only necessary to avoid/remove one of the components in each causal field.

A more pragmatic way of understanding causality in CVD was described by Austin Bradford Hill in 1965, known as Hill's criteria of causation. He described nine minimum conditions needed to establish a causal relationship between two items:

1. Temporal relationship: exposure always precedes the outcome. This is the only absolutely essential criterion and underlines the need for longitudinal cohort studies in epidemiology.
2. Strength: defined by the size of the association measured by appropriate statistical tests—the stronger the association the more likely the causal relationship. However, weak associations can still be causal (e.g. second-hand smoke and CHD).
3. Dose–response relationship—an increase in exposure increases the risk. However, the absence of a dose–response does not rule out causality, as a certain threshold for exposure can exist.
4. Consistency. If an association is causal it should be consistent across studies, geography, and time. This has been nicely demonstrated within CVD epidemiology because the same risk factors emerge in different studies at different times. On the other hand all studies could miss the same confounders, but this is unlikely in the case of established risk factors for CVD.
5. Plausibility. The association should agree with the currently accepted understanding of pathological processes. There needs to be a theoretical basis for the association. On the other hand, research that disagrees with established theory is not necessarily wrong, but can force a shift in the paradigm.
6. Consideration of alternative explanations. Other hypotheses should always be considered and discussed.
7. Experimental studies. If the condition can be prevented or ameliorated by an appropriate regimen the causal association is strengthened. This is one of the very strong criteria. Such experiments can be done in randomized clinical trials (e.g. lipid-lowering therapy reduces the occurrence of CHD).
8. Specificity: a single cause produces a specific effect. This condition is extremely seldom seen for CVD.
9. Coherence. The association should be compatible with existing theory and knowledge. It must be ascertained if any current knowledge has to be rejected in order to accept an association as causal.

Ideally, all these criteria can be used in an overall evaluation of possible causality for an exposure and the development of CVD, although this not always possible.

Major established risk factors for CHD

Smoking

The US Surgeon General's report of 1964 [17] suggested that smoking was a definite risk factor for lung cancer and chronic bronchitis, but was less emphatic in describing its relationship with CVD risk, suggesting that although risk increases in cigarette smokers the association had not been proven causal. However, over subsequent years a large body of evidence linking tobacco smoking to changes in inflammatory and thrombosis markers and with subclinical markers of atherosclerosis was accrued [18]. This evidence suggested a clear link between smoking and basic atherosclerotic disease mechanisms, increasing the risk of CHD by almost twofold. Important gender differences in risk exist, with women experiencing a higher risk of incident acute myocardial infarctions (MIs) than men [19–22] that is not easily explained by differences in smoking patterns or baseline risk [19]. Data from systematic reviews of tobacco cessation studies after MI showed marked reductions in risk of almost 40% within 2 years [23,24].

The harmful effects of second-hand smoke have been also solidly established, with a relative risk for CHD of 1.26 to 1.65 with exposure to second-hand smoke [25,26], and legislation banning smoking in public places and the workplace has rapidly decreased admissions for MI [27].

Blood lipids

An association between blood lipids and atheromatosis in animals was first suggested over 100 years ago by Virchow and then Anitschcov. Observational evidence from numerous migrant studies, the Seven Countries Study [3], and the Framingham Study [28,29] found the association in humans—confirmed later in the MRFIT [30], PROCAM [31], and ARIC [32] studies. The development of lipid reduction therapies, particularly HMG-CoA reductase inhibitors (statins) provided experimental evidence of causality [33,34].

Total cholesterol is clearly associated with CHD risk, with a 1 mmol/L reduction in total cholesterol being associated with reductions in CHD mortality ranging from about 50% in men and women aged 40–49 and 17% in those aged 70–79. This is across the range of cholesterol levels seen in most developed countries, and is a linear relationship with no evidence of a threshold [35].

Statins effectively reduce cholesterol levels by between 1.0 and 2.8 mmol/L (depending on drug, dose, and adherence). A reduction of 1 mmol/L is associated with an 11% reduction in risk of ischaemic heart disease, increasing to 36% after 5 years [33].

High-density lipoproteins (HDL) represent another important lipid subfraction; they are protective and have a strong inverse association with CHD events. Thus, an increase in HDL of 1 mg/dl is associated with a reduction of 2–3% in total CVD risk [36]. Interestingly, randomized clinical trials of novel drugs aimed to increase HDL levels have consistently failed to show any reduction in CVD risk [37].

Triglycerides have been associated with CVD risk, but their levels tend to reciprocate HDL concentrations. Their role as an independent risk factor remains controversial, and current control strategies only target them in special cases [38].

Dietary saturated fats are the main determinants of blood lipid levels, particularly total cholesterol [39]. However, not all dietary fats are harmful. Monounsaturated fatty acids (e.g. olive oil), polyunsaturated fatty acids (e.g. marine omega-3 fatty acids), and plant-based omega-6 fatty acids all consistently reduce CVD risk, particularly when they replace saturated fats or trans-fats [40–43].

Blood pressure

Numerous observational and experimental studies have linked high blood pressure with adverse cardiovascular outcomes, and the association has been characterized at both metabolic and functional levels [44,45].

Diastolic blood pressure (DBP) has been identified as an independent, graded, and important predictor of CVD risk in large, prospective cohort studies and randomized clinical trials [44–46]. However, later studies which focused on systolic blood pressure (SBP) and risk demonstrated an even stronger association. The PSC systematic review found that each difference of 20 mmHg in SBP was associated with almost a threefold difference in stroke mortality and a twofold difference in ischaemic heart disease mortality. Interestingly, the relationship was linear down to an SBP as low as 115 mmHg. Although the risk attenuated in those aged 80 years and above, the absolute difference in event rates was biggest at older ages. For stroke, DBP and SBP are equally important as determinants of risk up to age 62 years, whereas SBP is more important in older adults [46]. Reduction of blood pressure, and crucially SBP, significantly reduces vascular events and deaths in people who are free from vascular disease. The CVD and CHD risk associated with blood pressure has been also found in many other populations [47,48]. Antihypertensive treatments reduce CHD mortality by about 10–12%, and reduce stroke risk more substantially, with a 37% reduction in total events and a 36% reduction in fatal strokes [47,48].

Several factors determine blood pressure levels, including chronic stress [49], physical activity [50], and body weight [51,52]; but diet, and particularly salt intake, play a major role [53]. A large body of evidence suggests that salt consumption is probably the single most important factor determining blood pressure levels. The biological mechanisms have been explored in animal studies, and epidemiological evidence has been found in ecological studies like INTERSALT [54] or INTERMAP [55] and in the prospective cohort study EPIC-Norfolk [56]. INTERSALT estimated that the effect of a sodium intake higher by 100 mmol/day was to raise SBP by approximately 3–6 mmHg (SBP) and DBP by 0-3 mmHg. This relation prevailed for both men and women, for younger and older people, and for participants without hypertension [54]. The INTERMAP study, with improved exposure and outcome measurements, confirmed the association at the individual level in more detail, although for a more limited set of countries [55]. The EPIC-Norfolk study found that individuals with salt intakes below 5 g/day halved their risk of developing high blood pressure compared with those with high intakes (10 g/day or more) [56]. Interestingly, they also found that a high intake of dietary potassium was associated with lower blood pressure [56].

The effect of salt on cardiovascular outcomes has also been explored in randomized controlled trials. The THOP I and II studies [57] found that a reduction of salt intake resulted in a reduction in SBP of between 1.2 and 1.7 mmHg and a 25% reduction in risk of cardiovascular events over 10 to 15 years. An educational campaign on salt intake in two matched communities in Portugal [58] showed that the average blood pressure fell by 3.6/5.0 mmHg at 1 year and 5.0/5.1 mmHg at 2 years in the intervention community. Although other community intervention trials failed to observe changes in salt consumption, they also reported a lack of change in blood pressure levels.

The focus on salt reduction initiatives across entire populations has probably been one of the most important drivers in decreasing blood pressure levels in many populations [53,59,60].

Obesity

Obesity and overweight are conditions associated with an imbalance in energy intake and expenditure. The current physical, cultural, and marketing environments are a powerful determinant of the continuing increases in obesity prevalence reported in the late twentieth and early twenty-first centuries [61,62].

Adipose tissue is metabolically active and can release a host of mediators that control body weight homeostasis and insulin resistance. Crucially, it also influences inflammation and thrombotic pathways leading to endothelial dysfunction and atherosclerosis [63]. Not surprisingly, therefore, obesity is strongly associated with diabetes and elevated CVD risk factors [64] and is associated with excess mortality, mainly attributable to CVD and several common cancers [65–67].

However, the independent effect of obesity is probably small [68], suggesting that most of its associated risk is mediated by more proximal risk factors, like SBP, elevated cholesterol, and diabetes.

Diabetes mellitus

Diabetes mellitus (DM) is a risk factor for CHD, increasing risk by approximately 2.4 times in men and 5.1 times in women [69,70]. It also accelerates the onset of early atheroma formation at young ages [71] and negates the low risk otherwise experienced by premenopausal women [72]. Patients with diabetes have similar rates of events to patients with pre-existing CHD but without diabetes [73]. All levels of abnormal glucose metabolism are associated with CVD, primarily diabetes-induced arterial macrovascular atherosclerotic disease [43].

The mechanisms leading to enhanced development of atherosclerosis in people with diabetes are complex, and probably involve endothelial dysfunction, inflammatory mediators, modification of lipid metabolism, hypertension, and renal impairment [74,75]. This direct endothelial toxicity is further compounded by the fact that people with diabetes tend to have higher levels of other risk factors [76]. Not surprisingly, cardiovascular events are the main cause of death in adults with diabetes, with 80% of them attributable to CVD [77].

However, there is still substantial doubt about the benefits of controlling diabetes for cardiovascular risk. Epidemiological evidence suggests that diabetes is an important, strong, and independent risk factor. Yet, the results of randomized controlled trials on intensive glucose control strategies showed no effect on stroke outcomes or mortality, only a decrease in non-fatal MIs [78,79]. This lack of reversibility is interesting, as diabetes is considered to confer the same level of risk as in those with established CHD [73], but this perhaps partly reflects that many patients already have advanced atherosclerotic disease when they are diagnosed with diabetes. Screening for type 2 diabetes and intensive treatment do not reduce the incidence of CVD [80].

The evidence for diabetes prevention appears more encouraging. A growing body of evidence based on randomized clinical trials suggest that the incidence of diabetes could be halved relatively quickly with multiple interventions including changes to lifestyle and diet [81]. In the Diabetes Prevention Program study metformin was associated with a 31% reduction in the risk of diabetes, albeit less than the 58% risk reduction observed in the diet and lifestyle arm [82].

Physical inactivity

Physical inactivity has been recognized since the 1950s to be associated with total mortality and cardiovascular risk; however, most of the evidence base is observational. This body of evidence suggests that moving from a sedentary state to a sustained active lifestyle can reduce total mortality and CVD risk by about 20–35% [83]. There is often a graded response, and with additional benefits in other outcomes too, like mental health, diabetes, certain cancers, and osteoporosis [84]. Physical activity might prevent CVD through pathways mediated by other risk factors, such as increasing HDL levels [85], reducing blood pressure [86], improving insulin resistance and glucose tolerance, and reducing the risk of type 2 diabetes [87]. Recently even very low level activity has been shown to have a beneficial effect [88]; this has led to the introduction of 'sedentarism' (e.g. TV viewing, using a PC) as an independent risk factor [89,90], which may be mediated through lack of activation of the lipoprotein lipase (LPL) system (LPL is important for controlling plasma triglyceride catabolism, HDL cholesterol, and other metabolic risk factors) [91].

Despite controversies regarding exposure measurement and the complex causal pathways involved, physical inactivity seems to confer a similar risk in men and women, and is independent of the level of adiposity [92]. Interestingly, it seems as if it is mainly leisure time physical activity and not occupational physical activity that is beneficial in reducing CVD risk. There is a stronger protective effect for CHD than for stroke [93,94].

The built environment has a strong influence on physical activity. Aspects like housing, land use, housing density, open space, and patterns of compact development in city and community planning are associated with increased levels of physical activity but do not seem to affect body weight [95]. Transport policies, and multicomponent interventions in workplaces or schools can also increase levels of physical activity [96].

Physical activity is not included in any clinical risk scores. However, most primary prevention guidelines recommend periods of moderate to intense physical activity as an effective intervention to reduce cardiovascular risk [97].

Dietary patterns and other nutritional factors

We have already discussed the link between dietary factors and specific biological risk factors. However, substantial evidence to support the concept of cardioprotective nutrients and dietary patterns has been accumulated since the landmark Seven Countries Study [98]. Although many of the data are observational, causality can be established for beneficial effects of the intake of fruit and vegetables, nuts, wholegrains, and fish, and also for detrimental effects of trans-fatty acids, foods and beverages with high glycaemic index, and processed meat [98,99]. Furthermore, the 'Mediterranean diet pattern' and the DASH diet have shown beneficial effects confirmed in randomized controlled trial [98]. An analysis of diet patterns in the INTERHEART case–control study has found that higher levels of a 'prudent diet' (rich in fruits and vegetables) were powerfully associated with reduced risk of a first acute MI across participants in 52 countries [100]. In general, beneficial dietary patterns are associated with high levels of cardiovascular protective macronutrients and micronutrients [98].

Among nutritional risk factors, industrial trans-fats merit special attention. These are artificial fats used mainly in processed foods for commercial reasons and are not considered to have any nutritional value. They have a profound effect on increasing CHD risk. Replacing 1% of energy from trans-fat with unsaturated fats reduces CHD risk by approximately 12% (5.5–18.5%) [40]. Several countries have now successfully implemented the complete removal of industrial trans-fats from human food [101].

In summary, certain dietary patterns have established cardiometabolic benefits. These are diets that are higher in dietary fibre, healthy fatty acids, vitamins, antioxidants, potassium, other minerals, and phytochemicals and lower in refined carbohydrates, sugars, salt, saturated fatty acids, dietary cholesterol, and trans-fat. The role of other dietary supplements, micronutrients, and vitamins is complex and remains less than clear [99].

Alcohol

The relationship between alcohol intake and CHD risk is complex. The relationship has been described as 'J'-shaped, with increased risk at high alcohol consumption and zero consumption and a lower risk for low to moderate intake [102,103], or as 'L'-shaped, where a protective effect was observed for alcohol consumption at low to high levels but not for zero consumption. However, there are concerns about publication bias for low alcohol intake [102,104,105]. There is greater clarity about increased levels of mortality from stroke with increasing alcohol consumption [105–107].

An alcohol consumption of between 2.5 and 14.9 g/day was associated with a reduction in risk of about 14–35% for CVD mortality, and for incidence and mortality for CHD and strokes [105,106]. The intake of ethanol seems to be the most important factor, rather than any specific component of the alcoholic beverage such as beer or wine [108,109].

However, the pattern of drinking is more important. Regular low to moderate intake seems to be protective [108–111], while episodic immoderate ('binge') alcohol intake confers a considerable risk of incident MI and total mortality [109,112].

Furthermore, chronic heavy alcohol intake might have major consequences, as illustrated by the huge temporal variations in CVD mortality rates seen in Russia and other former soviet socialist republics after the breakdown of the Soviet Union in the 1990s [113]. It is clear now that this phenomenon is not caused by misclassification of the causes of death [113,114]. Although causality has not been established with experimental data, current guidelines in most countries recognize that while low to moderate intake of alcohol might be beneficial for CVD risk, higher intakes are harmful. Alcohol consumption is thus not recommended by the British Heart Foundation, the National Heart Forum, or the American Heart Association [115].

Other risk factors: social determinants, life-course influences, and genetic factors

The socioeconomic determinants of health are usually assessed as social gradients in mortality or morbidity. In the United Kingdom these patterns are readily visible, with substantial mortality gradients by socioeconomic levels or geographically across a north–south divide. For example, the mortality rate ratio between the most deprived quintile and the most affluent is 1.5 for both men and women, and almost 3 if we consider only premature deaths of people under 65 years of age [116,117]. In the United States, people without a high-school education lost almost three times as many life-years as more educated people, and CVD accounted for about 35% of this difference (CHD itself explained 11%) [118].

These gradients are also evident in the distribution of cardiovascular risk. For example, in the United States there are major differences in risk factor prevalence and combined cardiovascular risk by ethnicity [119,120] and other measures of socioeconomic status [121]. In several European countries, people in the lower socioeconomic strata are more frequently current smokers, diabetic, have a higher BMI, a higher intake of alcohol, and a lower intake of fruit and vegetables [122].

Worse socioeconomic conditions in childhood are frequently associated with increased CVD risk in adulthood [123,124]. This is possibly mediated by early life and childhood trajectories in risk factors, predicting cardiovascular risk factor levels in young adulthood [14,125].

Social and environmental influences in childhood may also have an important effect on CVD risk in adulthood. The timing of other exposures starting *in utero*—and even transgenerationally—is also important [126]. Perhaps the first evidence for early life influences on adult CHD risk was provided by Forsdahl [127], who found that infant mortality rates in the early twentieth century were strongly correlated with the CHD mortality rate seven decades later, suggesting that early childhood nutrition or perinatal phenomena might be linked to CHD risk.

The hypothesis of 'developmental origins' of CHD, as championed by Barker [128], suggests that many measures of foetal growth, as a proxy for the womb environment, have shown that *in utero* events are related to risk of CHD in adult life [129,130].

Perinatal and early childhood influences also are linked to later, pre-adulthood risk factor levels [125,129]. Moreover, substantial 'tracking' occurs; thus cholesterol, BMI, and SBP measured in childhood or adolescence predict CHD risk 50 years later [129].

However, the scale of life-course effects on causation of CHD remains unclear. Not least because such influences operating on individuals would be expected to operate at the population level as cohort effects [131]. Furthermore, potentially confounding socioeconomic effects can be difficult to disentangle. However, the decline in CHD in most high-income countries can be better explained by period effects than cohort effects [132].

Genetic factors also play a causal role in CHD. The Framingham Offspring Study suggests that heritability may be an important factor for premature CHD. Participants with a family history of premature CHD (defined as a history of CHD in first-degree relatives before the age of 55 in men and 65 in women) had twice the risk of those who did not, even after adjustment for classical risk factors [133]. Single-gene association and several candidate loci and gene sets have been identified in linkage and genome-wide association studies, usually associated with metabolic pathways related to lipid metabolism [134].

The interaction of environmental factors with particular genetic risk profiles may also be important in CHD. Thus, for example, APOE e4 high-risk alleles might not affect CHD risk in the absence of smoking [135]. Although Mendelian genetics or even genome-wide association studies fail to explain a substantial proportion of the burden of CHD, heritable and non-heritable epigenetic changes might occasionally play an important role in individual cases [136].

However, in general, the potential candidates have small effect sizes [137], low predictive power, and low population impact measures [137] compared with classical risk factors [138]. Genetic factors account for less than 20% of the variance in maintenance of ideal cardiovascular health (an aggregate risk factor package including total cholesterol < 200 mg/dl, blood pressure <120/<80 mmHg, and no diabetes). Behavioural and environmental factors thus have a far more powerful role in preservation or loss of optimal levels of health with ageing.

The rapid changes over time within countries and the marked differences in CHD mortality observed between countries, as discussed above, are powerful indicators of the major role of environmental factors and make it very implausible to attribute such trends to changes in the distribution of genetic determinants [139]. Moreover, the results from classical studies of migrants, particularly among Japanese populations, suggest that the risk of CHD and stroke increases substantially when populations are exposed to western dietary environments [140,141].

Psychosocial factors, particularly personality and chronic stress, have been described to be associated with cardiovascular risk. Although the association of personality type 'A' with CHD risk has been largely abandoned [142], hostility and rage are associated with an increased risk in people free of CHD [143]. The Whitehall II study showed that low job control, but not job demands or social support, was associated with increased risk of CHD [144]. Permanent work- or home-related stress was associated with the risk of incident MI in the MRFIT trial and the INTERHEART study [145,146].

Structural determinants

The causal web in Fig. 1.1 represents a complex interaction of multiple levels of causal factors. Most of our knowledge about cardiovascular epidemiology has been developed with the individual as the unit of analysis. However, a mounting evidence base suggests that 'structural' factors are as important as the traditional biological risk factors and are powerful determinants of burden of CVD, and probably in generating and maintaining social inequalities [147].

Current sociological theories have shown the complex interrelationship between levels of different determinants of cardiovascular risk and other non-communicable diseases. Individuals do not act in a vacuum but their behaviour is nested in a number of other layers. These layers are essentially a hierarchy from the micro level (e.g. individual choice, genetics) though intermediate levels (e.g. the workplace or healthcare) and macro levels (e.g. policy at city, state, or regional level) to the global level (e.g. national policies and global trade and markets) [148].

As we have already discussed, many of the major 'downstream' determinants of CVD explaining most of the disease burden can be traced back to lifestyle determinants (notably smoking, diet, and physical activity). In turn, these 'upstream' factors are heavily influenced by the political, economic, social, and built environment [27,62,149]. Thus, control strategies for the burden of CVD will be most effective when they take these complexities into account. Strategies aimed at the individual will focus on the micro level while prevention at a larger scale should focus on the intermediate and higher levels.

The story of tobacco control has provided public health professionals with a powerful understanding of how the interaction of public health and industry could evolve [62]. Education, legislation and regulation, and economic intervention have been shown to be effective not only for controlling smoking but also improving diet and physical activity [27,96]. Furthermore, these gains can be achieved very quickly [150].

Diet is a useful example of multiple nested determinants [148]. Mounting evidence suggests that industrialization of food production and distribution are also key factors influencing modern societies' excessive exposure to salt, saturated fats, trans-fats, and refined sugars [151]. This phenomenon can be characterized by the increasing concentration of food production and processing in the hands of transnational companies who have the remit to maximize profit for shareholders without any concern for potential public health effects. Furthermore, the health and other societal costs are passed to other actors [152]. Thus, the political and economic influences on food production, processing, and marketing are emerging as potential modifiable risk factors, amenable to public health interventions emulating previous successes in tobacco control [152]. Many of these activities have important empirical evidence of their effectiveness [98].

Incorporating all this into the web of causation of CHD is therefore important. There has recently been renewed debate on the focus of interventions from individual responsibility towards changing a harming social, political, economic, and physical environment [62,152].

In a political declaration at a high-level meeting of the United Nations (UN) General Assembly in 2011 on the prevention and control of non-communicable diseases [153], the General Assembly recognized:

- that non-communicable diseases are a threat to the economy of many member states, and may lead to increasing inequality
- the critical importance of reducing the level of exposure of individuals and populations to the common modifiable risk factors for non-communicable diseases, namely tobacco use, unhealthy diet, physical inactivity, and the harmful use of alcohol
- that effective non-communicable disease prevention and control require leadership and multisectoral approaches for health at the government level.

Evidence for stroke

The term CVD comprises a range of diseases including CHD, stroke, and peripheral vascular disease. Although a very heterogeneous category, the ischaemic forms of CVD are the predominant ones and share most of their determinants. However, some differences exist within the umbrella term CVD. We briefly consider stroke, as an example of another disease included with the CVD category.

Stroke is a heterogeneous disease, but is mainly composed of ischaemic and hypertension-related haemorrhagic strokes. However, the main burden is related to ischaemic stroke, which comprises about 80% of the disease burden [154].

Most of the risk factors for CHD are also risk factors for stroke, but the strength of the association is different. If we consider total stroke, hypertension is significantly more important for stroke than for CHD [population attributable risk fraction (PARF) 35% vs. 18%] as well as the ratio of apolipoprotein B/A1 (PARF 25% vs. 49%) [155].

As already discussed, heavy alcohol intake increases the risk of stroke, although there is still a more complex effect on CHD outcomes.

Certain heart conditions are specific risk factors for stroke, like atrial fibrillation, dilated cardiomyopathy, or congenital septal communication defects. These conditions increase the risk of cerebral embolism, a cause of ischaemic stroke. For example, individuals in the control group of large atrial fibrillation anticoagulation trials have a mean annual incidence of stroke of 4.5%, and half of those strokes resulted in death or severe disability [156–160], with risk increasing markedly with age [161].

The combined effects of the major cardiovascular risk factors are universal and explain most CHD

Studies seeking to replicate the Framingham findings have consistently showed that the classical cardiovascular risk factor levels are useful for grading risk in both western and non-western populations worldwide. Calibration remains an interesting issue across different populations [162,163]. The Prospective Studies Collaboration and the Asia Pacific Collaboration have also suggested that the risk conferred by the classical risk factor is similar across western and non-western populations [35,48,164].

However, some countries like France or Japan show unexpectedly low CHD mortality rates with relatively high levels of risk factors. This situation, often described as 'the French paradox', the 'Mediterranean paradox', or the 'Japanese paradox', might challenge the paradigm of 'universality of risk factors effects'. These paradoxes have been partly explained in terms of misclassification of cause of death, diet, the existence of additional protective risk factors, or by previously ignored lag times [12,165]. However, further work is clearly required.

The list of confirmed and potential risk factors for CHD and stroke includes more than just the 'classical' ones. Candidate factors include thrombotic and inflammatory biomarkers, lipid subfractions, and endothelial function measures. A huge body of literature and current research is focused on finding novel risk factors for CHD. This quest has been fuelled by the claim that 'only half' of CHD incidence can be explained by the classical, major biological risk factors, promoting a frantic search for new ones. However, the source of this erroneous statement is difficult to locate; it was discussed and demolished by Magnus and Beaglehole in a key paper published in 2002 [166].

This debate is essentially about finding new targets for intervention, and for this reason it is easier to focus on the importance of candidate novel risk factors based on relative risks. However, a better way to understand the impact of a risk factor can be summarized as the PARF, a variable that reflects both the frequency of the risk factor in the population and the strength of its association with CHD. One of the crucial assumptions of this concept is that the risk factor should be causally related to the outcome, because the PARF estimates the proportion of disease incidence that can be eliminated if the risk factor is completely removed from the population. By using the PARF approach, the INTERHEART study [146] estimated that the population-attributable fraction associated with lifestyle and diet-related risk factors is about 90%, suggesting that there is little room for significant 'novel' candidates, whatever strength they might have.

The importance of the crucial role of the major risk factors can be also illustrated by the 'low-risk concept'. Individuals at 'low risk' for CHD, defined in terms of people who have never smoked, do not have diabetes, and have normal or low blood pressure and blood lipids experience the lowest rates of CVD [167–169). Young individuals who maintain this ideal cardiovascular health profile into middle age experience dramatically lower lifetime risks for major CVD events [170] and lower non-CVD mortality [168]. This 'low-risk' profile now forms the cornerstone of the American Heart Association's 2020 Strategic Impact Goals [171].

A rapidly growing number of novel biomarkers are now emerging for evaluation [141,142]. C-reactive protein (CRP) offers an instructive example of an 'exciting' new risk factor which has waxed and now waned in perceived importance. For long championed as a novel risk factor, it now appears more useful simply as a measure of an individual's total burden of atheromatous disease, rather than having a substantial causal role [172,173].

Another important distinction is to differentiate causal risk factors from the identification of earlier, pre-clinical phases of an already established pathological process. The distinction between a risk factor and a risk marker is thus important, mainly because some disease control strategies involve the identification of individuals with subclinical disease. However, all of the emerging 'risk factors' identified by the US Preventive Services Task Force were found wanting in terms of their classification power and therapeutic potential, compared with current strategies to manage intermediate-risk patients using only the major classical risk factors [174], but novel strategies including multiple biomarkers from different pathophysiological pathways might prove useful in improving prediction for primary prevention purposes [175].

What can explain the CVD epidemic?

Recent global trends in the epidemiology of CVD are complex, suggesting that countries are at different stages of the epidemic. What drives these epidemics?

The availability of effective interventions for preventing and treating CHD was one of the key achievements of medicine in the twentieth century. The advent of coronary care units and coronary artery bypass grafting in the 1960s heralded the development of more powerful and effective therapies aimed at preventing or treating the clinical manifestations of CVD [176]. However, even at the beginning of the twenty-first century, treatments were still not being used to their full potential [177,178]. Although progress is unrelenting in terms of utilization, this suggests that their role in driving the declining trends in CVD does not explain the full story.

Risk factor changes have also been dramatic over the last 30 or 40 years [59,175,179]. In countries with a declining burden of CVD, significant declines in smoking, blood pressure, and cholesterol have been observed. In countries with increasing burden of disease, major risk factors are increasing, despite the adoption of many evidence-based medical and surgical interventions. The global increase in diabetes and obesity are probably heralding a new phase of the CVD epidemic.

Relatively few studies have systematically studied the relative contributions of evidence-based treatments and risk factors changes as drivers of the trends. Because this question cannot be practically addressed with randomized controlled trials, it has mainly been studied using observational designs and, more recently, modelling studies.

The MONICA project was an observational study that addressed this question explicitly. The objectives of the MONICA project were first to observe the trends in CVD mortality and morbidity and second to evaluate the extent to which these trends were related to changes in known risk factors, including daily living habits, healthcare, and major socioeconomic features. The study was conducted in 37 populations in 21 different countries beginning in 1980 and finalizing data collection by the late 1990s. The contribution of risk factors to CHD incidence rates was assessed by looking at the association between 10-year trends in major risk factors (smoking, blood pressure, and blood cholesterol) and 10-year trends in incidence (fatal and non-fatal events). Careful biochemical measurements and strict event ascertainment and death certification procedures were key features of this exemplar study. Almost 13 million people were monitored over 10 years, and more than 300 000 men and women were sampled and examined for risk factors. During the 10-year period 166 000 MIs were registered.

In the MONICA populations, CHD mortality rates fell by 4% per year. About two-thirds of the observed fall could be attributed to a fall in event rates, while one-third could be attributed to a fall in case fatality [180]. The effect of individual risk factors on risk was lower than observed in the cohort studies, but when corrected for dilution regression bias the results were comparable [181,182].

Modelling studies offer a unique opportunity to build on the extensive body of evidence on CVD causation. The US CHD Policy model is a state-transition, cell-based model developed in the 1980s [183]. It was initially used to examine trends in CHD mortality [184,185] and expected gains in life expectancy from risk factor modifications [186]. The model showed that in the US population and for the period 1980–90 risk factor changes made a 50% contribution to the mortality decline while treatments contributed 43%.

IMPACT is a cell-based model originally developed by Capewell and colleagues in 1996 [187]. It combines data from many sources on patient numbers, treatment uptake, treatment effectiveness, risk factor trends, and consequent mortality effects. The model can be used to estimate the proportion of change in mortality that is attributable to specific treatments or risk factor changes. It has been used to explore the contributions of risk factors and treatments in over 10 countries. In most of the studied countries (New Zealand, Scotland, England and Wales, Sweden, Italy, Spain, Iceland, the United States, and Canada) CHD mortality rates have been declining. The IMPACT model consistently found that about 40–72% of the fall in deaths could be attributed to changes in risk factors and 23–55% to treatments [177]. An interesting observation from IMPACT modelling related to the city of Beijing was that CHD trends were increasing, essentially driven by a huge increase in cholesterol levels. This might be related to the rapid adoption of a 'westernized' diet, rich in saturated fats [188].

Recent findings in central European populations are particularly interesting. Here rapid declines in mortality have been observed after decades of increasing rates, linked to profound socioeconomic changes resulting in substantial modification of exposure to CHD risk factors. The abrupt changes in mortality have been explained in terms of profound and population-wide changes in diet and lifestyle [189–191].

Finland experienced a marked decline in CHD mortality during the twentieth century, associated with the implementation of nationwide, population-level policies. Serum cholesterol declined significantly in both men and women over that period. Blood pressure declined up to 2002, but levelled afterward. Smoking followed a more complex pattern, declining in men but increasing in women until 2002, and levelling off since then. BMI increased in men throughout the period and in women it started to increase in 1982. Collectively, the changes in risk factors explain about 60% of the observed decline of 80% in CHD mortality [192].

Future trends

Trends in CHD mortality generally declined in most developed countries in the last part of the twentieth century, and more recently in central European countries after the collapse of the Soviet Union. However, in many low- and middle-income countries the epidemic is still increasing [193].

However, worrying adverse trends in risk factors might be heralding the start of a new phase of the epidemic. Obesity and diabetes have increased dramatically almost everywhere throughout the world [193,194]. In western countries declines in cigarette smoking have stalled in many places, particularly in the young [195], but there is frank expansion in low- and middle-income countries [196]. Similarly there is evidence that blood pressure levels have stopped declining in some countries, for example in women in the United States [197], and they are increasing in Oceania, east Africa, and south and southeast Asia for both genders [59]. Furthermore, CVD prevalence (or burden of disease) is likely to increase also over the next few decades due to the ageing of populations in many parts of the world (quite apart from any changes in risk factor levels or treatment uptakes) [198–200]. There is evidence from the United States, Australia, the United Kingdom, and elsewhere that the declining CHD mortality trends seen over the last 30 years or so have recently flattened in younger adults (and are possibly even increasing slightly), but at the moment these analyses are inevitably based on small numbers of deaths [117,201–204]. In Iceland, if the adverse recent (last 5–10 years) trends in risk factors continue, an increase in age- and sex-specific CVD incidence could occur (J. Critchley, personal communication, 2012).

Conclusions

The causes of CHD have been comprehensively studied over the last five decades. The relationship of occurrence of CVD (mainly CHD and stroke) with diet, smoking, and other lifestyle factors is now well established. The role of biological, downstream risk factors and their link with more upstream determinants has also been established with increasing confidence. Although still there is no definitive answer to the question of what drives trends in CVD morbidity and mortality, observational and modelling studies consistently suggest that both risk factors and medical treatments have made a substantial contribution to the observed trends in CHD mortality.

The fact that the current epidemics across the globe are at different stages and that rates are increasing in many countries makes current study of these trends pertinent, especially given the alarming increases in obesity and diabetes. Furthermore, developing our understanding of the multilevel nature of CHD causation is allowing us to identify powerful upstream and structural determinants of risk.

As a result, many potential targets for intervention acting at different levels of the CVD causal web exist and now form the basis for modern CVD prevention strategies. Furthermore, when deciding upon actions to control the future disease burden, the search for new risk factors might be considered an activity of secondary importance. The priority policy targets remain tobacco and alcohol control, poor diet, and physical inactivity.

Further reading

Beaglehole R, Magnus P. The search for new risk factors for coronary heart disease: occupational therapy for epidemiologists? *Int J Epidemiol* 2002; **31**: 1117–22.

Capewell S, Morrison CE, McMurray JJ. Contribution of modern cardiovascular treatment and risk factor changes to the decline in coronary heart disease mortality in Scotland between 1975 and 1994. *Heart* 1999; **81**: 380–6.

Hill AB. The environment and disease: association or causation? *Proc R Soc Med* 1965; **58**: 295–300.

Jørgensen T, Capewell S, Prescott E, et al. Population-level changes to promote cardiovascular health. *Eur J Prev Cardiol* 2013; **20**: 409–21.

Kuh D, Ben-Shlomo Y. *A life course approach to chronic disease epidemiology*, 2004. New York: Oxford University Press.

Lewington S, Whitlock G, Clarke R, et al. Blood cholesterol and vascular mortality by age, sex, and blood pressure: a meta-analysis of individual data from 61 prospective studies with 55,000 vascular deaths. *Lancet* 2007; **370**: 1829–39.

Mendis S, Puska P, Norrving B. *Global atlas on cardiovascular disease prevention and control*, 2011. Geneva: World Health Organization.

Rose G. *The strategy of preventive medicine*, 1992. Oxford: Oxford University Press.

Stuckler D, Nestle M. Big food, food systems, and global health. *PLoS Med* 2012; **9**: e1001242.

Tunstall-Pedoe H. (ed.). *MONICA. Monograph and Multimedia Sourcebook. World's largest study of heart disease, stroke, risk factors, and population trends 1979–2002*, 2003. Geneva: World Health Organization.

References

1 Mendis S, Puska P, Norrving B. (eds). *Global atlas on cardiovascular disease prevention and control*, 2011. Geneva: World Health Organization.

2 Dawber TR, Meadors GF, Moore FE Jr. Epidemiological approaches to heart disease: the Framingham Study. *Am J Public Health* 1951; **41**: 279–86.

3 Keys A, Menotti A, Aravanis C, et al. The seven countries study: 2,289 deaths in 15 years. *Prevent Med* 1984; **13**: 141–54.

4 Welin L, Tibblin G, Svardsudd K, et al. Prospective study of social influences on mortality. The study of men born in 1913 and 1923 1. *Lancet* 1985; **1**: 915–18.

5 Osler M, Linneberg A, Glumer C, et al. The cohorts at the Research Centre for Prevention and Health, formerly 'The Glostrup population studies'. *Int J Epidemiol* 2011; **40**: 602–10.

6 James AL, Palmer LJ, Kicic E, et al. Decline in lung function in the Busselton Health Study: the effects of asthma and cigarette smoking. *Am J Respir Crit Care Med* 2005; **171**: 109–14.

7 Clarke R, Emberson J, Fletcher A, et al. Life expectancy in relation to cardiovascular risk factors: 38 year follow-up of 19,000 men in the Whitehall study 3. *Br Med J* 2009; **339**: b3513.

8 Tunstall-Pedoe H. (ed.). *MONICA. Monograph and Multimedia Sourcebook. World's largest study of heart disease, stroke, risk factors, and population trends 1979–2002*, 2003. Geneva: World Health Organization.

9 Evans A, Salomaa V, Kulathinal S, et al. MORGAM (an international pooling of cardiovascular cohorts). *Int J Epidemiol* 2005; **34**: 21–7.

10 Kuulasmaa K, Tolonen H, Koponen P, et al. An overview of the European Health Examination Survey Pilot Joint Action. *Arch Publ Health* 2012; **70**: 20.

11 Berenson GS, Wattigney WA, Tracy RE, et al. Atherosclerosis of the aorta and coronary arteries and cardiovascular risk factors in persons aged 6 to 30 years and studied at necropsy (the Bogalusa Heart Study). *Am J Cardiol* 1992; **70**: 851–8.

12 Law M, Wald N, Stampfer M, et al. Why heart disease mortality is low in France: the time lag explanation. *Br Med J* 1999; **318**: 1471–80.

13 Rose G. Incubation period of coronary heart disease. *Int J Epidemiol* 2005; **34**: 242–4.

14 Labarthe DR, Dai S, Day RS, et al. Findings from Project HeartBeat!: their importance for CVD prevention. *Am J Prev Med* 2009; **37**: S105–S115.

15 Mackie JL. *The cement of the universe*, 1974. Oxford: Oxford University Press.

16 Rothman KJ. Causes. *Am J Epidemiol* 1976; **104**: 587–92.

17 US Department of Health. *Smoking and health: report of the Advisory Committee to the Surgeon General of the Public Health Service*, 1964. Washington, DC: Government Printing Office.

18 US Department of Health. *The health consequences of smoking: a report of the US Surgeon General*, 2004. Washington, DC: Government Printing Office.
19 Prescott E, Hippe M, Schnohr P, et al. Smoking and risk of myocardial infarction in women and men: longitudinal population study. *Br Med J* 1998; **316**: 1043.
20 Floderus B, Cederlöf R, Friberg L. Smoking and mortality: a 21-year follow-up based on the Swedish Twin Registry. *Int J Epidemiol* 1988; **17**: 332–40.
21 Janghorbani M, Hedley AJ, Jones RB, et al. Gender differential in all-cause and cardiovascular disease mortality. *Int J Epidemiol* 1993; **22**: 1056–63.
22 Njølstad I, Arnesen E, Lund-Larsen PG. Smoking, serum lipids, blood pressure, and sex differences in myocardial infarction. *Circulation* 1996; **93**: 450–6.
23 Critchley JA, Capewell S. Mortality risk reduction associated with smoking cessation in patients with coronary heart disease: a systematic review. *J Am Med Assoc* 2003; **290**: 86–97.
24 Wilson K, Gibson N, Willan A, et al. Effect of smoking cessation on mortality after myocardial infarction: meta-analysis of cohort studies. *Arch Intern Med* 2000; **160**: 939–44.
25 Lightwood JM, Coxson PG, Bibbins-Domingo K, et al. Coronary heart disease attributable to passive smoking: CHD policy model. *Am J Prev Med* 2009; **36**: 13–20.
26 Whincup PH, Gilg JA, Emberson JR, et al. Passive smoking and risk of coronary heart disease and stroke: prospective study with cotinine measurement. *Br Med J* 2004; **329**: 200.
27 Glantz S, Gonzalez M. Effective tobacco control is key to rapid progress in reduction of non-communicable diseases. *Lancet* 2012; **379**: 1269–71.
28 Kannel WB, Dawber TR, Friedman GD. Risk factors in coronary heart disease; an evaluation of several serum lipids as predictors of coronary heart disease. *Ann Intern Med* 1964; **61**: 888–99.
29 Kannel WB, Dawber TR, Kagan A, et al. Factors of risk in the development of coronary heart disease – six year follow-up experience; the Framingham Study. *Ann Intern Med* 1961; **55**: 33–50.
30 Neaton JD, Wentworth D. Serum cholesterol, blood pressure, cigarette smoking, and death from coronary heart disease overall findings and differences by age for 316 099 white men. *Arch Intern Med* 1992; **152**: 56–64.
31 Cullen P, Schulte H, Assmann G. The Münster Heart Study (PROCAM): total mortality in middle-aged men is increased at low total and LDL cholesterol concentrations in smokers but not in non-smokers. *Circulation* 1997; **96**: 2128–36.
32 Sharrett AR, Patsch W, Sorlie PD. Associations of lipoprotein cholesterols, apolipoproteins A-I and B, and triglycerides with carotid atherosclerosis and coronary heart disease. The Atherosclerosis Risk in Communities (ARIC) Study. *Arterioscler Thromb Vasc Biol* 1994; **14**: 1098–104.
33 Law MR, Wald NJ, Rudnicka AR. Quantifying effect of statins on low density lipoprotein cholesterol, ischaemic heart disease, and stroke: systematic review and meta-analysis. *Br Med J* 2003; **326**: 1423.
34 Taylor F, Ward K, Moore THM, et al. Statins for the primary prevention of cardiovascular disease. *Cochrane Database Syst Rev* 2011; (1): CD004816.
35 Lewington S, Whitlock G, Clarke R, et al. Blood cholesterol and vascular mortality by age, sex, and blood pressure: a meta-analysis of individual data from 61 prospective studies with 55,000 vascular deaths. *Lancet* 2007; **370**: 1829–39.
36 Forrester JS, Makkar R, Shah PK. Increasing high-density lipoprotein cholesterol in dyslipidemia by cholesteryl ester transfer protein inhibition: an update for clinicians. *Circulation* 2005; **111**: 1847–54.
37 Briel M, Ferreira-Gonzalez I, You JJ, et al. Association between change in high density lipoprotein cholesterol and cardiovascular disease morbidity and mortality: systematic review and meta-regression analysis. *Br Med J* 2009; **338**: b92.
38 Gandotra P, Miller M. The role of triglycerides in cardiovascular risk. *Curr Cardiol Rep* 2008; **10**: 505–11.
39 Clarke R, Frost C, Collins R, et al. Dietary lipids and blood cholesterol: quantitative meta-analysis of metabolic ward studies. *Br Med J* 1997; **314**: 112–16.
40 Mozaffarian D, Katan MB, Ascherio A, et al. Trans fatty acids and cardiovascular disease. *N Engl J Med* 2006; **354**: 1601–13.
41 Mozaffarian D, Micha R, Wallace S. Effects on coronary heart disease of increasing polyunsaturated fat in place of saturated fat: a systematic review and meta-analysis of randomized controlled trials. *PLoS Med* 2010; **7**: e1000252.
42 Saravanan P, Davidson NC, Schmidt EB, et al. Cardiovascular effects of marine omega-3 fatty acids. *Lancet* 2010; **376**: 540–50.
43 Wingard DL, Barrett-Connor EL, Scheidt-Nave C, et al. Prevalence of cardiovascular and renal complications in older adults with normal or impaired glucose tolerance or NIDDM. A population-based study. *Diabetes Care* 1993; **16**: 1022–5.
44 Landmesser U, Drexler H. Endothelial function and hypertension. *Curr Opin Cardiol* 2007; **22**: 316–20.
45 Schiffrin EL, Canadian Institutes of Health Research Multidisciplinary Research Group on Hypertension. Beyond blood pressure: the endothelium and atherosclerosis progression. *Am J Hypertens* 2002; **10**: 115S–122S.
46 Vishram JKK, Borglykke A, Andreasen AH, et al. Impact of age on the importance of systolic and diastolic blood pressures for stroke risk/novelty and significance. *Hypertension* 2012; **60**: 1117–23.
47 He J, Whelton PK. Elevated systolic blood pressure and risk of cardiovascular and renal disease: overview of evidence from observational epidemiologic studies and randomized controlled trials. *Am Heart J* 1999; **138**: S211–S219.
48 Lawes CM, Bennett DA, Parag V, et al. Blood pressure indices and cardiovascular disease in the Asia Pacific region: a pooled analysis. *Hypertension* 2003; **42**: 69–75.
49 Chandola T, Brunner E, Marmot M. Chronic stress at work and the metabolic syndrome: prospective study. *Br Med J* 2006; **332**: 521–5.
50 Whelton SP, Chin A, Xin X, et al. Effect of aerobic exercise on blood pressure: a meta-analysis of randomized, controlled trials. *Ann Intern Med* 2002; **136**: 493–503.
51 Stamler R, Stamler J, Riedlinger WF, et al. Weight and blood pressure. *J Am Med Assoc* 1978; **240**: 1607–10.
52 Dyer AR, Elliott P. The INTERSALT study: relations of body mass index to blood pressure. INTERSALT Co-operative Research Group. *J Hum Hypertens* 1989; **3**: 299–308.
53 He FJ, MacGregor GA. A comprehensive review on salt and health and current experience of worldwide salt reduction programmes. *J Hum Hypertens* 2009; **23**: 363–84.
54 Elliott P. The INTERSALT study: an addition to the evidence on salt and blood pressure, and some implications. *J Hum Hypertens* 1989; **3**: 289–98.
55 Zhou BF, Stamler J, Dennis B, et al. Nutrient intakes of middle-aged men and women in China, Japan, United Kingdom, and United States in the late 1990s: the INTERMAP study. *J Hum Hypertens* 2003; **17**: 623–30.
56 Khaw KT, Bingham S, Welch A, et al. Blood pressure and urinary sodium in men and women: the Norfolk cohort of the European Prospective Investigation into Cancer (EPIC-Norfolk). *Am J Clin Nutr* 2004; **80**: 1397–403.
57 Cook NR, Cutler JA, Obarzanek E, et al. Long term effects of dietary sodium reduction on cardiovascular disease outcomes: observational follow-up of the trials of hypertension prevention (TOHP). *Br Med J* 2007; **334**: 885–8.

58 Forte JG, Miguel JM, Miguel MJ, et al. Salt and blood pressure: a community trial. *J Hum Hypertens* 1989; **3**: 179–84.

59 Danaei G, Finucane MM, Lin JK, et al. National, regional, and global trends in systolic blood pressure since 1980: systematic analysis of health examination surveys and epidemiological studies with 786 country-years and 5.4 million participants. *Lancet* 2011; **377**: 568–77.

60 He FJ, MacGregor GA. Reducing population salt intake worldwide: from evidence to implementation. *Prog Cardiovasc Dis* 2010; **52**: 363–82.

61 Caballero B. The global epidemic of obesity: an overview. *Epidemiol Rev* 2007; **29**: 1–5.

62 Glickman D, Greenwood M, Purcell W. *Accelerating progress in obesity prevention: solving the weight of the nation*, 2012. Washington, DC: National Academies Press.

63 Van Gaal LF, Mertens IL, De Block CE. Mechanisms linking obesity with cardiovascular disease. *Nature* 2006; **444**: 875–80.

64 National Lung Heart and Blood Institute. Evaluation and Treatment of High Blood Cholesterol in Adults. Executive summary of the third report of The National Cholesterol Education Program (NCEP) Expert Panel on detection, evaluation, and treatment of high blood cholesterol in adults (Adult Treatment Panel III). *J Am Med Assoc* 2001; **285**: 2486–97.

65 Calle EE, Thun MJ, Petrelli JM, et al. Body-mass index and mortality in a prospective cohort of US adults. *N Engl J Med* 1999; **341**: 1097–105.

66 Flegal KM, Graubard BI, Williamson DF, et al. Excess deaths associated with underweight, overweight, and obesity. *J Am Med Assoc* 2005; **193**: 1861–7.

67 Fontaine KR, Redden DT, Wang C, et al. Years of life lost due to obesity. *J Am Med Assoc* 2003; **198**: 187–93.

68 The Emerging Risk Factors Collaboration. Separate and combined associations of body-mass index and abdominal adiposity with cardiovascular disease: collaborative analysis of 58 prospective studies. *Lancet* 2011; **377**: 1085–95.

69 Kannel WB. Lipids, diabetes, and coronary heart disease: insights from the Framingham Study. *Am Heart J* 1985; **110**: 1100–7.

70 Wilson PWF, D'Agostino RB, Levy D, et al. Prediction of coronary heart disease using risk factor categories. *Circulation* 1998; **97**: 1837–47.

71 McGill HC Jr, McMahan CA, Malcom GT, et al. Effects of serum lipoproteins and smoking on atherosclerosis in young men and women. The PDAY Research Group. Pathobiological Determinants of Atherosclerosis in Youth. *Arterioscler Thromb Vasc Biol* 1997; **17**: 95–106.

72 Brezina V, Padmos I. Coronary heart disease risk factors in women. *Eur Heart J* 1994; **15**: 1571–84.

73 Haffner SM, Lehto S, Rönnemaa T, et al. Mortality from coronary heart disease in subjects with type 2 diabetes and in nondiabetic subjects with and without prior myocardial infarction. *N Engl J Med* 1998; **339**: 229–34.

74 Hurst RT, Lee RW. Increased incidence of coronary atherosclerosis in type 2 diabetes mellitus: mechanisms and management. *Ann Intern Med* 2003; **139**: 824–34.

75 Nakagami H, Kaneda Y, Ogihara T, et al. Endothelial dysfunction in hyperglycemia as a trigger of atherosclerosis. *Curr Diabetes Rev* 2005; **1**: 59–63.

76 American Diabetes Association. Role of cardiovascular risk factors in prevention and treatment of macrovascular disease in diabetes. *Diabetes Care* 1989; **12**: 573–9.

77 Bonow RO, Bohannon N, Hazzard W. Risk stratification in coronary artery disease and special populations. *Am J Med* 1996; **101** (Suppl. 4A): 4A17S–22S.

78 Mannucci E, Monami M, Lamanna C, et al. Prevention of cardiovascular disease through glycemic control in type 2 diabetes: a meta-analysis of randomized clinical trials. *Nutr Metabol Cardiovasc Dis* 2009; **19**: 604–12.

79 Siebenhofer A, Jeitler K, Pieber TR, et al. Intensive glucose control and cardiovascular outcomes. *Lancet* 2009; **374**: 523.

80 Simmons RK, Sharp SJ, Sandbaek A, et al. Does early intensive multifactorial treatment reduce total cardiovascular burden in individuals with screen-detected diabetes? Findings from the ADDITION-Europe cluster-randomized trial. *Diabet Med* 2012; **29**: e409–e416.

81 Tuomilehto J, Lindström J. The major diabetes prevention trials. *Curr Diabetes Rep* 2003; **3**: 115–22.

82 Knowler WC, Barrett-Connor E, Fowler SE, et al. Reduction in the incidence of type 2 diabetes with lifestyle intervention or metformin. *N Engl J Med* 2002; **346**: 393–403.

83 Nocon M, Hiemann T, Müller-Riemenschneider F, et al. Association of physical activity with all-cause and cardiovascular mortality: a systematic review and meta-analysis. *Eur J Cardiovasc Prev Rehab* 2008; **15**: 239–46.

84 Warburton DER, Nicol CW, Bredin SSD. Health benefits of physical activity: the evidence. *Can Med Assoc J* 2006; **174**: 801–9.

85 Kelley GA, Kelley KS, Tran ZV. Exercise, lipids, and lipoproteins in older adults: a meta-analysis. *Prev Cardiol* 2005; **8**: 206–14.

86 Fagard RH. Exercise characteristics and the blood pressure response to dynamic physical training. *Med Sci Sports Exerc* 2001; **33**: 484–92.

87 Tuomilehto J, Lindström J, Eriksson JG, et al. Prevention of type 2 diabetes mellitus by changes in lifestyle among subjects with impaired glucose tolerance. *N Engl J Med* 2001; **344**: 1343–50.

88 Leitzmann MF, Park Y, Blair A, et al. Physical activity recommendations and decreased risk of mortality. *Arch Intern Med* 2007; **167**: 2453–60.

89 Katzmarzyk PT, Church TS, Craig CL, et al. Sitting time and mortality from all causes, cardiovascular disease, and cancer. *Med Sci Sports Exerc* 2009; **41**: 998–1005.

90 Dunstan DW, Barr EL, Healy GN, et al. Television viewing time and mortality: the Australian Diabetes, Obesity and Lifestyle Study (AusDiab). *Circulation* 2010; **121**: 384–91.

91 Hamilton MT, Hamilton DG, Zderic TW. Role of low energy expenditure and sitting in obesity, metabolic syndrome, type 2 diabetes, and cardiovascular disease. *Diabetes* 2007; **56**: 2655–67.

92 Katzmarzyk PT, Janssen I, Ardern CI. Physical inactivity, excess adiposity and premature mortality. *Obesity Rev* 2003; **4**: 257–90.

93 Li J, Siegrist J. Physical activity and risk of cardiovascular disease - a meta-analysis of prospective cohort studies. *Int J Environ Res Public Health* 2012; **9**: 391–407.

94 Holtermann A, Hansen JV, Burr H, et al. The health paradox of occupational and leisure-time physical activity. *Br J Sports Med* 2012; **46**: 291–5.

95 Durand CP, Andalib M, Dunton GF., A systematic review of built environment factors related to physical activity and obesity risk: implications for smart growth urban planning. *Obesity Rev* 2011; **12**: e173–e182.

96 Mozaffarian D, Afshin A, Benowitz NL, et al. Population approaches to improve diet, physical activity, and smoking habits. *Circulation* 2012; **126**: 1514–63.

97 Graham I, Atar D, Borch-Johnsen K, et al. European guidelines on cardiovascular disease prevention in clinical practice: executive summary. *Eur Heart J* 2007; **28**: 2375–414.

98 Mozaffarian D, Appel LJ, Van Horn L. Components of a cardioprotective diet. *Circulation* 2011; **123**: 2870–91.

99 Mente A, de Koning L, Shannon HS, et al. A systematic review of the evidence supporting a causal link between dietary factors and coronary heart disease. *Arch Intern Med* 2009; **169**: 659–69.

100 Iqbal R, Anand S, Ounpuu S, et al. Dietary patterns and the risk of acute myocardial infarction in 52 countries: results of the INTERHEART Study. *Circulation* 2008; **118**: 1929–37.

101 Stender S, Dyerberg J, Bysted A, et al. A trans world journey. *Atheroscler Suppl* 2006; **7**: 47–52.

102 Corrao G, Rubbiati L, Bagnardi V, et al. Alcohol and coronary heart disease: a meta-analysis. *Addiction* 2000; **95**: 1505–23.

103 Di Castelnuovo A, Costanzo S, Bagnardi V, et al. Alcohol dosing and total mortality in men and women: an updated meta-analysis of 34 prospective studies. *Arch Intern Med* 2006; **166**: 2437–45.

104 Maclure M. Demonstration of deductive meta-analysis: ethanol intake and risk of myocardial infarction. *Epidemiol Rev* 1993; **15**: 328–51.

105 Ronksley PE, Brien SE, Turner BJ, et al. Association of alcohol consumption with selected cardiovascular disease outcomes: a systematic review and meta-analysis. *Br Med J* 2011; **342**: d671.

106 O'Keefe JH, Bybee KA, Lavie CJ. Alcohol and cardiovascular health: the razor-sharp double-edged sword. *J Am Coll Cardiol* 2007; **50**: 1009–14.

107 Sacco RL, Elkind M, Boden-Albala B, et al. The protective effect of moderate alcohol consumption on ischemic stroke. *J Am Med Assoc* 1999; **281**: 53–60.

108 Mukamal KJ, Conigrave KM, Mittleman MA, et al. Roles of drinking pattern and type of alcohol consumed in coronary heart disease in men. *N Engl J Med* 2003; **348**: 109–18.

109 Mukamal KJ, Maclure M, Muller JE, et al. Binge drinking and mortality after acute myocardial infarction. *Circulation* 2005; **115**: 3839–45.

110 Mukamal KJ, Jensen MK, Grønbaek M, et al. Drinking frequency, mediating biomarkers, and risk of myocardial infarction in women and men. *Circulation* 2005; **112**: 1406–13.

111 Rehm J, Sempos CT, Trevisan M. Average volume of alcohol consumption, patterns of drinking and risk of coronary heart disease—a review. *J Cardiovasc Risk* 2003; **10**: 15–20.

112 Naimi TS, Brewer RD, Mokdad A, et al. Binge drinking among US adults. *J Am Med Assoc* 2003; **289**: 70–5.

113 Leon DA, Chenet L, Shkolnikov VM, et al. Huge variation in Russian mortality rates 1984-94: artefact, alcohol, or what? *Lancet* 1997; **350**: 383–8.

114 Leon DA, Shkolnikov VM, McKee M, et al. Alcohol increases circulatory disease mortality in Russia: acute and chronic effects or misattribution of cause? *Int J Epidemiol* 2010; **39**: 1279–90.

115 International Center for Alcohol Policies. *Drinking guidelines*. URL: <http://www.icap.org/PolicyIssues/DrinkingGuidelines/Guidelinestable/tabid/204/Defaults.aspx>.

116 British Heart Foundation. *Heart statistics*. URL: <http://www.bhf.org.uk/research/heart-statistics.aspx > (accessed 11 November 2014).

117 O'Flaherty M, Bishop J, Redpath A, et al. Coronary heart disease mortality among young adults in Scotland in relation to social inequalities: time trend study. *Br Med J* 2009; **339**: b2613.

118 Wong MD, Shapiro MF, Boscardin WJ, et al. Contribution of major diseases to disparities in mortality. *N Engl J Med* 2002; **347**: 1585–92.

119 Kurian AK, Cardarelli KM. Racial and ethnic differences in cardiovascular disease risk factors: a systematic review. *Ethn Dis* 2007; **17**: 143–52.

120 Mensah GA, Mokdad AH, Ford ES, et al. State of disparities in cardiovascular health in the United States. *Circulation* 2005; **111**: 1233–41.

121 Muennig P, Sohler N, Mahato B. Socioeconomic status as an independent predictor of physiological biomarkers of cardiovascular disease: evidence from NHANES. *Prev Med* 2007; **45**: 35–40.

122 Mackenbach JP, Cavelaars AEJM, Kunst AE, et al. Socioeconomic inequalities in cardiovascular disease mortality. An international study. *Eur Heart J* 2000; **21**: 1141–51.

123 Galobardes B, Smith GD, Lynch JW. Systematic review of the influence of childhood socioeconomic circumstances on risk for cardiovascular disease in adulthood. *Ann Epidemol* 2006; **16**: 91–104.

124 Pollitt R, Rose K, Kaufman J. Evaluating the evidence for models of life course socioeconomic factors and cardiovascular outcomes: a systematic review. *BMC Publ Health* 2005; **5**: 7.

125 Labarthe DR, Nichaman MZ, Harrist RB, et al. Development of cardiovascular risk factors from ages 8 to 18 in Project HeartBeat!: Study design and patterns of change in plasma total cholesterol concentration. *Circulation* 1997; **95**: 2636–42.

126 Lynch J, Smith GD. A life course approach to chronic disease epidemiology. *Ann Rev Publ Health* 2005; **26**: 1–35.

127 Forsdahl A. Are poor living conditions in childhood and adolescence an important risk factor for arteriosclerotic heart disease? *Br J Prev Soc Med* 1977; **31**: 91–5.

128 Barker DJP. Fetal origins of coronary heart disease. *Br Med J* 1995; **311**: 171–4.

129 Kuh D, Ben-Shlomo Y. *A life course approach to chronic disease epidemiology*, 2004. New York: Oxford University Press.

130 Leon DA, Lithell HO, Vâgerö D, et al. Reduced fetal growth rate and increased risk of death from ischaemic heart disease: cohort study of 15 000 Swedish men and women born 1915-29. *Br Med J* 1998; **317**: 241–5.

131 Barker DJP, Bagby SP. Developmental antecedents of cardiovascular disease: a historical perspective. *J Am Soc Nephrol* 2005; **16**: 2537–44.

132 Taylor R, Page A, Danquah J. The Australian epidemic of cardiovascular mortality 1935-2005: effects of period and birth cohort. *J Epidemiol Commun Health* 2012; **66**: e18.

133 Lloyd-Jones DM, Nam BH, D'Agostino RB, et al. Parental cardiovascular disease as a risk factor for cardiovascular disease in middle-aged adults. *J Am Med Assoc* 2004; **291**: 2204–11.

134 Musunuru K, Kathiresan S. Genetics of coronary artery disease. *Ann Rev Genom Hum Genet* 2010; **11**: 91–108.

135 Talmud PJ. How to identify gene-environment interactions in a multifactorial disease: CHD as an example. *Proc Nutr Soc* 2004; **63**: 5–10.

136 Smith GD. Epidemiology, epigenetics and the 'Gloomy Prospect': embracing randomness in population health research and practice. *Int J Epidemiol* 2011; **40**: 537–62.

137 Ioannidis JPA. Prediction of cardiovascular disease outcomes and established cardiovascular risk factors by genome-wide association markers. *Cardiovasc Genet* 2009; **2**: 7–15.

138 Samani NJ, Erdmann J, Hall AS, et al. Genomewide association analysis of coronary artery disease. *N Engl J Med* 2007; **357**: 443–53.

139 Jamison DT, Breman JG, Measham AR. *Prevention of chronic disease by means of diet and lifestyle changes*, 2006. Washington, DC: World Bank.

140 Sekikawa A, Horiuchi BY, Edmundowicz D, et al. A natural experiment in cardiovascular epidemiology in the early 21st century. *Heart* 2003; **89**: 255–7.

141 Syme SL, Marmot MG, Kagan A, et al. Epidemiologic studies of coronary heart disease and stroke in Japanese men living in Japan, Hawaii, and California. *Am J Epidemiol* 1975; **102**: 477–80.

142 Myrtek M. Meta-analyses of prospective studies on coronary heart disease, type A personality, and hostility. *Int J Cardiol* 2001; **79**: 245–51.

143 Chida Y, Steptoe A. The association of anger and hostility with future coronary heart disease: a meta-analytic review of prospective evidence. *J Am Coll Cardiol* 2009; **53**: 936–46.

144 Bosma H, Marmot MG, Hemingway H, et al. Low job control and risk of coronary heart disease in Whitehall II (prospective cohort) study. *Br Med J* 1997; **314**: 558–65.

145 Matthews KA, Gump BB. Chronic work stress and marital dissolution increase risk of posttrial mortality in men from the Multiple Risk Factor Intervention Trial. *Arch Intern Med* 2002; **162**: 309–15.
146 Yusuf S, Hawken S, Ounpuu S, et al. Effect of potentially modifiable risk factors associated with myocardial infarction in 52 countries (the INTERHEART study): case-control study. *Lancet* 2004; **364**: 937–52.
147 Whitehead M, Dahlgren G. What can be done about inequalities in health? *Lancet* 1991; **338**: 1059–63.
148 Jørgensen T, Capewell S, Prescott E, et al. Population-level changes to promote cardiovascular health. *Eur J Prev Cardiol* 2013; **20**: 409–21.
149 Barbour V, Clark J, Simpson P, et al. *PLoS Medicine* series on big food: the food industry is ripe for scrutiny. *PLoS Med* 2012; **9**: e1001246.
150 Capewell S, O'Flaherty M. Rapid mortality falls after risk-factor changes in populations. *Lancet* 2011; **378**: 752–3.
151 Stuckler D, Nestle M. Big food, food systems, and global health. PLoS Med 2012; **9**: e1001242.
152 Jahiel R. Corporation-induced diseases, upstream epidemiologic surveillance, and urban health. *J Urban Health* 2008; **85**: 517–31.
153 United Nations. *Resolution adopted by the General Assembly. Political declaration of the high-level meeting of the General Assembly on the prevention and control of non-communicable diseases*, 2012. Sixty-sixth session. Agenda item 117. URL: <http://www.who.int/nmh/events/un_ncd_summit2011/political_declaration_en.pdf>
154 Goldstein LB, Bushnell CD, Adams RJ, et al. Guidelines for the primary prevention of stroke: a guideline for healthcare professionals from the American Heart Association/American Stroke Association. *Stroke* 2011; **42**: 517–84.
155 Tu JV. Reducing the global burden of stroke: INTERSTROKE. *Lancet* 2010; **376**: 74–5.
156 Stroke Prevention in Atrial Fibrillation Investigators. Stroke Prevention in Atrial Fibrillation Study. Final results. *Circulation* 1991; **84**: 527–39.
157 Poller L, Aronow WS, Karalis DG, et al. The effect of low-dose warfarin on the risk of stroke in patients with nonrheumatic atrial fibrillation. *N Engl J Med* 1991; **325**: 129–32.
158 Go AS, Hylek EM, Chang Y, et al. Anticoagulation therapy for stroke prevention in atrial fibrillation. *J Am Med Assoc* 2003; **290**: 2685–92.
159 Ezekowitz MD, Bridgers SL, James KE, et al. Warfarin in the prevention of stroke associated with nonrheumatic atrial fibrillation. *N Engl J Med* 1992; **327**: 1406–12.
160 Petersen P, Godtfredsen J, Boysen G, et al. Placebo-controlled, randomised trial of warfarin and aspirin for prevention of thromboembolic complications in chronic atrial fibrillation: the Copenhagen AFASAK study. *Lancet* 1989; **333**: 175–9.
161 Singer DE, Albers GW, Dalen JE, et al. Antithrombotic therapy in atrial fibrillation: American College of Chest Physicians Evidence-Based Clinical Practice Guidelines (8th Edition). *Chest* 2008; 133 (Suppl. 6): 546S–592S.
162 Bitton A, Gaziano T. The Framingham Heart Study's impact on global risk assessment. *Prog Cardiovasc Dis* 2010; **53**: 68–78.
163 Eichler K, Puhan MA, Steurer J, et al. Prediction of first coronary events with the Framingham score: a systematic review. Am Heart J 2007; **153**: 722–31, 731.e1–8.
164 Lewington S, Clarke R, Qizilbash N, et al. Age-specific relevance of usual blood pressure to vascular mortality: a meta-analysis of individual data for one million adults in 61 prospective studies. *Lancet* 2002; **360**: 1903–13.
165 Sekikawa A, Kuller LH. Why heart disease mortality is low in France: miscoding may explain Japan's low mortality from coronary heart disease. *Br Med J* 1999; **319**: 255.
166 Beaglehole R, Magnus P. The search for new risk factors for coronary heart disease: occupational therapy for epidemiologists? *Int J Epidemiol* 2002; **31**: 1117–22.
167 Ford ES, Li C, Zhao G, et al. Trends in the prevalence of low risk factor burden for cardiovascular disease among United States adults. *Circulation* 2009; **120**: 1181–8.
168 Stamler J, Stamler R, Neaton JD, et al. Low risk-factor profile and long-term cardiovascular and noncardiovascular mortality and life expectancy: findings for 5 large cohorts of young adult and middle-aged men and women. *J Am Med Assoc* 1999; **282**: 2012–18.
169 Berry JD, Dyer A, Cai X, et al. Lifetime risks of cardiovascular disease. *N Engl J Med* 2012; **366**: 321–9.
170 Liu K, Daviglus ML, Loria CM, et al. Healthy lifestyle through young adulthood and the presence of low cardiovascular disease risk profile in middle age/clinical perspective. *Circulation* 2012; **125**: 996–1004.
171 Lloyd-Jones DM, Hong Y, Labarthe D, et al. Defining and setting national goals for cardiovascular health promotion and disease reduction. *Circulation* 2010; **121**: 586–613.
172 Elliott P. Genetic loci associated with c-reactive protein levels and risk of coronary heart disease. *J Am Med Assoc* 2009; **302**: 37–48.
173 The Emerging Risk Factor Collaboration. C-reactive protein concentration and risk of coronary heart disease, stroke, and mortality: an individual participant meta-analysis. *Lancet* 2010; **375**: 132–40.
174 Helfand M, Buckley DI, Freeman M, et al. Emerging risk factors for coronary heart disease: a summary of systematic reviews conducted for the US Preventive Services Task Force. *Ann Intern Med* 2009; **151**: 496–507.
175 Blankenberg S, Zeller T, Saarela O, et al. Contribution of 30 biomarkers to 10-year cardiovascular risk estimation in 2 population cohorts. The MONICA, Risk, Genetics, Archiving, and Monograph (MORGAM) Biomarker Project. *Circulation* 2010; **121**: 2388–97.
176 Nabel EG, Braunwald E. A tale of coronary artery disease and myocardial infarction. *N Engl J Med* 2012; **366**: 54–63.
177 Ford ES, Ajani UA, Croft JB, et al. Explaining the decrease in U.S. deaths from coronary disease, 1980–2000. *N Engl J Med* 2007; **356**: 2388–98.
178 Unal B, Critchley J, Capewell S. Explaining the decline in coronary heart disease mortality in England and Wales, 1981–2000. *Circulation* 2004; **109**: 1101–7.
179 Danaei G, Finucane MM, Lu Y, et al. National, regional, and global trends in fasting plasma glucose and diabetes prevalence since 1980: systematic analysis of health examination surveys and epidemiological studies with 370 country-years and 2.7 million participants. *Lancet* 2011; **378**: 31–40.
180 Tunstall-Pedoe H, Kuulasmaa K, Mahonen M, et al. Contribution of trends in survival and coronary-event rates to changes in coronary heart disease mortality: 10-year results from 37 WHO MONICA project populations. Monitoring trends and determinants in cardiovascular disease. *Lancet* 1999; **353**: 1547–57.
181 Laatikainen T, Critchley J, Vartiainen E, et al. Explaining the decline in coronary heart disease mortality in Finland between 1982 and 1997. *Am J Epidemiol* 2005; **162**: 764–73.
182 Magnus P, Beaglehole R. The real contribution of the major risk factors to the coronary epidemics: time to end the 'only-50%' myth. *Arch Intern Med* 2001; **161**: 2657–60.
183 Weinstein MC, Coxson PG, Williams LW, et al. Forecasting coronary heart disease incidence, mortality, and cost: the Coronary Heart Disease Policy Model. *Am J Public Health* 1987; **77**: 1417–26.

184 Hunink MGM, Goldman L, Tosteson ANA, et al. The recent decline in mortality from coronary heart disease, 1980–1990. *J Am Med Assoc* 1997; **277**: 535–42.

185 Goldman L, Phillips KA, Coxson P, et al. The effect of risk factor reductions between 1981 and 1990 on coronary heart disease incidence, prevalence, mortality and cost. *J Am Coll Cardiol* 2001; **38**: 1012–17.

186 Tsevat J, Weinstein MC, Williams LW, et al. Expected gains in life expectancy from various coronary heart disease risk factor modifications. *Circulation* 1991; **83**: 1194–201 [published erratum appears in *Circulation* 1991; **84**: 2610].

187 Capewell S, Morrison CE, McMurray JJ. Contribution of modern cardiovascular treatment and risk factor changes to the decline in coronary heart disease mortality in Scotland between 1975 and 1994. *Heart* 1999; **81**: 380–6.

188 Critchley J, Liu J, Zhao D, et al. Explaining the increase in coronary heart disease mortality in Beijing between 1984 and 1999. *Circulation* 2004; **110**: 1236–44.

189 Bandosz P, O'Flaherty M, Drygas W, et al. Decline in mortality from coronary heart disease in Poland after socioeconomic transformation: modelling study. *Br Med J* 2012; **344**: d8136.

190 Zatonski W, Campos H, Willett W. Rapid declines in coronary heart disease mortality in eastern Europe are associated with increased consumption of oils rich in alpha-linolenic acid. *Eur J Epidemiol* 2008; **23**: 3–10.

191 Zatonski WA, McMichael AJ, Powles JW. Ecological study of reasons for sharp decline in mortality from ischaemic heart disease in Poland since 1991. *Br Med J* 1998; **316**: 1047–51.

192 Vartiainen E, Laatikainen T, Peltonen M, et al. Thirty-five-year trends in cardiovascular risk factors in Finland. *Int J Epidemiol* 2010; **39**: 504–18.

193 Mirzaei M, Truswell AS, Taylor R, et al. Coronary heart disease epidemics: not all the same. *Heart* 2009; **95**: 740–6.

194 Finucane MM, Stevens GA, Cowan MJ, et al. National, regional, and global trends in body-mass index since 1980: systematic analysis of health examination surveys and epidemiological studies with 960 country-years and 9.1 million participants. *Lancet* 2011; **377**: 557–67.

195 Warren CW, Jones NR, Peruga A, et al. Global youth tobacco surveillance, 2000-2007. *MMWR Surveill Summ* 2008; **57**: 1–28.

196 Mackay J, Riksen M, Ross H. *The tobacco atlas*, 2012. Atlanta, GA: American Cancer Society.

197 Capewell S, Ford ES, Croft JB, et al. Cardiovascular risk factor trends and potential for reducing coronary heart disease mortality in the United States of America. *Bull World Health Org* 2010; **88**: 120–30.

198 Heidenreich PA, Trogdon JG, Khavjou OA, et al. Forecasting the future of cardiovascular disease in the United States. *Circulation* 2011; **123**: 933–44.

199 World Health Organization. *The global burden of disease: 2004 update*, 2008. URL: <http://www.who.int/healthinfo/global_burden_disease/gbd_report_2004update_covertoc.pdf>

200 Huovinen E, Härkänen T, Martelin T, et al. Predicting coronary heart disease mortality—assessing uncertainties in population forecasts and death probabilities by using Bayesian inference. *Int J Epidemiol* 2006; **35**: 1246–52.

201 Ford ES, Capewell S. Coronary heart disease mortality among young adults in the U.S. from 1980 through 2002: concealed leveling of mortality rates. *J Am Coll Cardiol* 2007; **50**: 2128–32.

202 O'Flaherty M, Allender S, Taylor R, et al. The decline in coronary heart disease mortality is slowing in young adults (Australia 1976-2006): a time trend analysis. *Int J Cardiol* 2012; **158**: 193–8.

203 O'Flaherty M, Ford E, Allender S, et al. Coronary heart disease trends in England and Wales from 1984 to 2004: concealed levelling of mortality rates among young adults. *Heart* 2008; **94**: 178–81.

204 Vaartjes I, O'Flaherty M, Grobbee DE, et al. Coronary heart disease mortality trends in the Netherlands 1972–2007. *Heart* 2011; **97**: 569–73.

PART 2

Aetiology and pathophysiology of atherosclerosis

CHAPTER 2

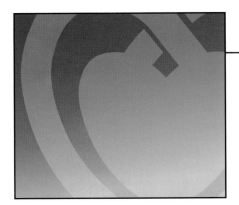

Genetic background of atherosclerosis and its risk factors

Lesca M. Holdt and Daniel Teupser

Contents

Summary

Atherosclerosis risk is modulated by a complex interplay between genetic and environmental factors. Recent genome-wide association studies have led to the identification of over 50 gene variants which modulate atherogenesis. Risk factors for atherosclerosis are in part also genetically determined: 40% of the variants contributing to atherogenesis overlap with gene variants modulating its risk factors, while the remaining 60% reside in regions which have previously not been related to atherosclerosis, suggesting that our knowledge about the pathophysiology of atherogenesis is incomplete. Despite these advances, the current relevance of these finding for clinical practice is limited. This is mainly due to the small effect sizes of identified risk variants with insufficient discriminatory power. In addition, a large portion of the genetic contribution to atherosclerosis is still unknown. The major promise therefore lies in understanding the pathophysiology of newly identified genes with the perspective of novel therapeutic approaches.

Heritability of atherosclerosis and its risk factors

Atherosclerosis is a complex genetic disease with a strong environmental component and significant gene–environment interaction (➲ Fig. 2.1). Complex genetic diseases are caused by a large number of genes and do not follow the classical pattern of Mendelian inheritance. It is also important to recognize that major risk factors for atherosclerosis, for example hyperlipidaemia, hypertension, and diabetes mellitus, are themselves complex genetic disorders. This all adds to the complicated nature of this common disease.

In population genetics, heritability is a measure that describes the contribution of genetic components to the variability of a trait in a defined population. The heritability for different end-points of atherosclerosis is approximately 50%, and it may be estimated from twin studies (➲ Table 2.1) [1]. In their classic work using the Swedish Twin Registry, Marenberg and colleagues [1,2] compared the concordance rate for monozygotic and dizygotic twins for myocardial infarction. They found that the risk of myocardial infarction was increased three-fold in female dizygotic twins (who share 50% of their genetic make-up) compared with 15-fold in female monozygotic twins (who share 100% of their genetic make-up) if their twin sister had previously suffered from myocardial infarction before the age of 55 years [2]. The genetic component for the risk of developing myocardial infarction appeared

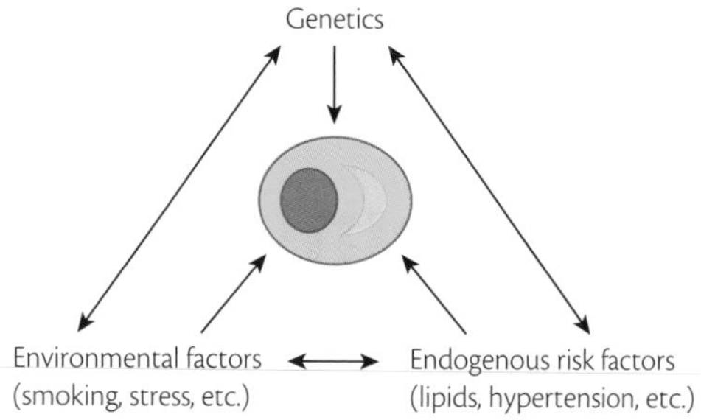

Fig. 2.1 Atherosclerosis is a complex genetic trait, driven by multiple genetic, environmental, and endogenous risk factors, and their interaction.

Table 2.1 Heritability estimates of atherosclerosis and its risk factors, and percentage of genetic variability explained by genome-wide association studies

Risk factor	Heritability	Number of loci identified by major GWAS	Genetic variability explained by major GWAS
Coronary artery disease/ myocardial infarction	40–50% [1]	46 [9]	6% [9]
Blood pressure	~30% [26]	28 [15]	0.9% [15]
Diabetes mellitus	26% [27]	63 [16]	~10% [16,28]
LDL cholesterol	45–60% [29,30]	36 [17]	~25–30% [17]
HDL cholesterol	47–62% [29,30]	47 [17]	~25–30% [17]
Lp(a)	65–94% [31,32]	4 [33]	~20% [33]
Addiction to smoking	~50% [34,35]	5 [18]	~1% [18]

GWAS, genome-wide association studies; LDL, low-density lipoprotein; HDL, high-density lipoprotein; Lp(a), lipoprotein(a).

to be particularly strong for younger individuals and declined with age [1,2]. Heritability has also been estimated for the major risk factors for atherosclerosis, and ranges from about 26% for diabetes mellitus to about 90% for plasma levels of lipoprotein(a) (➲ Table 2.1) [3]. A major limitation from the standpoint of causation is that heritability estimates only reveal the presence of a genetic component for a particular disease or risk factor but do not allow the genes responsible to be pinpointed.

Identification of the genetic factors for atherosclerosis

Several approaches have been used to identify genetic factors for atherosclerosis. A major breakthrough was achieved in 2007 with the advent of genome-wide association studies (GWAS) [4–7]. This type of study has made a significant contribution to the identification of the genetic components of atherosclerosis and its risk factors. GWAS have become possible as a result of major advances in microarray technology, allowing the simultaneous determination of >10^6 genetic variants from a single DNA sample and thus

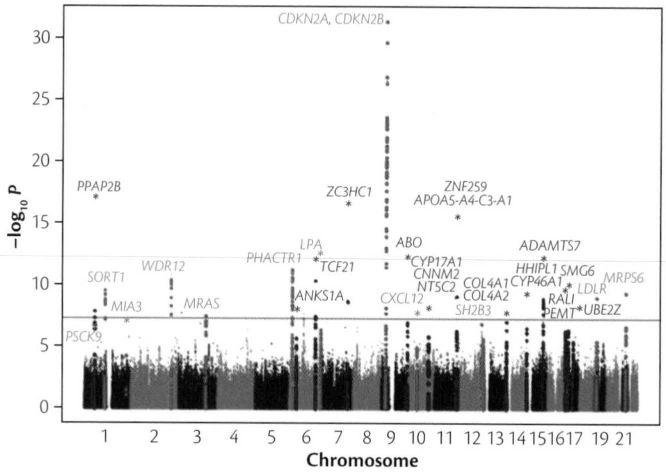

Fig. 2.2 Graphical summary of the results of genome-wide association studies for coronary artery disease from the CARDIoGRAM Consortium [8]. The –log *p* values of associations are plotted across the genome. Loci that were known at the time of the study (2011) are in red, novel loci found in the study are in blue.

Reprinted by permission from Macmillan Publishers Ltd: *Nature Genetics*, Schunkert, H. et al. Large-scale association analyses identifies 13 new susceptibility loci for coronary artery disease, *Nat Genet*. Mar 6, 2011; **43**(4): 333–338.

providing a representative picture of the variations present in an individual's genome. Application of this technology to large cohorts of cases with atherosclerosis and healthy controls allows systematic testing of how each of the >10^6 genetic variants is distributed between cases and controls. Differences in distribution are expressed as *p*-values, where small *p*-values indicate an association of a genomic variant with coronary artery disease. For easier overview, these *p*-values are usually plotted as negative decadic logarithms (–log *p*) across the genome (Manhattan plot). To reduce the chance of false positives, only *p*-values $< 5 \times 10^{-8}$ (based on a Bonferroni-corrected *p*-value of 0.05 for 10^6 tests, corresponding to $-\log p > 7.3$) are considered statistically significant. Since genetic effects tended to be small, it turned out that large cohorts were necessary to gain sufficient statistical power for the identification of causal variants. The largest study to date is a meta-analysis of several GWAS for coronary artery disease conducted by the CARDIoGRAM Consortium, involving 22 233 cases of coronary artery disease and 64 762 controls with a follow-up in 56 682 individuals [8]. The Manhattan plot of the results is shown in ➲ Fig. 2.2. This work was followed up by the CARDIoGRAM-plusC4D Consortium, which added additional cohorts, resulting in a total of 46 gene loci for coronary artery disease and providing by far the largest contribution to the field so far [9].

Genetics of different types of atherosclerotic cardiovascular disease

Atherosclerosis can occur in different vascular beds, leading to coronary artery disease, peripheral artery disease, and stroke as the three major types. Coronary artery disease has been the best studied of these, and more than 50 genetic variants identified by

GWAS are known to be involved [10]. In contrast, the only firmly established locus for peripheral artery disease is a locus on chromosome (Chr) 9p21 [11], which also modulates coronary artery disease and stroke [12]. For stroke, the METASTROKE Consortium identified three additional loci with genome-wide significance [13]. One of these loci, *histone deacetylase 9* (*HDAC9*), overlapped with coronary artery disease. Moreover, it has now become clear that there are marked differences in the genes responsible for the different subtypes of ischaemic stroke, related to differences in the underlying pathophysiology [13]. In summary, different types of atherosclerotic disease have certain genetic risk variants in common but also might differ in some specific genetic components.

New insights into the pathophysiology of atherosclerosis from GWAS

One of the major lessons from GWAS is that our current understanding of coronary artery disease is incomplete, since the majority of identified genes were not previously known to be involved. A good example is a locus on Chr9p21, which is the strongest genetic factor for atherosclerosis known today (2015). The locus resides in a 'gene desert'—a genomic region devoid of protein coding genes—which was not linked with atherosclerosis in the pre-GWAS era [12]. The association of Chr9p21 with atherosclerosis has been replicated in numerous studies, leaving no doubt that this locus plays a major role in atherogenesis. Functional studies have revealed that this region contains a long non-coding RNA, *antisense non-coding RNA at the INK4 locus* (*ANRIL*), which is not translated into a protein and is differentially regulated by the Chr9p21 risk genotype. Little is currently known about the mechanisms of such long non-coding RNAs, and functional studies suggest a role in epigenetic chromatin modification, thereby affecting key mechanisms of atherogenesis [14]. Taken together, GWAS have led to the identification of several genomic regions, but uncovering the functions of the responsible genes in atherogenesis will be a major challenge for the future.

Genetic modulation of atherosclerosis risk factors

GWAS approaches have also been applied to identify genes responsible for modulating the major risk factors of atherosclerosis. The largest single GWAS for blood pressure was conducted by a consortium of more than 300 authors in 200 000 individuals and it identified 28 genetic loci, of which 22 loci were, a priori, not strong candidates [15] (➲Table 2.1). For type 2 diabetes mellitus, a meta-GWAS with an effective sample size of 34 840 cases and 114 981 controls revealed 63 loci [16]. For blood lipids, 95 loci with genome-wide significance were reported in a meta-GWAS of more than 100 000 individuals. Fifty-nine of these loci were novel and showed significant genome-wide associations with lipid traits for the first time [17]. Intriguingly, the individual exposure

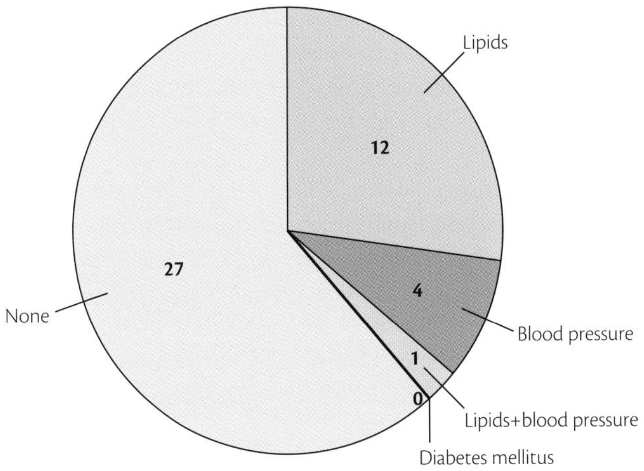

Fig. 2.3 Numbers of genetic variants for risk factors overlapping with genetic variants for coronary artery disease identified by the CARDIoGRAMplusC4D Consortium [9]. Total overlap is only 17 out of 44 (about 40%), suggesting that the majority of genetic risk is modulated by novel mechanisms unrelated to known risk factors for coronary artery disease.

to pro-atherogenic environmental conditions is—at least in part—also genetically driven. One such example is cigarette smoking, another major risk factor for atherosclerosis. While smoking might be considered as an environmental risk factor in the first place, addiction to smoking is a complex genetic trait [18,19]. Therefore, individuals carrying genetic risk variants are not only more prone to smoke but also to develop peripheral artery disease [19].

One approach to establishing causality between a risk factor and atherosclerosis is to look for overlaps between genetic variants which modulate risk factors and atherosclerosis at the same time. The CARDIoGRAMplusC4D Consortium identified such overlaps for 17 out of 44 loci (no data were available for two loci), corresponding to an overlap of 39% (➲ Fig. 2.3) [9]. On the other hand, 61% of genetic variants were *not* related to risk factors, thus holding the promise of new insights into the pathophysiology of atherogenesis.

Clinical implications

Even though a large number of loci related to atherosclerosis have been identified so far, the current relevance of these finding for clinical practice is limited. This is mainly due to the small effect sizes of the identified risk variants, each explaining <1% of the variability of the disease. Therefore, addition of the Chr9p21 risk variant—the largest frequent single genetic effect—to conventional risk factors has had no or only a marginal benefit for the prediction of coronary risk (for review see [12]). A multimarker approach, adding several dozen additional genetic variants with even smaller effect sizes, is not promising either since most individuals carry a mix of protective variants and risk variants, thus reducing the discriminative power. Moreover, the currently know gene loci explain only a small portion (<30%) of the genetic variability of atherosclerosis and its risk factors (➲ Table 2.1). The term 'missing heritability' has been coined for the large genetic contribution that is still unknown [20], and several strategies have been proposed to identify its causes [21]. Finally, we only are just beginning to understand gene–environment interactions [22], first proposed over 50 years ago in James Neel's 'thrifty gene hypothesis' [23].

The Joint European Society of Cardiology (ESC) guidelines on cardiovascular disease prevention in clinical practice (version 2012) conclude that 'the importance of the familial prevalence of early-onset CVD is not yet sufficiently understood in clinical practice' [24]. They currently do not see a value in DNA-based tests for common genetic variants (➲ Box 2.1), but encourage extended cascade screening for rare variants in cases of familial hypercholesterolaemia [24].

For the future, a risk score consisting of a very large number of small effects is expected to increase the area under the curve to 0.7 [25]. However, identifying and testing the effects of these variants in very large cohorts of a million individuals is a prerequisite [25] and currently prohibits this approach.

Box 2.1 ESC guidelines for genetic testing [24]

- DNA-based tests for common genetic polymorphisms do not currently add significantly to diagnosis, risk prediction, or patient management and cannot be recommended.
- The added value of genotyping, as an alternative or in addition to phenotyping, for better management of risk and early prevention in relatives cannot be recommended.

Conclusion

The lesson from recent GWAS is that atherosclerotic risk is modulated by a large number of genetic variants, each having only a very small effect, thus prohibiting clinical use at this point. The major promise lies in understanding the pathophysiology of newly identified genes, with the hope of novel therapeutic approaches.

Further reading

Holdt LM, Teupser D. Recent studies of the human chromosome 9p21 locus, which is associated with atherosclerosis in human populations. *Arterioscler Thromb Vasc Biol* 2012; **32**: 196–206.

Marenberg ME, Risch N, Berkman LF, et al. Genetic susceptibility to death from coronary heart disease in a study of twins. *N Engl J Med* 1994; **330**: 1041–6.

Perk J, De Backer G, Gohlke H, et al. European Guidelines on cardiovascular disease prevention in clinical practice (version 2012). The Fifth Joint Task Force of the European Society of Cardiology and Other Societies on Cardiovascular Disease Prevention in Clinical Practice (constituted by representatives of nine societies and by invited experts). *Eur Heart J* 2012; **33**: 1635–701.

Schunkert H, Konig IR, Kathiresan S, et al. Large-scale association analysis identifies 13 new susceptibility loci for coronary artery disease. *Nat Genet* 2011; **43**: 333–8.

The CARDIoGRAMplusC4D Consortium. Large-scale association analysis identifies new risk loci for coronary artery disease. *Nat Genet* 2013; **45**: 25–33.

References

1 Zdravkovic S, Wienke A, Pedersen NL, et al. Heritability of death from coronary heart disease: a 36-year follow-up of 20 966 Swedish twins. *J Intern Med* 2002; **252**: 247–54.

2 Marenberg ME, Risch N, Berkman LF, et al. Genetic susceptibility to death from coronary heart disease in a study of twins. *N Engl J Med* 1994; **330**: 1041–6.

3 Lusis AJ, Fogelman AM, Fonarow GC. Genetic basis of atherosclerosis: part I: new genes and pathways. *Circulation* 2004; **110**: 1868–73.

4 Helgadottir A, Thorleifsson G, Manolescu A, et al. A common variant on chromosome 9p21 affects the risk of myocardial infarction. *Science* 2007; **316**: 1491–3.

5 McPherson R, Pertsemlidis A, Kavaslar N, et al. A common allele on chromosome 9 associated with coronary heart disease. *Science* 2007; **316**: 1488–91.

6 Samani NJ, Erdmann J, Hall AS, et al. Genome-wide association analysis of coronary artery disease. *New Engl J Med* 2007; **357**: 443–53.

7 The Wellcome Trust Case Control Consortium. Genome-wide association study of 14,000 cases of seven common diseases and 3,000 shared controls. *Nature* 2007; **447**: 661–78.

8 Schunkert H, Konig IR, Kathiresan S, et al. Large-scale association analysis identifies 13 new susceptibility loci for coronary artery disease. *Nat Genet* 2011; **43**: 333–8.

9 The CARDIoGRAMplusC4D Consortium. Large-scale association analysis identifies new risk loci for coronary artery disease. *Nat Genet* 2013; **45**: 25–33.

10 Holdt LM, Teupser D. From genotype to phenotype in human atherosclerosis—recent findings. *Curr Opin Lipidol* 2013; **24**: 410–18.

11 Murabito JM, White CC, Kavousi M, et al. Association between chromosome 9p21 variants and the ankle-brachial index identified by a meta-analysis of 21 genome-wide association studies. *Circ Cardiovasc Genet* 2012; **5**: 100–12.

12 Holdt LM, Teupser D. Recent studies of the human chromosome 9p21 locus, which is associated with atherosclerosis in human populations. *Arterioscler Thromb Vasc Biol* 2012; **32**: 196–206.

13 Traylor M, Farrall M, Holliday EG, et al. Genetic risk factors for ischaemic stroke and its subtypes (the METASTROKE collaboration): a meta-analysis of genome-wide association studies. *Lancet Neurol* 2012; **11**: 951–62.

14 Holdt LM, Hoffmann S, Sass K, et al. Alu elements in ANRIL non-coding RNA at chromosome 9p21 modulate atherogenic cell functions through trans-regulation of gene networks. *PLoS Genet* 2013; **9**: e1003588.

15 International Consortium for Blood Pressure Genome-Wide Association Studies. Genetic variants in novel pathways influence blood pressure and cardiovascular disease risk. *Nature* 2011; **478**: 103–9.

16 Morris AP, Voight BF, Teslovich TM, et al. Large-scale association analysis provides insights into the genetic architecture and pathophysiology of type 2 diabetes. *Nat Genet* 2012; **44**: 981–90.

17 Teslovich TM, Musunuru K, Smith AV, et al. Biological, clinical and population relevance of 95 loci for blood lipids. *Nature* 2010; **466**: 707–13.

18 Tobacco and Genetics Consortium. Genome-wide meta-analyses identify multiple loci associated with smoking behavior. *Nat Genet* 2010; **42**: 441–7.

19 Thorgeirsson TE, Geller F, Sulem P, et al. A variant associated with nicotine dependence, lung cancer and peripheral arterial disease. *Nature* 2008; **452**: 638–42.

20 Manolio TA, Collins FS, Cox NJ, et al. Finding the missing heritability of complex diseases. *Nature* 2009; **461**: 747–53.

21 Eichler EE, Flint J, Gibson G, et al. Missing heritability and strategies for finding the underlying causes of complex disease. *Nat Rev Genet* 2010; **11**: 446–50.

22 Dempfle A, Scherag A, Hein R, et al. Gene-environment interactions for complex traits: definitions, methodological requirements and challenges. *Eur J Hum Genet* 2008; **16**: 1164–72.

23 Neel JV. Diabetes mellitus: a 'thrifty' genotype rendered detrimental by 'progress'? *Am J Hum Genet* 1962; **14**: 353–62.

24 Perk J, De Backer G, Gohlke H, et al. European Guidelines on cardiovascular disease prevention in clinical practice (version 2012). The Fifth Joint Task Force of the European Society of Cardiology and Other Societies on Cardiovascular Disease Prevention in Clinical Practice (constituted by representatives of nine societies and by invited experts). *Eur Heart J* 2012; **33**: 1635–701.

25 Chatterjee N, Wheeler B, Sampson J, et al. Projecting the performance of risk prediction based on polygenic analyses of genome-wide association studies. *Nat Genet* 2013; **45**: 400–5, 5e 1–3.

26 Miall WE, Oldham PD. The hereditary factor in arterial blood-pressure. *Br Med J* 1963; **1**: 75–80.

27 Poulsen P, Kyvik KO, Vaag A, et al. Heritability of type II (non-insulin-dependent) diabetes mellitus and abnormal glucose tolerance—a population-based twin study. *Diabetologia* 1999; **42**: 139–45.

28 Voight BF, Scott LJ, Steinthorsdottir V, et al. Twelve type 2 diabetes susceptibility loci identified through large-scale association analysis. *Nat Genet* 2010; **42**: 579–89.

29 Friedlander Y, Kark JD, Stein Y. Biological and environmental sources of variation in plasma lipids and lipoproteins: the Jerusalem Lipid Research Clinic. *Hum Hered* 1986; **36**: 143–53.

30 Perusse L, Despres JP, Tremblay A, et al. Genetic and environmental determinants of serum lipids and lipoproteins in French Canadian families. *Arteriosclerosis* 1989; **9**: 308–18.

31 Austin MA, Sandholzer C, Selby JV, et al. Lipoprotein(a) in women twins: heritability and relationship to apolipoprotein(a) phenotypes. *Am J Hum Genet* 1992; **51**: 829–40.

32 Scholz M, Kraft HG, Lingenhel A, et al. Genetic control of lipoprotein(a) concentrations is different in Africans and Caucasians. *Eur J Hum Genet* 1999; **7**: 169–78.

33 Qi Q, Workalemahu T, Zhang C, et al. Genetic variants, plasma lipoprotein(a) levels, and risk of cardiovascular morbidity and mortality among two prospective cohorts of type 2 diabetes. *Eur Heart J* 2012; **33**: 325–34.

34 Koopmans JR, Slutske WS, Heath AC, et al. The genetics of smoking initiation and quantity smoked in Dutch adolescent and young adult twins. *Behav Genet* 1999; **29**: 383–93.

35 Li MD, Cheng R, Ma JZ, et al. A meta-analysis of estimated genetic and environmental effects on smoking behavior in male and female adult twins. *Addiction* 2003; **98**: 23–31.

CHAPTER 3

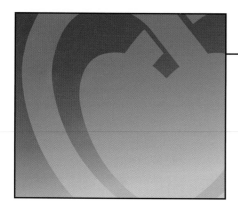

From risk factors to plaque development and plaque destabilization

Ulf Landmesser and Wolfgang Koenig

Contents

Summary

Over the last decades vascular research has unveiled the complex interaction between exposure to risk factors and pathological changes at the vessel wall. It has become clear that risk factors such as smoking or hyperlipidaemia first cause a pre-morbid phenotype with reversible dysfunction of flow-mediated vasodilation, referred to as endothelial dysfunction (ED). Although ED is not a disease in itself it was shown to be a negative prognostic indicator in patients with hypertension, diabetes, and stable coronary artery disease. If exposure to risk factor(s) does not cease, ED develops into the first morphological vascular changes that finally lead to atherosclerosis: through the expression of vascular adhesion factors, monocytes transmigrate into the subintimal space where they may transform into macrophages in the presence of lipid deposits. Cholesterol crystals are one of the mechanisms that have been shown to lead to pro-inflammatory activation of macrophages. Atherosclerotic plaques are characterized by lipid-laden macrophages, lymphocytes, and dendritic cells that release several pro-inflammatory factors such as cytokines and chemokines. The progression from stable coronary plaques to the plaque rupture that underlies the acute coronary syndrome occurs more frequently if a large necrotic core (a lipid-rich centre) is present. The thin fibrous cap that is disrupted is often infiltrated by foamy macrophages and has few smooth muscle cells. T-cell-derived interferon-gamma may limit collagen production by vascular smooth muscle cells, and T-cell-derived CD40 ligand can activate the release of collagenase from activated macrophages contributing to destabilization of the fibrous cap. The chapter provides a basic up-to-date concept of the development and progression of atherosclerosis and highlights the stages where preventive measures may still be effective.

The development of atherosclerotic plaques

Atherosclerosis is a complex multifocal disease of medium-sized and large arteries that is promoted both by modifiable risk factors, such as hypercholesterolaemia, smoking, obesity, diabetes, and hypertension, and by genetic susceptibility [1]. Numerous studies have suggested that atherosclerosis represents a maladaptive chronic vascular immune–inflammatory disease, involving innate and adaptive immune responses that are at least

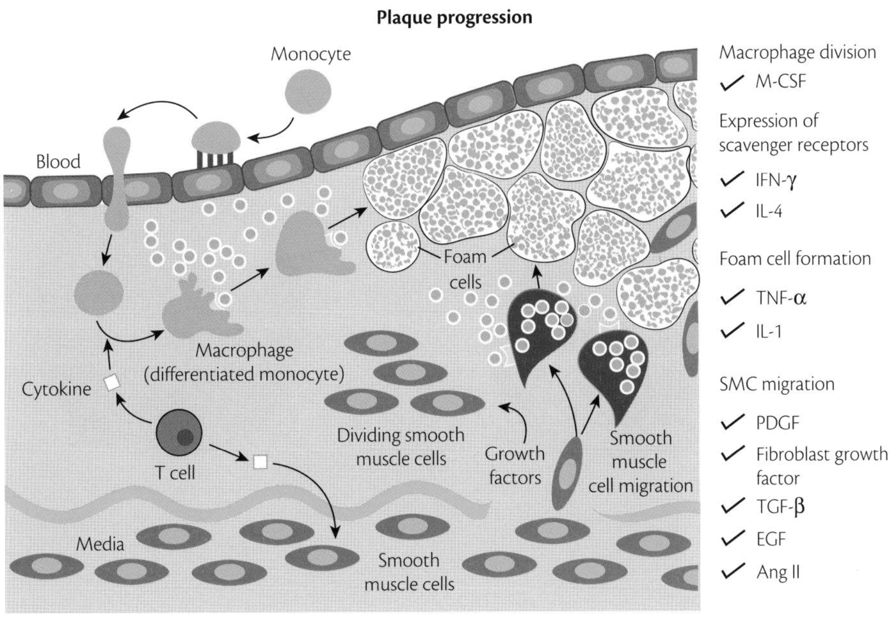

Fig. 3.1 Endothelial cell activation leads to monocyte adhesion and sub-endothelial LDL promotes foam cell formation. M-CSF, macrophage colony-stimulating factor; IFN-γ, interferon-gamma; TNF-α, tumour necrosis factor-alpha; SMC, smooth muscle cell; PDGF, platelet-derived growth factor.

partially driven by pro-atherogenic lipoproteins, in particular modified low-density lipoprotein (LDL) [2,3].

Moreover, endothelial cells in the arteries can be activated to express leucocyte adhesion molecules by all known cardiovascular risk factors, promoting leucocyte adhesion and infiltration that may subsequently lead to the development and progression of atherosclerotic plaque (➲ Fig. 3.1) [4]. Furthermore, cardiovascular risk factors reduce the availability to endothelial cells of nitric oxide derived from endothelial nitric oxide (NO) synthase that promotes a pro-inflammatory and pro-thrombotic phenotype of the endothelium.

Atherosclerotic plaques are particularly characterized by lipid-laden macrophages, lymphocytes, and dendritic cells that release several pro-inflammatory factors, such as cytokines and chemokines. Cholesterol crystals are one of the mechanisms that have been shown to lead to the pro-inflammatory activation of macrophages by stimulating the NLRP3 inflammasome and promoting the release of cytokines, in particular interleukin (IL)-1 beta [5]. Whereas modifications to LDL that promote its uptake by macrophages in the vascular wall have long been considered to be one of the mechanisms leading to arterial inflammation and atherosclerosis, more recent studies have suggested that in patients with cardiovascular risk factors, or who are at increased cardiovascular risk, the anti-atherogenic effects of high-density lipoproteins (HDLs) are impaired due to modifications that result, at least in part, from inflammatory activation. Modified HDL has been shown to promote vascular inflammation via the LOX-1 or TLR-2 receptor [6,7].

Clearly, both innate and adaptive immunological responses play a major role in the development and progression of atherosclerosis. Notably, both macrophages and T and B lymphocytes can either increase or limit vascular inflammatory responses. For T lymphocytes, the T helper (TH)-1 cell subset has been suggested to play a pro-atherogenic role, whereas regulatory T cells, a subpopulation of T cells functioning to maintain immune homeostasis by suppressing pathogenic immune responses, probably play an anti-atherogenic role [8,9]. Similarly, macrophages have different phenotypes (e.g. macrophage polarization into M1 or M2 macrophages) that can either promote or limit inflammation [10]. Recent experimental studies have suggested that atherosclerosis can also be promoted by mechanisms leading to retention of macrophages in the artery wall, i.e. preventing macrophages emigrating from atherosclerotic plaques [11].

A causal role for inflammatory mechanisms in the pathophysiology of atherosclerosis is further suggested by the results of recent large-scale genetic Mendelian randomization studies [12,13].

Destabilization of atherosclerotic plaques

Whereas the development of atherosclerotic plaque starts early in life, clinical manifestations of atherosclerotic coronary artery disease frequently appear later in life as either 'stable coronary disease' or, frequently, as an acute coronary syndrome, indicating a long 'asymptomatic' phase of the disease. In fact, it probably takes many years or decades to develop the advanced lesions responsible for clinical disease, offering great opportunities for detection and prevention.

The morphologies of coronary artery plaques observed in patients with acute coronary syndrome underlying thrombosis are primarily physically ruptured plaques and plaque erosions, with plaque rupture being the most frequent cause of acute coronary syndromes, particularly in men [14–16]. This was initially suggested as a result of autopsy studies, but has more recently been

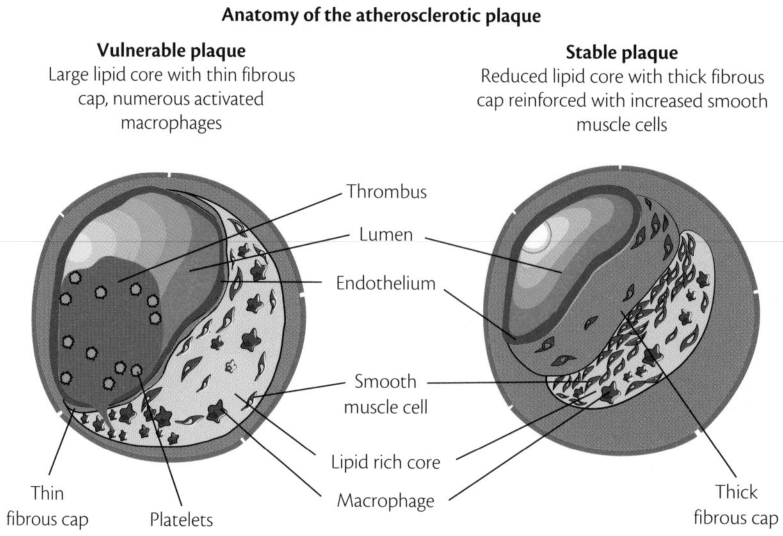

Fig. 3.2 Characteristics of a vulnerable rupture-prone atherosclerotic plaque compared with a stable plaque. The thin fibrous cap, large lipid core, and numerous activated macrophages are shown.

confirmed using high-resolution intracoronary imaging methods, such as optical coherence tomography imaging, in patients with an acute coronary syndrome [14–16].

Ruptured plaques frequently have a large necrotic core (a lipid-rich centre) and a thin fibrous cap that is disrupted, and they are often infiltrated by foamy macrophages and have few smooth muscle cells [14,15] (➲ Fig. 3.2). Several mechanisms can contribute to destabilization of the fibrous cap, for example T-cell-derived interferon-gamma may limit collagen production by vascular smooth muscle cells and T-cell-derived CD40 ligand can activate the release of collagenase from activated macrophages [14], indicating cross-talk between T cells (adaptive immune cells) and macrophages, the more frequent innate immune effector cells (➲ Fig. 3.3) [14].

Plaque erosion lesions are often rich in smooth muscle cells and proteoglycans with fewer signs of inflammation [15]. However, a recent study has suggested that plaque erosions are associated with higher levels of serum myeloperoxidase and a higher density of myeloperoxidase-positive cells in coronary thrombi [16].

Notably, statin therapy, which reduces the risk of acute coronary syndromes, has only a limited impact on the degree of coronary stenosis, suggesting that this treatment rather alters the biological features of the plaque to prevent intracoronary thrombus formation, termed 'plaque stabilization' [17].

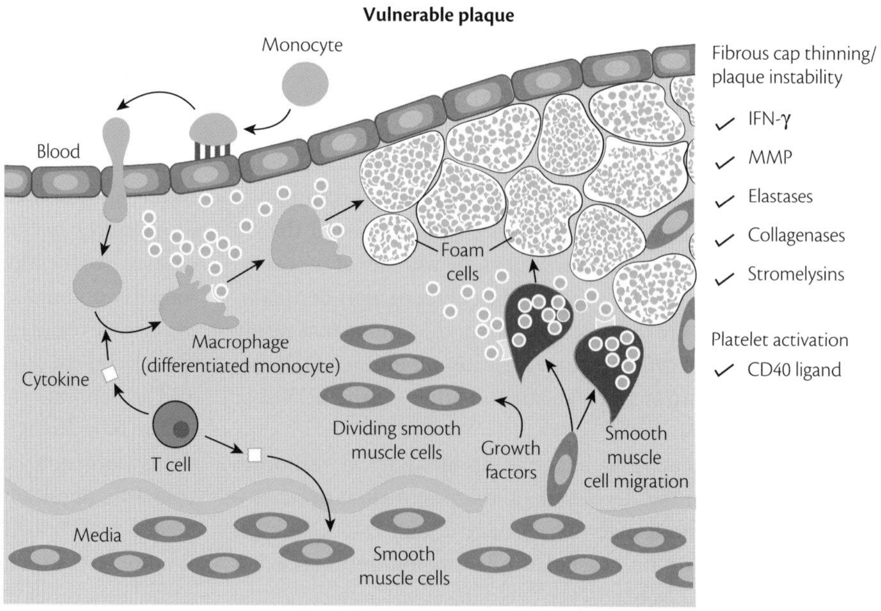

Fig. 3.3 TH1 lymphocytes release interferon-gamma that inhibits collagen syntheses by vascular smooth muscle cells and CD40 ligand leading to the release of collagenase from activated macrophages promoting destabilization of the atherosclerotic plaque. IFN-γ, interferon-gamma; MMP, matrix metalloproteinase.

References

1 Schunkert H, König IR, Kathiresan S, et al. Large-scale association analysis identifies 13 new susceptibility loci for coronary artery disease. *Nat Genet* 2011; **43**: 333–8.

2 Weber C, Noels H. Atherosclerosis: current pathogenesis and therapeutic options. *Nat Med* 2011; **17**: 1410–22.

3 Moore KJ, Tabas I. Macrophages in the pathogenesis of atherosclerosis. *Cell* 2011; **145**: 341–55.

4 Landmesser U, Hornig B, Drexler H. Endothelial function: a critical determinant in atherosclerosis? *Circulation* 2004; **109**: II27–II33.

5 Duewell P, Kono H, Rayner KJ, et al. NLRP3 inflammasomes are required for atherogenesis and activated by cholesterol crystals. *Nature* 2010; **464**: 1357–61.

6 Besler C, Heinrich H, Rohrer L, et al. Mechanisms underlying adverse effects of HDL on eNOS-activating pathways in patients with coronary artery disease. *J Clin Invest* 2011; **121**: 2693–708.

7 Speer T, Rohrer L, Blyszczuk P, et al. Abnormal high-density lipoprotein induces endothelial dysfunction via activation of Toll-like receptor-2. *Immunity* 2013; **38**: 754–68.

8 Lahoute C, Herbin O, Mallat Z, et al. Adaptive immunity in atherosclerosis: mechanisms and future therapeutic targets. *Nat Rev Cardiol* 2011; **8**: 348–58.

9 Klingenberg R, Gerdes N, Badeau RM, et al. Depletion of FOXP3 + regulatory T cells promotes hypercholesterolemia and atherosclerosis. *J Clin Invest* 2013; **123**: 1323–34.

10 Leitinger N, Schulman IG. Phenotypic polarization of macrophages in atherosclerosis. *Arterioscler Thromb Vasc Biol* 2013; **33**: 1120–6.

11 van Gils JM, Derby MC, Fernandes LR, et al. The neuroimmune guidance cue netrin-1 promotes atherosclerosis by inhibiting the emigration of macrophages from plaques. *Nat Immunol* 2012; **13**: 136–43.

12 Hingorani AD, Casas JP. The interleukin-6 receptor as a target for prevention of coronary heart disease: a mendelian randomisation analysis. *Lancet* 2012; **379**: 1214–24.

13 Sarwar N, Butterworth AS, Freitag DF, et al. Interleukin-6 receptor pathways in coronary heart disease: a collaborative meta-analysis of 82 studies. *Lancet* 2012; **379**: 1205–13.

14 Libby P. Mechanisms of acute coronary syndromes and their implications for therapy. *N Engl J Med* 2013; **368**: 2004–13.

15 Falk E, Nakano M, Bentzon JF, et al. Update on acute coronary syndromes: the pathologists' view. *Eur Heart J* 2013; **34**: 719–28.

16 Ferrante G, Nakano M, Prati F, et al. High levels of systemic myeloperoxidase are associated with coronary plaque erosion in patients with acute coronary syndromes: a clinicopathological study. *Circulation* 2010; **122**: 2505–13.

17 Ylä-Herttuala S, Bentzon JF, Daemen M, et al. Stabilisation of atherosclerotic plaques. Position paper of the European Society of Cardiology (ESC) Working Group on Atherosclerosis and Vascular Biology. *Thromb Haemost* 2011; **106**: 1–19.

CHAPTER 4

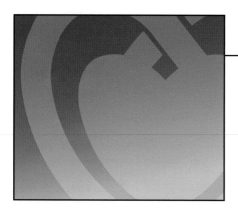

The role of thrombosis

Elena M. Faioni, Maddalena Lettino, and Marco Cattaneo

Contents

Summary

Acute thrombotic occlusions of arterial vessels are often due to fissure of an atherosclerotic plaque, with consequent activation of haemostasis and clot formation. Arterial thrombosis also plays a crucial role in accelerating the progression of atherosclerotic lesions, and it is becoming clear that mechanisms that sustain chronic inflammation and the development of atheroma share many features with those that sustain thrombosis of the plaque. Chronic activation of endothelium, platelets, and leucocytes leads to plaque formation, while acute events, related to a flare-up of inflammation, precipitate plaque fissure and thereby promote thrombus formation on the plaque, partial or total vessel occlusion, and flow disturbance. Thrombus-derived proteins stimulate plaque growth and progression, and the thrombus itself is incorporated into the plaque, further restricting the vessel lumen. A more detailed understanding of the various steps implicated in plaque thrombosis and progression and the related clinical manifestations is required for tailoring of individual therapy, identification of novel therapeutic targets, and increasing the success of primary and secondary prevention.

Introduction

Acute thrombotic occlusions of arterial vessels, which may precipitate myocardial infarction and/or stroke (major causes of mortality and morbidity in both developed and emerging countries), are often due to fissure of an atherosclerotic plaque, with consequent activation of haemostasis and clot formation [1]. Arterial thrombosis also plays a crucial role in accelerating the progression of atherosclerotic lesions; it is becoming clear that mechanisms that sustain chronic inflammation and the development of atheroma share many features with those that sustain thrombosis of the plaque. ➲ Figure 4.1 gives a schematic illustration of our current understanding of these events. Chronic activation of endothelium, platelets, and leucocytes leads to plaque formation. Acute events, related to a flare-up of inflammation, precipitate plaque fissure and thereby promote thrombus formation on the plaque, partial or total vessel occlusion, and flow disturbance. Thrombus-derived proteins stimulate plaque growth and progression, and the thrombus itself is incorporated into the plaque, further restricting the vessel lumen. This vicious cycle is extremely difficult to interrupt, as shown by the lack of decrease in morbidity and mortality beyond a fixed percentage with current therapeutic approaches [2]. A more detailed understanding of the various steps implicated in plaque

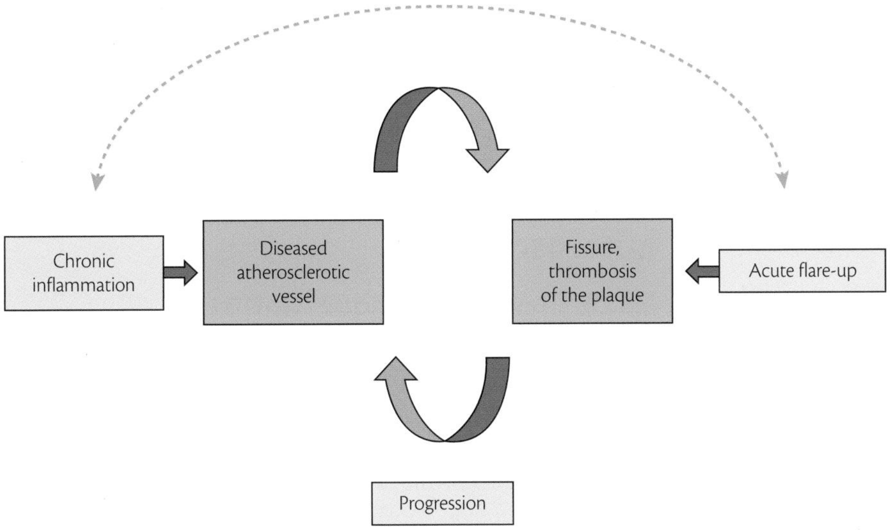

Fig. 4.1 Schematic representation of plaque formation, thrombosis, and progression. Chronic activation of adhesion molecules, endothelium, platelets, and leucocytes leads to plaque formation. Acute events, related to inflammation and coagulation, precipitate plaque fissure and thereby promote thrombus formation on the plaque and vessel occlusion. Thrombus-derived proteins stimulate plaque growth and progression.

thrombosis and progression and the related clinical manifestations is required to allow tailoring of individual therapy, identification of novel therapeutic targets, and increased success of primary and secondary prevention.

Pathogenic mechanisms of thrombosis on ruptured atherosclerotic plaques and plaque progression

Loss of the endothelial protective phenotype and the shift towards a thrombogenic surface

Normal endothelium is an anticoagulant, anti-inflammatory surface. Leucocytes and platelets do not adhere to resting endothelium and clotting is averted by the presence of receptors and molecules that prevent the amplification of haemostasis by thrombin. Glycosaminoglycans (GAGs) coat the surface of the endothelium and function as cofactors to antithrombin, a serine protease inhibitor with high specificity for thrombin and activated factor X [3]. A moderate but locally important reduction in antithrombin function may be caused by a reduction in the availability of GAGs at the endothelial surface [3]. Antithrombin also promotes the release of prostacyclin from endothelial cells *in vivo*, through its interaction with GAGs [4].

Thrombomodulin is expressed on the surface of quiescent endothelium. This is a receptor that acts as an important scavenger of the trace amounts of thrombin that are constantly generated physiologically and, by changing its substrate specificity, promotes activation of protein C, a pivotal anticoagulant [5]. Inflammatory mediators, such as tumour necrosis factor-alpha and interleukin (IL)-1, downregulate thrombomodulin, thus shutting down endogenous anticoagulant protection [6]. The same mediators can upregulate the expression of adhesion molecules for leucocytes [7]. The net result is a shift towards a pro-inflammatory, procoagulant phenotype which favours plaque formation.

Nitric oxide is a potent inhibitor of platelet activation, the first and essential step in arterial thrombus formation, through an increase in intracellular guanosine monophosphate; it is also a potent vasodilator [8]. It is produced by nitric oxide synthases, intracellular enzymes that are also present in endothelial cells and are downregulated by low-density lipoprotein (LDL) and oxidative stress [9]. Prostacyclin is another important inhibitor of platelet activation through increase of cyclic adenosine monophosphate [10]. Prostacyclin is derived from the metabolism of arachidonic acid, which is impaired by cigarette smoking [11]. Another factor protecting the endothelium is CD39, an ecto-ADPase, the function of which is to degrade adenosine diphosphate (ADP), a potent platelet agonist, released from cells [12].

Globally, a dysfunction of the endothelium predisposes to atherosclerosis and to a pro-thrombotic phenotype [13]. At some point, the plaque endothelium is eroded as a consequence of endothelial death, exposing the plaque core, rich in lipids, necrotic cells, and fibrous substances, and triggering haemostasis and thrombus formation.

Platelet adhesion and activation

Platelets adhere to collagen and von Willebrand factor in the subendothelium. Under conditions of high shear, such as those found in stenotic vessels, von Willebrand factor plays a major role in interaction between platelets and the sub-endothelium [14]. Platelets translocate over a specifically shear-stress conformed von Willebrand factor, which, together with other adhesive proteins, allows firm adhesion, followed by activation and secretion, leading to the formation of a platelet aggregate [14]. Secretion of substances stored in platelet granules, among which are platelet agonists such as ADP and serotonin, amplifies aggregation and further platelet recruitment, through specific receptors and signalling pathways [15].

Tissue factor, thrombin, and fibrin generation

Activation of platelets leads to exposure of phosphatidylserine, which promotes the assembly of coagulation complexes on the

Table 4.1 Main pro-coagulant, anticoagulant, and pro-inflammatory functions of thrombin

General functions	Specific functions
Amplification of coagulation and clot formation	Activates cofactors V and VIII Cleaves fibrinogen to fibrin Activates factor XIII
Platelet activation	Activates platelets through protease-activated receptors (PARs)
Inflammation	Chemoattractant for neutrophils Stimulates cell adhesion
Stimulation of cell proliferation	Growth factors from platelet and endothelium activation
Anticoagulant pathway	Activates protein C

plasma membrane, favouring thrombin formation [16]. Coagulation is also triggered by the release of sub-endothelial tissue factor [17]. Although plaque thrombosis is usually rich in platelets, the tail of the platelet thrombus (in the low-flow area) is fibrin rich [18]. The fibrin clot can extend if the endothelium surrounding the fissured plaque is dysfunctional and therefore lacks anticoagulant protection. Thrombin, an enzyme involved in the coagulation process, possesses pro-thrombotic and pro-inflammatory functions (summarized in ➲ Table 4.1), thus linking coagulation, inflammation, and plaque progression [19].

Factors responsible for plaque progression

Incorporation of the clot within the growing plaque is a frequent occurrence over time, and is one of the main mechanisms of plaque growth until the vessel is totally occluded by a thrombotic event associated with a clinically evident ischaemia [20]. Other mechanisms are responsible for plaque progression. Intraplaque haemorrhage, which triggers plaque development via activated coagulation factors and cell debris, can occur spontaneously or develop during anticoagulant and antiplatelet therapies (especially if they occur together) [21]. Another important aspect is the pro-inflammatory role of platelets [22]. Though most experimental evidence derives from animal studies, this aspect is becoming an interesting focus for targeted preventive strategies. Finally, perturbance of flow plays a major role in platelet adhesion: it has been shown that platelets are more adherent in conditions of impairment of laminar flow, such as that observed over plaques [23].

New players

Coagulation initiated by tissue factor is only one of the possible pathways for thrombin generation. Coagulation can be initiated by contact activation via factor XII. Recent work has shown that dense platelet granules store and release inorganic polyphosphates which directly bind and activate factor XII [24]. Mice lacking factor XII do not bleed, and at the same time are protected from thrombus formation and ischaemic stroke [25]. Additionally, a novel fusion protein with activated factor XII-inhibiting action protects mice from thrombus formation in an experimental model of carotid artery thrombosis, without inducing bleeding [26]. Though these results are preliminary, they provide new insights into the mechanisms of thrombus formation, as distinct from normal haemostasis, and suggest novel therapeutic strategies.

Thrombosis as a complication of atherosclerosis

Factors favouring plaque rupture

Rupture of high-risk, vulnerable plaque is responsible for coronary thrombosis, the main cause of unstable angina (UA), acute myocardial infarction, and sudden cardiac death. It has been suggested that the processes of atherosclerosis and thrombosis appear to be interdependent and could therefore come under the single term 'atherothrombosis', which includes atherosclerosis and its thrombotic complications [27]. Atherothrombosis usually involves non-stenotic atherosclerotic plaques—the plaque composition rather than its volume is considered the major determinant of the disease.

Plaques that are prone to rupture are called 'high-risk' or 'vulnerable' plaques. A written consensus from a group of experts has properly standardized these terms defining a vulnerable, high-risk plaque as a plaque that is at increased risk of thrombosis, while a ruptured plaque is an atherosclerotic vascular lesion with a deep injury and a real defect or gap in the fibrous cap that separates its lipid-rich atheromatous core from the flowing blood, thereby exposing the thrombogenic core of the plaque [28]. These plaques have a large core of extracellular lipids intermixed with areas of necrotic material, mainly deriving from apoptotic cells, covered by a thin fibrous cap. Lipids derive from the sub-endothelial accumulation of LDL particles (native and modified through oxidation), which induce endothelial secretion of chemotactic substances and the expression of adhesion receptors, including integrins and selectins, which favour the recruitment of monocytes into the arterial wall. Once monocytes reach the intimal space, they transform into macrophages and begin to take up LDL particles, accumulating huge amounts of lipids. Lipid-loaded cells, or 'foam cells', release cytokines, growth factors, and other enzymes such as matrix metalloproteinases (MMPs) that are capable of degrading the fibrous cap and the sub-endothelial basement membrane, promoting plaque rupture [29]. High-risk vulnerable plaques are therefore characterized by the significant activation of inflammation with high levels of pro-inflammatory markers and low levels of anti-inflammatory cytokines (especially IL-10), both in the blood and inside the plaque. Inflammation also contributes to increased oxygen demand inside the plaque, resulting in relative hypoxia, which acts as a most potent stimulus of neoangiogenesis. In atherosclerotic plaques inflammation and hypoxia synergistically stimulate the proliferation of vasa vasorum, promoting intimal invasion and progression of atherosclerosis. Thin-walled neovessels are fragile and prone to bleed inside the plaque, and lipid-rich red blood cell membranes and free haemoglobin accumulate and contribute to increased inflammation, lipid core volume, and oxidative stress [21].

Pathological studies have suggested that to favour plaque rupture a thin fibrous cap should be associated with a lipid-rich atheroma. A thin fibrous cap (maximum thickness less than 65 μm) is in fact easily digested by macrophages and MMPs, and was described by Burke et al. [30] in 95% of ruptured plaques in 113 patients with coronary artery disease complicated by sudden cardiac death. More recently, the PROSPECT prospective, multicentre study evaluated the natural history of coronary atherothrombosis, using multimodality intravascular imaging *in vivo* to identify the clinical and lesion-related factors that place patients with an acute coronary syndrome (ACS) at risk for adverse new cardiac events [31]. Six hundred and ninety-seven patients with ACS who had undergone three-vessel coronary angiography and percutaneous revascularization of the culprit lesion were followed up for a median time of 3.4 years, and subsequent major cardiovascular events were adjudicated to be related to either originally treated lesions or untreated ones. This study again demonstrated that most non-culprit lesions responsible for follow-up events were not angiographically stenosing at baseline: moreover a thin fibrous cap was documented to be one of the major independent predictors of events in association with other lesion characteristics [31].

Because an atherosclerotic plaque is subject to mechanical loadings due to blood pressure and flow, which could exceed its material strength, there are also physical causes that contribute to pathological plaque rupture. Experimental data suggest that the role of structural stresses in plaques is even more important in triggering rupture than the wall shear stress due to blood flow. It is well known that calcified plaques are stiffer than lipid-rich ones and that the fibrous cap rich in inflammatory cells is weaker and more susceptible to breakage than a hypocellular one. It has therefore been demonstrated that from a merely physical point of view, a lipid-rich atheroma with a high-volume lipid core and a superimposed thin fibrous cap is conceivably more prone to rupture than a fibrotic plaque, with a preferable break location in the highly cellular part of the cap itself [32].

A different form of coronary plaque rupture is erosion, characterized by the loss of endothelial coverage of atherosclerotic lesions with a thick cap rich in proteoglycans and smooth muscle cells, with minimal inflammatory infiltration. A necrotic core is frequently present, but it is far from the vessel lumen, close to the adventitia. Patients with this kind of vulnerable plaque are usually younger than those with ruptured lipid-rich plaques, and the narrowing of the vessel lumen at sites of thrombosis is frequently mild. Farb et al. [33] examined over 400 cases of sudden death, finding a coronary thrombosis in 60% of the patients; 55–60% of thrombi were superimposed over ruptured plaques with a lipid-rich core while 30–35% were over eroded plaques. Plaque erosion is associated with smoking, especially in women, accounting for more than 80% of sudden pre-menopausal coronary deaths [34].

Clinical manifestations of coronary thrombosis

ACS is the most common clinical manifestation of coronary thrombosis, and is still associated with consistent morbidity and mortality. Thrombosis is usually superimposed on ruptured or eroded plaques and is frequently associated with distal embolization. Myocardial ischaemia and necrosis both derive from occlusion of the lumen of an epicardial coronary vessel and from obliteration of the small and distal coronary branches by microemboli of platelets and red blood cells. A spectrum of diseases are included in the definition of ACS: UA, non-ST-segment elevation myocardial infarction (NSTEMI), ST-segment elevation myocardial infarction (STEMI), and sudden cardiac death. All these conditions are usually characterized by the abrupt occurrence of frank chest discomfort or pain associated with diaphoresis and unexplained fatigue, and sometimes with dyspnoea, nausea, and vomiting. Plaque rupture and coronary thrombosis can also occur without any associated clinical manifestation. Moreover, in ACS patients multiple plaque ruptures with different grades of superimposed thrombosis distinct from the culprit lesion have been documented *in vivo* [35].

When prolonged ischaemia produces myocardial infarction, patients are classified on the basis of the electrocardiogram (ECG) characteristics (➲ Fig. 4.2):

1. Patients with prolonged chest pain (>20 minutes) and persistent ST-segment elevation usually develop STEMI.
2. Patients with accessional chest pain or discomfort lasting less than 20 minutes, associated with dynamic deviation of the ST-segment on ECG, both as transient elevation and as depression, generally develop non-STEMI (NSTEMI). Other ECG abnormalities may associate with NSTEMI or unstable angina, like T-wave inversion, flat T-waves, or pseudo T-wave normalization.

Patients with NSTEMI and STEMI might differ in the type of thrombus superimposed on a ruptured plaque. A platelet-rich clot only partially occluding the artery is more common in UA and NSTEMI, while a fibrin-rich clot, frequently superimposed on a white one, totally occluding the coronary artery is more common in STEMI [36].

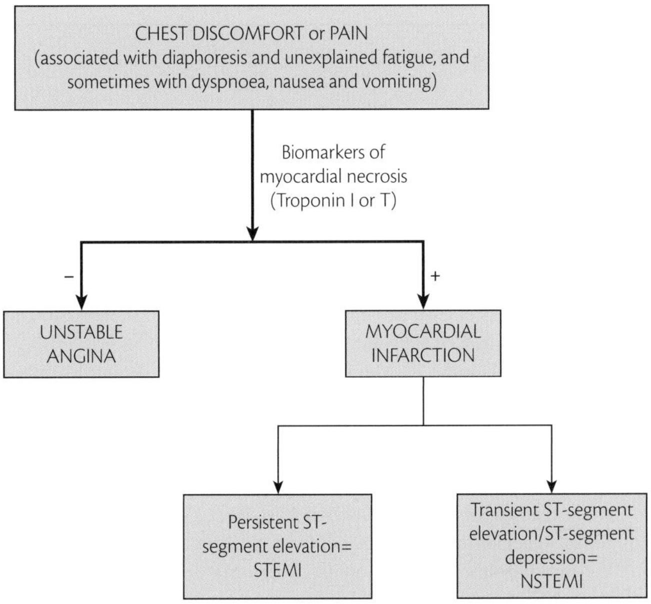

Fig. 4.2 Diagnosis and classification of acute coronary syndromes.

Differences in the type of thrombus also call for different risk stratification approaches to the patient and different therapy goals. Both UA/NSTEMI and STEMI are life-threatening diseases, but for patients with UA/NSTEMI different levels of risk of death or progression from those in STEMI should guide the physician to choose the best pharmacological treatment and revascularization strategy within a time span that could range from a few hours to some days. For STEMI patients, the priority is to open the occluded vessel as soon as possible, either by primary percutaneous coronary intervention (pPCI) or by thrombolysis, if the former is not available and the time from symptom onset to the first medical contact is not more than 12 hours.

Sudden cardiac death is a major problem in developed countries. It is defined as an unexpected death from a cardiac cause occurring within a short time in a person with or without pre-existing heart disease because of abrupt loss of heart function. Thirteen per cent of deaths reported by the Framingham Heart Study after a follow-up time of about 20 years were attributable to sudden cardiac death, and in 80% of cases a coronary artery disease was the main cause [37].

The annual incidence of ACS in Europe is in the range of 1 in 80 to 1 in 170 of the population, with a higher rate of NSTEMI than STEMI [38]. Even though death is more frequent during initial hospital stay for STEMI patients than NSTEMI ones, at 6 months the mortality rate becomes quite similar in both conditions. In the United States approximately 1.36 million hospitalizations have a discharge diagnosis of ACS; 61% of them are myocardial infarctions (MI) and two-thirds of MI patients have NSTEMI [39].

Several cardiovascular risk factors are associated with a high probability of developing ACS in patients with atherosclerosis, including male gender, age, cigarette smoking, hypertension, dyslipidaemia, and diabetes. Other clinical variables, including age, diabetes, non-cardiac comorbidities, and signs of heart failure, are associated with worse outcome in patients presenting with an ACS.

Further reading

Aate R, Cioni G, Ricci I, et al. Thrombosis and acute coronary syndrome. *Thromb Res* 2012; **129**: 235–40.

Braunwald E. Unstable angina and non-ST elevation myocardial infarction. *Am J Respir Crit Care Med* 2012; **185**: 924–32.

Institute of Medicine (US) Committee on Preventing the Global Epidemic of Cardiovascular Disease; Meeting the Challenges in Developing Countries. *Promoting cardiovascular health in the developing world: a critical challenge to achieve global health*, 2010. Washington, DC: The National Academies Press.

Davignon J, Ganz P. Role of endothelial dysfunction in atherosclerosis. *Circulation* 2004; **109**: III27–III32.

Esmon CT. Crosstalk between inflammation and thrombosis. *Maturitas* 2008; **61**: 122–31.

Falk E. Pathogenesis of atherosclerosis. *J Am Coll Cardiol* 2006; **47**: C7–C12.

Fuster V, Moreno PR, Fayad ZA, et al. Atherothrombosis and high-risk plaque. Part I: evolving concepts. *J Am Coll Cardiol* 2005; **46**: 937–54.

Hagedorn I, Vögtle T, Nieswandt B. Arterial thrombus formation. Novel mechanisms and targets. *Hämostaseologie* 2010; **30**: 127–35.

Jackson SP. Arterial thrombosis—insidious, unpredictable and deadly. *Nat Med* 2011; **17**: 1423–36.

Kumar A, Cannon C. Acute coronary syndromes: diagnosis and management, Part I. *Mayo Clinic Proc* 2009; **84**: 917–38.

Levy M, van der Poll T, Büller HR. Bidirectional relation between inflammation and coagulation. *Circulation* 2004; **109**: 2698–704.

Linden MD, Jackson DE. Platelets: pleiotropic roles in atherogenesis and atherothrombosis. *Int J Biocem Cell Biol* 2010; **42**: 1762–6.

Moreno PR, Purushothaman M, Purushothaman K-R. Plaque neovascularization: defense mechanisms, betrayal, or a war in progress. *Ann NY Acad Sci* 2012: **1254**: 7–17.

References

1 Institute of Medicine (US) Committee on Preventing the Global Epidemic of Cardiovascular Disease; Meeting the Challenges in Developing Countries. *Promoting cardiovascular health in the developing world: a critical challenge to achieve global health*, 2010. Washington, DC: The National Academies Press, p. 49.

2 Jackson SP. Arterial thrombosis—insidious, unpredictable and deadly. *Nat Med* 2011; **17**: 1423–36.

3 Opal SM, Kessler CM, Roemisch J, et al. Antithrombin, heparin, and heparin sulfate. *Crit Care Med* 2002; **30**: S325–S331.

4 Uchiba M, Okajima K, Murakami K, et al. Effects of antithrombin III (ATIII) and TRP49-modified ATIII on plasma level of 6-keto-PGF-1α in rats. *Thromb Res* 1995; **80**: 201–8.

5 van der Wower M, Collen D, Conway EM. Thrombomodulin-protein C-EPCR system: integrated to regulate coagulation and inflammation. *Arterioscler Thromb Vasc Biol* 2004; **24**: 1374–83.

6 Sohn RH, Deming CB, Johns DC, et al. Regulation of endothelial thrombomodulin expression by inflammatory cytokines is mediated by activation of nuclear factor-kappa B. *Blood* 2005; **105**: 3910–17.

7 Collins T, Read MA, Neish AS, et al. Transcriptional regulation of endothelial cell adhesion molecules: NF-kappa B and cytokine-inducible enhancers. *FASEB J* 1995; **9**: 899–909.

8 Massion PB, Feron O, Dessy C, et al. Nitric oxide and cardiac function. Ten years after, and continuing. *Circ Res* 2003; **93**: 388–98.

9 Chatterjee A, Black SM, Catravas JD. Endothelial nitric oxide (NO) and its pathophysiologic regulation. *Vascul Pharmacol* 2008; **49**: 134–40.

10 Arehart E, Gleim S, Kasza Z, et al. Prostacyclin, atherothrombosis, and cardiovascular disease. *Curr Med Chem* 2007; **14**: 2161–9.

11 Reinders JH, Brinkman HJ, van Mourik JA, et al. Cigarette smoke impairs endothelial cell prostacyclin production. *Arteriosclerosis* 1986; **6**: 15–23.

12 Goepfert C, Imai M, Brouard S, et al. CD39 modulates endothelial cell activation and apoptosis. *Mol Med* 2000; **6**: 591–603.

13 Davignon J, Ganz P. Role of endothelial dysfunction in atherosclerosis. *Circulation* 2004; **109**: III27–III32.

14 Di Stasio E, De Cristofaro R. The effect of shear stress on protein conformation: physical forces operating on biochemical systems: the case of von Willebrand factor. *Biophys Chem* 2010; **153**: 1–8.

15 Cattaneo M. Light transmission aggregometry and ATP release for the diagnostic assessment of platelet function. *Semin Thromb Hemost* 2009; **35**: 158–67.

16 Lhermusier T, Chap H, Payrastre B. Platelet membrane phospholipid asymmetry: from the characterization of a scramblase activity to the identification of an essential protein mutated in Scott syndrome. *J Thromb Haemost* 2011; **9**: 1883–91.

17 Eilertsen KE, Østerud B. Tissue factor: (patho)physiology and cellular biology. *Blood Coagul Fibrinolysis* 2004; **15**: 521–38.

18 Davies MJ. A macro and micro view of coronary vascular insult in ischemic heart disease. *Circulation* 1990; **82**: 1138–46.

19 Esmon CT. Crosstalk between inflammation and thrombosis. *Maturitas* 2004; **47**: 305–14.

20 Yokoya K, Takatsu H, Suzuki T, et al. Process of progression of coronary artery lesions from mild or moderate stenosis to moderate or severe stenosis: a study based on four serial coronary arteriograms per year. *Circulation* 1999; **100**: 903–9.

21 Kolodgie FD, Gold HK, Burke AP, et al. Intraplaque hemorrhage and progression of coronary atheroma. *N Engl J Med* 2003; **349**: 2316–25.

22 Lievens D, von Hundelshausen P. Platelets in atherosclerosis. *Thromb Haemost* 2011; **106**: 827–38.

23 Nesbitt WS, Westein E, Tovar-Lopez FJ, et al. A shear gradient-dependent platelet aggregation mechanism drives thrombus formation. *Nat Med* 2009; **15**: 665–73.

24 Müller F, Mutch NJ, Schenk WA, et al. Platelet polyphosphates are proinflammatory and procoagulant mediators *in vivo*. *Cell* 2009; **139**: 1143–56.

25 Renné T, Pozgajová M, Grüner S, et al. Defective thrombus formation in mice lacking coagulation factor XII. *J Exp Med* 2005; **202**: 271–81.

26 Hagedorn I, Schmidbauer S, Pleines I, et al. Factor XIIa inhibitor recombinant human albumin Infestin-4 abolishes occlusive arterial thrombus formation without affecting bleeding. *Circulation* 2010; **121**: 1510–17.

27 Viles-Gonzales JF, Fuster V, Badimon JJ. Atherothrombosis: a widespread disease with unpredictable and life-threatening consequences. *Eur Heart J* 2004; **25**: 1197–207.

28 Shaar JA, Muller JE, Falk E, et al. Terminology for high-risk and vulnerable coronary artery plaques. Report of a meeting on the vulnerable plaque, June 17 and 18, 2003, Santorini, Greece. *Eur Heart J* 2004; **25**: 1077–82.

29 Badimon L, Storey RF, Vilahur G. Update on lipids, inflammation and atherothrombosis. *Thromb Haemost* 2011; **105** (Suppl. 1): S34–S42.

30 Burke AP, Farb A, Malcom GT, et al. Coronary risk factors and plaque morphology in men with coronary disease who died suddenly. *N Engl J Med* 1997; **336**: 1276–82.

31 Stone GW, Maehara A, Lansky AJ, et al. for the PROSPECT Investigators. A prospective natural-history study of coronary atherosclerosis. *N Engl J Med* 2011; **364**: 226–35.

32 Sadat U, Teng Z, Gillard JH. Biochemical structural stresses of atherosclerotic plaques. *Expert Rev Cardiovasc Ther* 2010; **8**: 1469–81.

33 Farb A, Burke AP, Tang AL, et al. Coronary plaque erosion without rupture into a lipid core. A frequent cause of coronary thrombosis in sudden coronary death. *Circulation* 1996; **93**: 1354–63.

34 Virmani R, Kolodgie FD, Burke AP, et al. Lessons from sudden coronary death: a comprehensive morphological classification scheme for atherosclerotic lesions. *ATVB* 2000; **20**: 1262–75

35 Rioufol G, Finet G, Ginon I, et al. Multiple atherosclerotic plaque rupture in acute coronary syndrome: a three-vessel intravascular ultrasound study. *Circulation* 2002; **106**: 804–8.

36 Mizuno K, Satumo K, Miyamoto A, et al. Angioscopic evaluation of coronary artery thrombi in acute coronary syndromes. *N Engl J Med* 1992; **326**: 287–91.

37 Zipes DP, Wellens HJ. Sudden cardiac death. *Circulation* 1998; **98**: 2334–51.

38 Hasdai D, Behar S, Wallentin L, et al. A prospective survey of the characteristics, treatments and outcomes of patients with acute coronary syndromes in Europe and the Mediterranean basin: the Euro Heart Survey of Acute Coronary Syndromes (Euro Heart Survey ACS). *Eur Heart J* 2002; **23**: 1190–201.

39 Lloyd-Jones D, Adam R, Carnethon M, et al. American Heart Association Statistics Committee and Stroke Statistics Subcommittee. Heart disease and stroke statistics—2009 update, a report from the American Heart Association Statistics Committee and Stroke Statistics Subcommittee. *Circulation* 2009; **119**: 480–6.

PART 3

Components of preventive cardiology

CHAPTER 5

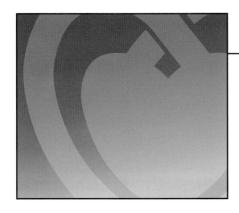

Risk stratification and risk assessment*

Ian Graham, Marie Therese Cooney, and Dirk De Bacquer

Contents

Summary

Cardiovascular disease (CVD) is the biggest cause of death worldwide. The underlying atherosclerosis starts in childhood and is often advanced when it becomes clinically apparent many years later, when it may kill without warning. CVD is manageable: it can be tackled by changes in lifestyle and risk factors and by therapy. Management of risk factors unequivocally reduces mortality and morbidity. In apparently healthy people, CVD risk is most frequently the result of multiple interacting risk factors. A risk estimation system such as SCORE (Systematic COronary Risk Evaluation) can assist in making logical management decisions, and may help to avoid both under- and over-treatment; however, certain individuals declare themselves to be at high CVD risk without the need for risk scoring and require immediate attention to all risk factors. In younger people a low absolute risk may conceal a very high relative risk, and use of a relative risk chart or calculating their 'risk age' may help in advising them of the need for intensive lifestyle modifications. While women appear to be at lower CVD risk than men, this is misleading as risk is deferred by approximately 10 years rather than avoided. All risk estimation systems are relatively crude and require attention to qualifying statements and additional factors affecting risk can be accommodated in electronic risk estimation systems such as HeartScore. The total risk approach allows flexibility: if perfection cannot be achieved with one risk factor, trying harder with others can still reduce risk.

Introduction

The atherosclerosis that causes cardiovascular disease (CVD) starts in childhood, or indeed *in utero*, and develops insidiously over many years. By the time that symptoms occur the underlying disease is often advanced. Furthermore, the first manifestation may be a fatal event. Thus conventional therapies are likely to only be palliative or indeed inapplicable if the person dies before help is available. This is the rationale for the preventive approach, which is underpinned by the fact that the major causes of atherosclerosis are known and by unequivocal evidence that modifying them reduces risk.

* This chapter is based on Section 3 of the 2012 Joint European Guidelines on cardiovascular disease prevention in clinical practice [1], with certain revisions and additions. This is to help promote compatibility with established guidance.

The preventive approach to CVD is ideally lifelong, starting at birth. In real life, preventive efforts are typically targeted at middle-aged or older people, especially men, with established CVD ('secondary prevention') or those at high risk of developing a first cardiovascular event because of a combination of risk factors such as smoking, elevated blood pressure (BP), diabetes, or dyslipidaemia ('primary prevention'). The terms primary and secondary prevention are now regarded as obsolete because they falsely dichotomize risk—the development of techniques that can detect subclinical atherosclerosis has shown its continuous and graded nature, from those with asymptomatic disease to those with symptomatic disease. Preventive efforts in the young, the very old, or those at mild to moderate risk are still limited. Indeed, while logical, evidence of their benefits from randomized controlled trials is limited. Nevertheless, it is likely that the benefits of preventive measures directed at these groups could be substantial.

Over 30 years ago, Geoffrey Rose [2] defined the differences between two approaches to CVD prevention: the population strategy and the high-risk strategy. The population strategy aims to reduce the incidence of CVD at the population level via lifestyle and environmental changes targeted at the population at large. Examples include measures to ban smoking in public places, to reduce the salt content of food, and to reduce consumption of saturated fat, and measures to promote activity and avoid overweight. This approach may bring large benefits to the population, although it may offer little to the individual—the 'prevention paradox' [3]. The impact of such an approach on the total number of cardiovascular events in the population may be large, because everyone is targeted and the majority of cardiovascular events occur in the very substantial group of people who are at only modest risk.

In the high-risk approach, preventive measures aim to reduce risk factor levels in those at the highest cardiovascular risk, either individuals without CVD in the upper part of the total cardiovascular risk distribution or those with established CVD. Although individuals targeted in this strategy are more likely to benefit from the preventive interventions, the impact at the population level is limited because there are few people at such high risk. Implicit in this approach is the need to identify high-risk individuals through opportunistic or systematic screening or through publicity to encourage those who may be at risk to seek a risk assessment.

The two approaches should be regarded as complementary rather than competitive, although a high-risk approach in isolation has a limited effect on the total burden of disease. The relative effects of each approach have been modelled in order to assist health planners [4].

The proposal to use total risk estimation as a central tool to identify those patients requiring prevention was a key recommendation of the first Joint European Societies Guidelines on CHD prevention published in 1994 [5]. This is because clinicians treat the whole person rather than individual risk factors, and total cardiovascular risk reflects a combination of several risk factors that may interact, sometimes multiplicatively. Having said that, the logical implication that total risk assessment is associated with improved clinical outcomes when compared with other strategies has not been adequately tested.

Although clinicians often ask for a threshold value at which to trigger an intervention, this is problematic: risk is a continuum and there is no exact point above which, for example, a drug is automatically indicated nor below which lifestyle advice may not usefully be offered. This issue is dealt with in more detail in other chapters, as is the issue of how to advise younger people at low absolute but high relative risk, and the fact that all elderly people will eventually be at high risk of death and may be over-exposed to drug treatments.

The priorities suggested in this chapter are to assist the physician in dealing with individual people and patients. As such, they acknowledge that individuals at the highest levels of risk gain most from risk factor management. As noted elsewhere, although such individuals gain most, the majority of deaths in a community are of those at lower levels of risk simply because they are more numerous than high-risk individuals who, paradoxically, develop fewer events in absolute terms [2]. Thus a strategy for individuals at high risk must be complemented by public health measures to reduce, as far as is practicable, population levels of cardiovascular risk factors and to encourage a healthy lifestyle.

Strategies

The term 'total cardiovascular risk' means the likelihood of a person developing an atherosclerotic cardiovascular event over a defined period of time. 'Total risk' implies the risk estimated by considering the effect of the major factors of age, gender, smoking, BP, and lipid levels. This term has become widely used; however, 'total risk' is not comprehensive because the effects of other risk factors are not considered, except as qualifying statements.

The importance of total risk estimation before management decisions are made is illustrated in ➲ Table 5.1 and ➲ Fig. 5.1. ➲ Figure 5.1 shows that the effect of lipid levels on risk is modest in women who are at otherwise low risk, and that the risk advantage of being female is lost by the combination of smoking and mild hypertension. ➲ Table 5.1 shows that a person with a cholesterol concentration of 8 mmol/L can be at one-tenth of the risk of someone with a cholesterol concentration of 5 mmol/L if the latter is a hypertensive

Table 5.1 Impact of combinations of risk factors on risk

Sex	Age (years)	Cholesterol (mmol/L)	BP (mmHg)	Smoker	Risk (%)
F	60	8	120	No	2
F	60	7	140	Yes	5
M	60	6	160	No	8
M	60	5	180	Yes	21

BP, blood pressure; F, female; M, male.

Reproduced from: Perk J, De Backer G, Gohlke H, et al. European Guidelines on cardiovascular disease prevention in clinical practice (version 2012): the Fifth Joint Task Force of the European Society of Cardiology and Other Societies on Cardiovascular Disease Prevention in Clinical Practice (constituted by representatives of nine societies and by invited experts). * Developed with the special contribution of the European Association for Cardiovascular Prevention and Rehabilitation (EACPR). *Eur J Prev Cardiol* 2012; **19**(4): 585–667.

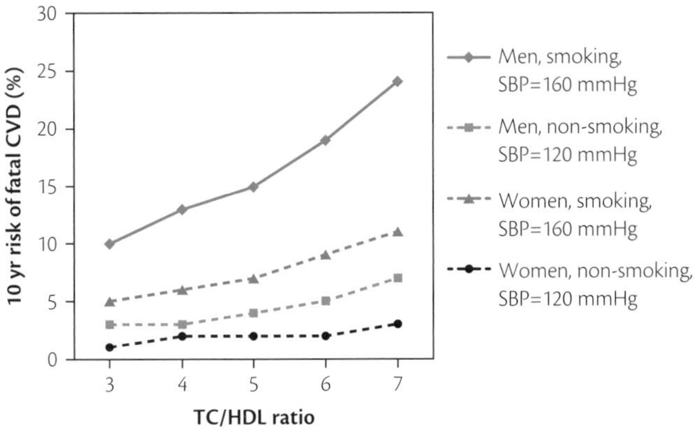

Fig. 5.1 Relationship between the ratio of total cholesterol (TC)/HDL cholesterol and 10-year fatal CVD events in men and women aged 60 years with and without risk factors, based on a risk function derived from the SCORE project.

Reproduced from: Perk J, De Backer G, Gohlke H, et al. European Guidelines on cardiovascular disease prevention in clinical practice (version 2012): the Fifth Joint Task Force of the European Society of Cardiology and Other Societies on Cardiovascular Disease Prevention in Clinical Practice (constituted by representatives of nine societies and by invited experts). * Developed with the special contribution of the European Association for Cardiovascular Prevention and Rehabilitation (EACPR). *Eur J Prev Cardiol* 2012; **19**(4): 585–667.

male smoker. While audits such as EUROASPIRE [5,6] suggest there is inadequate management of risk factors in very high-risk subjects, it is also likely that, in the context of low-risk subjects who have not had a vascular event, there is the potential for substantial overuse of drugs by inappropriate extrapolation of the results of trials conducted mostly in high-risk men to low-risk individuals. In general, women and old and young subjects have been under-represented in the classic drug trials that have informed guidelines to date.

For these considerations to have an impact on clinical practice it is essential for clinicians to be able to assess risk rapidly and with sufficient accuracy to allow logical management decisions. This realization led to the development of the risk chart used in the 1994 and 1998 guidelines [5,7]. This chart, developed from a concept pioneered by Anderson et al. [8] used age, sex, smoking status, blood cholesterol, and systolic blood pressure (SBP) to estimate the 10-year risk of a first fatal or non-fatal coronary heart disease (CHD) event. There were several problems with that chart, outlined in the fourth Joint Task Force Guidelines on prevention [9], which led to the currently recommended risk estimation system: SCORE (Systematic COronary Risk Evaluation).

Risk estimation

When do I assess total risk?

People with established CVD, diabetes, very high levels of individual risk factors, and moderate to severe renal impairment are already at high or very high risk of further events and need prompt attention to all risk factors. Total risk assessment systems such as SCORE are intended for use in apparently healthy people.

While the ideal scenario would be for all adults to have their risk of CVD assessed, this may not be practicable for many societies. This decision must be made by individual countries and will be dependent on resources. While outside the scope of this book, it is reasonable to suggest that school curricula should introduce the concepts of risk and of individual responsibility regarding the choice of an appropriate lifestyle.

Most people will visit their family doctor at least once over a 2-year period and this gives the opportunity for risk assessment. General practice databases may be of assistance. For clinicians, it is suggested that total risk assessment be offered during a consultation if:

1. The person asks for it.
2. One or more risk factors such as smoking, overweight, or hyperlipidaemia are known.
3. There is a family history of premature CVD or of major risk factors such as hyperlipidaemia.
4. There are symptoms suggestive of CVD, bearing in mind that the presence of CVD automatically places the person in the 'very high' risk category and should prompt immediate attention to all risk factors.

Special efforts should be made to assess risk in the socially deprived.

How do I assess risk?

Risk estimation systems in general

Risk is the product of several interacting risk factors, and it is recommended that a formal risk estimation system is used. There are several systems available for assessing total cardiovascular risk, including Framingham [10], SCORE [11], ASSIGN [12], QRISK [13], PROCAM [14], WHO/ISH [15], and the Reynolds score [16]. These have all been comprehensively reviewed [17–19]. ➲ Table 5.2 [17] outlines the criteria for a clinically useful risk assessment system and ➲ Table 5.3 [17] summarizes the characteristics of the cited risk estimation systems.

Certain conclusions may be drawn:

1. All risk estimation systems have drawn on the principles defined by the Framingham investigators.
2. The major determinants of CVD risk are age and gender, which will produce an area under the receiver operating curve (AUROC) of 60% or more (where 50% is chance, and 100% is perfect risk estimation).
3. The addition of risk factors will rarely achieve an AUROC of >85%.
4. Available risk estimation systems do not differ greatly in their performance if applied to a population that is recognizably similar to that from which the risk function was derived in terms of baseline risk and risk factor distributions.
5. Recalibration, using up to date local cause-specific mortality and risk factor prevalence data, can improve the performance of risk estimation systems when applied to different populations.
6. Risk will be over-estimated in populations in whom CVD is declining and underestimated in populations in which it is

Table 5.2 Criteria for a clinically useful risk estimation system

Appropriate statistical methods for derivation of the function
- Representative sample from the population from which the system is to be applied
- Sufficient power (large enough sample size)
- Accepted statistical methods
- The end-point predicted by the function should be defined in such a way that it is easily standardized across populations and relevant to the outcomes of RCTs of preventive measures

Performance of the function—internal and external validity

Discrimination—the ability of the function to separate those who will develop the end-point from those who will not

Often assessed using:
- Area under receiver operating characteristic curve (AUROC)—a means for expressing the maximum achievable sensitivity and specificity. An AUROC of 1 indicates perfect discrimination; 0.5 equates to chance. Values in the region of 0.9 are often achieved for diagnostic tests. Values rarely exceed 0.8 for risk estimation. Harrell's C statistic gives the same information but can be used with variable follow-up
- Sensitivity/specificity/positive predictive value/negative predictive value

Calibration—a measure of how closely predicted outcomes agree with actual outcomes

Often assessed using either:
- Hosmer–Lemeshow goodness of fit testing—lower values indicate better fit, values less than 20 generally considered good fit. Significant p-values indicate lack of fit
- Predicted to observed ratios—the closer the value to 1, the better the fit. Values greater than 1 indicate overestimation and vice versa

Reclassification
- Net reclassification index—a measure of the net percentage of those who do and who do not develop the end-point within the time period that are correctly reclassified to a different risk category when a new risk factor is added to the risk estimation system

Usability of the system
- The format affects the ease of use of the system. This will also impact on the uptake of the system by users

Inclusion of appropriate risk factors
- Most risk estimation systems include age, gender, and conventional risk factors including lipid levels, smoking, and blood pressure
- Inclusion of other factors may be important, especially if they have been shown to be powerful risk determinations and prevalent in the population to which the system is to be applied (e.g. social deprivation)
- Some advocate the use of only risk factors which are potentially modifiable, although most agree that risk factors to be included should be chosen based on whether they improve risk estimation because those identified as high risk can still modify their risk by favourably altering their other risk factors
- Systems using only easily measured non-laboratory measures have been developed recently

Has use of the system been shown to result in measurable health gains?

Reproduced from: Cooney MT, Dudina AL, Graham IM. Value and limitations of existing scores for the assessment of cardiovascular risk: a review for clinicians. *Journal of the American College of Cardiology* 2009; **54**: 1209–27.

increasing. This can be dealt with by recalibration. Examples of recalibrated SCORE charts can be viewed at <http://www.heartscore.org>.

7. The ROC expresses the overall performance of a risk estimation system. At the extremes of risk, management decisions will be obvious—what is needed is optimal performance close to a threshold at which one will make a management decision. This issue is addressed, if not completely solved, by the use of the net reclassification index.
8. Recent work has indicated that the β-coefficients associated with risk factors are not independent of age, and that current systems overestimate risk in older people, pointing to a need for ongoing large prospective cohort studies to calculate risk in 5–10-year age bands.

The SCORE risk estimation system

The 2003, 2007, and 2012 Joint European Guidelines on the prevention of CVD in clinical practice [1,9,20] as well as the 2011 European Society of Cardiology/European Atherosclerosis Society (ESC/EAS) Guidelines for the management of dyslipidaemias [21] have all used the ESC recommended SCORE chart for risk estimation [12], which is based on data from 12 European cohort studies. It includes 205 178 subjects examined at baseline between 1970 and 1988 with 2.7 million years of follow-up and 7934 cardiovascular deaths. The SCORE risk function has been externally validated [22]. ➲ Box 5.1 lists the advantages of using the SCORE risk charts.

Risk charts such as SCORE are intended to facilitate the estimation of risk in ostensibly healthy people. Patients who have had a clinical event such as an acute coronary syndrome (ACS) or stroke, or who have diabetes, renal impairment, or very high levels of individual risk factors have already declared themselves to be at high risk of a further event and automatically qualify for intensive risk factor evaluation and management.

SCORE differs from earlier risk estimation systems in several important ways, and was modified somewhat for the 2012 Joint European Guidelines on CVD prevention in clinical practice [1]. We will now discuss details of these differences and modifications.

Risk of fatal CVD events or total events

The SCORE system estimates the 10-year risk of a fatal atherosclerotic event, whether heart attack, stroke, aneurysm of the aorta, or others. All International Classification of Diseases (ICD) codes that could reasonably be assumed to be atherosclerotic are included. Many other systems only estimate the risk of CHD.

Table 5.3 Characteristics of current risk estimation systems

	Framingham [10]	SCORE [11]	ASSIGN—SCORE [12]	QRISK1 [13] and QRISK2 [3]	PROCAM [14]	WHO/ISH [15]	Reynolds risk score [16,42]
Data	Prospective studies: Framingham Heart Study and Framingham Offspring Study. Latest version includes both	Pooled prospective studies	SHHEC prospective study	QRESEARCH database	Prospective study	Methods differ from other risk estimation functions—not based on prospective data	Randomized controlled trials. Women: Women's Health study. Men: Physician's Health study II
Population	General population Framingham, MA, USA. Baselines: 1968–71, 1971–5, 1984–7	12 prospective studies from 11 European countries. Baselines: 1972–91	Random sample from general population in Scotland. Baseline 1984–7	Data collected from 1993 to 2008	Healthy employees. Baseline: 1978–95	Not applicable	Women: health service employees Baseline 1993–6 Men: physicians Baseline 1997
Sample type	Volunteer	Mostly random samples from general population, some occupational cohorts	Random	Health records of general practice attendees. Not random	Industrial employee volunteers. Not random	Not applicable	Health service employees—volunteer, not random
Sample size	3969 men and 4522 women	117 098 men and 88 080 women	6540 men and 6757 women	1.28 million (QRISK1) or 2.29 million (QRISK2)	18 460 men and 8515 women	Not applicable	24 558 women and 10 724 men
Statistical methods	Cox (earlier versions Weibull [8])	Cox and Weibull	Cox	Imputation of substantial missing data. Cox	Cox and Weibull. Exploratory analyses with neural networks also [43]	Relative risks associated with risk factors were taken from the comparative risk assessment project. These were combined with the estimated absolute risks for each WHO subregion based on the Global Burden of Disease study	Cox
Calculates	10-year risk of CHD events originally. Latest version: 10-year risk of CVD events	10-year risk of CVD mortality	10-year risk of CVD events	10-year risk of CVD events	Two separate scores calculate 10-year risks of major coronary events and cerebral ischaemic events	10-year risk of CVD events	10 year risk of incident MI, stroke, coronary revascularization, or cardiovascular death
Age range	30–75	40–65	30–74	35–74	20–75	40–79	45–80
Variables	Gender, age, total cholesterol, HDL cholesterol, SBP, smoking status, diabetes, hypertensive treatment	Gender, age, total cholesterol or total cholesterol/HDL cholesterol ratio, SBP, smoking status. Versions for use in high- and low-risk countries	Gender, age, total cholesterol, HDL cholesterol, SBP, smoking (no. of cigarettes), diabetes, area-based index of deprivation, family history	QRISK1: gender, age, total cholesterol to HDL cholesterol ratio, SBP, smoking status, diabetes, area-based index of deprivation, family history, BMI, antihypertensive treatment. QRISK2 also includes ethnicity and chronic diseases	Age, gender, LDL cholesterol, HDL cholesterol, diabetes, smoking, SBP	Gender, age, SBP, smoking status, diabetes ± total cholesterol. Different charts available for worldwide regions	Gender, age, SBP, smoking, hs-CRP, total cholesterol, HDL cholesterol, family history of premature MI (parent aged < 60), HbA1C if diabetic

(continued)

Table 5.3 Continued

	Framingham [10]	SCORE [11]	ASSIGN—SCORE [12]	QRISK1 [13] and QRISK2 [3]	PROCAM [14]	WHO/ISH [15]	Reynolds risk score [16,42]
Formats	Simplified scoring sheets. Colour charts have been generated for some guidelines, e.g. JBS and New Zealand guidelines. Online calculators. Portable calculators	Colour-coded charts, HeartScore (online and CD-based), stand-alone electronic versions	Online calculator	Online calculator	Simple scoring sheet and online calculators	Colour-coded charts	Online calculator
Developments	Latest version includes version based on non-laboratory values only, substituting BMI from lipid measurements	National, updated recalibrations		QRISK2 includes interaction terms to adjust for the interactions between age and some of the variables	Recent change in the methods (Weibull) allows extension of risk estimation to women and broader age range		-
Recommended by guidelines	NCEP guidelines [44]. Other national guidelines recommend adapted versions, including New Zealand [45]	European guidelines on CVD prevention [9]	Recommended by SIGN [46]	NICE guidelines on lipid modification [47]	International Task Force for Prevention of Coronary Disease guidelines	WHO guidelines on CVD prevention [15]	No
Website	Online and downloadable risk calculator available at: <http://www.nhlbi.nih.gov/guidelines/cholesterol/index/htm>	Online and downloadable risk calculators available at: <http://www.heartscore.org>	Online risk calculator available at: <www.assign-score.com>	Online risk calculator available at: <http://www.qrisk.org>	Online calculator available at: <http://www.chd-taskforce.com/procam_interactive.html>	Charts downloadable at: <http://www.who.int/cardiovascular_diseases/guidelines/Pocket_GL_information/en/index.html>	Online calculator: <http://www.reynoldsriskscore.com>
Internal validation—discrimination	AUROC: men 0.76 (0.75–0.78), women 0.79 (0.77–0.81)	AUROC high risk: 0.80 (0.80–0.82). AUROC low risk: 0.75 (0.73–0.77)	AUROC: men 0.73, women 0.77	QRISK2 AUROC: men 0.79 (0.79–0.79), women: 0.82 (0.81–0.82)	AUROC: 0.82 for coronary events, 0.78 for cerebral ischaemic events	Not specified	AUROC: women 0.808, men 0.708
Internal validation—calibration	Hosmer–Lemeshow goodness of fit testing (HL): men 13.48, women 7.79	Not specified	Observed 10-year CVD incidence rates: men 11.7%, women 6.4%. Median ASSIGN: men 11.7%, women: 6.2%	Good correlation between observed and predicted risks in both men and women—presented graphically only—in each decile of risk	Not specified	Not specified	Women 0.62, men 12.9
External validation—discrimination	PRIME study [48]: Belfast 0.68, France 0.66. Dutch study: 0.86 (0.84–0.88) [49]. Cleveland study: 0.57 [29]. China [50]: men 0.75 (0.72–0.78), women 0.79 (0.74–0.85). THIN (UK) [51]: men 0.74 (0.73–0.74), women 0.76 (0.76–0.76). EPIC Norfolk [52]: 0.71. UK women (BHHS) [53]: 0.66 (0.62–0.69)	Dutch study [49]: 0.85 (0.83–0.87). Cleveland study [29]: 0.73. Norwegian study [54] (range for different age groups): men 0.65–0.68, women 0.66–0.72. Austrian study [55]: men 0.76 (0.74–0.79), women 0.78 (0.74–0.82). Icelandic study [56]: 0.80 (0.78–0.82) (SCORE high); 0.80 (0.77–0.82) (SCORE low)	Not assessed	THIN database (UK). QRISK1 AUROC [51]: men 0.76 (0.76–0.77), women 0.79 (0.79–0.79)	PRIME study [48]: Belfast 0.61, France: 0.64	Not assessed	Not assessed

WHO/ISH, World Health Organization/International Society of Hypertension; SIGN, Scottish Intercollegiate Guidelines Network; MI, myocardial infarction; BMI, body mass index; hs-CRP, high-sensitivity CRP; HbA1C, glycated haemoglobin A1C; JBS, Joint British Societies; NCEP, National Cholesterol Education Program; NICE, National Institute for Health and Care Excellence; THIN, The Health Improvement Network; SHHEC, Scottish Heart Health Extended Cohort; BHHS, British Women's Heart and Health study; UK, United Kingdom.

Reproduced from: Cooney MT, Dudina AL, Graham IM. Value and limitations of existing scores for the assessment of cardiovascular risk: a review for clinicians. *Journal of the American College of Cardiology* 2009; **54**: 1209–27.

Box 5.1 Advantages of using the SCORE risk chart

- Intuitive, easy-to-use tool
- Takes account of the multifactorial nature of CVD
- Allows flexibility in management if an ideal risk factor level cannot be achieved; total risk can still be reduced by reducing other risk factors
- Allows a more objective assessment of risk over time
- Establishes a common language of risk for clinicians
- Shows how risk increases with age
- The new relative risk chart helps to illustrate how a young person with a low absolute risk may be at a substantially high and reducible relative risk
- Calculation of an individual's 'risk age' may also be of use in this situation

The choice of CVD mortality rather than total (fatal + non-fatal) events was deliberate, although not universally popular. Rates of non-fatal events are critically dependent upon definitions and the methods used in their ascertainment. Striking changes in both diagnostic tests and therapies have occurred since the SCORE cohorts were assembled. Critically, the use of mortality permits recalibration to allow for time-trends in CVD mortality, as we shall discuss. Nevertheless it is essential to address the issue of total risk.

In the 2003 guidelines [20], a 10-year risk of death from CVD of ≥5% was arbitrarily considered as 'high'. Yet this implies a 95% chance of *not* dying from CVD within 10 years—less than impressive when counselling patients. The new guideline nomenclature is that everyone with a 10-year risk of cardiovascular death of ≥5% has an *increased risk*. Clearly the risk of total fatal and non-fatal events is higher, and clinicians naturally wish for this to be quantified. The biggest contributor to the high-risk SCORE charts is FINRISK, which has data on non-fatal events defined according to the MONICA project [23]. Calculating total event rates from FINRISK suggests that, at the level (5%) at which risk management advice is likely to be intensified, total event risk is about 15%. This threefold multiplier is somewhat smaller in older people in whom a first event is more likely to be fatal. An examination of the Framingham estimates of risk of total CVD events results in similar conclusions: a 5% SCORE risk of CVD death equates to a 10–25% Framingham risk of total CVD, depending upon which of the Framingham functions is chosen. Again the lower end of the range applies to older people.

In summary, the reasons for retaining a system that estimates fatal as opposed to fatal + non-fatal CVD are:

- Death is a hard and reproducible end-point; a non-fatal event is variable and depends upon definitions, diagnostic criteria, and diagnostic tests, all of which may vary over time. Thus, the '20% total CVD (or CHD)' risk used to denote high risk in many guidelines is likely to be variable, unstable over time, and hard to validate.
- A high risk of CVD death automatically indicates a higher risk of total events.
- The multiplier to convert fatal to total CVD is similarly unstable and is often less than clinicians expect, since follow-up is terminated in all current systems with the *first* event and subsequent fatal or non-fatal events are not counted.
- The use of fatal CVD as the end-point allows accurate recalibration to other countries and cultures to adjust for time trends in mortality and in risk factor prevalence, an important consideration given the cultural diversity within Europe.

Risk thresholds

Clinicians often ask for thresholds to trigger certain interventions, but this is problematic since risk is a continuum and there is no threshold at which, for example, a drug is automatically indicated. A particular problem relates to young people with high levels of risk factors: a low absolute risk may conceal a very high relative risk requiring intensive lifestyle advice. In the 2003 guidelines [20] extrapolation of risk to age 60 was proposed to stress that a high absolute risk would eventually occur if preventive action were not taken earlier. It was not intended that such young people should be necessarily treated as if they were 60—a literal interpretation of this concept could lead to excessive drug treatment in younger people. A relative risk chart has now been added to the absolute risk charts to illustrate, particularly in younger people, how lifestyle changes can substantially reduce risk as well as reducing the increasing risk that comes with with ageing. A new approach to this problem of lifetime risk in these guidelines is the concept of cardiovascular risk age (see the section 'Cardiovascular risk age').

Age and gender

There is another problem that concerns older and elderly people. In some age categories the majority, especially men, will have estimated cardiovascular death risks exceeding the 5% level based on age (and gender) only, even when other cardiovascular risk factor levels are relatively low. This could lead to excessive use of drugs in these age groups.

High-density lipoprotein cholesterol, triglycerides, and newer risk factors

The role of high-density lipoprotein (HDL) cholesterol in risk estimation has been systematically re-examined using the SCORE database [24,25]. HDL cholesterol can make a substantial contribution to risk estimation if it is entered as an independent variable. For example, HDL cholesterol modifies risk at all levels of risk estimated from the SCORE total cholesterol charts [24]. Furthermore, this effect is seen in both sexes and in all age groups, including older women [25]. This is particularly important at levels of risk just below the ≥5% threshold for intensive risk modification—many of these subjects will qualify for intensive advice if their HDL cholesterol is low [24]. SCORE charts incorporating different levels of HDL cholesterol are included in the lipid guidelines [21]. The electronic, interactive version of SCORE—HeartScore (<http://www.heartscore.org>)—has been adjusted to allow for the inclusion of HDL cholesterol in calculating total CVD risk.

The role of raised plasma triglycerides as a predictor of CVD has been debated for many years. Fasting triglycerides relate to risk in univariate analyses but the effect is attenuated by adjustment for other factors, especially HDL cholesterol [26]. More recently, attention has focused on non-fasting triglycerides, which may be more strongly related to risk independent of the effects of HDL cholesterol [27–30].

Dealing with the impact of additional risk factors such as HDL cholesterol, body weight, family history, and newer risk markers is difficult within the constraint of a paper chart, and risk may also be higher than indicated in the charts in:

- sedentary individuals
- abdominal obesity
- socially deprived individuals
- ethnic minority groups
- pre-clinical atherosclerosis (e.g. carotid plaque)
- low HDL cholesterol
- increased triglycerides
- increased fibrinogen
- increased apolipoprotein B
- increased lipoprotein(a), especially in combination with familial hypercholesterolaemia
- impaired renal function.

HeartScore is not so constrained. It currently replicates SCORE in an electronic format but will be used to accommodate the results of new SCORE analyses, such as those relating to HDL cholesterol, as these are checked and validated. It should be stressed, however, that although many risk factors have been identified in addition to those included in the available risk functions [such as C-reactive protein (CRP) and homocysteine levels] their contribution to absolute cardiovascular risk estimations for individual patients (in addition to the classical risk factors) is generally modest [30].

The impact of self-reported diabetes has been re-examined. While there is heterogeneity between cohorts, the overall impact of diabetes on risk appears greater than in risk estimation systems based on the Framingham cohort, with relative risks of approximately five in women and three in men (unpublished data).

The SCORE risk charts are shown in ➲ Figs 5.2–5.4, including a chart of relative risks; instructions on their use and qualifiers are given in the remainder of the chapter.

Cardiovascular risk age

The risk age of a person with several cardiovascular risk factors is the age of a person with the same level of risk but with ideal levels of risk factors. Thus a high-risk 40-year-old may have a risk age of 60 years or more. Risk age is an intuitive and easily understood way of illustrating the likely reduction in life expectancy that a young person with a low absolute but high relative risk of CVD will be exposed to if preventive measures are not adopted.

Risk age can be estimated visually by looking at the SCORE chart (as illustrated in ➲ Fig. 5.5). Alternatively, to provide a more

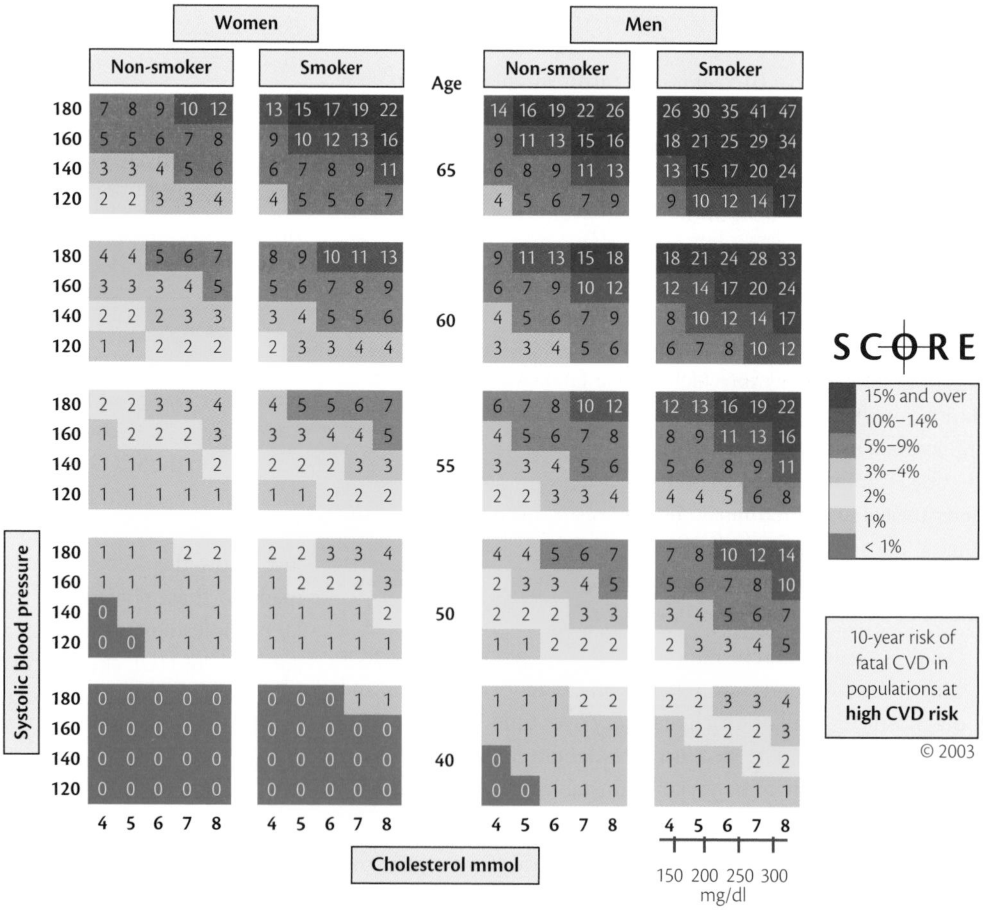

Fig. 5.2 SCORE chart: 10-year risk of fatal CVD in populations at high CVD risk based on the following risk factors: age, sex, smoking, systolic blood pressure, total cholesterol. Note that the risk of total (fatal + non-fatal) CVD events will be approximately three times higher than the figures given.
Reproduced from: Perk J, De Backer G, Gohlke H, et al. European Guidelines on cardiovascular disease prevention in clinical practice (version 2012): the Fifth Joint Task Force of the European Society of Cardiology and Other Societies on Cardiovascular Disease Prevention in Clinical Practice (constituted by representatives of nine societies and by invited experts). * Developed with the special contribution of the European Association for Cardiovascular Prevention and Rehabilitation (EACPR). *Eur J Prev Cardiol* 2012; **19**(4): 585–667.

Age	Systolic blood pressure	Women Non-smoker 4	5	6	7	8	Women Smoker 4	5	6	7	8	Men Non-smoker 4	5	6	7	8	Men Smoker 4	5	6	7	8
65	180	4	5	6	6	7	9	9	11	12	14	8	9	10	12	14	15	17	20	23	26
	160	3	3	4	4	5	6	6	7	8	10	5	6	7	8	10	10	12	14	16	19
	140	2	2	2	3	3	4	4	5	6	7	4	4	5	6	7	7	8	9	11	13
	120	1	1	2	2	2	3	3	3	4	4	2	3	3	4	5	5	5	6	8	9
60	180	3	3	3	4	4	5	5	6	7	8	5	6	7	8	9	10	11	13	15	18
	160	2	2	2	2	3	3	4	4	5	5	3	4	5	5	6	7	8	9	11	13
	140	1	1	1	2	2	2	2	3	3	4	2	3	3	4	4	5	5	6	7	9
	120	1	1	1	1	1	1	2	2	2	3	2	2	2	3	3	3	4	4	5	6
55	180	1	1	2	2	2	3	3	3	4	4	3	4	4	5	6	6	7	8	10	12
	160	1	1	1	1	1	2	2	2	3	3	2	2	3	3	4	4	5	6	7	8
	140	1	1	1	1	1	1	1	1	2	2	1	2	2	2	3	3	3	4	5	6
	120	0	0	1	1	1	1	1	1	1	1	1	1	1	2	2	2	2	3	3	4
50	180	1	1	1	1	1	1	1	2	2	2	2	2	3	3	4	4	4	5	6	7
	160	0	0	1	1	1	1	1	1	1	1	1	1	2	2	2	2	3	3	4	5
	140	0	0	0	0	0	1	1	1	1	1	1	1	1	1	2	2	2	2	3	3
	120	0	0	0	0	0	0	0	0	1	1	1	1	1	1	1	1	1	2	2	2
40	180	0	0	0	0	0	0	0	0	0	0	0	1	1	1	1	1	1	1	2	2
	160	0	0	0	0	0	0	0	0	0	0	0	0	0	1	1	1	1	1	1	1
	140	0	0	0	0	0	0	0	0	0	0	0	0	0	0	0	0	1	1	1	1
	120	0	0	0	0	0	0	0	0	0	0	0	0	0	0	0	0	0	0	1	1

Cholesterol mmol

150 200 250 300 mg/dl

SCORE

- 15% and over
- 10%–14%
- 5%–9%
- 3%–4%
- 2%
- 1%
- < 1%

10-year risk of fatal CVD in populations at **low CVD risk**

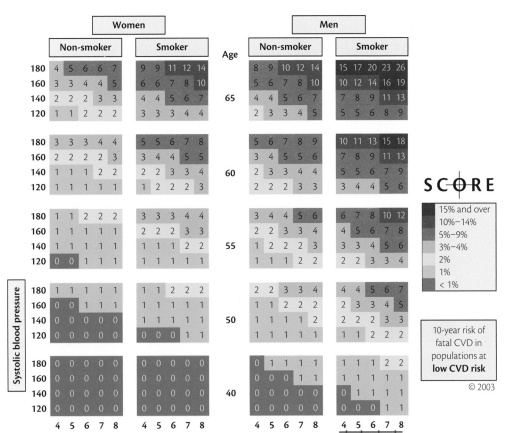

Fig. 5.3 SCORE chart: 10-year risk of fatal CVD in populations at low CVD risk based on the following risk factors: age, sex, smoking, systolic blood pressure, total cholesterol.
Reproduced from: Perk J, De Backer G, Gohlke H, et al. European Guidelines on cardiovascular disease prevention in clinical practice (version 2012): the Fifth Joint Task Force of the European Society of Cardiology and Other Societies on Cardiovascular Disease Prevention in Clinical Practice (constituted by representatives of nine societies and by invited experts). * Developed with the special contribution of the European Association for Cardiovascular Prevention and Rehabilitation (EACPR). *Eur J Prev Cardiol* 2012; **19**(4): 585–667.

Systolic blood pressure (mmHg)	Non-smoker 4	5	6	7	8	Smoker 4	5	6	7	8
180	3	3	4	5	6	6	7	8	10	12
160	2	3	3	4	4	4	5	6	7	8
140	1	2	2	2	3	3	3	4	5	6
120	1	1	1	2	2	2	2	3	3	4

Cholesterol (mmol/L)

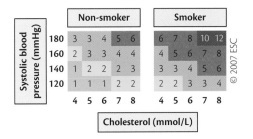

Fig. 5.4 Relative risk chart. Because this chart shows *relative* and not *absolute* risk a person in the top right-hand box has a risk that is 12 times higher than a person in the bottom left. This may be helpful when advising a young person with a low absolute but high relative risk of the need for lifestyle change.
Reproduced from: Perk J, De Backer G, Gohlke H, et al. European Guidelines on cardiovascular disease prevention in clinical practice (version 2012): the Fifth Joint Task Force of the European Society of Cardiology and Other Societies on Cardiovascular Disease Prevention in Clinical Practice (constituted by representatives of nine societies and by invited experts). * Developed with the special contribution of the European Association for Cardiovascular Prevention and Rehabilitation (EACPR). *Eur J Prev Cardiol* 2012; **19**(4): 585–667.

accurate estimation, a table of risk ages for different risk factor combinations is provided in ➲ Fig. 5.6. In this table the risk age is calculated compared with someone with ideal risk factor levels, which have been taken as non-smoking, total cholesterol of 4.0 mmol/L and a blood pressure of 120 mmHg [31]. Risk age is also automatically calculated as part of the latest revision of HeartScore.

Risk age has been shown to be independent of the cardiovascular end-point used [31], which by-passes the dilemma of whether to use a risk estimation system based on CVD mortality or on the more attractive, but less reliable, end-point of total CVD events. Risk age can be used in any population regardless of baseline risk and of secular changes in mortality and therefore also avoids the need for recalibration [32]. At present risk age is recommended for helping to communicate CVD risk, especially to younger people with a low absolute risk but a high relative risk. It is not currently recommended to base treatment decisions on risk age.

Other diseases with increased risk for CVD

Atherosclerosis is an inflammatory disease in which immune mechanisms interact with metabolic risk factors to initiate, propagate and activate lesions in the arterial tree [33]. Several diseases in which infection or non-infectious inflammatory processes determine the clinical picture are associated with an increased cardiovascular event rate (see ➲ Table 5.4). The optimal concept of prevention in these diseases is not established and randomized studies evaluating prognosis are not available. Optimal adjustment of all risk factors appears advisable even in the absence of randomized studies.

Low-risk and high-risk countries

The fact that CVD mortality has declined in many European countries means that more countries now fall into the low-risk

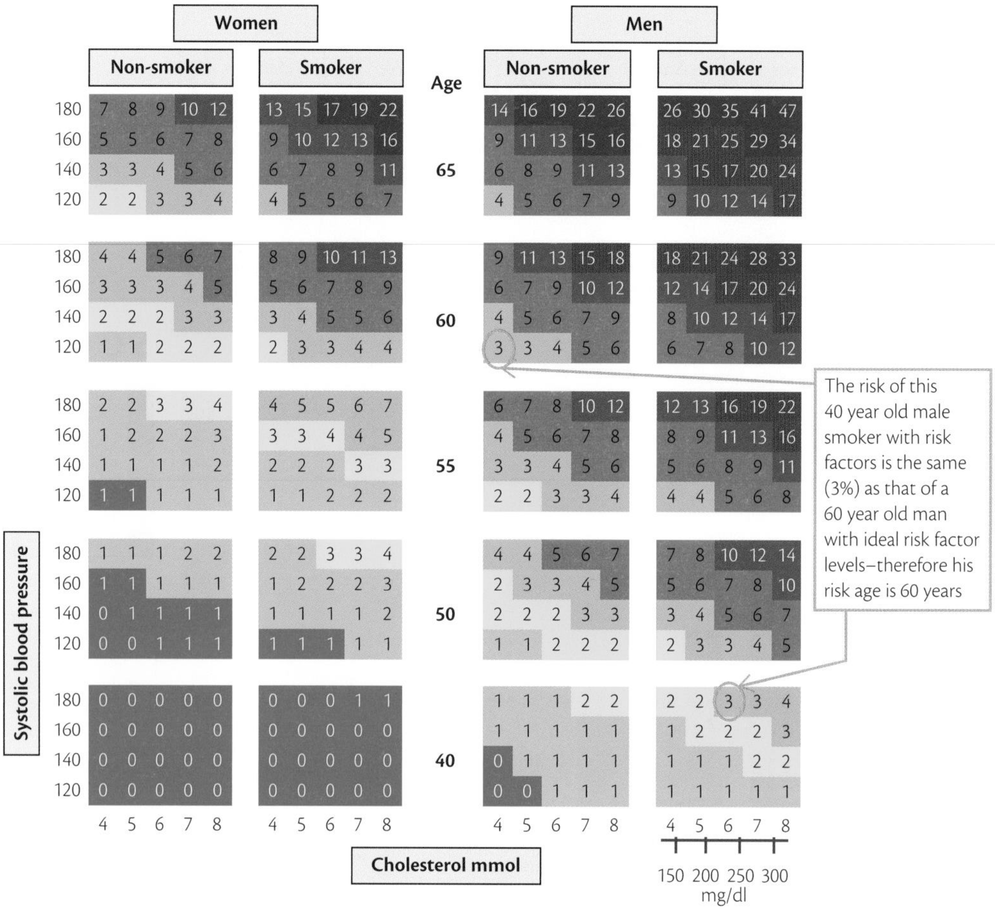

Fig. 5.5 SCORE chart for use in high-risk European regions illustrating how the approximate risk age can be read off the chart.

Reproduced from: Perk J, De Backer G, Gohlke H, et al. European Guidelines on cardiovascular disease prevention in clinical practice (version 2012): the Fifth Joint Task Force of the European Society of Cardiology and Other Societies on Cardiovascular Disease Prevention in Clinical Practice (constituted by representatives of nine societies and by invited experts). * Developed with the special contribution of the European Association for Cardiovascular Prevention and Rehabilitation (EACPR). *Eur J Prev Cardiol* 2012; **19**(4): 585–667.

category. While any cut point is arbitrary and open to debate, in the current (2012) European guidelines the cut points are based on CVD plus diabetes mortality for 2008 in those aged 45–74 years (220/100 000 for men and 160/100 000 for women) [34]. This defines 21 countries and marks a point at which there is an appreciable gap before the 22nd country (the Czech Republic). Using this definition, low-risk countries are (in ascending level of risk for men): France, Spain, Switzerland, the Netherlands, Italy, Iceland, Norway, Belgium, the United Kingdom, Sweden, Ireland, Denmark, Luxembourg, Portugal, Austria, Malta, Germany, Slovenia, Finland, Greece, and Cyprus.

This list is based on European countries that are members of the ESC. However, several European countries are not ESC members because they do not have a national cardiac society or because of their population size. In addition, the Joint Task Force felt it sensible to also look at Mediterranean countries that are ESC members but not strictly 'European' in WHO terminology. When this was done, Monaco, San Marino, Andorra, and Israel joined the 'low-risk' list. So, in alphabetical order for both sexes, the list of 25 low-risk counties becomes: Andorra, Austria, Belgium, Cyprus, Denmark, Finland, France, Germany, Greece, Iceland, Ireland, Israel, Italy, Luxembourg, Monaco, the Netherlands, Malta, Norway, Portugal, San Marino, Slovenia, Spain, Sweden, Switzerland, and the United Kingdom (➲ Fig. 5.7).

Some European countries have levels of risk that are more than double the CVD mortality of 220/100 000 in men used to define a low-risk country. The male:female ratio in these countries is smaller than in low-risk countries, suggesting a major problem for women, and even the high-risk charts may underestimate risk in these countries. Countries with a CVD mortality risk of >500/100,000 for men and >250/100,000 for women are: FYR Macedonia, Lithuania, Bulgaria, Latvia, Georgia, Moldova, Azerbaijan, Kyrgyzstan, Belarus, Armenia, Uzbekistan, Russia, Ukraine, and Kazakhstan (➲ Fig. 5.8).

How to use the risk estimation charts

- Use of the low-risk chart is recommended for the countries listed as low risk in the section 'What is a low-risk country?'. Use of the high-risk chart is recommended for all other European and Mediterranean countries. Note that several countries have undertaken national recalibrations to allow for time trends in mortality and risk factor distributions. Such charts are likely to better represent current risk levels.
- To estimate a person's 10-year risk of CVD death, find the correct table for their gender, smoking status and age. Within the table find the cell nearest to the person's BP and total cholesterol. Risk estimates will need to be adjusted upwards as the person approaches the next age category.

Age	Systolic blood pressure (mmHg)	Women, Non-smoker					Women, Smoker					Men, Non-smoker					Men, Smoker				
		4	5	6	7	8	4	5	6	7	8	4	5	6	7	8	4	5	6	7	8
	180	78	80	81	83	84	87	88	90	92	95	83	85	88	91	94	95	98	101	105	109
	160	73	75	76	78	80	81	83	85	87	89	76	79	81	84	87	88	90	94	97	101
65	140	69	70	72	74	76	76	78	80	82	84	70	73	75	78	81	81	83	86	90	93
	120	65	66	68	69	71	72	73	75	77	79	65	67	70	72	75	75	77	80	83	86
	180	72	73	75	76	78	79	81	83	85	87	76	78	81	84	87	87	90	93	97	100
	160	68	69	70	72	74	75	76	78	80	82	70	72	75	78	80	80	83	86	89	93
60	140	64	65	66	68	70	70	72	73	75	77	65	67	69	72	75	74	77	80	83	86
	120	60	61	63	64	66	66	68	69	71	73	60	62	64	67	69	69	71	74	77	80
	180	66	67	68	70	71	72	74	75	77	79	69	71	74	76	79	79	82	85	88	91
	160	62	63	64	66	67	68	69	71	73	74	64	66	68	71	74	73	76	79	82	85
55	140	58	59	61	61	64	64	65	67	69	70	59	61	63	66	68	68	70	73	76	79
	120	55	56	57	59	60	61	62	63	64	66	55	57	59	61	64	63	65	68	70	73
	180	59	60	62	63	64	65	66	68	69	71	62	64	67	69	72	71	74	77	80	83
	160	56	57	58	59	61	62	63	64	66	67	58	60	62	64	67	66	68	71	74	77
50	140	53	54	55	56	58	58	59	61	62	64	54	56	58	60	62	61	64	66	68	71
	120	50	51	52	53	55	55	56	57	59	60	50	52	54	56	58	57	59	61	64	66
	180	53	54	55	56	57	58	59	60	62	63	56	58	60	62	64	64	66	68	71	74
	160	50	51	52	53	54	55	56	57	59	60	52	54	55	57	60	59	61	63	66	68
40	140	48	48	49	50	52	52	53	54	55	57	48	50	52	54	56	55	57	59	61	64
	120	45	46	47	48	49	49	50	51	52	54	45	47	48	50	53	51	53	55	57	59
	180	47	48	49	50	51	51	52	53	54	55	49	51	52	54	56	56	58	60	62	65
	160	45	46	46	47	48	49	49	50	51	53	46	47	49	51	53	52	54	56	58	60
40	140	43	43	44	45	46	46	47	48	49	50	43	44	46	47	49	48	50	52	54	56
	120	40	41	42	43	44	44	45	45	46	48	40	41	43	44	46	45	47	49	51	52

Total Cholesterol (mmol/l)

Fig. 5.6 Risk ages for each risk factor combination in the SCORE chart.

Reproduced from: Perk J, De Backer G, Gohlke H, et al. European Guidelines on cardiovascular disease prevention in clinical practice (version 2012): the Fifth Joint Task Force of the European Society of Cardiology and Other Societies on Cardiovascular Disease Prevention in Clinical Practice (constituted by representatives of nine societies and by invited experts). * Developed with the special contribution of the European Association for Cardiovascular Prevention and Rehabilitation (EACPR). *Eur J Prev Cardiol* 2012; **19**(4): 585–667.

- People at low risk should be offered advice to maintain their low-risk status. While no threshold is universally applicable, the intensity of advice should increase with increasing risk. In general, those with a risk of CVD death of ≥5% qualify for intensive advice, and may benefit from drug treatment. At risk levels >10% drug treatment is more frequently required. In people aged over 60 these thresholds should be interpreted more leniently, because their age-specific risk is normally around these levels even when other cardiovascular risk factor levels are 'normal'. In particular, systematic initiation of drug treatment in all elderly individuals with risks greater than the 10% threshold should be discouraged.
- Relative risks may be unexpectedly high in young people even if absolute risk levels are low. The relative risk chart and estimation of risk age may be helpful in identifying and counselling such individuals.
- The charts may be used to give some indication of the effects of reducing risk factors, given that there will be a time lag before risk reduces and the results of randomized controlled trials (RCTs) in general give better estimates of benefits. A halving of risk is generally found in those who stop smoking.

Qualifiers

- The charts can assist in risk assessment and management but must be interpreted in the light of the clinician's knowledge and experience, especially with regard to local conditions.
- Risk will be overestimated in countries with a falling CVD mortality and underestimated in countries in which mortality is increasing.
- At any given age, risk estimates are lower for women than for men. This may be misleading because, eventually, at least as many women as men die from CVD. Inspection of the charts indicates that risk is merely deferred in women, with a 60-year-old woman resembling a 50-year-old man in terms of risk.

Table 5.4 Other diseases associated with increased risk for CVD

Influenza	Annual influenza vaccinations are recommended for patients with established CVD
Chronic kidney disease	Important determinant of risk as highlighted in the priorities (see ➲ Table 5.5). Hypertension, dyslipidaemia and diabetes mellitus are common among patients with chronic kidney disease, yet these patients tend to be less intensely treated than patients with normal renal function
Psoriasis	Risk greatest in younger patients with more severe disease
Rheumatoid arthritis	Patients with rheumatoid arthritis are twice as likely as the general population to suffer a myocardial infarction, increased CVD risk is possibly related to systemic inflammation and a pro-thrombotic state
Periodontitis	Periodontitis is associated with endothelial dysfunction, atherosclerosis, and an increased risk of myocardial infarction and stroke. Treatment of periodontitis is indicated and improvement of risk factors is advisable
Lupus erythematosus	Systemic lupus erythematosus is associated with endothelial dysfunction and an increased risk of CHD that is not fully explained by classic CHD risk factors
Vascular disease after radiation exposure	The incidence of ischaemic heart disease and stroke is increased many years after radiation exposure for treatment of lymphomas and for breast cancer, as well as for head and neck cancer
Vascular disease after transplantation	Cardiac allograft vasculopathy is the leading cause of late morbidity and mortality in heart transplant patients. Although it is a complex multifactorial process arising from immune and non-immune pathogenic mechanisms, the approach to cardiac allograft vasculopathy has been modification of underlying traditional risk factors and optimization of immune suppression

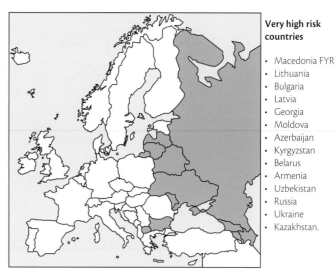

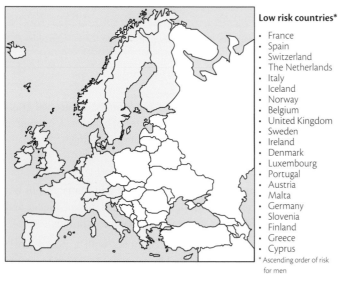

Fig. 5.7 New map of regions of Europe at low risk of CVD.

Priorities

Individuals at highest risk gain most from preventive efforts, which guides the priorities shown in ➲ Table 5.5. These risk categories, and hence priorities for intervention, are compatible with the joint ESC/EAS lipid guidelines [21]. The joint guidelines offer further advice on lipid intervention based on these risk categories. In addition, people with a strong family history of premature CVD or a family history of familial hyperlipidaemia deserve comprehensive risk assessment and, where necessary, treatment.

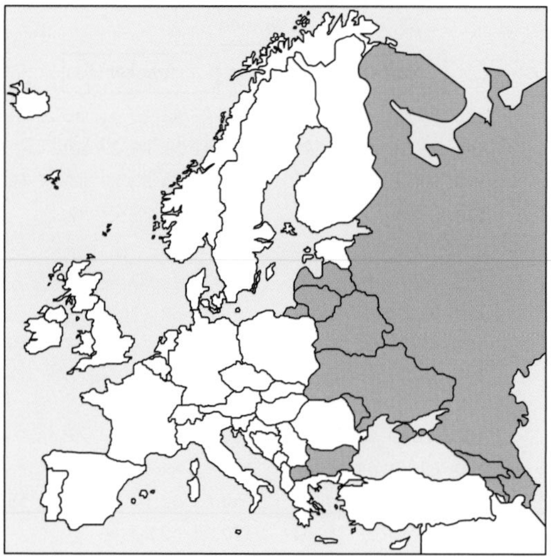

Fig. 5.8 Regions of Europe at very high risk of CVD (a CVD mortality risk of >500/100 000 for men and >250/100 000 for women, more than double the CVD mortality of 220/100 000 in men used to define low-risk countries). The male:female ratio is smaller than in low-risk countries, suggesting a major problem for women. Even the high-risk charts may underestimate risk in these countries.

Table 5.5 Priorities for CVD prevention

Very high risk	Subjects with any of the following: ◆ documented CVD ◆ type 2 diabetes, or type 1 diabetes and target organ damage such as microalbuminuria ◆ moderate to severe chronic kidney disease (GFR <60 ml/min/1.73 m^2) ◆ SCORE ≥10%
High risk	Markedly elevated single risk factors such as: ◆ familial dyslipidaemias ◆ severe hypertension SCORE ≥5% and <10%
Moderate risk	SCORE ≥1% and <5%, further modulated by: ◆ family history of premature CAD ◆ abdominal obesity ◆ low levels of physical activity ◆ low HDL cholesterol ◆ elevated triglycerides ◆ elevated hs-CRP ◆ social class
Low risk	SCORE <1% and free of qualifiers

GFR, glomerular filtration rate; CAD, coronary artery disease; hs-CRP, high-sensitivity CRP. Reproduced from: Perk J, De Backer G, Gohlke H, et al. European Guidelines on cardiovascular disease prevention in clinical practice (version 2012): The Fifth Joint Task Force of the European Society of Cardiology and Other Societies on Cardiovascular Disease Prevention in Clinical Practice (constituted by representatives of nine societies and by invited experts). * Developed with the special contribution of the European Association for Cardiovascular Prevention and Rehabilitation (EACPR). *Eur J Prev Cardiol* 2012; **19**(4): 585–667.

The latest guidelines

New guidelines on the prevention of CVD were issued in America in 2013 [22] and in the UK in 2014 [23].

The American AHA/ACC guidelines [22] included a new risk estimation system that was developed using pooled cohort data from four prospective studies: ARIC [24], the Cardiovascular Health Study [25], CARDIA [26], and the Framingham Original and Offspring studies [27]. This new system includes race-specific equations for non-Hispanic white Americans and African-Americans. However, probably due to the age of the cohorts, on external validation in the low-risk Physician's Health Study and Women's Health Study the new risk equation has been shown to over-estimate risk [22,28]. Thus far the applicability of the guidelines to Europe would seem limited.

The UK guidelines [23] include an innovative interactive risk estimation system. This is particularly aimed at UK citizens but the principles involved are widely applicable.

Conclusions

Total CVD risk estimation is a central tool for identifying those at highest multifactorial risk of developing CVD who should be targeted for lifestyle and risk factor management. The SCORE system has been updated with an estimate of total CVD risk as well as risk of CVD death. New information on diabetes is included. Information on relative as well as absolute risk has been added to facilitate the counselling of younger people whose low absolute risk may conceal a substantial and modifiable age-related risk.

The priorities defined in this chapter are for clinical use and reflect the fact that those at highest risk of a CVD event gain most from preventive measures. This approach should complement public actions to promote a healthy lifestyle and reduce levels of risk factors in the community as a whole.

The principles of risk estimation and the definition of priorities reflect an attempt to make complex issues simple and accessible. Their very simplicity makes them vulnerable to criticism. Above all they must be interpreted in the light of both the physician's detailed knowledge of their patient and associated conditions as well as local guidance.

Other issues relevant to total CVD risk assessment such as genetics, imaging for subclinical disease, the value of additional risk biomarkers, and psychosocial risk factors are discussed separately in ➲ Chapters 2, 6, 17, and 18, respectively.

Remaining gaps in the evidence

- Current systems of grading evidence give most weight to RCTs. While this is appropriate, many lifestyle measures are less amenable to such assessment than are drug treatments, which will therefore tend to receive a higher grade. The widely used Grading of Recommendations Assessment, Development, and Evaluation (GRADE) system attempts to address this issue, but more debate is needed.
- There are no recent RCTs of a total risk approach to risk assessment or risk management.
- The young, women, older people, and ethnic minorities continue to be under-represented in clinical trials.
- A systematic comparison of current international guidelines is needed to define areas of agreement and the reasons for discrepancies.

Further reading

Asmann G, Cullen P, Schulte H. Simple scoring scheme for calculating the risk of acute coronary events based on the 10-year follow-up of the prospective cardiovascular Munster (PROCAM) study. *Circulation* 2002; **105**: 310–15.

Conroy RM, Pyorala K, Fitzgerald AP, et al. Estimation of ten-year risk of fatal cardiovascular disease in Europe: the SCORE project. *Eur Heart J* 2003; **24**: 987–1003.

Cooney MT, Dudina AL, Graham IM. Value and limitations of existing scores for the assessment of cardiovascular risk: a review for clinicians. *J Am Coll Cardiol* 2009; **54**: 1209–27.

Cooney MT, Cooney HC, Dudina A, et al. Assessment of cardiovascular risk. *Curr Hypertens Rep* 2010; **12**: 384–93.

Cooney MT, Dudina A, De Bacquer D, et al. HDL cholesterol protects against cardiovascular disease in both genders, at all ages and at all levels of risk. *Atherosclerosis* 2009; **206**: 611–16.

Cooney MT, Vartiainen E, Laatikainen T, et al. Cardiovascular risk age: concepts and practicalities. *Heart* 2012; **98**: 941–6.

Cuende JI, Cuende N, Calaveras-Lagartos J. How to calculate vascular age with the SCORE project scales: a new method of cardiovascular risk evaluation. *Eur Heart J* 2010; **31**: 2351–8.

D'Agostino RB, Sr, Vasan RS, Pencina MJ, et al. General cardiovascular risk profile for use in primary care: the Framingham Heart Study. *Circulation* 2008; **117**: 743–53.

Hippisley-Cox J, Coupland C, Vinogradova Y, et al. Performance of the QRISK cardiovascular risk prediction algorithm in an independent UK sample of patients from general practice: a validation study. *Heart* 2008; **94**: 34–9.

Jenning C, Mead A, Jones J, et al. *Preventive cardiology—a practical manual*, 2009. Oxford Care Manuals. Oxford: Oxford University Press.

Jackson R, Lawes CM, Bennett DA, et al. Treatment with drugs to lower blood pressure and blood cholesterol based on an individual's absolute cardiovascular risk. *Lancet* 2005; **365**: 434–41.

Kotseva K, Wood D, De Backer G, et al. Cardiovascular prevention guidelines in daily practice: a comparison of EUROASPIRE I, II, and III surveys in eight European countries. *Lancet* 2009; **373**: 929–40.

Perk J, De Backer G, Gohlke H, et al. European Guidelines on cardiovascular disease prevention in clinical practice (version 2012): the Fifth Joint Task Force of the European Society of Cardiology and Other Societies on Cardiovascular Disease Prevention in Clinical Practice (constituted by representatives of nine societies and by invited experts). *Eur J Prev Cardiol* 2012; **19**: 585–667 (see also: <http://www.escardio.org/guidelines>).

Rose G. *The stategy of preventive medicine*, 1992. Oxford: Oxford University Press.

Rose G. Sick individuals and sick populations. *Int J Epidemiol* 1985; **14**: 32–8.

Reiner Z, Catapano AL, De Backer G, et al. ESC/EAS Guidelines for the management of dyslipidaemias: the Task Force for the management of dyslipidaemias of the European Society of cardiology (ESC) and the European Atherosclerosis Society (EAS). *Eur Heart J* 2011; **32**: 1769–818 (see also: <http://www.escardio.org/guidelines>).

Ridker PM, Buring JE, Rifai N, et al. Development and validation of improved algorithms for the assessment of global cardiovascular risk in women: the Reynolds Risk Score. *J Am Med Assoc* 2007; **297**: 611–19.

Scottish Intercollegiate Guidelines Network. *Risk estimation and the prevention of cardiovascular disease. A national clinical guideline*, 2007. Edinburgh: Scottish Intercollegiate Guidelines Network.

Woodward M, Brindle P, Tunstall-Pedoe H. Adding social deprivation and family history to cardiovascular risk assessment: the ASSIGN score from the Scottish Heart Health Extended Cohort (SHHEC). *Heart* 2007; **93**: 172–6.

World Health Organization. *Prevention of cardiovascular disease: guidelines for assessment and management of cardiovascular risk*, 2007. Geneva: World Health Organization.

References

1 Perk J, De Backer G, Gohlke H, et al. European Guidelines on cardiovascular disease prevention in clinical practice (version 2012): The Fifth Joint Task Force of the European Society of Cardiology and Other Societies on Cardiovascular Disease Prevention in Clinical Practice (constituted by representatives of nine societies and by invited experts. *Eur J Prev Cardiol* 2012; **19**: 585–667.

2 Rose G. Sick individuals and sick populations. *Int J Epidemiol* 1985; **14**: 32–8.

3 Hippisley-Cox J, Coupland C, Vinogradova Y, et al. Predicting cardiovascular risk in England and Wales: prospective derivation and validation of QRISK2. *Br Med J* 2008; **336**: 1475–82.

4 Cooney MT, Dudina A, Whincup P, et al. Re-evaluating the Rose approach: comparative benefits of the population and high-risk preventive strategies. *Eur J Cardiovasc Prev Rehabil* 2009; **16**: 541–9.

5 Pyorala K, De Backer G, Graham I, et al. Prevention of coronary heart disease in clinical practice. Recommendations of the Task Force of the European Society of Cardiology, European Atherosclerosis Society and European Society of Hypertension. *Eur Heart J* 1994; **15**: 1300–31.

6 Kotseva K, Wood D, De Backer G, et al. Cardiovascular prevention guidelines in daily practice: a comparison of EUROASPIRE I, II, and III surveys in eight European countries. *Lancet* 2009; **373**: 929–40.

7 Wood D, De Backer G, Faergeman O, et al. Prevention of coronary heart disease in clinical practice: recommendations of the Second Joint Task Force of European and other Societies on Coronary Prevention. *Atherosclerosis* 1998; **140**: 199–270.

8 Anderson KM, Odell PM, Wilson PW, Kannel WB. Cardiovascular disease risk profiles. *Am Heart J* 1991; **121**: 293–8.

9 Graham I, Atar D, Borch-Johnsen K, et al. European guidelines on cardiovascular disease prevention in clinical practice: full text. Fourth Joint Task Force of the European Society of Cardiology and other societies on cardiovascular disease prevention in clinical practice (constituted by representatives of nine societies and by invited experts). *Eur J Cardiovasc Prev Rehabil* 2007; **14**(Suppl. 2): S1–S113.

10 D'Agostino RB, Sr, Vasan RS, Pencina MJ, et al. General cardiovascular risk profile for use in primary care: the Framingham Heart Study. *Circulation* 2008; **117**: 743–53.

11 Conroy RM, Pyorala K, Fitzgerald AP, et al. Estimation of ten-year risk of fatal cardiovascular disease in Europe: the SCORE project. *Eur Heart J* 2003; **24**: 987–1003.

12 Woodward M, Brindle P, Tunstall-Pedoe H. Adding social deprivation and family history to cardiovascular risk assessment: the ASSIGN score from the Scottish Heart Health Extended Cohort (SHHEC). *Heart* 2007; **93**: 172–6.

13 Hippisley-Cox J, Coupland C, Vinogradova Y, et al. Derivation and validation of QRISK, a new cardiovascular disease risk score for the United Kingdom: prospective open cohort study. *Br Med J* 2007; **335**: 136.

14 Assmann G, Cullen P, Schulte H. Simple scoring scheme for calculating the risk of acute coronary events based on the 10-year follow-up of the prospective cardiovascular Munster (PROCAM) study. *Circulation* 2002; **105**: 310–15.

15 World Health Organization. *Prevention of cardiovascular disease: guidelines for assessment and management of cardiovascular risk*, 2007. Geneva: World Health Organization.

16 Ridker PM, Buring JE, Rifai N, et al. Development and validation of improved algorithms for the assessment of global cardiovascular risk in women: the Reynolds Risk Score. *J Am Med Assoc* 2007; **297**: 611–19.

17 Cooney MT, Dudina AL, Graham IM. Value and limitations of existing scores for the assessment of cardiovascular risk: a review for clinicians. *J Am Coll Cardiol* 2009; **54**: 1209–27.

18 Cooney MT, Cooney HC, Dudina A, et al. Assessment of cardiovascular risk. *Curr Hypertens Rep* 2010; **12**: 384–93.

19 Cooney MT, Vartiainen E, Laatikainen T, et al. Elevated resting heart rate is an independent risk factor for cardiovascular disease in healthy men and women. *Am Heart J* 2010; **159**: 612–19. e3.

20 De Backer G, Ambrosioni E, Borch-Johnsen K, et al. European guidelines on cardiovascular disease prevention in clinical practice: third joint task force of European and other societies on cardiovascular disease prevention in clinical practice (constituted by representatives of eight societies and by invited experts). *Eur J Cardiovasc Prev Rehabil* 2003; **10**: S1–S10.

21 Reiner Z, Catapano AL, De Backer G, et al. ESC/EAS Guidelines for the management of dyslipidaemias: the Task Force for the management of dyslipidaemias of the European Society of Cardiology (ESC) and the European Atherosclerosis Society (EAS). *Eur Heart J* 2011; **32**: 1769–818.

22 Goff DC, Jr, Lloyd-Jones DM, Bennett G, et al; American College of Cardiology/American Heart Association Task Force on Practice Guidelines 2013 ACC/AHA guideline on the assessment of cardiovascular risk: a report of the American College of Cardiology/American Heart Association Task Force on Practice Guidelines. *J Am Coll Cardiol* 2014; **63**: 2935–59.

23 Board of the JBS. Joint British Societies' consensus recommendations for the prevention of cardiovascular disease (JBS3). *Heart* 2014; **100**(Suppl. 2): ii1–ii67.

24 The Atherosclerosis Risk in Communities (ARIC) Study: design and objectives. The ARIC investigators. *Am J Epidemiol* 1989; **129**: 687–702.

25 Fried LP, Borhani NO, Enright P, et al. The Cardiovascular Health Study: design and rationale. *Ann Epidemiol* 1991; **1**: 263–76.

26 Friedman GD, Cutter GR, Donahue RP, et al. CARDIA: study design, recruitment, and some characteristics of the examined subjects. *J Clin Epidemiol* 1988; **41**: 1105–16.

27 Kannel WB, Feinleib M, McNamara PM, et al. An investigation of coronary heart disease in families. The Framingham Offspring Study. *Am J Epidemiol* 1979; **110**: 281–90.
28 Cook NR, Ridker PM. Response to Comment on the reports of overestimation of ASCVD risk using the 2013 AHA/ACC risk equation. *Circulation* 2014; **129**: 268–9.
29 Aktas MK, Ozduran V, Pothier CE, et al. Global risk scores and exercise testing for predicting all-cause mortality in a preventive medicine program. *J Am Med Assoc* 2004; **292**: 1462–8.
30 Vartiainen E, Jousilahti P, Alfthan G, et al. Cardiovascular risk factor changes in Finland, 1972–1997. *Int J Epidemiol* 2000; **29**: 49–56.
31 Cooney MT, Dudina A, De Bacquer D, et al. How much does HDL cholesterol add to risk estimation? A report from the SCORE Investigators. *Eur J Cardiovasc Prev Rehabil* 2009; **16**: 304–14.
32 Cooney MT, Dudina A, De Bacquer D, et al. HDL cholesterol protects against cardiovascular disease in both genders, at all ages and at all levels of risk. *Atherosclerosis* 2009; **206**: 611–16.
33 Gotto AM, Jr. Triglyceride as a risk factor for coronary artery disease. *Am J Cardiol* 1998; **82**: 22Q–25Q.
34 Ridker PM. Fasting versus nonfasting triglycerides and the prediction of cardiovascular risk: do we need to revisit the oral triglyceride tolerance test? *Clin Chem* 2008; **54**: 11–13.
35 Abdel-Maksoud MF, Hokanson JE. The complex role of triglycerides in cardiovascular disease. *Semin Vasc Med* 2002; **2**: 325–33.
36 Sarwar N, Danesh J, Eiriksdottir G, et al. Triglycerides and the risk of coronary heart disease: 10,158 incident cases among 262,525 participants in 29 Western prospective studies. *Circulation* 2007; **115**: 450–8.
37 Wilson P, Pencina M, Jacques P, et al. C-reactive protein and reclassification of cardiovascular risk in the Framingham Heart Study. *Circulation: Cardiovasc Qual Outcomes* 2008; **1**: 92–7.
38 Cooney MT, Vartiainen E, Laatikainen T, et al. Cardiovascular risk age: concepts and practicalities. *Heart* 2012; **98**: 941–6.
39 Cuende JI, Cuende N, Calaveras-Lagartos J. How to calculate vascular age with the SCORE project scales: a new method of cardiovascular risk evaluation. *Eur Heart J* 2010; **31**: 2351–8.
40 Hansson G. Inflammation, atherosclerosis and coronary artery disease. *N Engl J Med* 2005; **352**: 1685–95.
41 World Health Organization. *Global health observatory data repository*. URL: <http://apps.who.int/ghodata/> (accessed 2011).
42 Ridker PM, Paynter NP, Rifai N, et al. C-reactive protein and parental history improve global cardiovascular risk prediction: the Reynolds Risk Score for men. *Circulation* 2008; **118**: 2243–51 (and 4 pp. following 2251).
43 Voss R, Cullen P, Schulte H, et al. Prediction of risk of coronary events in middle-aged men in the Prospective Cardiovascular Munster Study (PROCAM) using neural networks. *Int J Epidemiol* 2002; **31**: 1253–62.
44 Grundy SM, Cleeman JI, Merz CN, et al. Implications of recent clinical trials for the National Cholesterol Education Program Adult Treatment Panel III guidelines. *Arterioscler Thromb Vasc Biol* 2004; **24**: e149–e161.
45 New Zealand Guidelines Group. *The assessment and management of cardiovascular risk*, 2003. Wellington: New Zealand Guidelines Group.
46 Scottish Intercollegiate Guidelines Network. *Risk estimation and the prevention of cardiovascular disease. A national clinical guideline*, 2007. Edinburgh: Scottish Intercollegiate Guidelines Network.
47 Jackson R, Lawes CM, Bennett DA, et al. Treatment with drugs to lower blood pressure and blood cholesterol based on an individual's absolute cardiovascular risk. *Lancet* 2005; **365**: 434–41.
48 Empana JP, Ducimetiere P, Arveiler D, et al. Are the Framingham and PROCAM coronary heart disease risk functions applicable to different European populations? The PRIME Study. *Eur Heart J* 2003; **24**: 1903–11.
49 Scheltens T, Verschuren WM, Boshuizen HC, et al. Estimation of cardiovascular risk: a comparison between the Framingham and the SCORE model in people under 60 years of age. *Eur J Cardiovasc Prev Rehabil* 2008; **15**: 562–6.
50 Barzi F, Patel A, Gu D, et al. Cardiovascular risk prediction tools for populations in Asia. *J Epidemiol Commun Health* 2007; **61**: 115–21.
51 Hippisley-Cox J, Coupland C, Vinogradova Y, et al. Performance of the QRISK cardiovascular risk prediction algorithm in an independent UK sample of patients from general practice: a validation study. *Heart* 2008; **94**: 34–9.
52 Simmons RK, Sharp S, Boekholdt SM, et al. Evaluation of the Framingham risk score in the European Prospective Investigation of Cancer-Norfolk cohort: does adding glycated hemoglobin improve the prediction of coronary heart disease events? *Arch Intern Med* 2008; **168**: 1209–16.
53 May M, Lawlor DA, Brindle P, et al. Cardiovascular disease risk assessment in older women: can we improve on Framingham? British Women's Heart and Health prospective cohort study. *Heart* 2006; **92**: 1396–401.
54 Lindman AS, Veierod MB, Pedersen JI, et al. The ability of the SCORE high-risk model to predict 10-year cardiovascular disease mortality in Norway. *Eur J Cardiovasc Prev Rehabil* 2007; **14**: 501–7.
55 Ulmer H, Kollerits B, Kelleher C, et al. Predictive accuracy of the SCORE risk function for cardiovascular disease in clinical practice: a prospective evaluation of 44 649 Austrian men and women. *Eur J Cardiovasc Prev Rehabil* 2005; **12**: 433–41.
56 Aspelund T, Thorgeirsson G, Sigurdsson G, et al. Estimation of 10-year risk of fatal cardiovascular disease and coronary heart disease in Iceland with results comparable with those of the Systematic Coronary Risk Evaluation project. *Eur J Cardiovasc Prev Rehabil* 2007; **14**: 761–8.

CHAPTER 6

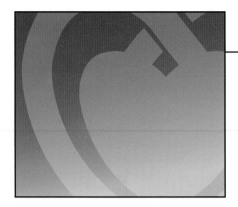

Imaging in cardiovascular prevention

Uwe Nixdorff, Stephan Achenbach, Frank Bengel, Pompilio Faggiano, Sara Fernández, Christian Heiss, Thomas Mengden, Gian Francesco Mureddu, Eike Nagel, Valentina Puntmann, and Jose Zamorano

Contents

Summary

Imaging tools in preventive cardiology can be divided into imaging modalities for assessing pre-clinical and clinical atherosclerosis and those for functional assessment of vascular function or vascular inflammation. Intima–media thickness as well as coronary calcium scoring are most frequently used to calculate the likelihood of pre-clinical atherosclerosis. However, beyond these two measurements there are other parameters derived by ultrasound and multi-detector computed tomography as well as magnetic resonance imaging and nuclear/molecular imaging. Functional tests include flow-mediated dilatation, pulse wave analysis, and ankle–brachial index. In clinical research other invasive measurements such as intravascular ultrasound/virtual histology/elastography, optical coherence tomography as well as thermography are being used. However, their value in clinical prevention still needs to be established.

Introduction

In cardiology, risk factors have a well-established causative role in initiating and accelerating the process of atherogenesis. Scoring systems like the European Society of Cardiology's (ESC) Systematic COronary Risk Evaluation (SCORE) aim to extract predictive information from the sum of established classical risk factors (global risk burden) to calculate the incidence of cardiovascular (CV) events like myocardial infarction (MI) [1]. These scores are based on large cohorts, i.e. they are population-based. Although this is helpful in CV risk stratification, and is even part of certain preventive workups (algorithms), there are certain limits to the individual approach to the patient at risk. Discrimination and calibration of population-based likelihoods for disease development are changing over time and may only be used in the ethnic/regional background for which the score was developed.

Pre-test probability and diagnostic assessment

In individualized prevention an objective assessment of atherosclerotic risk is therefore needed. A possible solution is direct imaging of the cardiovascular phenotype [2–4]. In low-risk individuals conventional diagnostic modalities (i.e. maximal exercise testing for ischaemia detection) are not useful because they operate best in individuals with medium pre-test

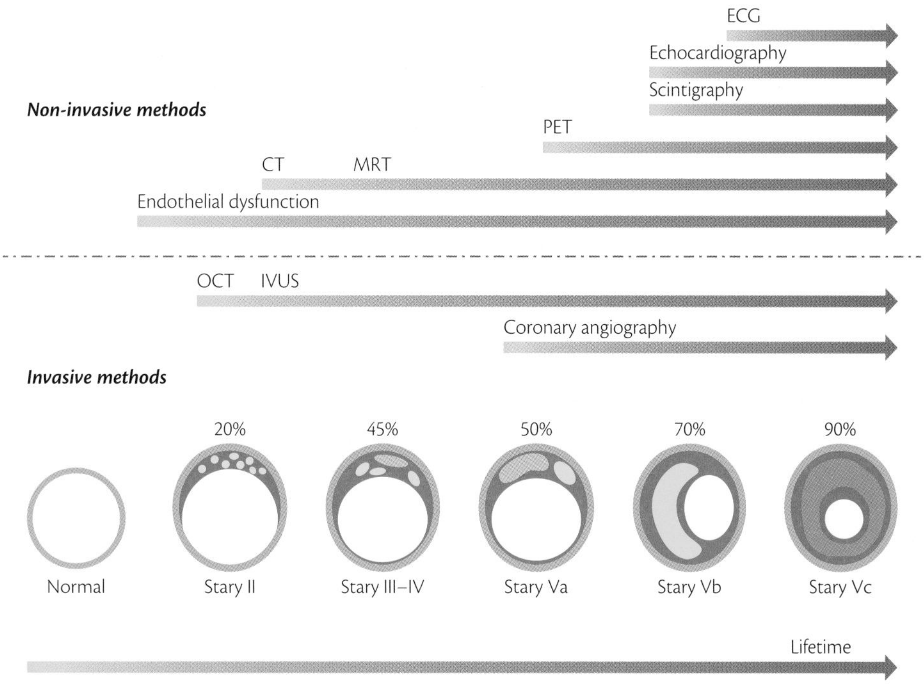

Fig. 6.1 Scheme of the development of coronary atherosclerosis including positive remodelling during increasing plaque burden and a list of invasive and non-invasive methods with regard to their ability to detect signs of atherosclerosis, starting with endothelial dysfunction and ending with signs of ischaemia in the ECG. Modified according to Erbel and Budoff [2] with permission.

probabilities of having a good diagnostic yield [5]. Using ergometry for the exclusion of significant coronary artery disease (CAD) in patients with low pre-test probability for the disease may result in a high rate of false positive results and unnecessary invasive examinations. A reasonable approach using Bayes' theorem to achieve a balanced relation of pre- and post-test probabilities requires imaging approaches that target the direct morphological substrate of atherosclerosis [3].

A further reason for detecting pre-clinical atherosclerosis by imaging is related to the fact that the vast majority of acute coronary events occur in haemodynamically insignificant (i.e. non-stenotic) plaques which are vulnerable and rupture-prone due to active inflammatory processes [6,7]. Because we have therapeutic strategies for halting the progression of atherosclerosis or minimizing atherothrombotic risks by lifestyle modification, high-dose statins [8], and platelet inhibition, imaging may open the door to effective therapeutic options.

Prognostically, risk prediction was shown to be improved by adding markers of subclinical organ damage to SCORE [9]. However, in addition to the need for reasonable discrimination [significant increases in the area under the curve (AUC), *c*-statistic, and receiver operator curve (ROC)] and calibration (varying with time and place) there should be some reclassification, measured as net reclassification improvement (NRI) [10] (approximately 10% more in addition to the usual risk scoring models is thought to be clinically relevant) [3].

The atherosclerotic continuum is the ideal pathophysiological process for pre-clinical detection and consecutive prevention because time lead bias [7] is not a significant concern. Sensitive, specific, and especially negative predictive imaging modalities have been developed for this purpose [2–4]. In this chapter we will focus on technologies that are available for patient care [3,4] (➲ Fig. 6.1; ➲ Tables 6.1 and 6.2). Others are still under development [11].

Table 6.1 Recommendations regarding imaging methods according to the European Guidelines on cardiovascular disease prevention in clinical practice (version 2012) [1]

Recommendations	Class of recommendation	Level of evidence	Grade
Measurement of carotid intima–media thickness and/or screening for atherosclerotic plaques by carotid artery scanning should be considered for cardiovascular risk assessment in asymptomatic adults at moderate risk	IIa	B	Strong
Measurement of ankle–brachial index should be considered for cardiovascular risk assessment in asymptomatic adults at moderate risk	IIa	B	Strong
Computed tomography for coronary calcium should be considered for cardiovascular risk assessment in asymptomatic adults at moderate risk	IIa	B	Weak
Exercise electrocardiography may be considered for cardiovascular risk assessment in moderate-risk asymptomatic adults (including sedentary adults considering starting a vigorous exercise programme), particularly when attention is paid to non-electrocardiogram markers such as exercise capacity	IIb	B	Strong

Reproduced from Perk J, De Backer G, Gohlke H, et al. European Guidelines on cardiovascular disease prevention in clinical practice (version 2012): The Fifth Joint Task Force of the European Society of Cardiology and Other Societies on Cardiovascular Disease Prevention in Clinical Practice (constituted by representatives of nine societies and by invited experts).
* Developed with the special contribution of the European Association for Cardiovascular Prevention and Rehabilitation (EACPR). *Eur J Prev Cardiol* 2012; **19**(4): 585–667.

Table 6.2 Schematic interpretation of the pros and cons of various diagnostic modalities (a)–(e) for pre-clinical detection of atherosclerosis

(a) Ultrasound of the vessel wall

	IMT	Plaque	Aneurysm	Targeted/therapeutic
CAD detection	–	–	–	–
CAD surrogate	+	+ +	+ +	+ +
Early timeline of atherosclerosis	+ + +	+ +	+	+
Evidence grade	+ +	+ +	+ +	–
Prognosis prediction	+ +	+ + (+)	+ +	–
Clinical decision making	(+)	+ + +	+ + +	+ + +
Variability	+ +	+	+	+ +
Cost-effectiveness	+ +	+ +	+ +	+
Availability	+ +	+ +	+ +	–
Expertise requirement	+ +	+ +	+	+ + +
Patient motivation/compliance enhancement	+	+ + +	+ +	+
Downstream testing	–	+	+ +	–
Side effects	–	–	–	+

–, no relevance; +/+ +/+ + +, low/intermediate/high relevance. IMT, intima-media thickness; CAD, coronary artery disease.

Table 6.2

(b) Echocardiography

	Coronary artery	Cardiac structure	LV function	Stress echo	MCE
CAD detection	+ +	–	–	+ + +	+ + +
CAD surrogate		+	+ +		
Early timeline of atherosclerosis	–	–	+	–	–
Evidence grade	+ +	–	+ + +	+ + +	+
Prognosis prediction	+ +	+	+ + +	+ + +	+ +
Clinical decision making	+ +	–	+ + +	+ + +	+ + +
Variability	+	+	+ +	+ +	+ +
Cost-effectiveness	+ +	+ +	+ +	+ +	+ +
Availability	+	+	+	+ +	–
Expertise requirement	+ + +	+ +	+ + +	+ + +	+ + +
Patient motivation/compliance enhancement	+ +	+	+ + +	+ + +	+ + +
Downstream testing	+ + +	(+)	+ +	+ + +	+ + +
Side effects	+	–	–	+	+

–, no relevance; +/+ +/+ + +, low/intermediate/high relevance. CAD, coronary artery disease; LV, left ventricle; MCE, myocardial contrast echocardiography.

Furthermore, algorithms for clinical pathways are only partly developed: scoring of particular CV risk factors (like ESC SCORE) as a fundamental basis for indicating any further imaging application, focusing especially on intermediate-risk patients, has been proposed [1,3]. Imaging tests may be used in middle-aged adults in order to identify pre-clinical atherosclerosis [12,13]. Awareness of the pathophysiological process may also help to improve adherence to lifestyle counselling and risk-modifying therapy [14–16].

Table 6.2

(c) Multi-detector computed tomography[a] and cardiac magnetic resonance imaging[b]

	CAC[a]	CTA[a]	Coronary artery[b]	LV function[b]	Ischaemia/ viability[b]	Plaque composition[b]
CAD detection	+ + +	+ + +	+ +	–	+ + +	–
CAD surrogate				+ +		+ +
Early timeline of atherosclerosis	+ +	+ (+)	–	–	–	+ +
Evidence grade	+ +	+ +	–	+ +	+ + +	+
Prognosis prediction	+ +	+ + +	+	+ + +	+ + +	+ +
Clinical decision making	+ + +	+ +	+	+ + +	+ + +	+ + +
Variability	+	+ +	+ +	+ +	+ +	+ +
Cost-effectiveness	+	+	–	–	+	+
Availability	–	–	–	–	–	–
Expertise requirement	+ +	+ + +	+ + +	+ + +	+ + +	+ + +
Patient motivation/compliance enhancement	+ + +	+ + +	+ +	+ +	+ +	+ + +
Downstream testing	+ +	+ +	+ +	+ +	+ + +	+ +
Side effects	+	+ +	(+)	(+)	(+)	(+)

–, no relevance; +/+ +/+ + +, low/intermediate/high relevance. CAD, coronary artery disease; CAC, coronary artery calcium; CTA, coronary CT angiography; LV, left ventricle.

Table 6.2

(d) Nuclear medicine and fundoscopy

	Plaque vulnerability	SPECT	Fusion Imaging	Fundoscopy
CAD detection	–	+ + +	+ +	–
CAD surrogate	+ +			(+)
Early timeline of atherosclerosis	+ +	–	+ +	+ +
Evidence grade	–	+ + +	–	+ +
Prognosis prediction	+	+ + +	+	+ +
Clinical decision making	+	+ + +	+	+
Variability	+	+ +	+ +	+ +
Cost-effectiveness	–	–	–	+
Availability	–	–	–	–
Expertise requirement	+ + +	+ +	+ + +	+ +
Patient motivation/compliance enhancement	+	+ +	+ +	+ +
Downstream testing	+ +	+ + +	+	+
Side effects	+ +	+ +	+ +	(+)

–, no relevance; +/+ +/+ + +, low/intermediate/high relevance. CAD, coronary artery disease; SPECT, single-photon emission computed tomography.

(continued)

Bias in screening for atherosclerosis

When applying imaging methods one should adhere to clear-cut criteria, for instance those published by the World Health Organization [17] (➲ Table 6.3). Screening tests have their biases and pitfalls: it is important that one is aware of the relevance of false positive and false negative results. The proportion of false positive and false negative results depends on the incidence of the disease. If a disease is rare, screening will produce more false positive results, which create a psychological burden for the individual patient and may mean unnecessary invasive tests. False negative results, on the other hand, may delay the diagnosis of potentially threatening diseases.

Table 6.2 (*continued*)

(e) Invasive procedures and functional testing

	IVUS/elastography	OCT	Thermography	FMD	PWA	ABI
CAD detection	+ + +	+ + +	+ + +	–	–	–
CAD surrogate				+ +	(+)	+
Early timeline of atherosclerosis	+ +	+ + +	+ + +	+ + +	+ + +	+ +
Evidence grade	+ +	–	–	–	+	+ +
Prognosis prediction	+	+	+	+	+ +	+ +
Clinical decision making	+ + +	+	+	+	+ +	+ +
Variability	+	+	+	+ + +	+ +	+
Cost-effectiveness	–	–	–	+	+	+ + +
Availability	–	–	–	–	+	+ + +
Expertise requirement	+ +	+ + +	+ + +	+ + +	+ +	+
Patient motivation/compliance enhancement	+ +	+ +	+ +	+ +	+ +	+
Downstream testing	+	+	+	+	+	+ +
Side effects	+ +	+ +	+ +	(+)	–	–

–, no relevance; +/+ +/+ + +, low/intermediate/high relevance; CAD, coronary artery disease; IVUS, intravascular ultrasound; OCT, optical coherence tomography; FMD, flow-mediated dilatation; PWA, pulse wave analysis; ABI, ankle–brachial index.

Table 6.3 WHO criteria for screening [17]

- The condition sought should be an important health problem for the individual and community
- There should be an accepted treatment or useful intervention for patients with the disease
- The natural history of the disease should be adequately understood
- There should be a latent or early symptomatic stage
- There should be a suitable and acceptable screening test or examination
- Facilities for diagnosis and treatment should be available
- There should be an agreed policy on whom to treat as patients
- Treatment started at an early stage should be of more benefit than treatment started later
- The cost should be economically balanced in relation to possible expenditure on medical care as a whole
- Case finding should be a continuing process and not a once and for all project

Data from Wilson JMG, Jungner G. Principles and practice of screening for disease. *WHO Chronicle* 1968; **22**: 473.

Other potential sources of bias include:

- Selection bias, which implies a specific bias in individual screening.
- Adherence or compliance bias; this might be introduced in those individuals who adhere very strictly to therapies and are thereby more willing to undergo screening, improving the apparent impact of the screening strategy.
- Lead-time bias overestimates the effectiveness of a screening test by detecting the disease at a much earlier stage; therefore, the time between diagnosis and disease/death will be prolonged, giving an artificial prolongation of 'survival with disease'.
- Length-time bias might work if screening performs better in detecting diseases with more favourable outcomes.

Ultrasound of vessel walls

Intima–media thickness (IMT)

High-resolution B-mode ultrasonography has a number of inherent methodological advantages: it is non-invasive, readily available, cost-effective, and does not involve radiation exposure. The carotid arteries are ideal for assessment due to their short distance from the skin and the carotid intima–media thickness (CIMT) is usually measured (➲ Fig. 6.2). Measurement of the IMT is defined according to the leading edge method as the distance between the lumen–intima border and the media–adventitia border. IMT

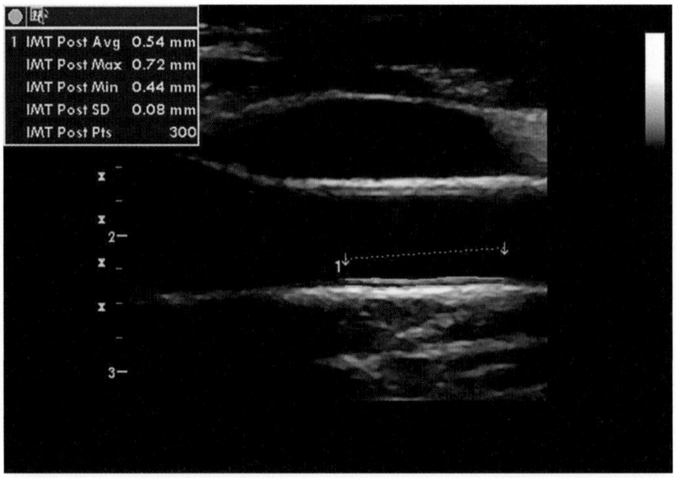

Fig. 6.2 Ultrasound scan of the common carotid artery with a high-frequency transducer, automatic contouring and measurement of the intima-media thickness (IMT) approximately 1 cm distal to the bulb. Note the average measurement result of 0.54 mm and the standard deviation of 0.08 mm in an individual assessment.

measurements are performed during diastole due to lower variability than in systole and might be restricted to the medial wall which has lower variability than the lateral wall. Automatic contour detection programs (about 150 measurements in < 0.1 s) are preferred [18,19] (➲ Fig. 6.2). IMT values imply predictive information on future events such as stroke and MI [20], as confirmed in a meta-analysis [21]. The detection of plaque increases the risk up to a hazard ratio (HR) of 2.3 [22]. According to the Rotterdam Study, a reclassification of Framingham risk score (FRS) was possible by CIMT to an NRI of 8.2% in women (less in men) [23]. The ARIC study found an NRI of 9.9% irrespective of gender [24]. Based on data from the ARIC trial [20] and the Nixdorf recall study, nomograms exist that enable calculation of age- and gender-referenced percentiles as well as biological age [25] (a calculator can be downloaded at <http://www.uk-essen.de/recall-studie/>). Commonly an IMT value is considered to be elevated if it is higher than the population-based 75th percentile. IMT values are linearly related to a number of established CV risk factors; however, interestingly this linearity is less clear with increasing age, demonstrating an age dependence [26]. IMT may also be useful as a follow-up parameter to assess the vascular effects of positive changes in risk profile: A meta-analysis on antihypertensive drugs comparing calcium channel blockers and angiotensin-converting enzyme (ACE) inhibitors demonstrated a significant decrease of IMT after therapy with calcium channel blockers [27]. In the placebo-controlled METEOR study high-dose rosuvastatin therapy prevented progression of IMT (i.e. increased thickening) over a 2-year follow-up [28]. In the REGRESS study a regression of IMT after 2 years of pravastatin therapy was confirmed [29].

Based on these convincing data the American Heart Association (AHA) guideline for assessment of CV risk in asymptomatic adults [4] recommends IMT measurement as a class IIa diagnostic assessment saying that

> measurement of CIMT is reasonable for CV assessment in asymptomatic adults at intermediate risk. Published recommendations on required equipment, technical approach, and operator training and experience for performance of the test must be carefully followed to achieve high-quality results (Level of Evidence: B).

In spite of this, the reliability of CIMT in single-patient risk assessment is still controversial due to high variability and relatively low intra-individual reproducibility. Otherwise, limitations can now be overcome by using newer radiofrequency systems (➲ Fig. 6.2).

Echo particle image velocimetry (EPIV) is a new technique that measures shear wall stress (in dyne/cm^2) through vector analysis of blood velocities at the wall at the carotid bifurcation by combining contrast with conventional two-dimensional (2D) ultrasound [30].

Plaque definition

In carotid artery ultrasound, plaques characteristically appear as a circumscript thickening with a more echogenic tissue composition (probably signifying calcification). Plaques may also be more echolucent (probably signifying soft plaque). Some lesions are borderline for which definitions of the Mannheim consensus are useful [18]. A plaque is a focal structure that protrudes into the lumen by ≥ 0.5 mm, or is 50% of the approximate IMT, or is > 1.5 mm from the media–adventitia/intima–lumen border. However, there are intermediate stages between elevated IMT values and plaque without any clear differentiation by ultrasound and even histology. Reporting of plaque findings by ultrasound should contain quantitative measures of length and brightness dimensions as well as thickness, but also characterization of plaque composition such as echolucent, calcified, homogeneous, heterogeneous, smooth, or irregular. Echolucent plaque imply an increased risk of CV events as compared with more calcified plaque. The prognostic implication of plaque formation is beyond that of a merely elevated IMT [22], although the latter still gives additional predictive information [18].

Aneurysm definition

Because of their frequently bad prognosis [31] aneurysms should be detected during a carotid ultrasound assessment. All imaging modalities able to image arterial vessels are capable of detecting aneurysms; cerebral aneurysms, due to their anatomical position, are better imaged by magnetic resonance imaging (MRI). However, the more frequent findings of abdominal aortic aneurysms (AAA) (more than 95% being located infrarenally) or great arterial vessel aneurysms can be conveniently imaged by less elaborate modalities like ultrasound. An aneurysm is a localized, blood-filled dilatation of the vessel mostly caused by atherosclerosis. The neck of the circumscript dilatation is always wider than its top (aneurysm verum). At the aorta dilatation is defined as a diameter of ≥ 3 cm, and the risk of rupture increases exponentially with the diameter of the dilatation. The ADAM study recommended surgical repair for aneurysms with a diameter >5.5 cm in men and >4.5 cm in women [32]. However, interventional endovascular procedures (e.g. stent-assisted Dacron® prostheses) should always to be considered as they carry a lower mortality. Otherwise, serial measurements might be important because accelerated increases in diameter (>1 cm/year) imply a high risk of rupture. Of note, about 70% of patients with aneurysms die of CVDs like MI and stroke.

Screening for AAAs was recommended by the American College of Preventive Medicine for ever-smoking men aged 65–75 years [33], by the American College of Cardiology (ACC)/AHA for men aged 60 years with a sibling or offspring who had an AAA [4], and by the Surgeon Vascular Society and the Society for Vascular Medicine and Biology for all men aged 60–85 years and women aged 60–95 years with CV risk factors or all individuals aged 50 years with a family history of AAA [34].

Targeted imaging of plaques and therapeutic ultrasound

Contrast ultrasound used with molecular imaging by site-targeted modification of the contrast bubble shell provides the ability to interact with activated inflammatory cells or with activated vascular endothelium [35]. For this purpose a gas-filled microbubble with intercellular adhesion molecule-1 (ICAM-1) antibodies on the shell has been developed for endothelial cell binding. Because expression of ICAM-1 by endothelial cells is associated with early atherosclerosis this could be used for the diagnosis of pre-clinical atherosclerosis [36].

Recent studies in animals have shown a potential use for microbubbles in therapeutic applications such as drug delivery. The interaction of the bubbles with high-pressure ultrasound generates their destruction by exaggerated oscillation, releasing the transported drug [37]. Microbubble disruption, together with the effect of ultrasound on the endothelium [38], increases cell permeability, allowing the passage of bubbles and drugs to the interstitial space. The same mechanism is used for gene delivery: genes bound to microbubbles can be carried to the target tissue without being digested [36], and once they reach it they are released by destruction of the bubbles by a high-mechanical-index ultrasound pulse.

Ultrasound contrast agents have also been used in the treatment of thrombosis in the presence or absence of fibrinolytic therapy [39]. A positive correlation between the use of ultrasound and the rate of thrombolysis was found in most, but not all, the studies. High-power, low-frequency ultrasound was associated with more effective clot lysis [40].

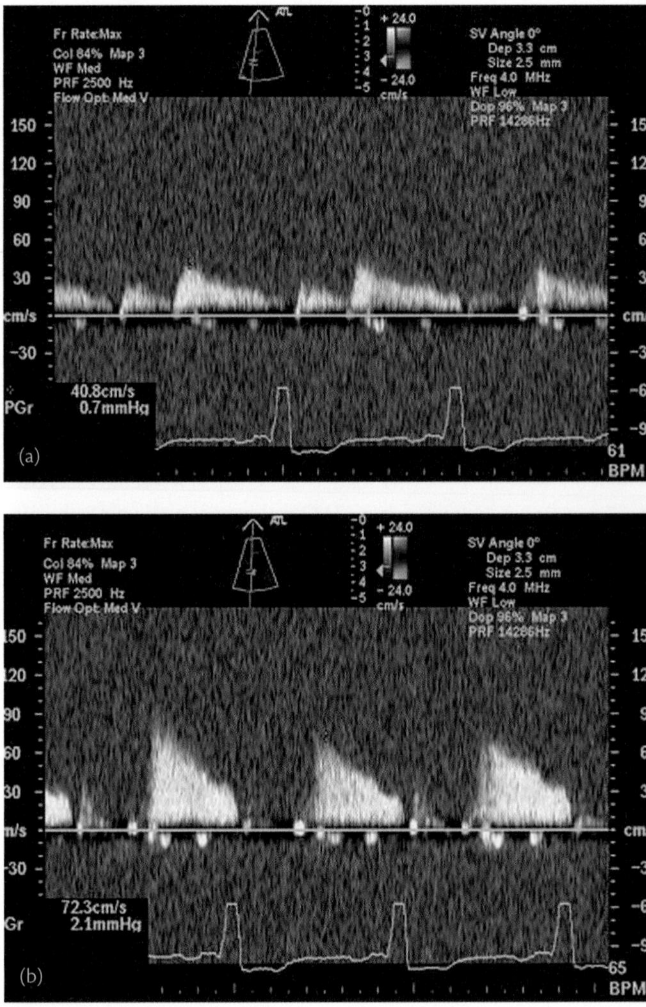

Fig. 6.3 Assessment of coronary flow by pulsed Doppler ultrasound showing peak diastolic flow velocities before (a) and after (b) administration of dipyridamole.

Echocardiography including tissue Doppler techniques

Coronary artery imaging

Transthoracic echocardiography (TTE)

The development of ultrasound technology, mainly second-harmonic imaging and the use of contrast agents, now allows direct visualization of epicardial coronary arteries by 2D TTE [41]. Although imaging of coronary arteries is technically demanding [37], blood flow in the left anterior descending coronary artery (LAD) can be assessed in most patients [37,42,43], while the posterior descending coronary artery can be visualized in 43 to 81% of patients [44–46] and the left circumflex coronary artery (CX) in 38% of patients [47]. Scanning of coronary arteries requires higher probe delivery frequencies than when studying apical segments; this is particularly the case for distal LAD imaging, due to its higher resolution. However, the better penetration of lower-frequency transducers is desirable, despite the lower resolution, for colour and pulsed Doppler examinations and for visualization of the other coronary arteries. In asymptomatic patients, LAD wall thickness and external diameter were observed as potential markers of subclinical coronary atherosclerosis [48]. Flow in coronary arteries is typically forward and biphasic with dome-like systolic and diastolic components; the latter predominates and in normal coronary circulation is principally responsible for coronary flow due to the high intramural pressure during systole.

Coronary artery flow velocity reserve (CFR) is the ratio between the peak diastolic flow velocity during maximal vasodilation (achieved with adenosine, dipyridamole, or physiological stress) and the basal diastolic flow velocity [46] (➲ Fig. 6.3). This ratio is not only influenced by the diameter of epicardial coronary arteries but also by the total cross-sectional area of the coronary resistance vessels, which is proportional to the microcirculatory bed. The maximum vasodilatation capacity depends on the basal tone of epicardial and microcirculatory arteries. In many disorders, for example hypertension, left ventricular (LV) hypertrophy, valvular diseases, and CAD, progressive vasodilatation may occur to maintain the stability of the coronary perfusion pressure. In these patients, CFR will be reduced because their ability to vasodilate after exercise or pharmacological stimulus is diminished. Although there is no consensus, it has been suggested that CFR values less than 2 indicate an altered CFR [47]. TTE has been applied to estimate the functional severity of intermediate coronary stenosis, reserving intervention for those patients with a reduced CFR [49], for the follow-up of percutaneous coronary interventions (PCIs) [50,51], and for the assessment of coronary recanalization in acute MI [52].

Calcification of cardiac structures

Identification of calcium deposits at the aortic valve (➲ Fig. 6.4) and/or the mitral apparatus (annulus, leaflets, papillary muscles) or a relevant thickening of ascending aorta walls, as detected by conventional TTE, was associated with higher CV morbidity and mortality rates in several prospective studies [53–55]. Furthermore, valvular calcifications are frequently detected in people with significant coronary atherosclerosis and carotid plaques,

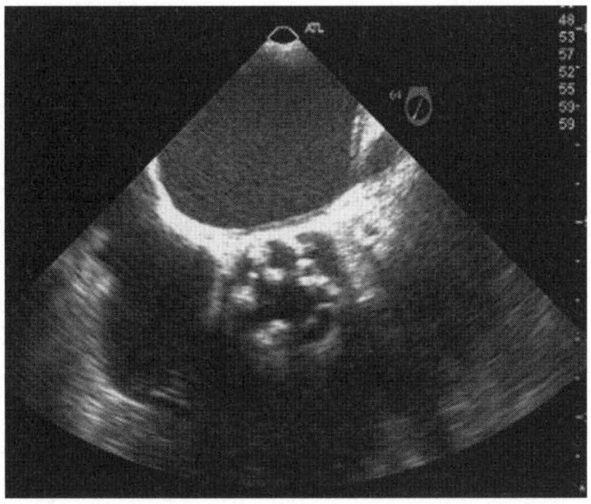

Fig. 6.4 Trans-oesophageal echocardiogram showing severe aortic valve calcification.

suggesting a similar pathogenic process [55,56]. Even though image acquisition is relatively simple and rapid, the approach is still qualitative or semi-quantitative. Although no data on any improvement in reclassification are currently available for large intermediate-risk populations, an echocardiographic calcium score (ECS) or calcification score index (CSI) assessed by TTE has been demonstrated to correlate with the FRS, the Duke score, and the LV mass index providing a simple, radiation-free index of cardiovascular disease (CVD) in patients with known or suspected CAD [56]. In a study by Nucifora et al. [55] ECS was associated with coronary calcium score > 400 [odds ratio (OR) 3.6; 95% confidence interval (CI) 2.4–5.5; $p < 0.001$]. Similarly, only ECS (OR 1.8; 95% CI 1.4–2.4; $p < 0.001$) and pre-test likelihood of CAD (OR 1.7; 95% CI 1.0–2.8; $p = 0.04$) were associated with obstructive CAD. After ROC curve analysis, ECS > 3 had the highest sensitivity and specificity for identification of patients with severe coronary artery calcification (87% for both) and obstructive CAD (74% and 82%; respectively) (AUC = 0.90; 95% CI 0.84–0.95; SEE = 0.03%; $p < 0.001$). The ability of ECS to predict obstructive CAD was similar to that of the coronary artery calcium (CAC) score obtained by electron beam computed tomography (AUC = 0.85; 95% CI 0.78–0.90; SEE = 0.03%; $p < 0.001$). In the cohort of 2723 American Indians participating in the Strong Heart Study, mitral annular calcification (MAC) but not aortic valve sclerosis was related to an increased incidence of stroke [risk ratio (RR) = 3.12; 95% CI 1.77–5.25], even after adjustment for clinical variables and C-reactive protein and fibrinogen (HR = 2.42; 95% CI 1.39–4.21) or the echocardiographic covariates left ventricular hypertrophy (LVH) and left atrial (LA) enlargement (HR = 1.89; 95% CI 1.04–3.41).

Subtle left ventricular dysfunction

Tissue Doppler imaging, strain and strain rate imaging, and speckle tracking

Strain (St) and strain rate (SR) are relatively new parameters for evaluating myocardial deformation with a large potential for clinical application. While St measures the longitudinal, radial, and circumferential deformation of myocardial tissue, reflecting the regional ejection fraction (EF), SR reflects the change in strain with respect to time, which is a parameter related to contractility. St and SR can both be measured using tissue Doppler, a mode that measures simultaneous myocardial velocities at different points, detecting wall motion abnormalities (WMA) more objectively and earlier than by conventional TTE (➲ Fig. 6.5). The second technique for assessing St and SR is speckle tracking, based on the search for ultrasound reflectors ('speckles') in the myocardium, which can be tracked frame by frame during the cardiac cycle. This technique allows St, SR, tissue velocity, and LV rotation to be assessed without the inconvenience of alignment sensitivity needed for tissue Doppler. Some studies report that St imaging is more sensitive than wall motion examination for detecting acute ischaemia [57]. Experimental work has shown that the most sensitive and specific parameters for detecting the presence of acute myocardial ischaemia are a reduction in SR (mainly longitudinal deformation), time to relaxation, and post-systolic thickening, defined as myocardial contraction after aortic valve closure [58]. The clinical applications of SR imaging are myocardial viability,

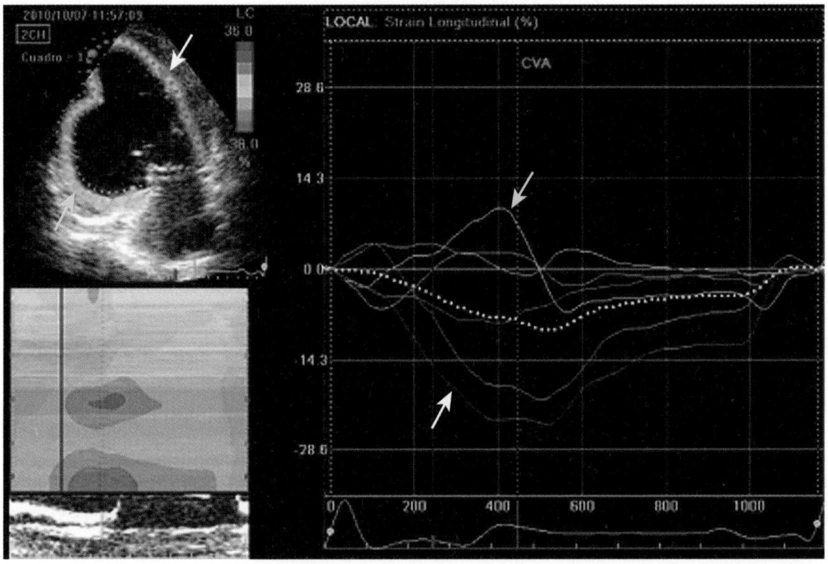

Fig. 6.5 A postero-inferior aneurysm evaluated by strain rate technique. Longitudinal strain is negative in the apical and anterior segments (white arrow) showing normal systolic contraction, while the inferior and posterior segments exhibit positive longitudinal strain (yellow arrow) due to the dyssynergic movement of the aneurysmatic area.

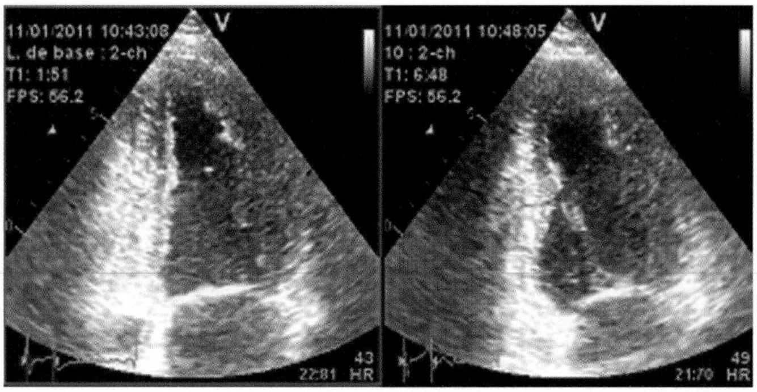

Fig. 6.6 Stress echocardiography protocol showing inferior hypokinesis after dobutamine infusion.

ventricular dyssynchrony, and the early detection of subclinical LV dysfunction. More work is still needed to determine the real value of this imaging tool.

Trans-oesophageal echocardiography (TEE)

The use of TEE for coronary artery imaging can provide information about coronary artery anomalies and proximal coronary disease [mainly the LAD and left main coronary artery (LMCA)] and measure flow reserve. Identification of LMCA stenosis by Doppler colour is feasible due to its parallel position with respect to the echo beam. By adjusting appropriate Nyquist limits to avoid areas of aliasing flow with no stenosis, the sensitivity and specificity of the technique for the diagnosis of significant CAD have reached 100% in some studies. The unfavourable position for Doppler pulse examination of the CX and right coronary artery (RCA) makes it difficult to apply and evaluate this technique [59]. A limitation of TEE is its evaluation of proximal segments, where the flow can be perfectly normal despite the presence of a distal stenosis; this is one of the reasons for the abandonment of TEE in the study of CFR [47].

Stress echocardiography

Stress echocardiography is an easy technique based on the indirect detection of myocardial ischaemia by visually assessing provoked WMA. The stress needed to produce ischaemia in these areas with a lower CFR can be achieved by physical exertion or pharmacological agents such as dobutamine or dipyridamole. Exercise stress (either a bike or treadmill) is preferred because of its lower rate of complications and a better physiological profile. The high sensitivity, specificity [60], and negative predictive value for ischaemia [61] of stress echocardiography (80–85, 85, and 98%, respectively) make it a valuable test for the detection of myocardial ischaemia (➲ Fig. 6.6), especially in patients with an intermediate pre-test probability of CAD. In preventive settings the very high negative predictive value may be important for excluding disease and predicting the uneventful survival rate (events being even higher in unexamined controls obtained from life tables) [62], which in most studies is < 1% per year.

Myocardial contrast echocardiography

Myocardial contrast echocardiography (MCE) is a valuable tool for assessing the presence of CAD due to the physical properties of contrast agents. The signal enhancement produced by this technique is caused by oscillation of contrast microbubbles interacting with ultrasound. Bubble vibration amplifies echo-producing signals at multiples of their frequency, termed harmonics [63], resulting in an increased blood–tissue interface. LV cavity opacification allows a better definition of endocardial borders thus increasing the accuracy of detection of segmentary contractility defects. Other applications of MCE include perfusion studies that show filling defects in LV walls in the presence of microcirculation or epicardial disease. The combined use of both these techniques during stress testing has demonstrated to increase true-positive test results by >50% compared with isolated WMA criteria [64].

Multi-detector computed tomography

Computed tomography (CT) imaging has made substantial technical progress in recent years. Wide detector coverage and improved spatial and temporal resolution as well as the ability to synchronize image acquisition or image reconstruction with the patient's electrocardiogram (ECG) has made it possible to utilize multi-detector CT (MDCT) for cardiac imaging. One of the most prominent applications has been coronary artery imaging. Coronary arteries can be depicted without contrast injection in order to identify and quantify coronary calcification, or the coronary arteries can be visualized after intravenous injection of contrast agent in order to perform 'coronary CT angiography' (CTA).

Coronary artery calcium scoring

With the exception of patients in renal failure, CAC is exclusively present in the context of atherosclerosis and it reflects a rough estimate of the total atherosclerotic burden [65]. The presence of CAC is usually assumed if a density exceeding 130 HU is found in non-enhanced CT images of the coronary arteries (➲ Fig. 6.7). The most frequently used method for quantification is the 'Agatston score', which is found by measuring the area and peak density of calcified plaque. Alternative measures of CAC exist, such as the calcified volume or the calcium mass, but since the majority of scientific data have been generated with the Agatston score it remains the most frequently used tool for quantification and reporting.

In the general population, CAC scores increase with age, and on average are higher in men than women [66]. Age- and gender-specific percentiles exist for various populations [66–68]. Nomograms permit the calculation of age- and gender-referenced percentiles as well as biological age (adopted from the Nixdorf recall study calculator <http://www.uk-essen.de/recall-studie/>). Since the presence and amount of CAC is tied to the presence and amount of coronary atherosclerotic plaque, and CAD events are typically caused by plaque rupture and erosion, it is fair to assume that coronary calcification is related to an individual's risk for death and coronary events. In asymptomatic individuals the absence of CAC is associated with a very low (<1% per year) risk of major CV events over the next 3 to 5 years, whereas an up to 11-fold increase in relative risk of major cardiac events has been reported in asymptomatic subjects with extensive coronary calcification

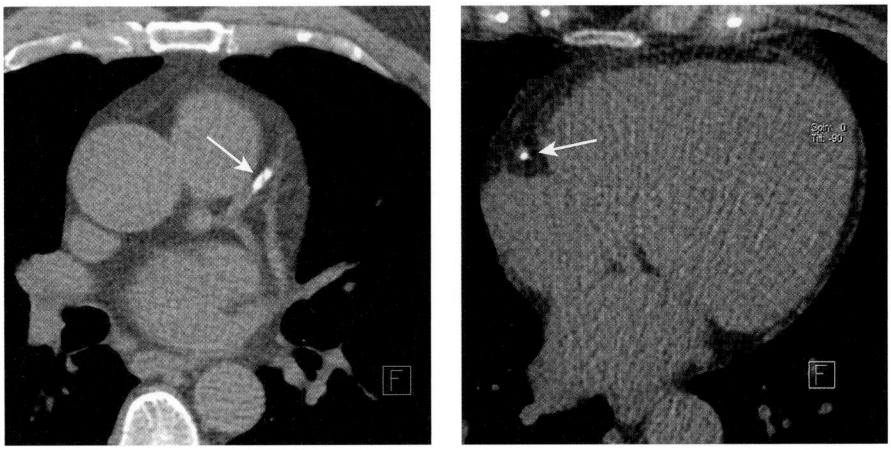

Fig. 6.7 Detection of coronary calcium in non-enhanced cardiac CT. Calcium in the left anterior descending coronary artery (left image, arrow), and in the right coronary artery (right image, arrow).

[69–73]. Two of the most prominent prospective large-scale trials which have convincingly demonstrated that measurement of CAC by CT has incremental prognostic information beyond assessment of traditional risk factors are the Nixdorf recall study [73] and the MESA trial [67,69] (➲ Table 6.4). Both have convincingly demonstrated that the presence of certain amount of CAC will reclassify individuals who seem to be at low or intermediate risk based on traditional risk factors to a high-risk category, and that this may mandate more intense modification of risk factors. Furthermore, several studies were able to demonstrate that CAC allows better risk stratification than other novel markers of risk, such as C-reactive protein [74] or IMT [75].

CAC increases progressively over time [76]. The rate of progression is correlated with non-coronary atherosclerosis [77], is related to cardiovascular risk factors [78], and shows a genetic association [79]. One study has observed a higher CAD event rate in individuals who displayed more rapid progression of CAC [80]. A number of trials have evaluated the influence of lipid-lowering therapy on the progression of CAC but have reported conflicting results [81–87]. Since, in addition, interscan variability is high, especially for low scores, no sufficiently strong data support the clinical use of repeated CAC scans.

Table 6.4 Risk of coronary events (adjusted for risk factors) that was associated with an increasing 'Agatston score' (a measure of the amount of calcium) in a population sample of 6722 individuals without coronary artery disease at study entry, followed for a mean period of 3.8 years [5]

Agatston score	Hazard ratio (major coronary events)	Number of individuals	
		With events	Total
0	1	8	3409
1–100	3.89	25	1728
101–300	7.08	24	752
≥ 301	6.84	32	833

Data from McClelland RL, Chung H, Detrano R, Post W, Kronmal RA. Distribution of coronary artery calcium by race, gender, and age. Results from the Multi-Ethnic Study of Atherosclerosis (MESA). *Circulation* 2006; **113**: 30–7 and Detrano R, Guerci AD, Carr JJ, Bild DE, Burke G, Folsom AR, Liu K, Shea S, Szklo M, Bluemke DA, O'Leary DH, Tracy R, Watson K, Wong ND, Kronmal RA. Coronary calcium as a predictor of coronary events in four racial or ethnic groups. *N Engl J Med* 2008; **358**: 1336–45.

In summary, the predictive value of CAC for the occurrence of future CVD events in asymptomatic individuals is widely accepted [88–91]. Current European guidelines on CVD prevention state that 'computed tomography for coronary calcium should be considered for cardiovascular risk assessment in asymptomatic adults at moderate risk' and provide it with a class IIa recommendation [1]. In clinical practice it is not quite clear which patients or individuals will profit from having a CAC scan performed. Most recommendations support a potential role for assessment of CAC in further risk stratification if patients have an intermediate Framingham or PROCAM risk:

> ... clinical decision-making could potentially be altered by coronary artery calcium measurement in patients initially judged to be at intermediate risk (10% to 20% in 10 years). The accumulating evidence suggests that asymptomatic individuals with an intermediate Framingham Risk Score may be reasonable candidates for ... testing using coronary artery calcium as a potential means of modifying risk prediction and altering therapy. [89]

In patients at high or very low risk it is currently assumed that CAC imaging will not be clinically reasonable since the result is unlikely to influence treatment decisions:

> ... the current literature on coronary artery calcium does not provide support for the concept that high-risk asymptomatic individuals can safely be excluded from medical therapy for coronary heart disease even if [the] coronary artery calcium score is 0. [20]

Unselected 'screening' or patient self-referral is uniformly not recommended [89–91].

Coronary CT angiography

After injection of contrast agent, CT imaging allows visualization of the coronary artery lumen ('coronary CT angiography', CTA). The image quality of CTA depends on many factors, but in selected patients high accuracy for stenosis detection can be achieved (➲ Fig. 6.8). In addition, CTA allows the detection of both calcified and also non-calcified plaque components (➲ Fig. 6.9). With some limitations, and under the prerequisite of excellent image quality, plaque quantification and characterization is possible. It has recently been shown that some characteristics determined by CT in coronary atherosclerotic plaques, such as positive remodelling and low CT attenuation of the atherosclerotic material, are

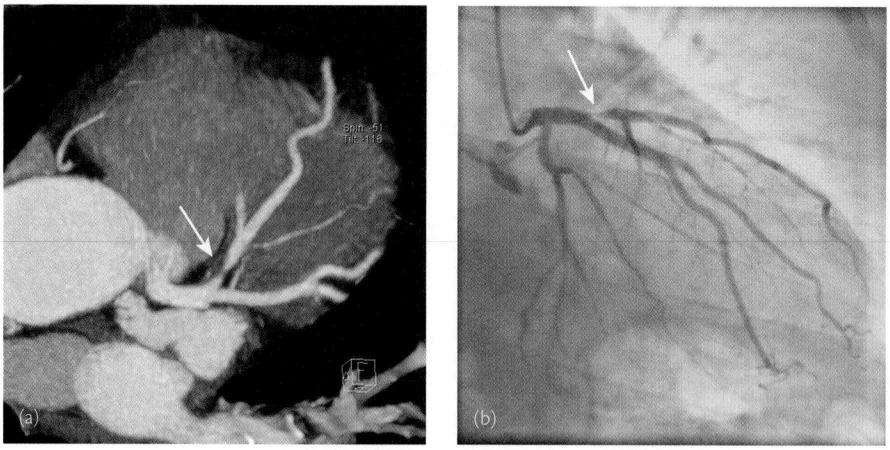

Fig. 6.8 Coronary CT angiography permits the identification of coronary artery stenosis. Here, a stenosis is present at the ostium of the left anterior descending coronary artery. Coronary CT angiography (a) demonstrates not only the lumen reduction but also the atherosclerotic material of the plaque that causes the stenosis, which is mainly non-calcified (arrow). The stenosis is confirmed by invasive coronary angiography (b, arrow).

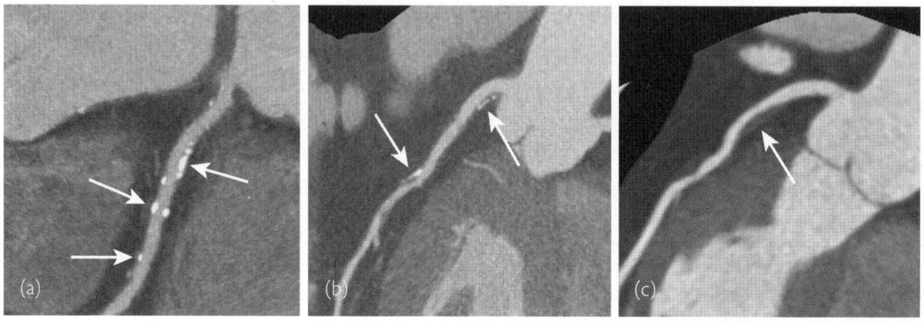

Fig. 6.9 Detection of non-obstructive coronary atherosclerotic plaque in contrast-enhanced coronary CT angiography: (a) completely calcified plaque, (b) partly calcified plaque; (c) completely non-calcified plaque.

associated with the occurrence of future acute coronary syndromes [92] (➲ Table 6.5). Recently, several studies and data based on large registries have been able to demonstrate a prognostic value of atherosclerotic lesions detected by CTA in both symptomatic and asymptomatic individuals. Min et al. [93] demonstrated increased overall mortality in patients with atherosclerotic lesions in more than five coronary artery segments while Ostrom et al. [94] demonstrated an increased mortality in patients with non-obstructive lesions in all three coronary arteries, or in patients who had obstructive lesions. A recently published analysis of a registry including more than 23 000 patients confirmed the prognostic value of CTA, when the presence of coronary stenoses but also the presence of non-obstructive plaque was associated with an increased risk of mortality [95]. However, the HR for non-obstructive plaque was relatively low (HR = 1.6; 95% CI 1.2–2.2). Another analysis of the same registry was unable to demonstrate for this mostly symptomatic patient group an incremental prognostic value of contrast-enhanced CTA over coronary calcium measurements, which can be performed without contrast and at a substantially lower radiation exposure [96]. Therefore, CTA, while a useful clinical tool for ruling out coronary artery stenosis in selected individuals with stable or acute chest pain [91,97], is currently not recommended for risk assessment purposes in asymptomatic individuals [91].

Table 6.5 Results of a prospective study by Motoyama et al. [92]. In this study 1059 patients were followed for a mean period of 27 months after a clinically indicated coronary CT angiogram. Coronary atherosclerotic plaques were identified and evaluated with regard to the presence of positive remodelling and low CT attenuation (attenuation values < 30 HU). The rate of acute coronary syndromes (ACS) during follow-up was substantially higher in patients with plaques that demonstrated positive remodelling and low CT attenuation than in patients with other types of plaque or without plaque

Finding at baseline	Total number of patients	ACS during follow-up	No ACS during follow-up
Plaques with positive remodelling *and* CT attenuation < 30 HU	45	10 (22%)	35 (78%)
Plaques with positive remodelling *or* CT attenuation < 30 HU	27	1 (4%)	26 (96%)
Plaques with *neither* positive remodelling *nor* CT attenuation < 30 HU	822	4 (0.5%)	816 (99%)
No plaque	167	0 (0%)	167 (100%)

Data from Motoyama S, Sarai M, Harigaya H, Anno H, Inoue K, Hara T, Naruse H, Ishii J, Hishida H, Wong ND, Virmani R, Kondo T, Ozaki Y, Narula J. Computed tomographic angiography characteristics of atherosclerotic plaques subsequently resulting in acute coronary syndrome. *J Am Coll Cardiol* 2009; **54**: 49–57.

Magnetic resonance imaging

Cardiac magnetic resonance imaging (CMR) is a technique that is sufficiently accurate and versatile to replicate complex (patho-) physiology in a variety of CV conditions (➲ Fig. 6.10). As a non-invasive, radiation-free imaging modality with high diagnostic yield it is well suited for investigating the presence of subclinical disease in an asymptomatic population. Faster imaging and increased availability of equipment and local expertise now allow

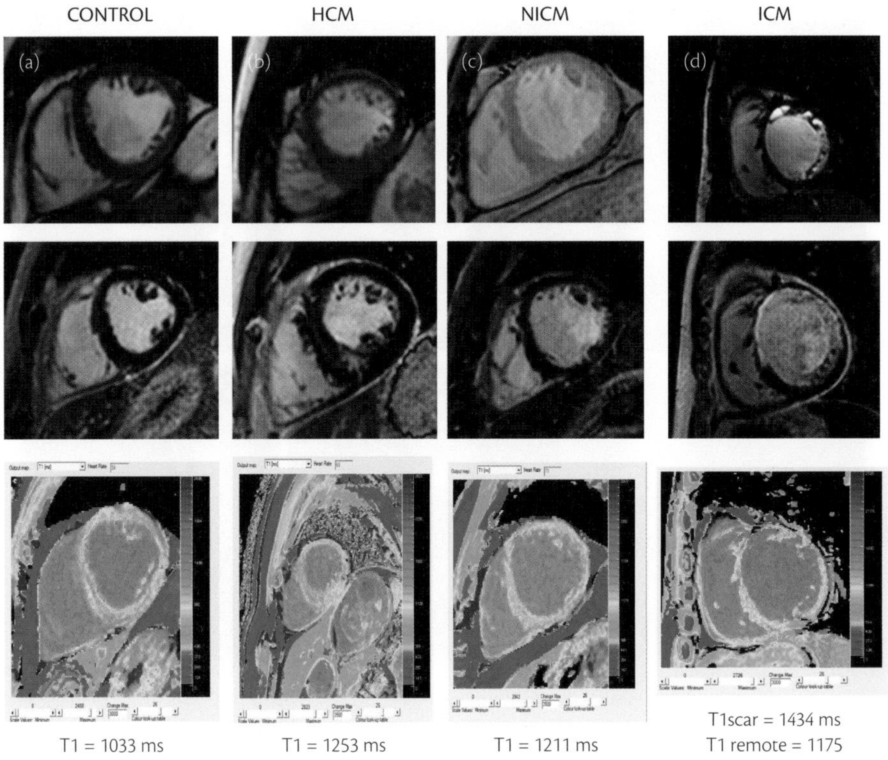

Fig. 6.10 Cardiomyopathy screening: examples of a healthy control (A), a patient with hypertrophic cardiomyopathy (B), a patient with idiopathic non-ischaemic (C) and ischaemic dilative cardiomyopathy (D). Upper panel: cine imaging reveals the structure and function and gives information about regional wall motion abnormalities. Middle panel: late gadolinium enhancement provides information on regional fibrosis. Lower panel: T_1 mapping as an increasingly promising tool to differentiate normal from abnormal myocardium and examples of native T_1 imaging in the corresponding cases.

for the use of this modality early in the diagnostic cascade. High costs are commonly offset by the reduced need for other imaging to reach the diagnosis [98]. Despite its obvious potential, evidence that CMR adds to patients' management in subclinical disease and primary prevention remains scarce. As the number of overall clinical indications is increasing, the evolving role of CMR is likely to gain importance by virtue of exclusion of disease and within the growing area of secondary prevention.

Coronary arteries

CMR is able to image the proximal course of the coronary arteries and exclude the presence of significant proximal CAD [99]. Clearly, CMR images of the coronary arteries are less crisp and detailed than those obtained with coronary artery imaging using modern multidetector CT scanners [100]. As both modalities suffer from artefacts due to calcifications in significant CAD (drop-out artefacts in CMR, white spillage artefacts in CTA), both are relatively unreliable for determining the significance of a coronary stenosis without additional perfusion imaging. Visualization of the proximal coronary arteries with CMR is also helpful for excluding an abnormal course [101].

Left and right ventricular volumes and function

Owing to its high accuracy, interstudy reproducibility, and low inter- and intra-observer variability CMR is the established reference standard for the assessment of cardiac volumes and function, and also LV mass [102]. This allows CMR to detect relatively small changes in volume and mass. Independent of imaging windows and planes, CMR is also invaluable in assessment of the right ventricle [103]. Because it depicts the right ventricular free wall it is able to provide information about global as well as regional function.

Myocardial ischaemia

Adenosine stress perfusion imaging by CMR is a widely used application and has low procedural risk [104]. It is probably the most accurate non-invasive technique in the current clinical routine for ruling out myocardial ischaemia and has been shown to be superior to single-photon emission computed tomography (SPECT) in a single-centre setting and not inferior to SPECT in a multicentre setting [105,106]. Similarly, dobutamine-stress magnetic resonance imaging (DSMRI), with or without stress perfusion, is also highly sensitive (like dobutamine stress echocardiography; DSE) [107]. However, as it has a higher procedural risk and the required expertise is less widely available it is used somewhat less frequently than DSE.

Myocardial tissue characterization and viability

Late gadolinium enhancement (LGE) marks an enlarged distribution volume and corresponds to histological substrates such as oedema or fibrosis [108]. Commonly called 'scar imaging', it is used for visualization of the post-infarct myocardial scar and prediction of recovery with revascularization [109]. It also identifies oedema and the area at risk in acute infarct and in the diffuse inflammation of myocarditis [110].

Great vessels and plaque composition

CMR is excellently suited for investigating the anatomical relations between vessel conduits and the chambers of the heart, to assess dimensions and blood flow within the great vessels. In addition,

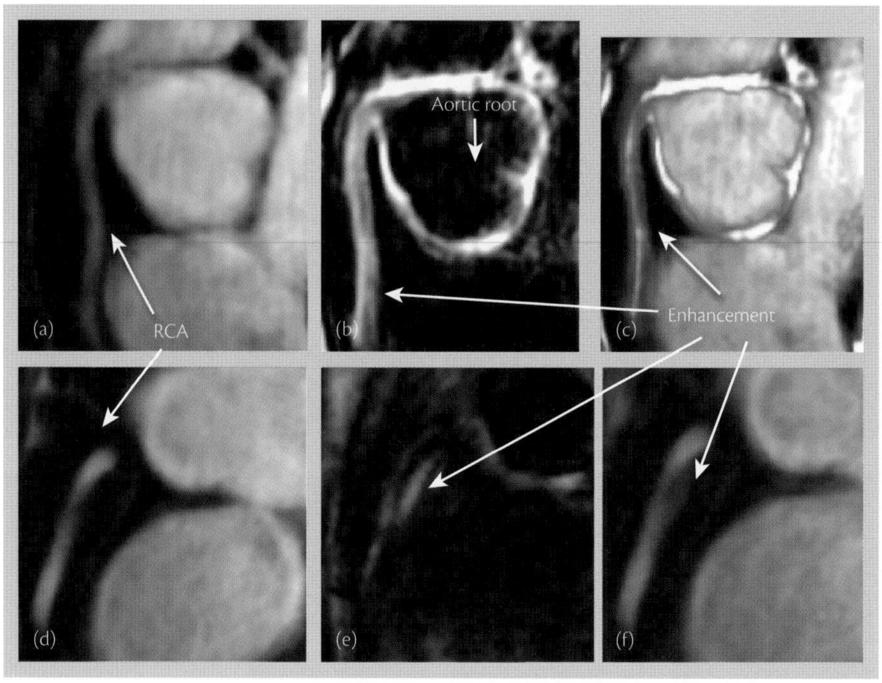

Fig. 6.11 Coronary enhancement imaging. Representative images of the right coronary artery (RCA) from a 38-year-old woman with systemic lupus erythematosus (A–C) and from an age/gender-matched healthy subject (D–F).
(A), (D) CMR coronary angiography with luminogram is used to measure the vessel length and lumen diameter.
(B), (E) Inversion recovery contrast-enhanced images with black-blood pre-pulse reveals the enhancement within the aortic and coronary vessel walls.
(C), (F) fused images of both coronary angiography and inversion-recovery contrast-enhanced images to depict the enhancement (purple) in relation to the vessel lumen (bright signal).

multicontrast applications can be used to assess atherosclerotic burden in carotid arteries and the abdominal aorta [111–113]. Flow and cine imaging with high temporal resolution can yield accurate information about aortic stiffness, by central aortic pulse wave velocity and distensibility, respectively [114,115]. The use of sophisticated sequences and fusion capabilities enables direct pathoanatomical imaging of active atherosclerosis of the vessels (➲ Fig. 6.11).

MRI also discriminates the composition of carotid plaque [116] by detection of the lipid core, carotid wall thickening, and intraplaque haemorrhage. Intraplaque haemorrhage is associated with hypertension and current smoking, while the presence of a lipid core is related to hypercholesterolaemia [117]. Measurement of the lipid core can be used to monitor plaque regression with antilipid therapy [118]. In 191 diabetic patients with moderate to high-grade carotid artery stenosis, there was a 92% concordance between MRI and 36 specimens obtained during carotid endarterectomy, irrespective of the degree of stenosis [119].

More recent developments include imaging of plaques with MR contrast agents, such as gadolinium chelates [120] or superparamagnetic iron oxide nanoparticles to mark inflammation [121]. In combination with positron emission tomography (PET), new molecular tracers have been developed to better understand the different phases of plaque development and vulnerability [122].

Nuclear/molecular imaging

CV molecular imaging promises to become a key diagnostic modality in CV medicine by visualizing specific targets and pathways that precede or underlie changes in morphology, physiology, and function. For earlier detection of disease, molecular imaging techniques are currently primarily focused on two areas: the vulnerable plaque, which precedes MI, and LV remodelling, which precedes heart failure.

Clinical observations that acute coronary events often result from rupture of atherosclerotic plaques at sites with no or minor luminal narrowing have stimulated the search for techniques to identify vulnerable, rupture-prone lesions [123]. Those may show characteristic morphological features, but they may still differ in their biology and their activity, which ultimately leads to rupture. Molecular-targeted approaches aim at identifying plaque inflammation, apoptosis, extracellular matrix activation, or platelet binding. Clinically, the most advanced approach is the use of the glucose analogue ^{18}F-fluorodeoxyglucose (FDG) and PET in order to identify elevated glucose metabolism in activated monocytes of vulnerable atherosclerotic lesions. This technique is based on a readily available FDA-approved tracer and has been validated against histology [124]. It has been shown to be reproducible [125], appears to be sensitive to therapy-induced changes (➲ Fig. 6.12), and has recently been used as an end-point in randomized trials [122].

There are several alternative approaches [126], many at the preclinical or very early clinical level, suggesting that the field remains a work in progress. Challenges related to the best targeting approach, to translation of animal model results to the clinical setting, to adequate imaging methodology for visualization of coronary artery biology, and to a suitable target patient population need to be overcome. The final goal of these efforts is improved clinical risk assessment through *in vivo* assessment of vascular biology.

Fundoscopy

There is evidence that microangiographic abnormalities of the retina correlate with CV risk factors in the metabolic syndrome [127] and age and arterial hypertension [128]. The fundus carries

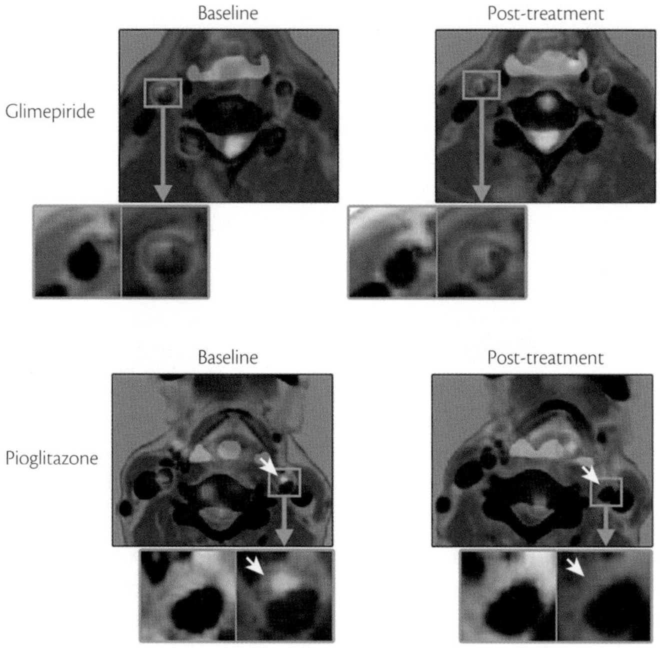

Fig. 6.12 Effects of treatment with pioglitazone and glimepiride on ^{18}F-fluorodeoxyglucose (FDG) uptake in atherosclerotic plaques. Representative FDG positron emission tomography/computed tomography with contrast media images (left) at baseline and (right) after 4-months' treatment with pioglitazone or glimepiride. Note the reduction in FDG uptake in the atherosclerotic plaque with pioglitazone treatment (arrows). Reprinted from Mizoguchi, et al. *JACC Cardiovasc Imaging* 2011; **4**: 1110–18, with permission from Elsevier.

predictive information not only for stroke [129,130] but also MI [131]. Pre-clinical findings are narrowing of the focal retinal arterioles or/and generalized changes to the retinal arterioles measured as arteriovenous ratio (AV ratio). There are age-referenced nomograms for AV ratios. Scanning laser Doppler flowmetry enables assessment of the wall-to-lumen ratio, thereby enabling functional imaging like flow-mediated dilatation (FMD) of the brachial artery [see the subsection 'Flow-mediated dilatation (FMD) (endothelial dysfunction)'] [132]. The availability of standard fundus cameras means that digital photography of the retina without mydriasis is possible for telemedical evaluation, enabling integration in CV pathways without the need for an attending ophthalmologist at assessing clinics and practices.

Invasive modalities (prevention research)

Invasive approaches are not relevant to practical preventive settings because pre-clinical examinations in asymptomatic individuals will not justify modalities that carry a certain risk. Thus, in the field of preventive cardiology these approaches are exclusively used in research programmes. However, there are potential applications for pathophysiological investigations (e.g. vulnerable plaque, vessel remodelling), series for controlling preventive interventions [e.g. the effects of statins on atheroma burden investigated by intravascular ultrasound (IVUS)], or the validation of non-invasive modalities (e.g. validation of the findings of multidetector CT by IVUS).

Intravascular ultrasound/virtual histology/ elastography

IVUS is an invasive imaging modality using a specially designed catheter with a miniaturized ultrasound probe attached to its distal end that is introduced to the coronary arteries. Due to a very short scanning distance the coronary wall is imaged with very high-frequency transducers (20–40 MHz) enabling high resolution. Thus, it has excellent determination and quantification of atheromatous plaques at the epicardial coronary artery as well as the vessel remodelling process known as the Glagov effect [133]. As this is not possible with conventional coronary angiography, IVUS is a valuable complementary method in interventional cardiology but also in more preventive areas. As well as quantitative plaque size, qualitative plaque composition may also be assessed, as may the effects of medications that interfere with the pathophysiological process of atherogenesis, such as statins. The ASTEROID trial [134] used IVUS to demonstrate the potential for atheroma regression induced by high-dose statins.

Methods to estimate plaque vulnerability rather than just morphology are also available. Based on the success of IVUS, various tools have been proposed to determine the composition of atheroma. One modality uses radiofrequency backscatter spectral analysis, also known as virtual histology, to provide information of plaque composition; the generated IVUS signals are visualized in colour-coded maps overlaying traditional grey-scale IVUS [135]. Information about compliance can also be obtained using ultrasonic tissue characterization as a second modality that depicts the lumen perimeter as colour-coded congruent lines. Those 'palpograms' are able to identify lesions with different elasticities independently of echogenicity contrast [136].

Optical coherence tomography

Optical coherence tomography (OCT) is an optical signal acquisition and processing method that captures micrometre-resolution (700–900 nm) three-dimensional images from optical scattering media like the coronary vessel wall using near-infrared light [137]. Coronary arteries can then be examined in order to detect vulnerable lipid-rich plaques that are differentiated from plaque erosions as well as calcified nodules [138]. Nanoparticles are now being used to improve the labelling of vascular adhesion molecules such as vascular cell adhesion molecule-1 (VCAM-1) [139]. In general, this method is still only used for research purposes.

Thermography

Thermal wires are able to measure the sites of maximum temperature with IVUS. The inflammatory process in vulnerable plaques may thus be detected. In fact, temperature measurements of coronary plaques enable accurate localization of the culprit lesion in patients with acute MI [140]. However, this method is still also used for research.

Functional testing

Flow-mediated dilatation (endothelial dysfunction)

Physiological functions of the vascular endothelium

The endothelium maintains vascular homeostasis via multiple complex interactions with cells in the vessel wall and lumen. It regulates vascular tone by balancing the production of vasodilators, most importantly nitric oxide (NO) but also prostaglandins and endothelium-derived hyperpolarizing factor, and constrictors, including endothelin-1. Endothelium-derived NO also participates in systemic physiological functions of the endothelium, such as the control of vascular tone and blood clotting. Furthermore, the endothelium controls blood fluidity and coagulation through the production of factors that regulate platelet activity, the clotting cascade, and the fibrinolytic system. Finally, the endothelium has the capacity to produce cytokines and adhesion molecules that regulate and direct inflammatory and regenerative processes. Thereby the endothelium modulates the structure and physicomechanical properties of the vessel walls over time.

Arterial endothelial function as a 'barometer' of cardiovascular health

In the presence of risk factors for CVD, together with a genetic disposition and environmental factors, the arterial endothelium loses its normal regulatory function for vessel wall homeostasis—a concept called 'endothelial dysfunction' [141]. The development and clinical manifestations of atherosclerosis include stable and unstable angina, acute MI, claudication, and stroke. These outcomes correlate with and are preceded by a loss of endothelial control of vascular tone, thrombosis, and the composition of the vascular wall. The severity of endothelial dysfunction relates to a patient's risk of experiencing an initial or recurrent CV event [142,143].

Both traditional and novel CV risk factors initiate a chronic inflammatory process that is accompanied by a loss of vasodilator and antithrombotic factors and an increase in vasoconstrictor and pro-thrombotic factors. Risk factors as diverse as smoking (active and passive), ageing, hypercholesterolaemia, hypertension, hyperglycaemia, and a family history of premature atherosclerotic disease are all associated with attenuation or loss of endothelium-dependent vasodilation in both adults and children. More recently recognized risk factors such as obesity, elevated C-reactive protein, postprandial state, hyperhomocysteinaemia, and chronic systemic infection are also associated with endothelial dysfunction. A growing number of interventions known to decrease CV risk, including a diet rich in fruits and vegetables, exercise, smoking cessation, weight reduction, or medication with ACE inhibitors and statin administration, will also improve endothelial function. Therefore, endothelial function is viewed as a 'barometer' for CV health that can be used for the evaluation of new therapeutic strategies.

Using FMD as a non-invasive tool to assess endothelial function in humans

While atherosclerosis is associated with a broad alteration in endothelial phenotype, assessment of the endothelium-dependent vasodilator function of peripheral arteries has emerged as an accessible indicator of endothelial health. In particular, stimuli that increase production of endothelium-derived NO have proven useful in assessing endothelium-dependent vasodilation in humans. Such stimuli include increased shear stress resulting from increased blood flow and receptor-dependent agonists, such as acetylcholine, bradykinin, or substance P. In healthy individuals, the endothelium responds to these stimuli by releasing vasodilator factors, particularly NO. Early studies demonstrated that patients with angiographically proven CAD display impaired FMD and a vasoconstrictor response to acetylcholine rather than the normal vasodilator response, probably reflecting loss of NO and unopposed constrictor effects of acetylcholine on vascular smooth muscle. Correlations exist between the endothelial function of peripheral and coronary arteries. Due to the ready accessibility of the brachial artery there has been considerable interest in non-invasive examination of endothelium-dependent FMD of the peripheral arteries using vascular ultrasound.

Prognostic value of FMD

A total of 23 studies including 14 753 subjects have addressed the predictive value of endothelial function as measured by brachial artery FMD [143]. For studies reporting continuous risk estimates, the pooled overall CVD risk was 0.92 (95% CI 0.88–0.95) for each 1% increase in FMD. The observed association seemed stronger ($p < 0.01$) in diseased populations than in asymptomatic populations [0.87 (95% CI 0.83–0.92) and 0.96 (95% CI 0.92–1.00) per 1% increase in FMD, respectively]. For studies reporting categorical risk estimates, the pooled overall CVD risk for high versus low FMD was on average 0.49 (95% CI 0.39–0.62). However, the incremental value of FMD measurements in addition to classical CV risk prediction models including the FRS or Heart SCORE has only been evaluated in a limited number of studies [142]. In one study of intermediate-risk male subjects the addition of FMD using 4.75% as a cut-off value increased the AUC (*c*-statistic) from 0.68 to 0.76. In the Cardiovascular Health Study and Multi-Ethnic Study of Atherosclerosis (MESA), no changes in the *c*-statistic were reported after the addition of FMD to the basic prediction model. The MESA study showed that the addition of FMD to the model reclassified 29% of the individuals into appropriate risk categories ($p < 0.0001$), mostly those at intermediate risk (NRI in the intermediate risk group was 28%; $p < 0.0001$). The authors concluded that these results need to be replicated in other cohorts and that the inter-observer and intra-observer variability of FMD measurements should decrease before implementation of FMD as a formal screening tool for CVD risk could be justified.

Technical issues with FMD

Briefly, FMD represents the percentage increase in diameter calculated on the basis of measurements of the diameter of the brachial artery pre- and post-ischaemia (and following reactive hyperaemia) [144] (➲ Fig. 6.13). In this context, ischaemia is induced through vessel occlusion by inflating a blood pressure cuff around the forearm or upper arm. Ischaemic dilation of downstream resistance vessels leads to increased flow in the upstream conduit brachial artery. Shear stress stimulates endothelial NO synthase and NO dilates the smooth muscle cells of the underlying vessel wall via activation of guanylate cyclase. Under standard conditions, brachial artery FMD is in large parts mediated by NO synthesis and is therefore used as a functional NO readout [145]. The absolute values may vary depending on a number of factors, including the position of the cuff, the site of artery used to measure diameter, time of ischaemia, and the time point of measurement after ischaemia. Comparisons of FMD values should be made with caution and ideally referred to values of a control group measured with an identical setup. This technique can safely be applied to large and diverse groups of patients. Repeated measurements can be made over time without side effects. As in the coronary circulation, endothelial function in the brachial circulation is impaired in the setting of traditional and novel risk factors and responds to interventions known to reduce CVD risk. Studies suggesting that endothelial function detected non-invasively in the brachial artery correlates with function in other conduit arteries, including the coronary arteries, demonstrate the systemic nature of endothelial dysfunction. When using FMD as a clinical read-out of NO bioactivity, several determinants of FMD and limitations of this method have to be taken into account when evaluating the results of FMD in clinical studies. Although the resolution of ultrasound and image analysis systems has greatly improved, one of the major limitations of FMD is its considerable dependence on the observer, requiring well-trained personnel to perform and critically review ultrasound images.

Pulse wave analysis (vascular stiffness)

Measurement of arterial stiffness as a tissue biomarker was included for the first time in the 2007 Guidelines of the European Hypertension Society [146].

The elastic properties of arteries depend on the molecular, cellular, and histological structure of the vessel wall. These change from proximal to distal in the aorta. Consequently, a physiological loss of aortic elasticity from proximal to distal occurs even in young healthy subjects, i.e. the distal aorta becomes stiffer [147]. The arterial elasticity or distensibility (the opposite of stiffness) is defined as a relative change in volume ($\delta V/V$) in relation to changes in pressure (P) [148]:

$$\text{elasticity} = \left(\delta V/V\right)/\delta P$$

For aortic stiffness, this means that ever fewer volume changes occur with increasing stiffness of the aorta. This also reduces the Windkessel function.

Stiffness of the aorta is a very suitable tissue biomarker since the aorta is one of the first organs in the body to age. Ageing processes in the vascular media are characterized inter alia by an increase in collagen as well as a decrease in elastin content, elastin fractures,

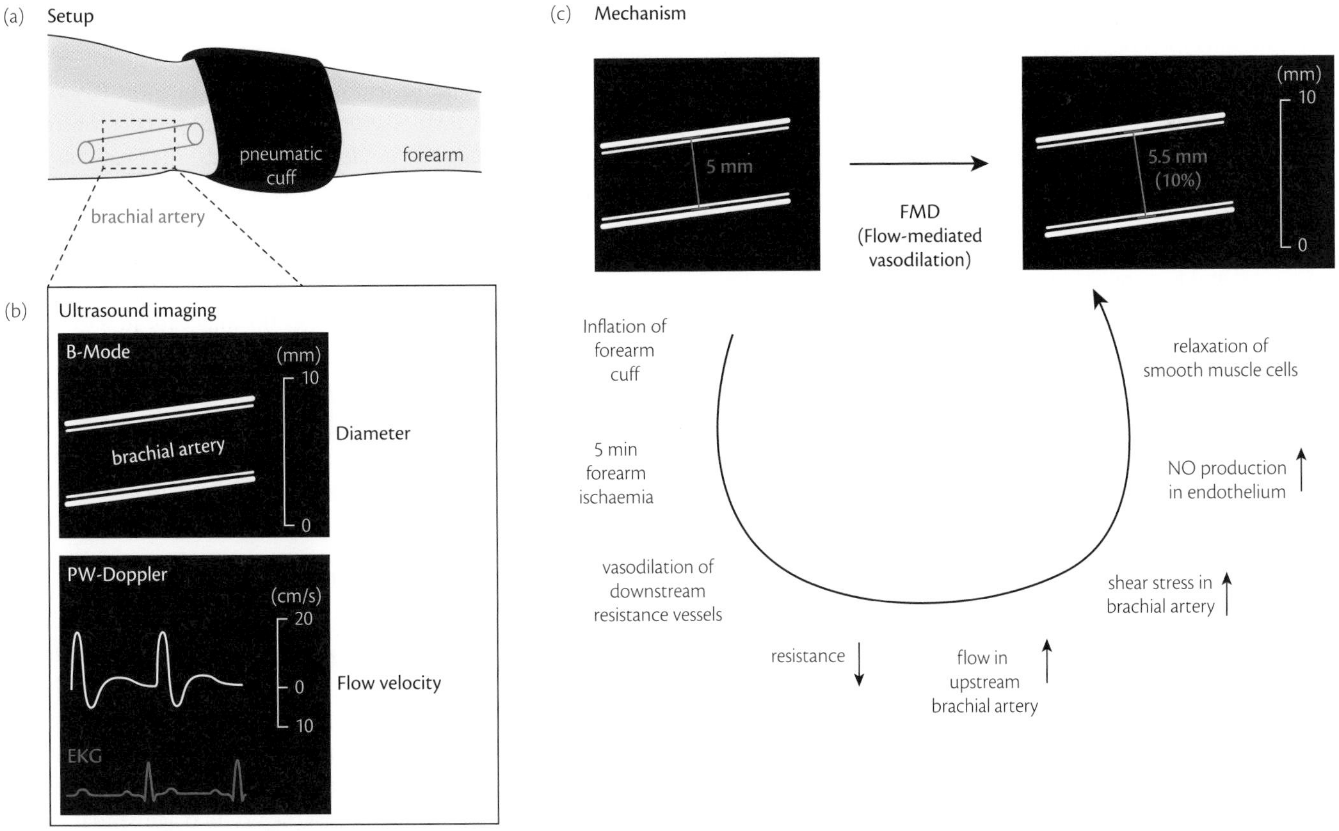

Fig. 6.13 Setup and mechanisms of flow-mediated vasodilation.

changes in the spatial organization and mechanical interactions between elastin, collagen, and smooth muscle cells, and ultimately calcifications [149]. These physiological ageing processes are speeded up under pathological conditions such as arterial hypertension, hyperlipidaemia, renal failure, diabetes mellitus, and lack of exercise as well as a high salt intake. This is referred to as accelerated vascular ageing or early vascular ageing (EVA) [150]. EVA is accompanied inter alia by increasing stiffness of the aorta and loss of the Windkessel function, manifested clinically as raised pulse pressure. In contrast to the classical CV risk factors such as arterial hypertension, hyperlipidaemia, or diabetes mellitus, arterial stiffness is a cumulative measure of the vessel-damaging effect of the risk factors over time that is similar to CIMT.

Methods of measurement

Arterial stiffness can be measured systemically, regionally, or locally [148,151]. ➲ Table 6.6 gives an overview of the most important methods of measuring vascular stiffness and pulse wave reflection.

Local stiffness in the carotid artery can be measured during an ultrasound investigation of the carotid arteries, for example. Special echotracking methods allow non-invasive measurement of the changes in vessel diameter and its correlation with changes in blood pressure. From these local measurements, arterial stiffness parameters such as elasticity, pulse wave velocity (PWV), and other local stiffness parameters can be determined [148]. The disadvantage of this method is that risk factors for vessel damage such as diabetes mellitus have different effects on vessels in different regions. Consequently, arterial stiffness parameters determined locally do not always reflect the changes taking place in the aorta.

The arterial stiffness of the aorta itself can be measured using elaborate MRI methods, but also regional measurements of arterial stiffness such as PWV (➲ Table 6.6). The aortic PWV is a direct measure of the stiffness of the aorta [152].

In the ascending aorta, the normal PWV is 4–5 m/s, in the abdominal aorta 5–6 m/s, and in the iliac and femoral arteries 8–9 m/s [148]. These different PWVs are a result of the 'stiffness gradient' in the normal aorta. The velocity of the pulse wave between the carotid and femoral arteries (cfPWV) has been investigated in numerous epidemiological studies and was shown to be an independent parameter predicting CV events. A disadvantage of this method is that the actual distance covered by the pressure wave is not known and can only be estimated [151].

Table 6.6 An overview of the most important methods of measuring vascular stiffness and pulse wave reflection

	Method	Site of measurement
Regional stiffness	Tonometer	Aortic PWV
	Mechanotransducer	Aortic PWV
	Echotracking	Aortic PWV
	Doppler Probes	Aortic PWV
Local stiffness	Echotracking	ACC, AFC, AB, AR
	Cine MRI	Aorta
Pulse wave reflection	Tonometer	All superficial arteries
	Oscillometry	AB
	Photoplethysmography	

PWV, pulse wave velocity; ACC, common carotid artery; AFC, common femoral artery; AB, brachial artery; AR, radial artery.

Additive predictive value of arterial stiffness compared with classical risk factors

A recently published meta-analysis listed a total of 17 risk factors. It showed that the simple measurement of regional aortic PWV (i.e. cfPWV) has an independent prognostic value above and beyond that of classical CV risk factors [153]. PWV is a direct measure of arterial stiffness, but indirect parameters such as pulse wave reflection (augmentation index, AIX) and central blood pressure are also used to characterize the damage to arterial vessels. The AIX is a measure of pulse wave reflection, for example at the aorta itself, at branching points in the arterial system itself (e.g. at the aortic bifurcation) and at pre-arteriolar resistance vessels (the 'true reflection point' is not known).

Central blood pressure can be determined non-invasively using several direct and indirect methods and is often used as an indirect parameter of arterial stiffness. In rising PWV due to increasing stiffness of the aorta there is a more rapid and earlier return of the reflected pulse wave (not in diastole but already in late systole). This leads to 'augmentation' and increase of the central pressure. However, besides its dependence on vascular stiffness, central blood pressure depends on a large number of other factors (mean arterial pressure, LV function, ejection time, heart rate, ventriculovascular coupling, pulse wave reflection, peripheral resistance, and the person's height). However, the evidence for the predictive prognostic relevance of central blood pressure and the AIX is weaker than that for aortic stiffness [146,148].

The independent additive prognostic value of aortic PWV over and beyond classical risk factors (e.g. the FRS) was demonstrated in two separate studies [154]. In the first study, 1045 patients with hypertension were investigated for 6 years for the incidence of CAD. The predictive value of PWV for coronary events was highest in the patient group with the lowest FRS (first tertile FRS). This finding, as well as that of other studies, shows that the appraisal of the CV risk only reflects incompletely the total exposure to vascular damage since it is the snapshot of CV risk factors.

Even when vascular damage parameters such as ankle–brachial index (ABI), CIMT, and brachial pulse pressure are used for risk stratification, a further superior predictive value of the PWV remains [154]. Measurement of cfPWV is regarded as the gold standard for determining aortic stiffness [151].

Normal values and instrument validation

A recently published meta-analysis calculated age- and blood pressure-related normal values for aortic PWV [155]. The systemic pressure obtained at the time of PWV measurement must always be considered in the interpretation, since the transmural pressure, and thus the transmural wall tension, is a major determinant of arterial stiffness. Age-adjusted percentiles for PWV (analogous to CAC score) have the advantage that the vascular age of an individual can be determined independently of chronological age. Other recommendations are to lay down an age-independent threshold value of 10 m/s for cfPWV [151]. Similar to the normal values for peripheral blood pressure measurements on the arm, the question arises as to whether the reference value for aortic PWV should be orientated to young healthy individuals where median values of 6.1 m/s (10th and 90th percentiles 5.3–7.1 m/s) are reported [156]. Even in elderly patients with manifest CV disease, PWV of 5–7 m/s are frequently attained with optimal blood pressure controls.

With regard to target values, we recommend orienting to the normal values of young healthy people (5.3–7.1 m/s). Since most currently available instruments are not validated according to any international validation protocol, we recommend systems of PWV determination that measure cfPWV directly and have in addition demonstrated their additive practical relevance in epidemiological and prognostic studies.

Ankle–brachial index

The ankle–brachial index (ABI) is a practical, very simple measurement for detecting peripheral artery disease as a surrogate of systemic atherosclerosis. Blood pressure is measured with a non-imaging Doppler probe at the posterior tibial artery/dorsalis pedis artery as well as the brachial artery. According to the getABI study the ratio of both measurements is defined as the ABI. An ABI < 0.9 is highly predictive of stenosis between the aorta and the distal leg arteries of over 50% [157]. Accuracy is very high compared with angiography (sensitivity 97%, specificity 100%) [158]. Notably, 50–89% of patients showing an ABI < 0.9 do not suffer any claudication, making the measurement a valuable tool in preventive cardiology. Prognostically, peripheral artery disease coincides with coronary events as well as strokes [159], and even patients with already proven CAD are at enhanced risk if ABI is reduced. In general, asymptomatic peripheral vascular disease detected by a positive ABI has been found to be associated with an incidence of CVD in men of about 20% at 10 years [158]. Both the ESC [1] and the ACC/AHA prevention guidelines [4] recommend the measurement of ABI for CV risk assessment in asymptomatic adults with intermediate risk (evidence class IIa).

Conclusions

Scoring systems are population-based and have several limitations in the assessment of asymptomatic individuals for CV risk. Imaging of pre-clinical atherosclerosis enables a quantitative assessment of the position of an individual along the pathophysiological continuum of atherosclerosis as a result of lifetime exposure to causative risk factors. There is an armamentarium of new but already sufficiently validated imaging methods capable of directly identifying pre-clinical atherosclerosis. They differ from more established modalities for diagnosing haemodynamically relevant disease, which due to Bayes' theorem are often not reasonable for preventive tasks. It is already clear that these new methods provide additional predictive information beyond risk factor scoring, and may be useful for supporting lifestyle modifications and monitoring the efficacy of these and drug treatment. The relative indications for the modalities are not yet well defined by algorithms; however, pathways from risk factor scoring to execution of particular imaging modalities have gathered some evidence to date. It is in intermediate-risk individuals that there is a reasonable expectation of reclassifying predictive information.

Further reading

Blumenthal R, Foody J, Wong ND. *Preventive cardiology: companion to Braunwald's heart disease: expert consult*, 2011. Philadelphia, PA: Saunders.

Greenland P, Alpert JS, Beller GA, et al; American College of Cardiology Foundation/American Heart Association Task Force on Practice Guidelines. 2010 ACCF/AHA guideline for assessment of cardiovascular risk in asymptomatic adults: a report of the American College of Cardiology Foundation/American Heart Association Task Force on Practice Guidelines. *Circulation* 2010; **122**: e584–e636.

Mureddu GF, Brandimarte F, Faggiano P, et al. Between risk charts and imaging: how should we stratify cardiovascular risk in clinical practice? *Eur Heart J Cardiovasc Imaging* 2013; **14**: 401–16.

Naghavi M. *Asymptomatic atherosclerosis. Pathophysiology, detection and treatment*, 2010. New York: Springer.

Perk J, de Backer G, Gohlke H, et al. European Association for Cardiovascular Prevention and Rehabilitation (EACPR); ESC Committee for Practice Guideline (cPG). European Guideline on cardiovascular disease prevention in clinical practice (version 2012). The Fifth Joint Task Force of the European Society of Cardiology and Other Societies on Cardiovascular Disease Prevention in Clinical Practice. *Eur Heart J* 2012; **33**: 1635–701.

References

1 Perk J, de Backer G, Gohlke H, et al; European Association for Cardiovascular Prevention and Rehabilitation (EACPR); ESC Committee for Practice Guideline (cPG). European Guideline on cardiovascular disease prevention in clinical practice (version 2012). The Fifth Joint Task Force of the European Society of Cardiology and Other Societies on Cardiovascular Disease Prevention in Clinical Practice. *Eur Heart J* 2012; **33**: 1635–701.

2 Erbel R, Budoff M. Improvement of cardiovascular risk prediction using coronary imaging: subclinical atherosclerosis: the memory of lifetime risk factor exposure. *Eur Heart J* 2012; **33**: 1201–17.

3 Mureddu GF, Brandimarte F, Faggiano P, et al. Between risk charts and imaging: how should we stratify cardiovascular risk in clinical practice? *Eur Heart J Cardiovasc Imaging* 2013; **14**: 401–16.

4 Greenland P, Alpert JS, Beller GA, et al; American College of Cardiology Foundation/American Heart Association Task Force on Practice Guidelines. 2010 ACCF/AHA guideline for assessment of cardiovascular risk in asymptomatic adults: a report of the American College of Cardiology Foundation/American Heart Association Task Force on Practice Guidelines. *Circulation* 2010; **122**: e584–e636.
5 Diamond GA, Forrester JS. Analysis of probability as an aid in the clinical diagnosis of coronary-artery disease. *N Engl J Med* 1979; **300**: 1350–8.
6 Falk E, Shah PK, Fuster V. Coronary plaque disruption. *Circulation* 1995; **92**: 657–71.
7 Naghavi M, Libby R, Falk E, et al. From vulnerable plaque to vulnerable patient: a call for new definitions and risk assessment strategies: Part I. *Circulation* 2003; **108**: 1664–72.
8 Puri R, Nissen SE, Ballantyne CM, et al. Factors underlying regression of coronary atheroma with potent statin therapy. *Eur Heart J* 2013; **34**: 1818–25.
9 Camici PG, Rimoldi OE, Gaemperli O, Libby P. Non-invasive anatomic and functional imaging of vascular inflammation and unstable plaque. *Eur Heart J* 2012; **33**: 1309–17.
10 Pencina MJ, D'Agostino RB Sr, D'Agostino RB Jr, et al. Evaluating the added predictive ability of a new marker: from area under the ROC curve to reclassification and beyond. *Stat Med* 2008; **27**: 157–72.
11 Ferket BS, Genders TS, Colkesen EB, et al. Systematic review of guidelines on imaging of asymptomatic coronary artery disease. *J Am Coll Cardiol* 2011; **57**: 1591–600.
12 Naghavi M, Falk E, Hecht HS, et al., SHAPE Task Force. From vulnerable plaque to vulnerable patient—Part III: Executive summary of the Screening for Heart Attack Prevention and Education (SHAPE) Task Force report. *Am J Cardiol* 2006; **98**: 2H–15H.
13 Lloyd-Jones DM. Cardiovascular risk prediction. Basic concepts, current status, and future directions. *Circulation* 2012; **121**: 1768–77.
14 Shah PK. Screening asymptomatic subjects for subclinical atherosclerosis: can we, does it matter, and should we? *J Am Coll Cardiol* 2010; **56**: 98–105.
15 Wong ND, Detrano RC, Diamond G, et al. Does coronary artery screening by electron beam computed tomography motivate potentially beneficial lifestyle behaviours? *Am J Cardiol* 1996; **78**: 1220–3.
16 Bovert P, Perret F, Cornuz J, et al. Improved smoking cessation in smokers given ultrasound photographs of their own atherosclerotic plaques. *Prev Med* 2002; **34**: 215–20.
17 Wilson JMG, Jungner G.Principles and practice of screening for disease. *WHO Chronicle* 1968; **22**: 473.
18 Touboul P-J, Hennerici MG, Meairs S, et al. Mannheim carotid intima-media thickness consensus (2004–2006). *Cerebrovasc Dis* 2007; **23**: 75–80.
19 Polak JF, Pencina MJ, O'Leary DH, et al. Common carotid artery intima-media thickness (IMT) progression as a predictor of stroke in MESA (Multi-Ethnic Study of Atherosclerosis). *Stroke* 2011; **42**: 3017–21.
20 O'Leary DH, Polak JF, Kronmal RA, et al. Carotid-artery intima and media thickness as a risk factor for myocardial infarction and stroke in older adults. Cardiovascular Health Study Collaborative Research Group. *N Engl J Med* 1999; **340**: 14–22.
21 Lorenz MW, Markus HS, Bots ML, et al. Prediction of clinical cardiovascular events with carotid intima-media thickness: a systemic review and meta-analysis. *Circulation* 2007; **115**: 459–67.
22 Mancia G, Laurent S, Agabiti-Rosei E, et al; European Society of Hypertension. Reappraisal of European guidelines on hypertensive management: a European Society of Hypertension Task Force document. *J Hypertens* 2009; **27**: 121–58.
23 Elias-Smale SE, Kavousi M, Verwoert GC, et al. Common carotid intima-media thickness in cardiovascular risk stratification of older people: the Rotterdam Study. *Eur J Rev Cardiol* 2012; **19**: 698–705.
24 Nambi V, Chambless L, Folsom A, et al. Carotid intima-media thickness and the presence or absence of plaque improves prediction of coronary heart disease risk: the ARIC (Atherosclerosis Risk in Communities) study. *J Am Coll Cardiol* 2010; **55**: 1600–7.
25 Bauer M, Möhlenkamp S, Lehmann N, et al. The effect of age and risk factors on coronary and carotid artery atherosclerotic burden in males—results of the Heinz Nixdorf Recall Study. *Atherosclerosis* 2009; **205**: 595–602.
26 Touboul PJ, Vicaut E, Labreuche J, et al; PARC study participating physicians. Correlation between the Framingham risk score and intima media thickness: the Paroi Artérielle et Risque Cardiovasculaire (PARC) study. *Atherosclerosis* 2007; **192**: 363–9.
27 Wang JG, Staessen JA, Li Y, et al. Carotid intima-media thickness and antihypertensive treatment: a meta-analysis of randomized controlled trials. *Stroke* 2006; **37**: 1933–40.
28 Crouse JR 3rd, Raichlen JS, Riley WA, et al; METEOR Study Group. Effect of rosuvastatin on progression of carotid intima-media thickness in low-risk individuals with subclinical atherosclerosis: the METEOR Trial. *J Am Med Assoc* 2007; **297**: 1344–53.
29 de Groot E, Jukema JW, Montauban van Swijndregt AD, et al. B-mode ultrasound assessment of pravastatin treatment effect on carotid and femoral artery walls and its correlations with coronary arteriographic findings: a report of the Regression Growth Evaluation Statin Study (REGRESS). *J Am Coll Cardiol* 1998; **31**: 1561–7.
30 Calermajer DS, Sorensen KE, Gooch VM, et al. Non-invasive detection of endothelial dysfunction in children and adults at risk for atherosclerosis. *Lancet* 1992; **340**: 1111–15.
31 Kim LG, P Scott RA, Ashton HA, et al. Multicentre Aneurysm Screening Study Group. A sustained mortality benefit from screening for abdominal aortic aneurysm. *Ann Intern Med* 2007; **146**: 699–706.
32 Lederle FA, Johnson GR, Wilson SE, et al. Prevalence and associations of abdominal aortic aneurysm detected through screening. Aneurysm Detection and Management (ADAM) Veterans Affairs Cooperative Study Group. *Ann Intern Med* 1997; **126**: 441–9.
33 Lim HS, Haq N, Mahmood S, et al.; the ACPM Prevention Practice Committee. Atherosclerotic cardiovascular disease screening in adults. American College of Preventive Medicine position statement on preventive practice. *Am J Prev Med* 2011; **40**: 380–1.
34 Kent KC, Zwolak RM, Jaff MR, et al; Society of Vascular Surgery, American Association of Vascular Surgery, Society for Vascular Medicine and Biology. Screening for abdominal aortic aneurysm: a consensus statement. *J Vasc Surg* 2004; **39**: 267–9.
35 Christiansen JP, Leong-Poi H, Klibanov AL, et al. Noninvasive imaging of myocardial reperfusion injury using leucocyte-targeted contrast echocardiography. *Circulation* 2002; **105**: 1764–7.
36 Villanueva FS, Jankowski RJ, Klibanov S, et al. Microbubbles targeted to intercellular adhesion molecule-1 bind to activated coronary endothelial cells. *Circulation* 1998; **98**: 1–5.
37 Krzanowaki M, Bodzon W, Petkow P. Imaging of all three coronary arteries by transthoracic echocardiography. An illustrated guide. *Cardiovasc Ultrasound* 2003; **1**: 16.
38 Nixdorff U, Schmidt A, Morant T, et al. Dose-dependent disintegration of human endothelial monolayers by contrast echocardiography. *Life Sci* 2005; **77**: 1493–501.
39 Dijkmans P, Juffermans L, Musters R, et al. Microbubbles and ultrasound: from diagnosis to therapy. *Eur J Echocardiogr* 2004; **5**: 245–6.
40 Schäfer S, Kliner S, Klinghammer L, et al. Influence of ultrasound operating parameters on ultrasound-induced thromboloysis *in vitro*. *Ultrasound Med Biol* 2005; **31**: 841–7.

41 Rigo F, Murer B, Ossena G, et al. Transthoracic echocardiography imaging of coronary arteries: tips, traps, and pitfalls. *Cardiovasc Ultrasound* 2008; **6**: 7.
42 Hozumi T, Yoshida K, Ogata Y, et al. Noninvasive assessment of significant left anterior descending coronary artery stenosis by coronary flow velocity reserve with transthoracic color Doppler echocardiography. *Circulation* 1998; **97**: 1557–62.
43 Hozumi T, Yoshida K, Akaasaka T, et al. Noninvasive assessment of coronary flow reserve in the anterior descending coronary artery by Doppler echocardiography: comparison with invasive technique. *J Am Coll Cardiol* 1998; **32**: 1251–9.
44 Caiati C, Montaldo C, Zedda N, et al. Validation of a non-invasive method (contrast enhanced transthoracic second harmonic echo Doppler) for the evaluation of coronary flow reserve: comparison with intra coronary Doppler flow wire. *J Am Coll Cardiol* 1999; **34**: 1193–200.
45 Lethen H, Tries H, Kersting S, et al. Validation of non-invasive assessment of coronary flow velocity reserve in the right coronary artery: comparison of transthoracic echocardiographic results with intracoronary Doppler flow measurements. *Eur Heart J* 2003; **24**: 1567–75.
46 Meimoun P, Sayah S, Maitre B. Mesure du flux et de la reserve coronaire par échographie transthoracique: un vieux concept, un outil modern, des intérets multiples. *Ann Cardiol Angéiol* 2004; **53**: 325–34.
47 Paolo Voci P, Pizzuto F, Romeo F. Coronary flow: a new asset for the echo lab? *Eur Heart J* 2004; **25**: 1867–79.
48 Gradus-Pizlo I, Sawada SG, Wright D, et al. Detection of subclinical coronary atherosclerosis using two-dimensional, high resolution transthoracic echocardiography. *J Am Coll Cardiol* 2001; **37**: 1422–9.
49 Ferrrari M, Schnell B, Werner GS, et al. Safety of deferring angioplasty in patients with normal coronary flow velocity reserve. *J Am Coll Cardiol* 1999; **33**: 82–7.
50 Ruscazio M, Montisci R, Colonna P, et al. Detection of coronary restenosis after coronary angioplasty by contrast-enhanced transthoracic echocardiographic Doppler assessment of coronary flow velocity reserve. *J Am Coll Cardiol* 2002; **40**: 896–903.
51 Pizzuto F, Voci P, Mariano E, et al. Non-invasive coronary flow reserve assessed by transthoracic coronary Doppler ultrasound in patients with left anterior descending coronary artery stents. *Am J Cardiol* 2003; **97**: 522–6.
52 Voci P, Mariano E, Pizzuto F, et al. Coronary recanalization in anterior myocardial infarction. The open perforator hypothesis. *J Am Coll Cardiol* 2002; **40**: 1205–13.
53 Otto CM, Lind BK, Kitzman DW, et al. Association of aortic valve sclerosis with cardiovascular mortality and morbidity in the elderly. *N Engl J Med* 1999; **341**: 142–7.
54 Faggiano P, D'Aloia A, Antonini-Canterin F, et al. Usefulness of cardiac calcification on two-dimensional echocardiography for distinguishing ischaemic from nonischaemic dilated cardiomyopathy: a preliminary report. *J Cardiovasc Med* 2007; **7**: 182–7.
55 Nucifora G, Schuijf JD, van Werkhoven JM, et al. Usefulness of echocardiographic assessment of cardiac and ascending aorta calcific deposits to predict coronary artery calcium and presence and severity of obstructive coronary artery disease. *Am J Cardiol* 2009; **103**: 1045–50.
56 Corciu AI, Siciliano V, Poggianti E, et al. Cardiac calcification by transthoracic echocardiography in patients with known or suspected coronary artery disease. *Int J Cardiol* 2010; **142**: 288–95.
57 Cabrera F. *Ecocardiografía*, 1st edn, 2011. Madrid: Panamericana.
58 Marwick T. Measurement of strain and strain rate by echocardiography. Ready for prime time? *J Am Coll Cardiol* 2006; **47**: 1313–27.
59 Youn H, Foster E. Transesophageal echocardiography (TEE) in the evaluation of the coronary arteries. *Cardiol Clin* 2000; **18**: 833–48.
60 Fox K, García MA, Ardissino D, et al; Task Force on the Management of Stable Angina Pectoris of the European Society of Cardiology; ESC Committee for Practice Guidelines (CPG). Guidelines on the management of stable angina pectoris: executive summary: The Task Force on the Management of Stable Angina Pectoris of the European Society of Cardiology. *Eur Heart J* 2006; **27**: 1341–81.
61 Metz LD, Beattie M, Hom R, et al. The prognostic value of normal exercise myocardial perfusion imaging and exercise echocardiography: a meta-analysis. *J Am Coll Cardiol* 2007; **49**: 227–37.
62 McCully R, Roger VL, Mahoney DW, et al. Outcome after normal exercise echocardiography and predictors of subsequent cardiac events: follow-up of 1,325 patients. *J Am Coll Cardiol* 1998; **31**: 144–9.
63 Schrope B, Newhouse VL, Uhlendorf V. Simulated capillary blood flow measurement using a nonlinear ultrasonic contrast agent. *Ultrasound Imaging* 1992; **14**: 134–58.
64 Gaibazzi N, Reverberi C, Squeri A. Contrast stress echocardiography for the diagnosis of coronary artery disease in patients with chest pain but without acute coronary syndrome: incremental value of myocardial perfusion. *J Am Soc Echocardiogr* 2009; **22**: 404–10.
65 Rumberger JA, Simons DB, Fitzpaterick LA, et al. Coronary artery calcium area by electron-beam computed tomography and coronary atherosclerotic plaque area: a histopathologic correlative study. *Circulation* 1995; **92**: 2157–62.
66 Hoff JA, Chomka EV, Krainik AJ, et al. Age and gender distribution of coronary artery calcium detected by electron beam tomography. *Am J Cardiol* 2001; **87**: 1335–9.
67 McClelland RL, Chung H, Detrano R, et al. Distribution of coronary artery calcium by race, gender, and age. Results from the Multi-Ethnic Study of Atherosclerosis (MESA). *Circulation* 2006; **113**: 30–7.
68 Schmermund A, Mohlenkamp S, Berenbein S, et al. Population-based assessment of subclinical coronary atherosclerosis using electron-beam computed tomography. *Atherosclerosis* 2006; **185**: 117–82.
69 Detrano R, Guerci AD, Carr JJ, et al. Coronary calcium as a predictor of coronary events in four racial or ethnic groups. *N Engl J Med* 2008; **358**: 1336–45.
70 Sarwar A, Shaw LJ, Shapiro MD, et al. Diagnostic and prognostic value of absence of coronary artery calcification. *JACC Cardiovasc Imaging* 2009; **2**: 675–88.
71 Taylor AJ, Bindeman J, Feuerstein I, et al. Coronary calcium independently predicts incident premature coronary heart disease over measured cardiovascular risk factors: mean three-year outcomes in the Prospective Army Coronary Calcium (PACC) project. *J Am Coll Cardiol* 2005; **46**: 807–14.
72 Greenland P, LaBree L, Azen SP, et al. Coronary artery calcium score combined with Framingham score for risk prediction in asymptomatic individuals. *J Am Med Assoc* 2004; **291**: 210–15.
73 Erbel R, Möhlenkamp S, Moebus S, et al; Heinz Nixdorf Recall Study Investigative Group. Coronary risk stratification, discrimination, and reclassification improvement based on quantification of subclinical coronary atherosclerosis: the Heinz Nixdorf Recall study. *J Am Coll Cardiol* 2010; **56**: 1397–406.
74 Park R, Detrano R, Xiang M, et al. Combined use of computed tomography coronary calcium scores and C-reactive protein levels in predicting cardiovascular events in non-diabetic individuals. *Circulation* 2002; **106**: 2073–7.
75 Folsom AR, Kronmal RA, Detrano RC, et al. Coronary artery calcification compared with carotid intima-media thickness in the prediction of cardiovascular disease incidence: the Multi-Ethnic Study of Atherosclerosis (MESA). *Arch Intern Med* 2008; **168**: 1333–9.
76 Schmermund A, Baumgart D, Möhlenkamp S, et al. Natural history and topographic pattern of progression of coronary calcification in symptomatic patients. *Arterioscler Thromb Vasc Biol* 2001; **21**: 421–6.

77 Taylor AJ, Bindeman J, Le TP, et al. Progression of calcified coronary atherosclerosis: relationship to coronary risk factors and carotid intima-media thickness. *Atherosclerosis* 2008; **197**: 339–45.
78 Kronmal RA, McClelland RL, Detrano R, et al. Risk factors for the progression of coronary artery calcification in asymptomatic subjects: results from the Multi-Ethnic Study of Atherosclerosis (MESA). *Circulation* 2007; **115**: 2722–30.
79 Cassidy-Bushrow AE, Bielak LF, Sheedy PF 2nd, et al. Coronary artery calcification progression is heritable. *Circulation* 2007; **116**: 25–31.
80 Raggi P, Callister TQ, Shaw LJ. Progression of coronary artery calcium and risk of first myocardial infarction in patients receiving cholesterol-lowering therapy. *Arterioscler Thromb Vasc Biol* 2004; **24**: 1272–7.
81 Callister TQ, Raggi P, Cooil B, et al. Effect of HmG-CoA reductase inhibitors on coronary artery disease as assessed by electron-beam computed tomography. *N Engl J Med* 1998; **339**: 1972–8.
82 Achenbach S, Ropers D, Pohle K, et al. Influence of lipid-lowering therapy on the progression of coronary artery calcification: a prospective evaluation. *Circulation* 2002; **106**: 1077–82.
83 Budoff MJ, Lane KL, Bakhsheshi H, et al. Rates of progression of coronary calcium by electron beam tomography. *Am J Cardiol* 2000; **86**: 8–11.
84 Raggi P, Davidson M, Callister TQ, et al. Aggressive versus moderate lipid-lowering therapy in hypercholesterolemic postmenopausal women: Beyond Endorsed Lipid Lowering with EBT Scanning (BELLES). *Circulation* 2005; **112**: 563–71.
85 Schmermund A, Achenbach S, Budde T, et al. Effect of intensive versus standard lipid-lowering treatment with atorvastatin on the progression of calcified coronary atherosclerosis over 12 months: a multicenter, randomized, double-blind trial. *Circulation* 2006; **113**: 427–37.
86 Arad Y, Spadaro LA, Roth M, et al. Treatment of asymptomatic adults with elevated coronary calcium scores with atorvastatin, vitamin C, and vitamin E: the St. Francis Heart Study randomized clinical trial. *J Am Coll Cardiol* 2005; **46**: 166–72.
87 Terry JG, Carr JJ, Kouba EO, et al. Effect of simvastatin (80 mg) on coronary and abdominal aortic arterial calcium (from the coronary artery calcification treatment with Zocor [CATZ] study). *Am J Cardiol* 2007; **99**: 1714–17.
88 Budoff MJ, Achenbach S, Blumenthal RS, et al; American Heart Association Committee on Cardiovascular Imaging and Intervention; American Heart Association Council on Cardiovascular Radiology and Intervention; American Heart Association Committee on Cardiac Imaging, Council on Clinical Cardiology. Assessment of coronary artery disease by cardiac computed tomography: a scientific statement from the American Heart Association Committee on Cardiovascular Imaging and Intervention, Council on Cardiovascular Radiology and Intervention, and Committee on Cardiac Imaging, Council on Clinical Cardiology. *Circulation* 2006; **114**: 1761–91.
89 Greenland P, Bonow RO, Brundage BH, et al; American College of Cardiology Foundation Clinical Expert Consensus Task Force (ACCF/AHA Writing Committee to Update the 2000 Expert Consensus Document on Electron Beam Computed Tomography); Society of Atherosclerosis Imaging and Prevention; Society of Cardiovascular Computed Tomography. ACCF/AHA 2007 clinical expert consensus document on coronary artery calcium scoring by computed tomography in global cardiovascular risk assessment and in evaluation of patients with chest pain: a report of the American College of Cardiology Foundation Clinical Expert Consensus Task Force (ACCF/AHA Writing Committee to Update the 2000 Expert Consensus Document on Electron Beam Computed Tomography). *Circulation* 2007; **115**: 402–26.
90 Schroeder S, Achenbach S, Bengel F, et al. Cardiac computed tomography: indications, applications, limitations, and training requirements: report of a Writing Group deployed by the Working Group Nuclear Cardiology and Cardiac CT of the European Society of Cardiology and the European Council of Nuclear Cardiology. *Eur Heart J* 2008; **29**: 531–56.
91 Taylor AJ, Cerqueira M, Hodgson JM, et al. American College of Cardiology Foundation Appropriate Use Criteria Task Force; Society of Cardiovascular Computed Tomography; American College of Radiology; American Heart Association; American Society of Echocardiography; American Society of Nuclear Cardiology; North American Society for Cardiovascular Imaging; Society for Cardiovascular Angiography and Interventions; Society for Cardiovascular Magnetic Resonance. ACCF/SCCT/ACR/AHA/ASE/ASNC/NASCI/SCAI/SCMR 2010 Appropriate use criteria for cardiac computed tomography. A Report of the American College of Cardiology Foundation Appropriate Use Criteria Task Force, the Society of Cardiovascular Computed Tomography, the American College of Radiology, the American Heart Association, the American Society of Echocardiography, the American Society of Nuclear Cardiology, the North American Society for Cardiovascular Imaging, the Society for Cardiovascular Angiography and Interventions, and the Society for Cardiovascular Magnetic Resonance. *J Cardiovasc Comput Tomogr* 2010; **4**: 407.e1–407.e33.
92 Motoyama S, Sarai M, Harigaya H, et al. Computed tomographic angiography characteristics of atherosclerotic plaques subsequently resulting in acute coronary syndrome. *J Am Coll Cardiol* 2009; **54**: 49–57.
93 Min JK, Shaw LJ, Devereux RB, et al. Prognostic value of multidetector coronary computed tomographic angiography for prediction of all-cause mortality. *J Am Coll Cardiol* 2007; **50**: 1161–70.
94 Ostrom MP, Gopal A, Ahmadi N, et al. Mortality incidence and the severity of coronary atherosclerosis assessed by computed tomography angiography. *J Am Coll Cardiol* 2008; **52**: 1335–43.
95 Min JK, Dunning A, Lin FY, et al; CONFIRM Investigators. Age- and sex-related differences in all-cause mortality risk based on coronary computed tomography angiography findings results from the International Multicenter CONFIRM (Coronary CT Angiography Evaluation for Clinical Outcomes: an International Multicenter Registry) of 23,854 patients without known coronary artery disease. *J Am Coll Cardiol* 2011; **58**: 849–60.
96 Cho I, Chang HJ, Sung JM, et al; CONFIRM Investigators. Coronary computed tomographic angiography and risk of all-cause mortality and nonfatal myocardial infarction in subjects without chest pain syndrome from the CONFIRM Registry (Coronary CT Angiography Evaluation for Clinical Outcomes: an International Multicenter Registry). *Circulation* 2012; **126**: 304–13.
97 Hamm CW, Bassand JP, Agewall S, et al; ESC Committee for Practice Guidelines, Bax JJ, Auricchio A, Baumgartner H, et al; Document Reviewers, Windecker S, Achenbach S, Badimon L, et al. ESC Guidelines for the management of acute coronary syndromes in patients presenting without persistent ST-segment elevation: the Task Force for the Management of Acute Coronary Syndromes (ACS) in Patients Presenting Without Persistent ST-segment Elevation of the European Society of Cardiology (ESC). *Eur Heart J* 2011; **32**: 2999–3054.
98 Bruder O, Schneider S, Nothnagel D, et al. EuroCMR (European Cardiovascular Magnetic Resonance) registry: results of the German pilot phase. *J Am Coll Cardiol* 2009; **54**: 1457–66.
99 Kim WY, Danias PG, Stuber M, et al. Coronary magnetic resonance angiography for the detection of coronary stenoses. *N Engl J Med* 2001; **345**: 1863–9.
100 Beanlands RS, Chow BJ, Dick A, et al. CCS/CAR/CANM/CNCS/CanSCMR joint position statement on advanced noninvasive cardiac imaging using positron emission tomography, magnetic

resonance imaging and multi-detector computed tomographic angiography in the diagnosis and evaluation of ischemic heart disease—executive summary. *Can J Cardiol* 2007; **23**: 107–19.
101 Douard H, Barat JL, Laurent F, et al. Magnetic resonance imaging of an anomalous origin of the left coronary artery from the pulmonary artery. *Eur Heart J* 1988; **9**: 1356–60.
102 Bellenger NG, Davies LC, Francis JM, et al. Reduction in sample size for studies of remodelling in heart failure by the use of cardiovascular magnetic resonance. *J Cardiovasc Magn Reson* 2000; **2**: 271–8.
103 Marcus FI, McKenna WJ, Sherrill D, et al. Diagnosis of arrhythmogenic right ventricular cardiomyopathy/dysplasia: proposed modification of the Task Force Criteria. *Eur Heart J* 2010; **31**: 806–14.
104 Nagel E, Klein C, Paetsch I, et al. Magnetic resonance perfusion measurements for the noninvasive detection of coronary artery disease. *Circulation* 2003; **108**: 432–7.
105 Greenwood JP, Maredia N, Younger JF, et al. Cardiovascular magnetic resonance and single-photon emission computed tomography for diagnosis of coronary heart disease (CE-MARC): a prospective trial. *Lancet* 2012; **379**: 453–60.
106 Jaarsma C, Leiner T, Bekkers SC, et al. Diagnostic performance of noninvasive myocardial perfusion imaging using single-photon emission computed tomography, cardiac magnetic resonance, and positron emission tomography imaging for the detection of obstructive coronary artery disease: a meta-analysis. *J Am Coll Cardiol* 2012; **59**: 1719–28.
107 Nagel E, Lehmkuhl HB, Bocksch W, et al. Noninvasive diagnosis of ischemia-induced wall motion abnormalities with the use of high-dose dobutamine stress MRI: comparison with dobutamine stress echocardiography. *Circulation* 1999; **99**: 763–70.
107 Rehwald WG, Fieno DS, Chen EL, et al. Myocardial magnetic resonance imaging contrast agent concentrations after reversible and irreversible ischemic injury. *Circulation* 2002; **105**: 224–9.
109 Kim RJ, Wu E, Rafael A, et al. The use of contrast-enhanced magnetic resonance imaging to identify reversible myocardial dysfunction. *N Engl J Med* 2000; **343**: 1445–53.
110 Friedrich MG, Sechtem U, Schulz-Menger J, et al; International Consensus Group on Cardiovascular Magnetic Resonance in Myocarditis. Cardiovascular magnetic resonance in myocarditis: a JACC White Paper. *J Am Coll Cardiol* 2009; **53**: 1475–87.
111 Yuan C, Kerwin WS, Ferguson MS, et al. Contrast-enhanced high resolution MRI for atherosclerotic carotid artery tissue characterization. *J Magn Reson Imaging* 2002; **15**: 62–7.
112 Wasserman BA, Smith WI, Trout HH, et al. Carotid artery atherosclerosis: in vivo morphologic characterization with gadolinium-enhanced double-oblique MR imaging initial results. *Radiology* 2002; **223**: 566–73.
113 Mohiaddin RH, Burman ED, Prasad SK, et al. Glagov remodeling of the atherosclerotic aorta demonstrated by cardiovascular magnetic resonance: the CORDA asymptomatic subject plaque assessment research (CASPAR) project. *J Cardiovasc Magn Reson* 2004; **6**: 517–25.
114 Grotenhuis HB, Westenberg JJ, Steendijk P, et al. Validation and reproducibility of aortic pulse wave velocity as assessed with velocity-encoded MRI. *J Magn Reson Imaging* 2009; **30**: 521–6.
115 Westenberg JJ, de Roos A, Grotenhuis HB, et al. Improved aortic pulse wave velocity assessment from multislice two-directional in-plane velocity-encoded magnetic resonance imaging. *J Magn Reson Imaging* 2010; **32**: 1086–94.
116 Yuan C, Mitsumori LM, Ferguson MS, et al. *In vivo* accuracy of multispectral magnetic resonance imaging for identifying lipid-rich necrotic cores and intraplaque hemorrhage in advanced human carotid plaques. *Circulation* 2001; **104**: 2051–6.
117 van den Bouwhuijsen QJ, Vernooij MW, Hofman A, et al. Determinants of magnetic resonance imaging detected carotid plaque components: the Rotterdam Study. *Eur Heart J* 2012; **33**: 221–9.
118 Zhao XQ, Dong L, Hatsukami T, et al. MR imaging of carotid plaque composition during lipid-lowering therapy: a prospective assessment of effect and time course. *JACC Cardiovasc Imaging* 2011; **4**: 977–86.
119 Esposito L, Saam T, Heider P, et al. MRI plaque imaging reveals high-risk carotid plaques especially in diabetic patients. *BMC Med Imaging* 2010; **10**: 27.
120 Ronald JA, Chen Y, Belisle AJ, et al. Comparison of gadofluorine-M and Gd-DTPA for noninvasive staging of atherosclerotic plaque stability using MRI. *Circ Cardiovasc Imaging* 2009; **3**: 226–34.
121 Wagner S, Schnorr J, Ludwig A, et al. Contrast-enhanced MR imaging of atherosclerosis using citrate-coated superparamagnetic iron oxide nanoparticles: calcifying microvesicles as imaging target for plaque characterization. *Int J Nanomedicine* 2013; **8**: 767–79.
122 Fayad ZA, Mani V, Woodward M, et al.; dal-PLAQUE Investigators. Safety and efficacy of dalcetrapib on atherosclerotic disease using novel non-invasive multimodality imaging (dal-PLAQUE): a randomized clinical trial. *Lancet* 2011; **378**: 1547–59.
123 Bengel FM. Atherosclerosis imaging on the molecular level. *J Nucl Cardiol* 2006; **13**: 111–18.
124 Tawakol A, Migrino RQ, Bashian GG, et al. In vivo ^{18}F-fluorodeoxyglucose positron emission tomography imaging provides a non-invasive measure of carotid plaque inflammation in patients. *J Am Coll Cardiol* 2006; **48**: 1818–24.
125 Rudd JH, Myers KS, Bansilal S, et al. (18)Fluorodeoxyglucose positron emission tomography imaging of atherosclerotic plaque inflammation is highly reproducible: implications for atherosclerosis therapy trials. *J Am Coll Cardiol* 2007; **50**: 892–6.
126 Sadeghi MM, Glover DK, Lanza GM, et al. Imaging atherosclerosis and vulnerable plaque. *J Nucl Med* 2010; 51 (Suppl. 1): 51S–65S.
127 Wong TY, Duncan BB, Golden SH, et al. Associations between the metabolic syndrome and retinal microvascular signs: the Atherosclerosis Risk In Communities study. *Invest Ophthalmol Vis Sci* 2004; **45**: 2949–54.
128 Leung H, Wang JJ, Rochtchina E, et al. Relationships between age, blood pressure, and retinal vessel diameters in an older population. *Invest Ophthalmol Vis Sci* 2003; **44**: 2900–4.
129 Wong TY, Klein P, Couper DJ, et al. Retinal microvascular abnormalities and incident stroke: the Atherosclerosis Risk in Communities Study. *Lancet* 2004; **358**: 1134–40.
130 Kobayashi S, Okada K, Koide H, et al. Subcortical silent brain infarction as a risk factor for clinical stroke. *Stroke* 1997; **28**: 1932–9.
131 Wong TY, Klein R, Nieto F, et al. Retinal microvascular abnormalities and 10-year cardiovascular mortality: a population-based case-control study. *Ophthalmology* 2003; **110**: 933–40.
132 Michelson G, Wärntges S, Baleanu D, et al. Morphometric age-related evaluation of small retinal vessels by scanning laser Doppler flowmetry: determination of a vessel wall index. *Retina* 2007; **27**: 490–8.
133 Zarins CK, Weisenberg E, Kolettis G, et al. Differential enlargement of artery segments in response to enlarging atherosclerotic plaques. *J Vasc Surg* 1988; **7**: 386–94.
134 Nissen SE, Nicholls SJ, Sipahi I, et al; ASTEROID Investigators. Effect of very high-intensity statin therapy on regression of coronary atherosclerosis: the ASTEROID trial. *J Am Med Assoc* 2006; **295**: 1556–65.
135 Taguchi I, Oda K, Yoneda S, et al. Evaluation of serial changes in tissue characteristics during statin-induced plaque regression using virtual histology-intravascular ultrasound studies. *Am J Cardiol* 2013; **111**: 1246–52.
136 Céspedes EI, de Korte CL, van der Steen AF. Intraluminal ultrasonic palpation: assessment of local and cross-sectional tissue stiffness. *Ultrasound Med Biol* 2000; **26**: 385–96.

137 Bezerra HG, Costa MA, Guagliumi G, et al. Intracoronary optical coherence tomography: a comprehensive review. *JACC Cardiovasc Interven* 2009; **2**: 1035–46.

138 Jia H, Abtahian F, Aguirre AD, et al. *In vivo* diagnosis of plaque erosion and calcified nodule in patients with acute coronary syndrome by intravascular optical coherence tomography. *J Am Coll Cardiol* 2013; **62**: 1748–58.

139 Nahrendorf M, Jaffer FA, Kelly KA, et al. Noninvasive vascular cell adhesion molecule 1 imaging identifies inflammatory activation of cells in atherosclerosis. *Circulation* 2006; **114**: 1504–11.

140 Takumi T, Lee S, Hamasaki S, et al. Limitation of angiography to identify the culprit plaque in acute myocardial infarction with coronary total occlusion utility of coronary plaque temperature measurement to identify the culprit plaque. *J Am Coll Cardiol* 2007; **50**: 197–203.

141 Widlansky ME, Gokce N, Keaney JF Jr, et al. The clinical implications of endothelial dysfunction. *J Am Coll Cardiol* 2003; **42**: 1149–60.

142 Peters SA, den Ruijter HM, Bots ML. The incremental value of brachial flow-mediated dilation measurements in risk stratification for incident cardiovascular events: a systematic review. *Ann Med* 2012; **44**: 305–12.

143 Ras RT, Streppel MT, Draijer R, et al. Flow-mediated dilation and cardiovascular risk prediction: a systematic review with meta-analysis. *Int J Cardiol* 2013; **168**: 344–51.

144 Charakida M, Masi S, Luscher TF, et al. Assessment of atherosclerosis: the role of flow-mediated dilatation. *Eur Heart J* 2010; **31**: 2854–61.

145 Green DJ, Jones H, Thijssen D, et al. Flow-mediated dilation and cardiovascular event prediction: does nitric oxide matter? *Hypertension* 2011; **57**: 363–9.

146 Mancia G, de Backer G, Cifkova R, et al. Guidelines for the management of arterial hypertension: the Task Force for the Management of Arterial Hypertension of the European Society of Cardiology (ESC) and of the European Society of Hypertension (ESH). *J Hypertens* 2007; **25**: 1105–87.

147 Laurent S, Hayoz D, Trazzi S, et al. Isobaric compliance of the radial artery is increased in patients with essential hypertension. *J Hypertens* 1993; **11**: 89–98.

148 Laurent S, Cockcroft J, Van Bortel L, et al., for the European Network for Non-invasive Investigation of Large Arteries. Expert consensus document on arterial stiffness: methodological issues and clinical applications. *Eur Heart J* 2006; **27**: 2588–605.

149 Lakatta EG, Levy D. Arterial and cardiac aging: major shareholders in cardiovascular enterprises: Part I. *Circulation* 2003; **107**: 139–46.

150 Nilsson P, Boutouyrie P, Laurent S. Vascular aging: a tale of EVA and ADAM in cardiovascular risk assessment and prevention. *Hypertension* 2009; **54**: 3–10.

151 Van Bortel LM, Laurent S, Boutouyrie P, et al; Artery Society; European Society of Hypertension Working Group on Vascular Structure and Function; European Network for Noninvasive Investigation of Large Arteries. Expert consensus document on the measurement of aortic stiffness in daily practice using carotid-femoral pulse wave velocity. *J Hypertens* 2012; **30**: 445–8.

152 Bramwell JC, Hill AV. The velocity of the pulse wave in man. *Proc R Soc Lond B* 1922; **93**: 298–306.

153 Wilkinson IB, McEniery CM, Schillaci G, et al., on behalf of the ARTERY Society. ARTERY Society guidelines for validation of non-invasive haemodynamic measurement devices: part 1, arterial pulse wave velocity. *Artery Res* 2010; **4**: 34–40.

154 Mattace-Raso FU, van der Cammen TJ, Hofman A, et al. Arterial stiffness and risk of coronary heart disease and stroke: the Rotterdam Study. *Circulation* 2006; **113**: 657–63.

155 The Reference Values for Arterial Stiffness Collaboration. Determinants of pulse wave velocity in healthy people and in the presence of cardiovascular risk factors: establishing normal and reference values. *Eur Heart J* 2010; **31**: 2338–50.

156 Vlachopoulos C, Aznaouridis K, Stefanadis C. Prediction of cardiovascular events and all-cause mortality with arterial stiffness: a systematic review and meta-analysis. *J Am Coll Cardiol* 2010; **55**: 1318–27.

157 Diehm C, Schuster A, Allenberg JR, et al. High prevalence of peripheral arterial disease and co-morbidity in 6880 primary care patients: cross-sectional study. *Atherosclerosis* 2004; **172**: 95–105.

158 Fowkes GF and the Ankle Brachial Index Collaboration. Ankle brachial index combined with Framingham risk score to predict cardiovascular events and mortality: a meta-analysis. *J Am Med Assoc* 2008; **300**: 197–200.

159 Hiatt WR. Medical treatment of peripheral arterial disease and claudication. *N Engl J Med* 2001; **344**: 1608–21.

CHAPTER 7

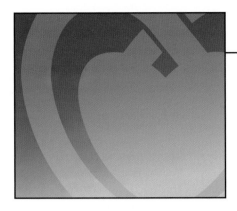

Primary prevention: principles and practice

Diego Vanuzzo and Simona Giampaoli

Contents

Summary

Cardiovascular primary prevention may be defined as a coordinated set of actions, at community and individual level, aimed at eradicating, eliminating, or compressing to later ages the impact of cardiovascular diseases and their related disability. It aims at healthy ageing. Cardiovascular epidemiology has elucidated the role of risk factors at individual and community level that predict the occurrence of heart attack and stroke in apparently healthy individuals and form the basis of strategies to reduce cardiovascular risk and subsequent diseases. There is now evidence that cardiovascular primary prevention works if three strategies are implemented together: (1) a population strategy (particularly through widespread adoption of healthy lifestyles, i.e. no smoking, a healthy diet, sufficient exercise, avoidance of overweight) that aims to keep everyone at low risk from infancy and reduce the cardiovascular risk profile of the whole community; (2) a strategy for individuals at high-risk, involving lifestyle changes and use of prophylactic evidence-based drugs if necessary; and (3) a strategy for individuals at intermediate risk who may benefit from non-invasive assessment of subclinical disease and end organ damage.

Introduction

What is cardiovascular primary prevention?

> 'It is better to be healthy than ill or dead. That is the beginning and the end of the only real argument for preventive medicine. It is sufficient' [1].

This concise and clear statement by Geoffrey Rose is still the best way to introduce the concept of primary prevention. Cardiovascular prevention as a whole may be defined, adapting Last's terminology [2], as a coordinated set of actions, at community and individual level, aimed at eradicating, eliminating, or minimizing the impact of cardiovascular diseases (CVD) and their related disability. In particular, cardiovascular primary prevention can be defined as the actions taken prior to the onset of CVD which remove the possibility that the disease will ever occur or at least delay its occurrence to older ages. More pragmatically the American Heart Association (AHA) considers CVD primary prevention as 'interventions designed to modify adverse levels of risk factors once present with the goal of preventing an initial CVD event' [3,4]. Cardiovascular primary prevention has had its basis in cardiovascular epidemiology and evidence-based medicine since the investigators in the Framingham Heart Study showed in 1961 that overtly healthy subjects with hypertension and hypercholesterolaemia were at higher risk of developing an acute myocardial infarction [5]. They coined the term 'coronary risk factors' [6]. There is evidence that unhealthy lifestyles are responsible for the levels of certain risk factors such as high blood pressure, lipids, and glucose [7,8]. In the following years other concepts have evolved in CVD prevention following the finding of the predictive value of coronary risk factors for other atherosclerotic diseases like stroke and peripheral artery disease [9], and so these factors are now termed 'cardiovascular risk factors'. Rose [1,10] proposed two complementary approaches to CVD prevention—a 'population strategy' and a strategy for 'high-risk' individuals—and Strasser [11] added the concept of 'primordial prevention' from the time of conception through early childhood and young adulthood to prevent the development of unhealthy lifestyles and related risk factors. More recently attention has been drawn to the positive long-term consequences of a favourable risk profile, and the value of maintaining a low cardiovascular risk at all ages, as proposed by Stamler et al. [12]. These concepts will be addressed and developed in this chapter, but the starting point is the real goal of CVD primary prevention—how to consider it in the wider context of prevention of non-communicable diseases (NCDs) and the conceptual framework which defines principles and practice.

Healthy ageing

One of the aims of CVD primary prevention is to contribute substantially to healthy ageing. Healthy ageing is a lifelong process that optimizes opportunities for improving and preserving health and physical, social, and mental wellbeing, independence, and quality of life and for enhancing successful life-course transitions [13]. CVD primary prevention can contribute to healthy ageing [14–19]. In 2005 Peel et al. [13] published a systematic review of the literature aimed at documenting the evidence for modifiable behavioural risk factors that predict healthy living in older cohorts. They found that determinants of healthy ageing included not smoking, being physically active, maintaining weight within normal ranges, and moderate alcohol consumption. It is noteworthy that the behavioural determinants of healthy ageing are cardiovascular risk factors amenable to primary prevention.

Gaining health

As many established risk factors for CVD are also predictive of some other NCDs, particularly type 2 diabetes, lung diseases, and common cancers, the concept of primary prevention of NCDs has emerged [20]. There are estimates that almost 60% of the disease burden in Europe, as measured by DALYs (disability-adjusted life years), is accounted for by seven leading risk factors: high blood pressure (12.8%); tobacco (12.3%); alcohol (10.1%); high blood cholesterol (8.7%); overweight (7.8%); low fruit and vegetable intake (4.4%); and physical inactivity (3.5%) [20]. Preventing and reducing these risk factors has the greatest potential for gain in health at a population and individual level.

A conceptual framework for CVD primary prevention

➲ Figure 7.1 illustrates a conceptual framework for CVD primary prevention [3,21]. It is known that unfavourable social and environmental conditions are directly linked to poor health [22], and to shared CVD/NCD risk factors like tobacco use, a diet high in fat, cholesterol, salt, and sugar, physical inactivity, and excessive alcohol intake. Social and economic health determinants are influenced by poverty, trade agreements, agriculture and transportation policies, capital flows, and activities of multinational companies. Agricultural subsidies and trade and capital market liberalization have contributed to reduce the prices and increase the availability of unhealthy products [23]. Although they are considered as 'causes of the causes' of CVD, the social and economic determinants of heart health call for political action which is mainly outside everyday clinical practice; however, physicians as a professional group can act through advocacy for primordial prevention.

Primary CVD prevention deals with healthy lifestyles and the control of risk factors at community and individual level. As already mentioned, many epidemiological and prevention studies have provided the scientific evidence base for effective preventive actions. The continuous relationship between levels of many risk factors and the risk of CVD is now widely accepted, to the extent that risk is now recognized as a continuum in the population [1]. Therefore those at high risk are considered an extreme of the distribution and definitions of high risk are generally arbitrary, though necessary for clinical intervention [1]. This approach, coupled with the observation that CVD risk factors cluster and interact multiplicatively to promote CVD risk [23], has led to the development of cardiovascular risk charts and scores [24–28] which recognize both the continuum of risk and the possibility that small elevations of many risk factors may confer a higher total CVD risk than a more marked increase of a single factor. From these considerations it is understandable that a large number of people at moderate risk may give rise to more cases of CVD than a small number of people at high risk, just because they are more of them [1]. Moreover there is a relationship between the population mean or median of a risk factor and the prevalence of high-risk subjects, as demonstrated in the INTERSALT study [29], and there is also a correlation between the average annual percentage change in CVD risk scores and the subsequent (4 years) percentage change in coronary-event rate, as shown in the MONICA study [30,31] (➲ Fig. 7.2). These data illustrate the rationale for combining a population and high-risk approach to CVD primary prevention, sustained over time to get lasting results.

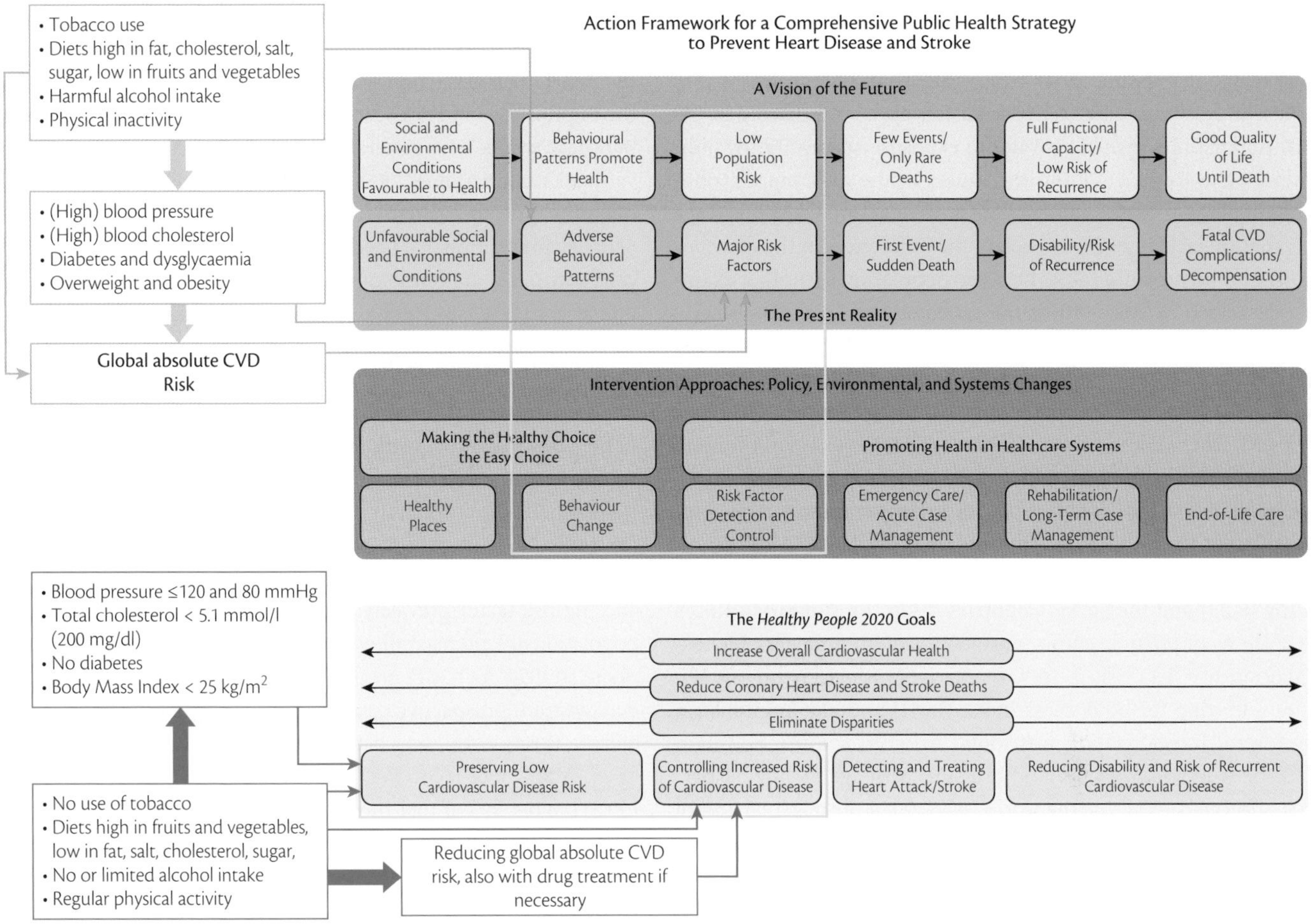

Fig. 7.1 A framework for cardiovascular primary prevention, at population and individual level. The areas covered by primary prevention are in the yellow frames. The lifestyles and risk factors conducive to high CVD risk and CVD occurrence are in the orange frames, and those maintaining a low CVD risk are in the green frames.

Modified from Weintraub W S et al. *Circulation* 2011; **124**: 967–990, and from Labarthe D et al. *Am J Prev Med* 2005; **29**(Suppl. 1): 146–151.

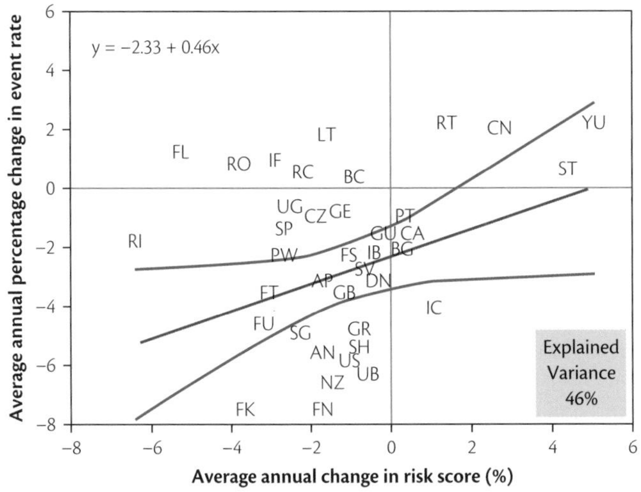

Fig. 7.2 The MONICA project. Regression of change in coronary-event rate on change in risk score. Lagged event period 4 years, men. The letter codes refer to the participating populations. For full details see <http://whqlibdoc.who.int/publications/2003/9241562234_p-i-xix.pdf>.

WHO MONICA Project; *Lancet* 2000: **355**: 675–687.

Principles of cardiovascular primary prevention

Strategies for cardiovascular primary prevention

In the abstract of his seminal paper 'Sick individuals and sick populations' [10], published in 1985, Rose assumes that the major determinants of population variation in a disease (the incidence rate) may not be the main cause of the disease. When evaluating the aetiological force of a given risk factor in individuals (the main focus of clinical medicine) the concept of relative risk is generally used, i.e. the risk in exposed individuals relative to the risk in non-exposed individuals; however, this may not be useful when considering community outcomes. For example, Rose investigated why some individuals have hypertension, and why some populations, like London civil servants [32], have a high frequency of hypertension and others, like Kenyan nomads [33], a low frequency. In the two settings the question of why some individuals have hypertension is the same, but looking at the blood pressure distributions, the proportion of people with hypertension, (e.g. a systolic blood pressure equal to or greater than 140 mmHg) is very different. So the causes of hypertension may be the same in the two populations (genetic variation, exposure susceptibility, individual behaviours, etc.), but the causes of the different distributions of blood pressure values could be diverse and widespread at a population level in order to explain the differences in the distribution of blood pressure values between populations. Another example described by Rose [10] is the distribution of total cholesterol observed in the Seven Countries study [7], which included the United States, former Yugoslavia, Japan, Finland, Italy, the Netherlands, and Greece. The distributions barely overlapped when east Finland, where coronary heart disease (CHD) was very common, was compared with Japan, where the incidence rate was low [34]. Here again the individual causes of hypercholesterolaemia may be different from those determining the prevalence in the populations. The two quoted observational studies, the INTERSALT study [8,29] and the Seven Countries study [7], supported Rose's hypothesis of possible community causes of an unfavourable distribution of CVD risk factors. In the INTERSALT study [8,29], after adjusting for body mass index (BMI) and alcohol intake, a significant linear relation was found between sodium excretion and the slope of systolic blood pressure with age for the 52 participating centres across the world ($b = 0.0034$ mmHg/year/mmol sodium; $p < 0.001$). In the Seven Countries study [7], Keys showed strong associations between population mean values for saturated fat intake versus serum cholesterol levels, and between population median values of cholesterol versus CHD mortality. Considering the population determinants of an unfavourable rightward shift in the population blood pressure and cholesterol distributions at an individual level, Rose suggested that genetic heterogeneity seems greater within than between populations, the opposite situation to that seen for environmental factors. Thus migrants tend to acquire the disease rates of their adopted country [10]. The two epidemiological approaches to aetiology, the individual and the population-based, have their counterparts in prevention. Rose [10] coined the terms and analysed the 'high-risk strategy' versus the 'population strategy'. The limited potential of the high-risk strategy for primary CVD prevention [10] derives from the weakness of predictive tools based on relative risk statistics to predict future disease for individuals as opposed to groups. Given the rightward distribution of risk factors in populations at major risk, 'a large number of people at a small risk may give rise to more cases of disease than the small number who are at a high risk' [10]. The major disadvantage of the population strategy is the so-called 'prevention paradox', i.e. 'a preventive measure which brings much benefit to the population [but] offers little to each participating individual' [10]. The majority of individuals in a population find this difficult to accept [10]:

> Mostly people act for substantial and immediate rewards, and the medical motivation for health education is inherently weak. Their health next year is not likely to be much better if they accept our advice or if they reject it. Much more powerful as motivators for health education are the social rewards of enhanced self esteem and social approval.

After 30 years Rose's words are still topical. From his original paper onward, volumes have been written on this subject, and the debate is still current. Recently some authors have evaluated the implications of Rose's strategies for CVD prevention [35–39], but these works were generally based on simulations from observational studies and yielded conflicting conclusions. To solve the dilemma, and to evaluate the evidence for the practice of CVD primary prevention, we need to consider two issues addressed recently by CVD epidemiology: the concepts of population-attributable risk (PAR) and global absolute CVD risk estimation.

Population-attributable risk

There are many definitions of PAR. It can be defined as an estimate of the proportion (or fraction) of the disease incidence which is attributable to the risk factor considered and which could be reduced if the modifiable and causal risk factor was eliminated. In prospective studies, PAR incorporates the relative risk conferred by the risk factor considered (generally the same in almost all the populations) and the risk factor prevalence (which can vary greatly in different populations). Understanding of the PAR can influence the appropriate strategy for CVD primary prevention, but it should only be derived from prospective cohort studies. These considerations may enlarge Rose's distinction between population and high-risk strategies. Many recent studies, in particular the MONICA project [30,31], have shown that the important distinction is not between the causes of incidence and the causes of cases—rather it is between the causes of incidence and the causes of population variation. In particular, a near-ubiquitous risk factor [e.g. high cholesterol of say ≥ 5.17 mmol/L (200 mg/dl)] can be an important cause of incidence in the population and of individual cases of disease, but may explain little of the population variation if it is considered alone, and, in this context, it may not be a useful means of identifying high-risk individuals within a particular population. These considerations have led to the concept of total or absolute CVD risk estimation as a tool for implementing comprehensive CVD primary prevention.

Total CVD risk estimation

It is now well known that atherosclerotic CVD is rarely the result of a single risk factor but is generally the final outcome of the combined effect of several risk factors. Specific tools are therefore necessary to evaluate the cumulative effect of the various combinations of risk factors, derived from longitudinal studies like the Framingham Study [24,28], the SCORE (Systematic COronary Risk Evaluation) study [26], or the CUORE study [40]. The absolute CVD risk represents the likelihood of developing CVD over a defined period of time, based on the values of several risk factors. This is discussed further in ➲ Chapter 5. Here it is important to underline that the availability of robust and easy to use tools of estimation of total CVD risk is fundamental not only in clinical practice but also for designing an appropriate primary prevention strategy directed at the whole population as well as people at intermediate and high risk. This was the experience of the Italian CUORE study [27,40]. ➲ Figure 7.3 shows the results obtained by reapplication of the CUORE risk score to participants in the CUORE study, after subdivision into CVD risk deciles. The dotted

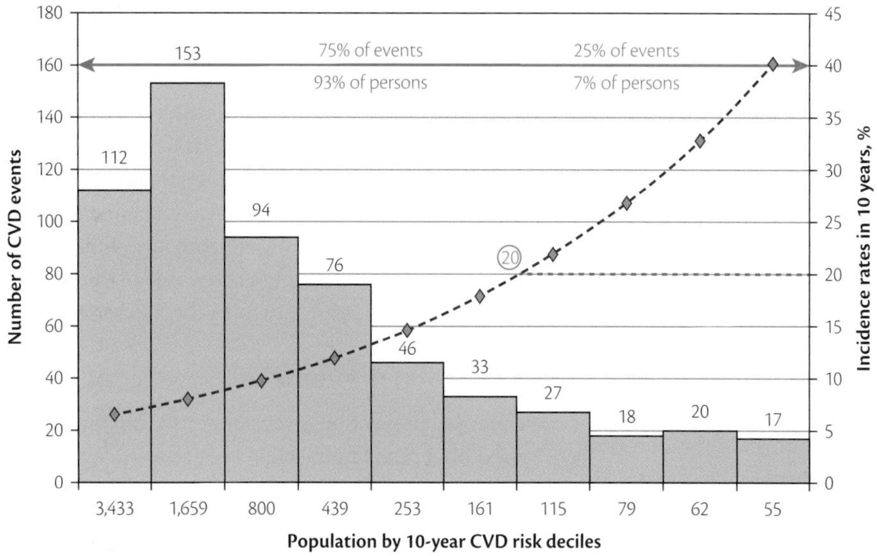

Fig. 7.3 Distribution of population and CVD events by 10-year CVD risk deciles for men aged 35–69 years in the Italian CUORE project. The bars represent the absolute number of men who had an incident CVD event in the risk decile (scale on left-hand axis). The dashed line, interpreted exponentially, indicates the percentage incident rate in 10 years for each decile (scale on right-hand axis). The line on the top of the figure refers to the contribution of high-risk subjects (7% with a CUORE risk ≥ 20%) to total events (25%) compared with subjects at a lesser risk.

line connects the mean decile incidence of disease, which is a measure of absolute risk. Men who are defined at high risk with a CUORE score of 20% or more in 10 years (which corresponds to 5% CVD mortality) represent 7% of the population and produce 25% of overall events. Seventy-five per cent of the events are therefore yielded by 93% of men at intermediate and low-risk. This pattern is more marked in women, where only 1% are at high risk, producing 4% of the events, while 99% are at intermediate and low risk, producing 96% of the events [40].

The CUORE study also evaluated the fate of individuals with a so-called favourable risk profile (or 'low-risk individuals'), with regard to both fatal and non-fatal CHD [41] and cerebrovascular disease (CBVD) events [42] as end-points. 'Low risk individuals' included people with all the following characteristics: total cholesterol < 5.17 mmol/L (< 200 mg/dl), systolic blood pressure (SBP) ≤ 120 mmHg, diastolic blood pressure (DBP) ≤ 80 mmHg, no antihypertensive medication, BMI < 25.0 kg/m^2, no diabetes, no smoking, i.e. favourable levels of all readily measured modifiable major CVD risk factors. 'Unfavourable but not high-risk individuals' included people with one or more of the following: total cholesterol 5.17–6.18 mmol/L (200–239 mg/dl), SBP 121–139 mmHg, DBP 81–89 mmHg (no antihypertensive medication), BMI 25.0–29.9 kg/m^2, no diabetes, no smoking. 'High-risk individuals' included people with one or more of the following: total cholesterol ≥ 6.19 mmol/L (≥ 240 mg/dl), SBP ≥ 140 mmHg, DBP ≥ 90 mmHg, need for antihypertensive medication, BMI ≥ 30.0 kg/m^2, diabetes, smoking. Only 3% of the cohort were low-risk at baseline, and they had virtually no CHD or CBVD in the following 10 years. The rates for unfavourable but not high-risk individuals (17% of the CUORE cohort) and high-risk individuals (80% of the cohort) were higher and with a graded increase to one, two, and three or more risk factors, as shown in ➲ Fig. 7.4.

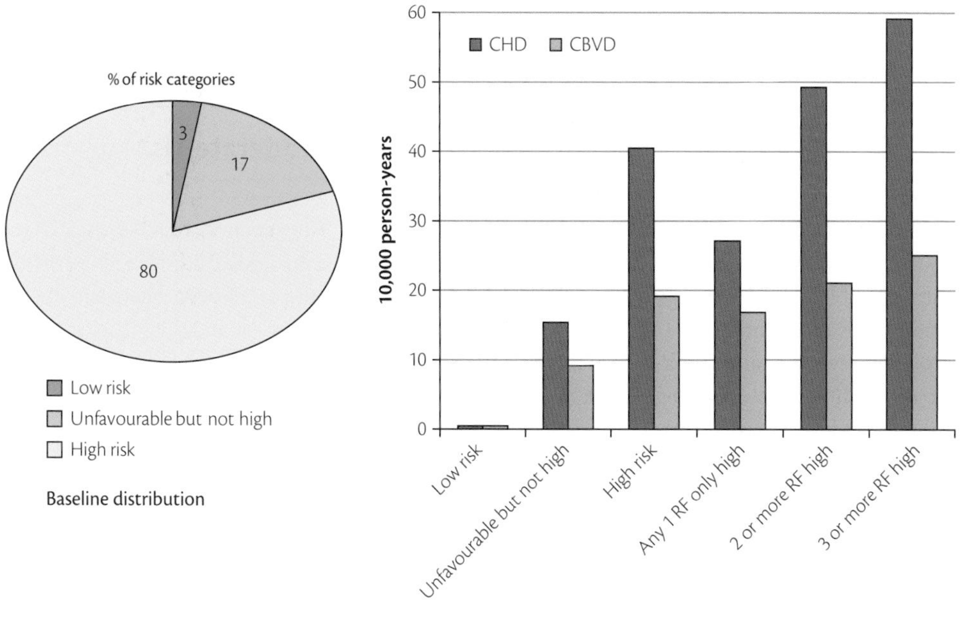

Fig. 7.4 Ten-year incidence of coronary heart disease (CHD) and cerebrovascular disease (CBVD) in low-risk individuals versus unfavourable and high-risk individuals, and baseline distribution, in the Italian CUORE study (sex-averaged, age-adjusted rate per 10 000 person-years, men and women combined; RF, risk factor).

Considering the risk distribution of the CUORE score, and applying to the same cohort Stamler et al.'s [12] definitions of low risk, unfavourable but not high risk, and high risk, it is evident that to achieve effective CVD primary prevention both a population and high-risk strategy need to be implemented simultaneously, with particular focus on maintaining at low risk those individuals with that profile.

Community heart health promotion

Since the 1970s many community programmes have been launched to prevent CVD, in particular the North Karelia project [43], which began in Finland in 1972. In 1974 the European Office of the WHO initiated the Comprehensive Cardiovascular Community Control Programmes (CCCCP) to expand this experience, enrolling nine European countries [44]. In the 1980s CCCCP evolved into the Countrywide Integrated Noncommunicable Disease Prevention Program (CINDI), with the aim of enlarging the community programme to other chronic diseases sharing the same risk factors [45]. These experiences were used in developing the WHO strategy to prevent and control NCDs [46]. In the United States three major demonstration programmes were started in the 1980s: the Stanford Five-City Project [47], the Minnesota Heart Health Program [48], and the Pawtucket Heart Health Program [49]. Many of those programmes were able to reduce CVD risk and some also reduced CVD incidence or mortality. In 2010 a systematic review was published evaluating 36 relevant community programmes conducted between 1970 and 2008 [50]. These programmes were multifaceted interventions employing combinations of media, screening, counselling activities, and environmental changes and were primarily evaluated using controlled before–after studies. Twelve studies reported changes in CVD/total mortality rates and they all showed a reduction, but were largely non-significant. In 22 studies, investigators reported changes in physiological CVD risk factors, and there was a positive trend in the total CVD risk score. The average net reduction in 10-year CVD risk was 0.65%. The discrepancy of results among these studies can be explained by the so-called 'community preventive dose': because most of the projects in larger communities had only very limited resources, and were restricted to educational and health service-based interventions over a number of years, the dose of the intervention was therefore small. An exception was the North Karelia Project [43], which was perhaps the most 'community based', i.e. it broadly influenced the physical and social environment of the community. A public health strategy was developed to reduce the population levels of the main CVD risk factors (elevated serum cholesterol, hypertension, and smoking). Great emphasis was put on promoting cholesterol-lowering dietary changes. A comprehensive community-level approach was adopted, involving health and other services, voluntary organizations, local media, businesses, and public policy. The high-risk approach was also implemented, but much of the high-risk strategy was implemented by dietary and other lifestyle changes, not just the use of drugs [51]. It is easier for a high-risk subject to comply with a healthier lifestyle if his/her family and social network share the same health values and behaviours. In this context we can conclude that integrated primary CVD prevention works and extends its effects to other NCDs as demonstrated in North Karelia, where at the end of the 1960s not only CHD mortality rates but also lung cancer mortality rates were higher than in the rest of Finland. When the North Karelia Project was extended to the whole of Finland in 1977, these gaps in CHD and lung cancer mortality virtually disappeared even though the whole of Finland experienced a declining trend in mortality from these diseases [52].

Primordial prevention

Primordial prevention, a term first used by Strasser [11], was conceived on a population-wide basis as a strategy to prevent whole societies from experiencing epidemics of the risk factors causing disease. The corresponding strategy at the individual level is to prevent the development of risk factors in the first place. The concept of promoting healthy behaviours for this purpose is well recognized and common to many guidelines and recommendations for CVD prevention, especially those that focus on actions during pregnancy and in childhood and adolescence [53]. The 'low risk' evaluation, discussed previously forms the scientific basis for endorsing this strategy, which should be offered to all children and adolescents.

High-risk primary prevention

Primary CVD prevention seeks to identify individuals at high risk for cardiovascular events through screening and the use of CVD risk assessment tools, and target them for additional evaluation, stratification, and intensive educational and drug treatments. Guidelines [54,55] concentrate on maximizing the use of these steps to produce the greatest reduction in clinical events and increases in quality of life and survival. Throughout the past four decades, the increasing expansion of this high-risk approach has been rewarding. In the United States it was estimated that for every 10% rise in treatments for elevated LDL-cholesterol in people younger than 80 years, approximately 8000 deaths could be prevented annually, and for a 10% rise in hypertension treatment, about 14 000 deaths per annum would be averted [56].

Intermediate-risk (or moderate-risk) primary prevention

Using CVD risk evaluation tools such as SCORE and CUORE [26,40] individuals with a SCORE risk ≥ 1 and $< 5\%$ at 10 years or a CUORE risk ≥ 5 and $< 20\%$ at 10 years represent the large majority of the population (➲ Figs 7.3 and 7.4). The first issue is the identification of those individuals at intermediate or moderate risk, and here the role of primary care is of paramount importance. General practitioners, occupational medicine specialists, general practice nurses, community nurses, pharmacists, and transfusion-centre personnel may use the CVD risk prediction tools routinely with every subject or patient they meet, but the barriers to this fundamental health approach are many and difficult to overcome [54]. Secondly, this strategy is largely based on lifestyle education (non-smoking, regular physical activity, a diet rich in vegetables, fruit, and fish, a low intake of fat, cholesterol and refined sugars, and correction of overweight if present) and primary care professionals must learn and practice these skills to reduce the CVD risk effectively. Thirdly, in resistant cases prophylactic therapy, especially with statins, antihypertensive drugs, or metformin may be considered. In these cases the issue of risk reclassification may be important, and is addressed in ➲ Chapter 5. In both the European [54] and American [55] guidelines other investigations are proposed in this group of individuals: measurement of carotid intima–media thickness and/or screening for atherosclerotic plaques by carotid artery scanning, measurement of ankle–brachial index (ABI), and computed tomography for coronary calcium, but there is conflicting evidence and divergence of opinion, especially regarding the measurement of coronary calcium. The big effort being made to reduce moderate risk through healthy lifestyles is certainly worthwhile, given the expected rise of mass disability from CVD in the coming decades [54], and, in particular, the increasing trends in obesity, which is becoming a worldwide epidemic in both children and adults [54].

Evidence of the effectiveness of CVD primary prevention

There are important randomized controlled trials documenting the effectiveness of CVD primary prevention in the adult population. In particular the MRFIT study [57], the Goteborg trial [58], the Oslo trial [59], and the WHO collaborative group trial [60], including the Belgian heart disease prevention project [61], have yielded some conflicting results. However, Kornitzer and De Backer [62] were able to demonstrate a correlation between the net difference in CV risk profile between the intervention and control groups and the net difference in coronary mortality (see ➲ Fig. 7.5), confirming that a difference in incident cases of CHD between intervention and control groups can only be expected to the extent that a difference in CV risk profile has been achieved.

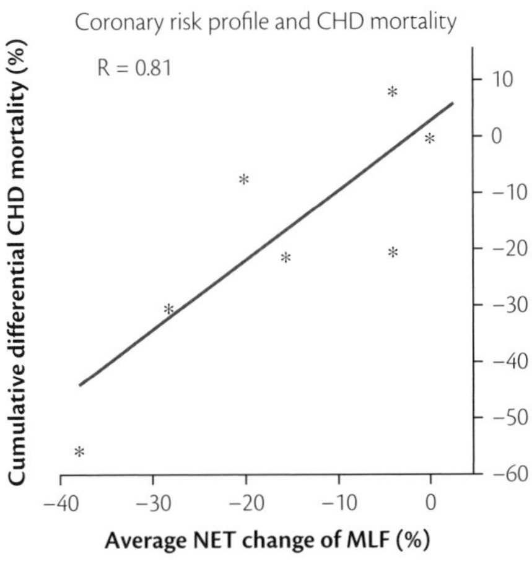

Fig. 7.5 Relation between the net difference in CV risk profile (MLF) and the net difference in coronary mortality in the Oslo trial, the Gothenburg trial, MRFIT, and the WHO European Collaborative Group Trial.
Modified from Kornitzer M, De Backer G. *Acta Clin Belg* 1986; **41**: 79–82.

Cardiovascular primary prevention in practice

Now we have considered the principles of CVD primary prevention it is easier to understand the various and integrated practices for its implementation.

Population-level changes to promote a healthy lifestyle

In May 2012, Jørgensen and collaborators [63] published a position paper on behalf of the Prevention, Epidemiology, and Population Science (PEP) section of the European Association for Cardiovascular Prevention and Rehabilitation, a constituent body of the European Society of Cardiology (ESC). The paper summarizes the best available scientific evidence for the effect of population-level changes on risk factors for CVD. The recommendations address the established risk factors for CVD, and are valid for some other NCDs that share the same risk factors, particularly type 2 diabetes, lung diseases, and common cancers. The focus is on unhealthy nutrition, smoking, physical inactivity, and excessive alcohol, which all can be modified through population-based strategies. The main conclusions and recommendations are shown in ➲ Table 7.1.

Table 7.1 Population-level changes to prevent CVD: main conclusions and recommendations

- CVD causes more than 4.3 million deaths per year in Europe and costs at least €190 billion
- Important modifiable risk factors for CVD (unhealthy diet, smoking, alcohol, and physical inactivity) all respond to structural changes in society
- Population-level interventions aim at small changes in the whole population, which can have a higher impact on overall CVD burden than changes among high-risk individuals
- Responsibility for structural changes should be shared between politicians, administrative authorities, and health professionals. Changes should be at international, national, and local levels
- Healthy dietary habits will be supported by changes in agricultural policies, tax on products with free sugar and saturated fat and subsidies for fruit and vegetables, reduction of salt and trans-fatty acids in processed foods, clear labelling of foods, and limiting advertising for junk food
- Completely smoke-free environments are the only way to protect non-smokers. Smoking and second-hand smoking can be regulated by taxation, restrictions in sale and use, banning advertising, plain packaging, and warning labels
- Physical activities should be integrated into daily life by subsidies to public transport and reallocating of road space to cycle and footpath lanes. Changes in schools, worksites, and the built environment can make physical activity a more natural part of daily life
- Alcohol intake can be reduced by taxation, low availability, regulation of advertising, and low social and legal tolerance of drink driving
- It is estimated that such population-level changes can halve CVD mortality rates
- In a complex, modern society there is an interaction between personal choices, production, and marketing. To secure a real free choice for citizens, health authorities need to ensure healthy defaults, thus balancing the vested interests of corporations, who are not responsible for public health

Source data from Jørgensen T, Capewell S, Prescott E, Allender S, Sans S, Zdrojewski T, De Bacquer D, de Sutter J, Franco OH, Løgstrup S, Volpe M, Malyutina S, Marques-Vidal P, Reiner Z, Tell GS, Verschuren WM, Vanuzzo D. Population-level changes to promote cardiovascular health. *Eur J Prev Cardiol*. 2013; **20**: 409–21.

All health professionals who practise CVD primary prevention should be aware of the enormous potential of promoting and encouraging healthy lifestyles. They can act in several ways.

1. Advocating, through their professional and scientific associations, for the legislative adoption of effective population structural changes promoting health. The ESC acted in this way, participating in the launch of the European Heart Health Charter at the European Parliament in Brussels, on 12 June 2007 [64,65] and promoting the European Chronic Disease Alliance which includes ten medical organizations covering diabetes, respiratory diseases, and cancer, representing over 100 000 health professionals [66].
2. Promoting healthy lifestyles in the four areas mentioned (smoking, nutrition, alcohol, physical activity) in all the subjects and patients they meet in their practice. Among doctors, evidence of a sizeable effect exists for smoking [67] and alcohol [68], but for the other areas the evidence is scantier [69]. Similar evidence exists for nurses, in whom their intervention in smoking cessation was found to be effective [70], but results on weight control were more controversial [71]. To be effective at community level, behavioural counselling practices need to be adopted and administered by the majority of health professionals, after effective training, as the experience on smoking cessation demonstrates [72].
3. Personally engaging in healthy lifestyles to familiarize themselves with the issues involved in maintaining lifelong healthy behaviours and to set a positive example for patients and the community. This was particularly underlined for physical activity and smoking [73].

Maintaining low-risk individuals throughout their life (primordial prevention)

Primordial CVD prevention must involve the maintenance of individual behavioural and lifestyle characteristics that achieve a level of health that prevents lifestyle-related risk factors from developing. The American Heart Association (AHA) incorporated the powerful principle of primordial prevention in defining 'ideal cardiovascular health' as part of the goal of reducing cardiac and stroke mortality by 20% by 2020 [74]. Ideal cardiovascular health consists of the absence of cardiovascular disease, a healthy lifestyle (sufficient exercise, a superior diet score, absence of smoking, and BMI < 25 kg/m²), and ideal health factors (untreated normal values of blood pressure, cholesterol, and fasting glucose). These parameters, termed Life's Simple 7™, are presented on an AHA educational website (<http://mylifecheck.heart.org/>), which promotes primordial prevention. The European guidelines on cardiovascular disease prevention in clinical practice (version 2012) [54], endorsing the European Heart Health Charter [64], define the characteristics of people who tend to stay healthy. The two profiles are shown in ➲ Table 7.2.

The similarity is evident, apart from one notable exception concerning blood pressure and cholesterol levels and some differences in the diet—stricter in the AHA formulation which explicitly proposes a DASH (dietary approaches to stop hypertension)-type eating plan [75]. Concerning the major risk factors, the AHA proposal is the same as that defining Stamler's [12] low-risk category. The AHA document [74] also defines ideal cardiovascular health for children, and this is important because in many countries paediatricians care for children and can act specifically in the childhood setting to promote primordial and primary prevention [76].

Table 7.2 Ideal cardiovascular health as defined by the American Heart Association and the European Society of Cardiology and other societies endorsing the 2012 CVD prevention guidelines

American Heart Association's Life's Simple 7™	European Heart Health Charter and 2012 guidelines
1. Not smoking or quitting over 1 year ago.	No use of tobacco
2. A body mass index < 25 kg/m²	No overweight (normal BMI 18.5–24.9 kg/m²)
3. Exercising at a moderate intensity ≥ 150 min (or 75 min at vigorous intensity) each week	Adequate physical activity: at least 30 min five times a week
4. Eating a 'healthy diet': adhering to four to five important dietary components (for a 2000 kcal daily diet, to be adapted): ◆ 4.5 cups or more of fruits and vegetables/day ◆ three or more 1-oz (31 g) servings of fibre-rich wholegrains/day (≥ 1.1 g of fibre per 10 g of carbohydrate) ◆ two or more 3.5-oz (109 g) servings of oily fish/week ◆ sodium intake < 1.5 g/day (= salt 4 g/day) ◆ sugar-sweetened beverage intake ≤ 450 kcal (36 oz, 1 litre) weekly Secondary dietary components are the following: ◆ nuts, legumes, and seeds: ≥ 4 servings/week ◆ processed meats: none or ≤ 2 servings/week ◆ saturated fat: < 7% of total energy intake	Healthy eating habits: ◆ saturated fatty acids to account for < 10% of total energy intake, through replacement by polyunsaturated fatty acids ◆ trans-unsaturated fatty acids: as little as possible, preferably no intake from processed food, and < 1% of total energy intake from natural origin ◆ < 5 g of salt per day (= 2 g of sodium) ◆ 30–45 g of fibre per day, from wholegrain products, fruits, and vegetables ◆ 200 g of fruit per day (2–3 servings) ◆ 200 g of vegetables per day (2–3 servings) ◆ fish at least twice a week, one of which to be oily fish ◆ consumption of alcoholic beverages should be limited to two glasses per day (20 g/day of alcohol) for men and one glass per day (10 g/day of alcohol) for women
5. Maintaining total cholesterol < 200 mg/dl (5.17 mmol/L)	Blood cholesterol below 5 mmol/L (190 mg/dl)
6. Keeping blood pressure < 120/80 mmHg	Blood pressure below 140/90 mmHg
7. Keeping fasting plasma glucose < 100 mg/dl (5.5 mmol/L)	Normal glucose metabolism [fasting plasma glucose < 5.6 mmol/L (100 mg/dl)]
	Avoidance of excessive stress

Source data from Perk J, De Backer G, et al. European Guidelines on cardiovascular disease prevention in clinical practice (version 2012). *Eur Heart J* 2012; **33**: 1635–1701, Lloyd-Jones DM, Hong Y, Labarthe D, et al. and American Heart Association Strategic Planning Task Force and Statistics Committee. Defining and Setting National Goals for Cardiovascular Health Promotion and Disease Reduction: The American Heart Association's Strategic Impact Goal Through 2020 and Beyond. *Circulation* 2010; **121**: 586–613.

Reducing the risk of intermediate-risk individuals

The practice of this strategy is perhaps one of the most difficult, because it requires the active involvement of health personnel, especially in the primary care setting, necessitating a reorganization of their work in order to follow some fundamental procedures [77], described in ➲ Table 7.3. Reorienting the health system and practices to carry out effective CVD primary prevention, though very important, has many barriers (➲ Table 7.3), as evaluated in various studies quoted in the 2012 European guidelines [54] and in other reviews [77].

Table 7.3 Primary CVD prevention: steps to identify and treat subjects at moderate and high risk in primary care

Steps	Actions	Barriers
1 Identifying subjects at risk	Risk factor screening including the lipid profile may be considered in adult men aged 40 or more and in women aged 50 or more or post-menopausal. The physician in general practice is the key person to initiate, coordinate, and provide long-term follow-up for CVD prevention	Health system: ◆ limited reimbursement ◆ increased liability ◆ inadequate staffing resource ◆ lack of specialist support ◆ budgetary concerns
2 Estimating CVD risk	High-risk subjects with any of the following: ◆ markedly elevated single risk factors such as familial dyslipidaemias and severe hypertension ◆ diabetes mellitus (type 1 or type 2) but without CV risk factors or target organ damage ◆ moderate chronic kidney disease (GFR 30–59 ml/min/1.73 m^2) ◆ A calculated SCORE of ≥ 5% and < 10% for 10-year risk of fatal CVD Moderate risk: subjects are considered to be at moderate risk when their SCORE is ≥ 1 and < 5% at 10 years	Health personnel: ◆ risk scoring is considered to be time consuming, simplifying a complex situation, and may result in overmedication
3 Evaluating lifestyles	This is a neglected issue, but simple evaluations according to the guidelines may give a quick reliable assessment, also useful for the intervention. For example, one question for smoking, one question for alcohol, five questions for diet, one question for physical activity may be enough and take 3–5 minutes	Health personnel: ◆ this activity is perceived as time-consuming and substantially useless, given the difficulties of changing behaviours for the evaluated subjects Subjects/patients: ◆ lifestyle questions perceived as too intrusive
3 Helping subjects (patients) to understand their personal risk	Providing patients with their CVD risk score is a useful means of motivating patients towards healthy behaviours. As a guide, physicians might wish to consider the following areas for communication with their patients: ◆ probability: focus on the relative risk faced by that particular patient ◆ exposure: communicate that everyone faces the risk of CVD ◆ hazard: emphasize the modifiable risk factors the patient can control ◆ create a mental picture of CVD events, without creating fear, because this can influence whether a patient takes prescribed medications	Health personnel: ◆ not trained in a difficult skill ◆ time constraints Subjects/patients: ◆ poor understanding/ awareness of personal disease risk
4 Developing a comprehensive management strategy for the individual subject (patient)	An effective management strategy for CVD should contain elements of lifestyle modification as well as pharmaceutical intervention, where appropriate As a first step in the management of their overall CVD risk, patients should be encouraged to adhere to healthy lifestyle habits. They should be informed of the benefits of smoking cessation, exercise, diet modification, and weight loss. In many subjects at moderate-risk, this may be sufficient In high-risk subjects, where lifestyle changes are insufficient, therapy is advised. This should include a range of interventions such as treatment of hypertension, dyslipidaemia, and diabetes It is important that the physician and patient closely collaborate to develop a management strategy that will suit the individual patient. It is also important to reiterate the need for adherence to both lifestyle changes and medications	Health personnel: ◆ not trained ◆ lack of critical evaluation of guidelines/confusion or lack of belief in contradictory guidelines ◆ time constraints ◆ aversion to polypharmacy ◆ inertia to changing medical practice Subjects/patients ◆ poor long-term adherence to lifestyle changes and poor adherence with CV risk-reducing medications ◆ aversion to polypharmacy ◆ lack of compliance ◆ side effects of medications ◆ cost of medications if not reimbursed
5 Providing continuous follow-up support	The aims of patient follow-up support should be to assess and communicate to the patient the success of intervention strategies in order to ◆ maintain patient motivation ◆ identify problems in adherence to the disease management strategy (there is a very real difference between obtaining a prescription for a medication and actually taking it) ◆ provide further disease/therapy information	

GFR, glomerular filtration rate.

Source data from Perk J, De Backer G, et al. European Guidelines on cardiovascular disease prevention in clinical practice (version 2012). *Eur Heart J* 2012; **33**: 1635–1701 and Erhardt L, Moller R, Puig JG. Comprehensive cardiovascular risk management—what does it mean in practice? *Vasc Health Risk Manag* 2007; **3**(5): 587–603.

One of the major barriers is the need for specific training of general practitioners and other primary care personnel to acquire the skills needed to evaluate global CVD risk and lifestyles, to communicate risk results to the subjects/patients, and organize behavioural counselling and follow-up programmes. In Italy we demonstrated that it is possible to launch initiatives to overcome these potential barriers [78,79]. The Italian national prevention plan 2005–2013 included a 10-year CVD risk assessment of the general population aged 35–69 years using the CUORE risk score [78]. Through the regional health authorities, general practitioners (GPs) were trained to assess global cardiovascular risk and encouraged to collect data on risk factors and the CUORE score in their patients and to contribute to the Cardiovascular Risk Observatory (CRO). Data were collected using cuore.exe software, easily and freely downloadable by GPs from the CUORE project website (<http://www.cuore.iss.it/>). From January 2007 to May 2010, 2858 GPs downloaded cuore.exe and 139 269 risk assessments on 117 345 people were sent to the CRO. Among those with at least two risk assessments, 8% (95% CI 7–9%) shifted to a lower risk class after 1 year. Although these are good results, there are about 46 000 Italian GPs and only 6% participated in the CRO project. The REACHOUT study [80] in nine European countries, enrolling 1103 patients, yielded similar results, while the cross-sectional EURIKA study [81], conducted in 12 European countries, showed that in Europe a large proportion of patients in primary prevention had CVD risk factors that remained uncontrolled, and lifestyle counselling was not well implemented.

Reducing the risk of high-risk individuals

At the primary care level the steps considered for moderate-risk individuals are the same for high-risk subjects (➲ Table 7.3). This practice, together with the possible further investigation of some categories of moderate-risk subjects, for example those with positive family history of premature CVD, can also rely on cardiologists, especially if working out of hospital [54] or in CVD prevention centres or in cardiac rehabilitation units. According to the 2012 European guidelines [54], those cardiologists have an essential role in CVD prevention, acting as consultants to general practitioners and general internists. They may serve as advisors in cases where there is uncertainty over the use of preventive medications or when the usual preventive options are difficult to apply (e.g. nicotine addiction, resistant obesity, side effects or insufficient efficacy of medication). A complete examination by a preventive cardiologist will often include an assessment of exercise capacity with stress testing, measurement of the ABI, echocardiographic evaluation, in particular to detect left ventricular hypertrophy, and assessment of pre-clinical atherosclerosis by vascular ultrasound at various sites (carotid, vertebral, and subclavian arteries, abdominal aorta and iliac arteries, arteries of the lower limbs). If some of these tests performed in asymptomatic subjects identify some pre-clinical condition, many patients with apparently low risk will experience a profound change in perception of their risk [54]. However, it should be noted that, at least in smokers, the communication of formerly unknown asymptomatic atherosclerosis did not alter the rate of quitting at 12 months [82]. Therefore cardiologists must also learn the basic skills for motivating the patients referred to them to better adhere to healthy lifestyles and drug treatment driven by their specialist assessment.

Conclusion

After considering the principles and practice of CVD primary prevention, a couple of basic questions remain: does CVD primary prevention work in the long run, and does it make a substantial contribution to the global reduction of CVD mortality compared with secondary prevention?

The answer is yes to both questions, based on two very important studies, the MONICA study [30,31,83,84] and the IMPACT study, both undertaken across many countries [85,86]. According to MONICA data, in men CHD mortality rates decreased in 25 populations and increased in 11 populations; in women CHD mortality rates decreased in 22 populations and increased in 13 populations. The MONICA project demonstrated the substantial contribution of both decreased incidence and increased survival and changes in the prevalence of risk factors to the declining trend of mortality: one-third of the decline in mortality was explained by changes in case fatality rates related to advancements in coronary care and two-thirds by declining incidence of coronary events partly explained by the reduction of classical risk factors [30,31,83,84].

Using information on changes in coronary risk factors and the effects of treatments, as estimated from the results of randomized controlled trials, the IMPACT model [85] estimates the expected influences on CHD mortality by age and gender. This study is considered in detail in ➲ Chapter 1, but here it is important to note that the IMPACT model was tested in different countries and gave similar results [86]. Beneficial reductions in major risk factors—in particular smoking, blood pressure, and cholesterol—at the population level accounted for 50–75% of the decrease in CHD deaths, although these favourable trends were counteracted by an increase in the prevalence of obesity and type 2 diabetes. Twenty-five to 50% of the decline in CHD death rates was attributed to treatments (antihypertensive drugs and statins) for patients at high risk or in secondary prevention, and to better treatments of acute myocardial infarction, heart failure, and other cardiac conditions.

In the continuum of CVD prevention, from primordial prevention to secondary prevention and rehabilitation, primary CVD prevention is playing the major role in the decline in CVD mortality in many populations. However, its potential is much greater—through also reducing non-fatal CVD events and premature and late disability, and therefore ensuring healthy ageing for the majority of people.

Further reading

Intersalt Cooperative Research Group. Intersalt: an international study of electrolyte excretion and blood pressure. Results for 24 hour urinary sodium and potassium excretion. *Br Med J* 1988; **297**: 319–28.

Jørgensen T, Capewell S, Prescott E, et al. Population-level changes to promote cardiovascular health. *Eur J Prev Cardiol* 2013; **20**: 409–21.

Keys A, Aravanis C, Blackburn H, et al. *Seven countries. A multivariate analysis of death and coronary heart disease*, 1980. Cambridge, MA: Harvard University Press.

Kuulasmaa K, Tunstall-Pedoe H, Dobson A, et al. Estimation of contribution of changes in classic risk factors to trends in coronary-event rates across the WHO MONICA project populations. *Lancet* 2000; **355**: 675–87.

Lloyd-Jones DM, Hong Y, Labarthe D, et al. American Heart Association Strategic Planning Task Force and Statistics Committee. Defining and setting national goals for cardiovascular health promotion and disease reduction: The American Heart Association's strategic impact goal through 2020 and beyond. *Circulation* 2010; **121**: 586–613.

Palmieri L, Donfrancesco C, Giampaoli S, et al. Favorable cardiovascular risk profile and 10-year coronary heart disease incidence in women and men: results from the Progetto CUORE. *Eur J Cardiovasc Prev Rehabil* 2006; **13**: 562–70.

Rose G. Sick individuals and sick populations. *Int J Epidemiol* 1985; **14**: 32–8.

Rose G. *Rose's strategy of preventive medicine* [with commentary by Kay-Tee Khaw and Michael Marmot], 2008. Oxford: Oxford University Press.

Stamler J, Neaton JD, Garside DB, et al. Current status: six established major risk factors—and low risk. In: Marmot M, Elliott P (eds) *Coronary heart disease epidemiology: from aetiology to public health*, 2005, pp. 46–54. Oxford: Oxford University Press.

Weintraub WS, Daniels SR, Burke LE, et al. on behalf of the American Heart Association Advocacy Coordinating Committee. Value of primordial and primary prevention for cardiovascular disease: a policy statement from the American Heart Association. *Circulation* 2011; **124**: 967–90.

References

1 Rose G. *Rose's strategy of preventive medicine* [with commentary by Kay-Tee Khaw and Michael Marmot], 2008. Oxford: Oxford University Press.

2 Last JM (ed.) *A dictionary of epidemiology*, 4th edn, 2001. New York: Oxford University Press.

3 Weintraub WS, Daniels SR, Burke LE, et al. on behalf of the American Heart Association Advocacy Coordinating Committee. Value of primordial and primary prevention for cardiovascular disease: a policy statement from the American Heart Association. *Circulation* 2011; **124**: 967–90.

4 Kavey RE, Daniels SR, Lauer RM, et al. American Heart Association guidelines for primary prevention of atherosclerotic cardiovascular disease beginning in childhood. *Circulation* 2003; **107**: 1562–6.

5 Kannel WB, Dawber TR, Kagan A, et al. Factors of risk in the development of coronary heart disease—six-year follow-up experience. The Framingham Study. *Ann Intern Med* 1961; **55**: 33–50.

6 Braunwald E. The rise of cardiovascular medicine. *Eur Heart J* 2012; **33**: 838–45.

7 Keys A, Aravanis C, Blackburn H, et al. *Seven countries. A multivariate analysis of death and coronary heart disease*, 1980. Cambridge, MA: Harvard University Press.

8 Intersalt Cooperative Research Group. Intersalt: an international study of electrolyte excretion and blood pressure. Results for 24 hour urinary sodium and potassium excretion. *Br Med J* 1988; **297**: 319–28.

9 Kannel WB. An overview of the risk factors for cardiovascular disease. In: Kaplan NM, Stamler J (eds) *Prevention of coronary heart disease*, 1983, pp. 1–19. Philadelphia, PA: WB Saunders.

10 Rose G. Sick individuals and sick populations. *Int J Epidemiol* 1985; **14**: 32–8.

11 Strasser T. Reflections on cardiovascular diseases. *Interdiscip Sci Rev* 1978; **3**: 225–30.

12 Stamler J, Neaton JD, Garside DB, et al. Current status: six established major risk factors—and low risk. In: Marmot M, Elliott P (eds) *Coronary heart disease epidemiology: from aetiology to public health*, 2005, pp. 46–54, Oxford: Oxford University Press.

13 Peel NM, McClure RJ, Bartlett HP. Behavioral determinants of healthy aging. *Am J Prev Med* 2005; **28**: 298–304.

14 Burke GL, Arnold AM, Bild DE, et al. for the CHS Collaborative Research Group. Factors associated with healthy aging: the Cardiovascular Health Study. *J Am Geriatr Soc* 2001; **49**: 254–62.

15 Haveman-Nies A, de Groot LC, van Staveren WA. Dietary quality, lifestyle factors and healthy ageing in Europe: the SENECA study. *Age Ageing* 2003; **32**: 427–34.

16 Vita AJ, Terry RB, Hubert HB, et al. Aging, health risks, and cumulative disability. *N Engl J Med* 1998; **338**: 1035–41.

17 Daviglus ML, Liu K, Pirzada A, et al. Favorable cardiovascular risk profile in middle age and health-related quality of life in older age. *Arch Intern Med* 2003; **163**: 2460–8.

18 Stamler J, Stamler R, Neaton JD, et al. Low-risk factor profile and long-term cardiovascular and noncardiovascular mortality and life expectancy: findings for 5 large cohorts of young adult and middle-aged men and women. *J Am Med Assoc* 1999; **282**: 2012–18.

19 Daviglus ML, Liu K, Greenland P, et al. Benefit of a favorable cardiovascular risk factor profile in middle age with respect to Medicare costs. *N Engl J Med* 1998; **339**: 1122–9.

20 WHO Europe. *Gaining health. The European Strategy for the Prevention and Control of Noncommunicable Diseases*, 2006. Copenhagen: WHO Regional Office for Europe.

21 Labarthe DR, Biggers A, Goff DC, Jr, et al. Translating a plan into action: a public health action plan to prevent heart disease and stroke. *Am J Prev Med* 2005; **29** (Suppl. 1): 146–51.

22 Commission on Social Determinants of Health. *Closing the gap in a generation: health equity through action on the social determinants of health. Final report of the Commission on Social Determinants of Health,* 2008. Geneva: World Health Organization.

23 Beaglehole R, Bonita R, Horton R, et al. Priority actions for the non-communicable disease crisis. *Lancet* 2011; **377**: 1438–47.

24 Anderson KM, Odell PM, Wilson PW, et al. Cardiovascular disease risk profiles. *Am Heart J* 1991; **121**: 293–8.

25 Jackson R, Lawes CM, Bennett DA, et al. Treatment with drugs to lower blood pressure and blood cholesterol based on an individual's absolute cardiovascular risk. *Lancet* 2005; **365**: 434–41.

26 Conroy RM, Pyorala K, Fitzgerald AP, et al. for the SCORE Project Group. Estimation of ten-year risk of fatal cardiovascular disease in Europe: the SCORE Project. *Eur Heart J* 2003; **24**: 987–1003.

27 Ferrario M, Chiodini P, Chambless LE, et al. Prediction of coronary events in a low incidence population: assessing accuracy of the CUORE cohort study prediction equation. *Int J Epidemiol* 2005; **34**: 413–21.

28 D'Agostino RB, Sr., Vasan RS, Pencina MJ, et al. General cardiovascular risk profile for use in primary care: the Framingham Heart Study. *Circulation* 2008; **117**: 743–53.

29 Rose G, Day S. The population mean predicts the number of deviant individuals. *Br Med J* 1990; **301**: 1031–4.

30 Kuulasmaa K, Tunstall-Pedoe H, Dobson A, et al. Estimation of contribution of changes in classic risk factors to trends in coronary-event rates across the WHO MONICA project populations. *Lancet* 2000; **355**: 675–87.

31 Tunstall-Pedoe H (ed.) *MONICA monograph and multimedia sourcebook*, 2003. Geneva: World Health Organization.

32 Reid DD, Brett GZ, Hamilton PJS, et al. Cardiorespiratory disease and diabetes among middle-aged male civil servants. *Lancet* 1974; **1**: 469–73.

33 Shaper AG. Blood pressure studies in East Africa. In: Stamler J, Stamler R, Pullman TN (eds) *The epidemiology of hypertension*, 1967, pp. 139–45. New York: Grune and Stratten.

34 WHO Expert Committee on Prevention of Coronary Artery Disease. Prevention of coronary artery disease. Report of a WHO Expert Committee. *WHO Technical Report Series* 678, 1982. Geneva: World Health Organization.

35 Manuel DG, Lim J, Tanuseputro P, et al. Revisiting Rose: strategies for reducing coronary heart disease. *Br Med J* 2006; **332**: 659–62.

36 Emberson J, Whincup P, Morris R, et al. Evaluating the impact of population and high-risk strategies for the primary prevention of cardiovascular disease. *Eur Heart J* 2004; **25**: 484–91.

37 McLaren L, McIntyre L, Kirkpatrick S. Rose's population strategy of prevention need not increase social inequalities in health. *Int J Epidemiol* 2010; **39**: 372–7.

38 Doyle YG, Furey A, Flowers J. Sick individuals and sick populations: 20 years later. *J Epidemiol Commun Health* 2006; **60**: 396–8.

39 Manuel DG, Rosella LC. Commentary: assessing population (baseline) risk is a cornerstone of population health planning—looking forward to address new challenges. *Int J Epidemiol* 2010; **39**: 380–2.

40 Giampaoli S, Palmieri L, Donfrancesco C, et al., on behalf of the CUORE project research group. Cardiovascular risk assessment in Italy: the CUORE project risk score and risk chart. *Ital J Publ Health* 2007; **4**: 102–9.

41 Palmieri L, Donfrancesco C, Giampaoli S, et al. Favorable cardiovascular risk profile and 10-year coronary heart disease incidence in women and men: results from the Progetto CUORE. *Eur J Cardiovasc Prev Rehabil* 2006; **13**: 562–70.

42 Giampaoli S, Palmieri L, Panico S, et al. Favorable cardiovascular risk profile (low risk) and 10-year stroke incidence in women and men: findings from 12 Italian population samples. *Am J Epidemiol* 2006; **163**: 893–902.

43 Puska P, et al. *Community control of cardiovascular diseases: the North Karelia project. Evaluation of a comprehensive community programme for control of cardiovascular diseases in North Karelia, Finland 1972-1977*, 1981. Copenhagen: WHO Regional Office for Europe.

44 Puska P, Leparski E. World Health Organization Regional Office for Europe. Comprehensive cardiovascular community control programmes in Europe. *EURO Report and Studies*, 106, 1988. Copenhagen: World Health Organization Regional Office for Europe.

45 World Health Organization Regional Office for Europe. *A strategy to prevent chronic disease in Europe. A focus on public health action. The CINDI vision*, 2004. Copenhagen: World Health Organization Regional Office for Europe.

46 World Health Organization. *Global strategy for the prevention and control of noncommunicable diseases: report by the Director-General*, 1999. Geneva: World Health Organization.

47 Farquhar JW, Fortmann SP, Flora JA, et al. Effects of communitywide education on cardiovascular disease risk factors. The Stanford five-city project. *J Am Med Assoc* 1990; **264**: 359–65.

48 Luepker RV, Murray DM, Jacobs DR, Jr, et al. Community education for cardiovascular disease prevention: risk factor changes in the Minnesota heart health program. *Am J Publ Health* 1994; **84**: 1383–93.

49 Carleton RA, Lasater TM, Assaf AR, et al. The Pawtucket heart health program: community changes in cardiovascular risk factors and projected disease risk. *Am J Publ Health* 1995; **85**: 777–85.

50 Pennant M, Davenport C, Bayliss S, et al. Community programs for the prevention of cardiovascular disease: a systematic review. *Am J Epidemiol* 2010; **172**: 501–16.

51 Jousilahti P, Vartiainen E, Pekkanen J, et al. Serum cholesterol distribution and coronary heart disease risk. Observations and predictions among middle-aged population in eastern Finland. *Circulation* 1998; **97**: 1087–94.

52 Puska P, Vartiainen E, Tuomilehto J, et al. Changes in premature deaths in Finland: successful long-term prevention of cardiovascular diseases. *Bull World Health Org* 1998; **76**: 419–25.

53 Kavey RE, Daniels SR, Lauer RM, et al. American Heart Association guidelines for primary prevention of atherosclerotic cardiovascular disease beginning in childhood. *Circulation* 2003; **107**: 1562–6.

54 Perk J, De Backer G, Gohlke H, et al. European guidelines on cardiovascular disease prevention in clinical practice (version 2012). *Eur Heart J* 2012; **33**: 1635–701.

55 Greenland P, Alpert JS, Beller GA, et al. ACCF/AHA guideline for assessment of cardiovascular risk in asymptomatic adults: a report of the American College of Cardiology Foundation/American Heart Association Task Force on Practice Guidelines. *Circulation* 2010; **122**: e584–e636.

56 Farley TA, Dalal MA, Mostashari F, et al. Deaths preventable in the US by improvements in use of clinical preventive services. *Am J Prev Med* 2010; **38**: 684–5.

57 Stamler J, Neaton JD, Cohen JD, et al.; MRFIT Research Group. Multiple risk factor intervention trial revisited: a new perspective based on nonfatal and fatal composite endpoints, coronary and cardiovascular, during the trial. *J Am Heart Assoc* 2012; **1**(5): e003640.

58 Wilhelmsen L, Berglund G, Elmfeldt D, et al. The multifactor primary prevention trial in Göteborg, Sweden. *Eur Heart J* 1986; **7**: 279–88.

59 Hjermann I, Velve Byre K, Holme I, et al. Effect of diet and smoking intervention on the incidence of coronary heart disease. Report from the Oslo Study Group of a randomised trial in healthy men. *Lancet* 1981; **2**: 1303–10.

60 World Health Organization European Collaborative Group. Multifactorial trial in the prevention of coronary heart disease: 3. Incidence and mortality results. *Eur Heart J* 1983; **4**: 141–7.

61 Kornitzer M, De Backer G, Dramaix M, et al. Belgian heart disease prevention project: incidence and mortality results. *Lancet* 1983; **1**: 1066–70.

62 Kornitzer M, De Backer G. Cardiovascular epidemiology: lessons from the community trials. *Acta Clin Belg* 1986; **41**: 79–82.

63 Jørgensen T, Capewell S, Prescott E, et al. Population-level changes to promote cardiovascular health. *Eur J Prev Cardiol* 2013; **20**: 409–21.

64 The European Heart Health Charter. URL: http://www.heartcharter.org/ (accessed 11 June 2013).

65 O'Kelly S, Ryden L. The political power of heart doctors: with the European Heart Health Charter towards a European policy on cardiovascular disease. *Eur J Cardiovasc Prev Rehabil* 2009; **16** (Suppl. 2): S58–S60.

66 O'Kelly S, Andersen K, Capewell S, et al. Bringing prevention to the population: an important role for cardiologists in policy-making. *Eur Heart J* 2011; **32**: 1964–7.

67 Stead LF, Bergson G, Lancaster T. Physician advice for smoking cessation. *Cochrane Database Syst Rev* 2008; (2): CD000165.

68 Kaner EF, Beyer F, Dickinson HO, et al. Effectiveness of brief alcohol interventions in primary care populations. *Cochrane Database Syst Rev* 2007; (2): CD004148.

69 Bock C, Diehl K, Schneider S, et al. Behavioral counseling for cardiovascular disease prevention in primary care settings: a systematic review of practice and associated factors. *Med Care Res Rev* 2012; **69**: 495–518.

70 Rice VH, Stead LF. Nursing interventions for smoking cessation. *Cochrane Database Syst Rev* 2008; (1): CD001188.

71 Flodgren G, Deane K, Dickinson HO, et al. Interventions to change the behaviour of health professionals and the organisation of care to promote weight reduction in overweight and obese adults. *Cochrane Database Syst Rev* 2010; (3): CD000984.

72 Carson KV, Verbiest MEA, Crone MR, et al. Training health professionals in smoking cessation. *Cochrane Database Syst Rev* 2012; (5): CD000214.

73 Thompson PD, Buchner D, Pina IL, et al. Exercise and physical activity in the prevention and treatment of atherosclerotic cardiovascular disease: a statement from the Council on Clinical Cardiology (Subcommittee on Exercise, Rehabilitation, and Prevention) and the Council on Nutrition, Physical Activity, and Metabolism (Subcommittee on Physical Activity). *Arterioscler Thromb Vasc Biol* 2003; **23**: e42–e49.

74 Lloyd-Jones DM, Hong Y, Labarthe D, et al. American Heart Association Strategic Planning Task Force and Statistics Committee. Defining and setting national goals for cardiovascular health promotion and disease reduction: the American Heart Association's strategic impact goal through 2020 and beyond. *Circulation* 2010; **121**: 586–613.

75 Appel LJ, Brands MW, Daniels SR, et al. Dietary approaches to prevent and treat hypertension: a scientific statement from the American Heart Association. *Hypertension* 2006; **47**: 296–308.

76 Expert Panel on Integrated Guidelines for Cardiovascular Health and Risk Reduction in Children and Adolescents; National Heart, Lung, and Blood Institute. Expert panel on integrated guidelines for cardiovascular health and risk reduction in children and adolescents: summary report. *Pediatrics* 2011; **128** (Suppl. 5): S213–S256.

77 Erhardt L, Moller R, Puig JG. Comprehensive cardiovascular risk management—what does it mean in practice? *Vasc Health Risk Manag* 2007; **3**: 587–603.

78 Giampaoli S. CUORE: a sustainable cardiovascular disease prevention strategy. *Eur J Cardiovasc Prev Rehabil* 2007; **14**: 161–2.

79 Palmieri L, Rielli R, Demattè L, et al. CUORE project: implementation of the 10-year risk score. *Eur J Cardiovasc Prev Rehabil* 2011; **18**: 642–9.

80 Benner JS, Erhardt L, Flammer M, et al.; REACH OUT Investigators. A novel programme to evaluate and communicate 10-year risk of CHD reduces predicted risk and improves patients' modifiable risk factor profile. *Int J Clin Pract* 2008; **62**: 1484–98.

81 Banegas JR, López-García E, Dallongeville J, et al. Achievement of treatment goals for primary prevention of cardiovascular disease in clinical practice across Europe: the EURIKA study. *Eur Heart J* 2011; **32**: 2143–52.

82 Rodondi N, Collet TH, Nanchen D, et al. Impact of carotid plaque screening on smoking cessation and other cardiovascular risk factors: a randomized controlled trial. *Arch Intern Med* 2012; **172**: 344–52.

83 Tunstall-Pedoe H, Vanuzzo D, Hobbs M, et al. Estimation of contribution of changes in coronary care to improving survival, event rates, and coronary heart disease mortality across the WHO MONICA project populations. *Lancet* 2000; **355**: 688–700.

84 Tunstall-Pedoe H, Kuulasmaa K, Mahonen M, et al. Contribution of trends in survival and coronary-event rates to changes in coronary heart disease mortality: 10-year results from 37 WHO MONICA project populations. Monitoring trends and determinants in cardiovascular disease. *Lancet* 1999; **353**: 1547–57.

85 Unal B, Critchley JA, Capewell S. Explaining the decline in coronary heart disease mortality in England and Wales between 1981 and 2000. *Circulation* 2004; **109**: 1101–7.

86 Di Chiara A, Vanuzzo D. Does surveillance impact on cardiovascular prevention? *Eur Heart J* 2009; **30**: 1027–9.

CHAPTER 8

Secondary prevention and cardiac rehabilitation: principles and practice

Massimo F. Piepoli and Pantaleo Giannuzzi

Contents

Summary

Secondary prevention through cardiac rehabilitation (CR) is the intervention that has the best scientific evidence for decreasing morbidity and mortality in coronary artery disease, in particular after myocardial infarction, but also after cardiac interventions in chronic stable heart disease. Cardiac patients with chronic heart disease and/or after an acute event deserve special care to improve their quality of life and to maintain or restore their functional capacity. They require counselling to avoid recurrence by adhering to a medication plan and adopting a healthy lifestyle. These secondary prevention targets are included in the overall goal of CR. CR can be viewed as the clinical application of preventive care by means of a professional integrated multidisciplinary approach for comprehensive risk reduction and global long-term care of cardiac patients. The CR approach comprises several integrated components and is delivered in tandem with a flexible follow-up strategy and easy access to a team of specialists. Components include patient assessment, physical activity counselling, exercise training, diet/nutritional counselling, weight control management, lipid management, blood pressure monitoring, smoking cessation, and psychosocial management. However, many of the risk factors can be mediated through exercise training programmes. Physical activity counselling and exercise training are the central components in all rehabilitation and preventive interventions. This chapter reviews the key components of a CR programme and summarizes current evidence-based best practice for the wide range of interventions of interest to the general cardiology community.

Clinical case: Mr X

- Three days ago, at 23:50, a 46-year-old man was hospitalized for severe, typical worsening chest pain, which had started around 50 minutes previously. He is a heavy-goods vehicle driver, lives with his wife and a teenage son, and has no previous relevant clinical history, but he has never consulted his GP, and he smokes and is overweight (BMI of 34 kg/m^2) with sedentary habits.
- In the emergency department the ECG showed acute anterior 'S-T segment elevation myocardial infarction'.

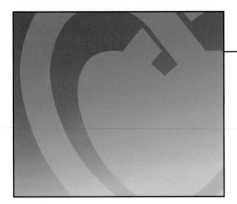

Clinical management

An emergency coronary angiogram documented a single proximal left anterior descending occlusion that was treated immediately with primary percutaneous coronary angioplasty and implantation of a drug-eluting stent. Subsequently the clinical course was uneventful, without complications, and Mr X felt all right. An echocardiogram performed on day 3 showed anterior-septal hypokinesia with moderately reduced ejection fraction (left ventricular ejection fraction 40%). Mr X was discharged on the same day with a diagnosis of 'S-T elevation myocardial infarction, due to proximal left anterior descending occlusion with residual impaired left ventricular function'. The following therapy was prescribed:

- aspirin 100 mg/day
- clopidogrel 75 mg/day
- atorvastatin 80 mg/day
- bisoprolol 1.25 mg/day
- ramipril 1.25 mg/day

and the recommendation was for an outpatient visit at 1–3 months.

Principles

Definition and aims

In recent years there has been impressive progress in pharmacological therapies and in sophisticated technology-based diagnostic and therapeutic procedures for cardiovascular diseases (CVD). As a consequence, a greater number of people now survive acute events but with a heavier burden of chronic conditions and limitations on their daily activities.

A management approach based on interventional cardiology and medication only is thus not effective—as the European Heart Health Charter [1], article 7, states: '... the burden of established cardiovascular disease may also be reduced by early diagnosis, appropriate disease management, rehabilitation and prevention, including structured lifestyle counselling'. After an acute event or with a chronic heart condition patients need structured support to restore their quality of life and to maintain or improve functional capacity. They require counselling to prevent recurrence by adhering to a medication plan and adopting a healthy lifestyle.

In secondary prevention, preventive cardiology equates to cardiac rehabilitation (CR), defined as a multifaceted and multidisciplinary intervention, affecting clinical status, functional capacity, recovery, and psychological wellbeing [2]. CR can be viewed as the clinical application of secondary prevention by means of a professional integrated multidisciplinary approach for comprehensive risk reduction and global long-term care of cardiac patients. This is accompanied by a flexible follow-up strategy, and easy access to a team of specialists. Thus, CR programmes are recommended (class I) by the European Society of Cardiology [3,4] and the American Heart Association and American College of Cardiology [5, 6, 7] in the treatment of patients with coronary artery disease (CAD) and chronic heart failure (CHF) [8, 9, 10]. Moreover, CR is considered a cost-effective intervention following an acute coronary event and CHF since it improves prognosis by reducing recurrent events and healthcare expenditure while prolonging life [11,12].

Despite its well-documented benefits, CR is vastly underutilized. Only about a third of coronary patients in Europe receives any form of CR [13,14]. The results of the EUROASPIRE audits of preventive care for coronary patients over the last 20 years show adverse lifestyle trends and an increasing prevalence of cardiovascular risk factors in these patients [15]. Moreover, even when implemented, most CR programmes are short-term interventions. Some recent studies on prevention and CR (e.g. EuroAction [16] and GOSPEL [17]) have the specific aim of maintaining beneficial longer-term life changes and improving prognosis in cardiac patients.

Indications

There is substantial evidence to conclude that a CR programme should be initiated in hospital and continued within 1 to 3 weeks after hospital discharge in an outpatient setting. Patients who are considered eligible include those who have experienced one or more of the conditions listed as a primary diagnosis some time within the previous 12 months and who have not already participated in an early outpatient CR/secondary prevention programme for the qualifying event/diagnosis:

- acute and chronic CAD
- recent cardiovascular surgery and intervention (coronary arteries or structural heart disease including heart valves)
- CHF
- cardiac transplantation
- peripheral arterial disease (PAD) and surgery/intervention to the great vessels
- receipt of a ventricular assist device (VAD)
- receipt of a pacemaker, cardiac resynchronization therapy, or implantable cardioverter defibrillator.

Phases and settings

Each individual affected by CVD can benefit from either an inpatient or outpatient CR programme divided into three phases.

Phase 1

Phase 1 is the earliest intervention during the stay in an acute hospital, including early mobilization and prevention of complications secondary to immobilization.

Phase 2

Phase 2 is the intervention performed following an index CVD event with the aim of clinical stabilization, risk stratification, and promotion of a long-term healthy status. It may be performed in inpatient or outpatient settings.

Structured inpatient (residential) CR programme

This type of programme should be considered as a transition phase for high-risk patients to promote stabilization before starting a longer-term outpatient CR programme (which is the main scenario for promoting long-term adherence). High-risk subjects include:

- patients with persistent clinical instability because of complications after an acute event or serious concomitant disease(s)
- patients with advanced HF (New York Heart Association functional classification class III–IV) needing intermittent or continuous drug infusion and/or mechanical support
- patients with a recent heart transplant
- patients discharged very early after the acute event, even if uncomplicated, and at high risk of instability (i.e. age, comorbidities)
- patients unable to attend a formal outpatient CR programme for any logistical reason.

Outpatient CR programme

An outpatient CR programme promotes and delivers preventive and rehabilitative services to more independent subjects in the outpatient setting early after a CVD event, generally within the first 1 to 3 months, but continues in a more flexible model preferably for as much as a year. It should be characterized by regular clinical control of adherence and risk factor management, performed by a multidisciplinary team held in an out-of-hospital clinic setting or in a specialized centre.

Home-based programme

This is delivered at the patient's home, prescribed and monitored at a distance by the multidisciplinary team with the support of educational materials, periodic visits to a centre, and contact with the team. The programme's components and activities are similar to those of an early outpatient CR programme.

Phase 3

Phase 3 is a long-term outpatient CR programme which provides longer-term delivery of preventive and rehabilitative services in the outpatient setting and/or in the community.

Practice: planning the individual rehabilitation process

Core components: principles and means of implementation common to all clinical conditions

In practical terms the implementation of a secondary prevention programme requires the identification of the core components for CR (➲ Table 8.1). In agreement with recent European statements [2] these have been classified as:

- clinical and risk assessment
- counselling about physical activity
- prescription of exercise training
- diet/nutritional counselling
- weight management
- lipid management
- blood pressure management,
- smoking cessation
- psychosocial management
- vocational support.

Table 8.1 Core components of cardiac rehabilitation with objectives common to all clinical conditions

Components	Method of application
Clinical and risk assessment	Evaluation: ◆ Clinical history: cardiovascular diagnoses and procedures, risk factors, comorbidities and disabilities, psychological stress, educational barriers, and preferences, vocational situation ◆ Symptoms: NYHA functional class for dyspnoea and CCS class for symptoms of angina ◆ Adherence: to medical regime and self-monitoring (weight, BP, symptoms) ◆ Physical examination: general health status, cardiovascular and pulmonary systems (i.e. cardiac and carotid murmurs, pulse HR, BP control, extremities for presence of arterial pulses), cardiovascular accidents with/without neurological sequelae, cognitive function ◆ ECG: HR, rhythm, repolarization ◆ Cardiac imaging (2D and Doppler echocardiography): ventricular function, valvular heart disease, presence of effusion where appropriate ◆ Blood testing: for routine biochemical assay including full blood count, electrolytes, renal and liver function, fasting blood glucose (haemoglobin A1C if fasting blood glucose is elevated or known diabetic), total cholesterol, LDL-C, HDL-C, triglycerides Intervention: ◆ Formulation of 'tailored' patient-specific plan of the CR programme, with priority short-term goals ◆ Discussion and provision of the initial and follow-up plans to the patient in collaboration with family members and primary healthcare providers and with clear, comprehensible information on the basic purpose of the CR programme and the role of each component (including optimal compliance with medical therapy) ◆ Education of the patient and family members on self-monitoring (weight, BP, warning symptoms and signs of instability e.g. angina, dyspnoea) and self management Expected outcomes: ◆ Evidence of patient treatment plan, outcome report, and discharge plan, including long-term management programme

Table 8.1 (*continued*) Core components of cardiac rehabilitation with objectives common to all clinical conditions

Components	Method of application
Physical activity counselling	Evaluation: ◆ Physical activity level by history; domestic, occupational, and recreational habits; activities relevant to age, gender, and daily life; readiness to change behaviour; self-confidence; barriers to increased physical activity, and social support in making positive changes Intervention: ◆ Education: sedentary lifestyle as risk factor and the benefits of physical activity—any increase in activity has a positive health benefit. Underline how benefits may be achieved and the need for lifelong continuation. If interruption of physical activity has occurred, physical, social, and psychological barriers should be explored, and alternative approaches suggested. Provide educational materials as part of counselling efforts ◆ Advice: individualize physical activity according to the patient's age, past habits, comorbidities, preferences, and goals. Caution patients to avoid performing unaccustomed vigorous physical activity (e.g. racquet sports and shovelling snow) ◆ Reassure regarding the safety of the recommended protocol ◆ Encourage involvement in leisure activities which are enjoyable and in group exercise training programmes as patients tend to revert to previous sedentary habits over time ◆ Recommend gradual increases in daily lifestyle activities over time, and how to incorporate them into a daily routine. A minimum of 30–60 min/session of moderately intense aerobic activity, preferably daily, at least 3–4 times a week Expected outcomes: ◆ Increased participation in domestic, occupational, and recreational activities ◆ Improved psychosocial wellbeing, prevention of disability, and enhancement of opportunities for independent self-care ◆ Improved aerobic fitness ◆ Improved prognosis
Exercise training (ET)	ET is defined as a sub-category of physical activity in which planned, structured, and repetitive bodily movements are performed to maintain or improve physical fitness and thus it is a structured intervention over a defined period of time. It should be integrated within the physical activity intervention (see 'Physical activity counselling') Evaluation: ◆ Peak exercise capacity: symptom-limited exercise testing, either on a bicycle ergometer or a treadmill. If this is not feasible (e.g. because of recent surgery), sub-maximal exercise evaluation and/or 6-minute walk test should be considered Intervention: ◆ Develop an individualized exercise prescription for aerobic and resistance training that is based on individual findings, risk stratification, comorbidities, and patient goals ◆ Recommend: (1) sub-maximal endurance training, i.e. starting at 50–60% of maximal work load or maximal oxygen uptake if available and gradually increasing according to the subjective feeling of exertion; (2) expand physical activity to include weight/resistance training twice a week ◆ During the initial supervised phases, an in-hospital ET programme may be appropriate in unstable and more fragile patients to verify individual responses and tolerability and promptly identify signs and symptoms indicating the need to modify or terminate the programme. The supervision should include physical examination, monitoring of HR, BP, and rhythm before, during, and after ET. The supervised period should be prolonged in patients with new symptoms, signs, BP abnormalities, and increased supraventricular or ventricular ectopy during exercise Expected outcomes: ◆ Increased cardiorespiratory fitness and enhanced flexibility, muscular endurance, and strength (by 5–10%) ◆ Reduction of symptoms, attenuated physiological responses to physical challenges, and improved psychosocial wellbeing
Diet/ nutritional counselling	Evaluation: ◆ Daily caloric intake and dietary content of fat, saturated fat, sodium, and other nutrients ◆ Assess eating habits ◆ Determine target areas of intervention as outlined for the core components of weight, diabetes, as well as HF, kidney disease, and other comorbidities Intervention: ◆ Education of patient (and family members) regarding dietary goals and how to attain them; salt, lipid, and water content of common foods ◆ Prescribe specific dietary modifications with the aim of reducing saturated fat intake. Recommendations should be sensitive and relevant to cultural preferences ◆ Healthy food choices: • wide variety of foods; low-salt foods • Mediterranean diet: fruits, vegetables, wholegrain cereals and bread, fish (especially oily), lean meat, low-fat dairy products • replace saturated fat with the above foods and with monounsaturated and polyunsaturated fats from vegetable (oleic acid as in olive oil and rapeseed oil) and marine sources to reduce total fat to <30% of energy, of which less than a third is saturated • Avoid: overweight and particularly beverages and foods with added sugars and salty food ◆ Integrate: behaviour-change models and compliance strategies in counselling sessions Expected outcome: ◆ A plan has been provided to address problems with eating behaviour ◆ The patient understands the basic principles of dietary content ◆ Patient adherence to the prescribed diet is improved

(*continued*)

Table 8.1 (*continued*) Core components of cardiac rehabilitation with objectives common to all clinical conditions

Components	Method of application
Weight control management	Evaluation: ◆ Measure weight, height, waist circumference, calculate BMI Intervention: ◆ Manage BMI: on each patient visit it is useful to consistently encourage weight control through an appropriate balance of physical activity, caloric intake, and formal behavioural programmes when indicated to achieve and maintain healthy BMI (18.5–24.9 kg/m^2) ◆ Manage waist circumference: if waist circumference is ≥ 89 cm in women or ≥ 103 cm in men it is beneficial to initiate lifestyle changes and consider treatment strategies for metabolic syndrome as indicated. Some men can develop multiple metabolic risk factors when the waist circumference is only marginally increased (e.g. 94–102 cm). They may have a strong genetic contribution to insulin resistance and could benefit from changes in life habits, similar to men with categorical increases in waist circumference ◆ Develop a combined diet, physical activity/exercise, and behavioural programme designed to reduce total caloric intake, maintain appropriate intake of nutrients and fibre, and increase energy expenditure. The exercise component should strive to include daily longer distance/duration walking (e.g. 60–90 min). Expected outcomes: ◆ Elaboration of an individualized strategy to lose 5–10% of body weight in 6 months and modification of associated risk factors if needed ◆ Continue to assess and modify interventions until progressive weight loss is achieved and modification of associated risk factors has occurred, if necessary ◆ In the long term the patient should adhere to diet and physical activity and an exercise programme aimed to achieve the established weight goal ◆ Where the goal is not attained, consider referring the patient to a specialist obesity clinic
Lipid management	Evaluation: ◆ Lipid profile: fasting measure of total cholesterol, HDL, LDL, and triglycerides. In those with abnormal levels, obtain a detailed history to determine whether diet, drug, and/or other conditions that may affect lipid levels can be altered ◆ Assess current therapy and compliance. Assess creatine kinase levels and liver function in patients taking lipid-lowering medications ◆ Repeat lipid profiles at 2 months after initiation or changes in lipid-lowering medications Intervention: ◆ Provide nutritional and physical activity counselling, as well as weight management ◆ Add or intensify drug treatment if necessary Expected outcomes: ◆ Total plasma cholesterol should be <5 mmol/L (<190 mg/dl) ◆ LDL-C should be <3 mmol/L (<115 mg/dl). LDL-C level 1.8 mmmol/L (<70 mg/dl) in all patients with established coronary disease
Blood pressure management	Evaluation: ◆ Measure seated resting BP on more than two visits ◆ Measure BP on both arms at programme entry ◆ To rule out orthostatic hypotension, measure lying, seated, and standing BP ◆ Assess current therapy and compliance Intervention ◆ Education: recommend lifestyle modifications—exercise, weight management, sodium restriction, and moderation of alcohol intake (i.e. 1-3 units daily: a unit equates to about 80 mL of wine, 250 mL of normal strength beer, and 30–50 mL of spirits) according to the DASH diet (<http://dashdiet.org/>); if patient has diabetes or chronic renal or cardiovascular disease, consider drug therapy ◆ If resting systolic BP is ≥ 140 mmHg or diastolic BP is ≥ 90 mmHg despite lifestyle changes, initiate drug therapy, considering total cardiovascular risk Expected outcomes: ◆ Continue to monitor and modify intervention until normalization of BP
Smoking cessation	Evaluation: ◆ Structured approaches to be used, e.g. the 5As (Ask, Advise, Assess, Assist, Arrange) ◆ Ask the patient about his/her smoking status and use of other tobacco products. Specify both the amount of smoking (cigarettes per day) and duration of smoking (number of years) ◆ Determine readiness to change; if ready, choose a date for quitting ◆ Assess for psychosocial factors that may impede success Intervention: ◆ All smokers should be professionally advised and encouraged to permanently stop smoking all forms of tobacco ◆ Provide structured follow-up, referral to special programmes. Behavioural advice and group or individual counselling and/or pharmacotherapy (including nicotine replacement) are recommended, as is a stepwise strategy for smoking cessation. Consider nicotine replacement therapy, combined with bupropion or varenicline if not contraindicated Expected outcome: ◆ Short term: patient will demonstrate readiness to change by initially expressing a decision to quit and selecting a quit date. Subsequently, patient will quit smoking and all tobacco use and adherence to pharmacological therapy ◆ Long-term abstinence from smoking

Table 8.1 (*continued*) Core components of cardiac rehabilitation with objectives common to all clinical conditions

Components	Method of application
Psychosocial management	Evaluation: ◆ Screen for psychological distress as indicated by clinically significant levels of depression, anxiety, anger or hostility, social isolation, occupational distress, marital/family distress, sexual dysfunction/adjustment, and substance abuse of alcohol and/or other psychotropic agents. Use interview and/or other standardized measurement tools. As guide, routine screening questions to be asked of every patient are: Over the past 2 weeks, have you felt down, depressed, or hopeless? Over the past 2 weeks, have you felt little interest or pleasure in doing things? In case of positive answers, assessment by a psychologist is needed ◆ Identify use of psychotropic medications Intervention: ◆ Offer individual and/or small-group education and counselling on adjustment to heart disease, stress management, and health-related lifestyle change (i.e. profession, car driving, and sexual activity), relaxation techniques ◆ Whenever possible, offer spouses and other family members, domestic partners, and/or significant others access to information sessions. Teach and support self-help strategies and ability to obtain effective social support. Provide vocational counselling in case of work-related stress Expected outcome: ◆ Absence of clinically significant psychosocial problems and acquisition of stress management skills ◆ Improved health-related quality of life
Vocational advice	Evaluation: ◆ Before discharge, return to prior activities must be discussed with patients and their partners and return to prior activities must be promoted, unless there is a medical contraindication ◆ The presence of any barriers an individual may face when returning to work following illness should be assessed Intervention: ◆ All procedures to help individuals to overcome barriers to returning to work and so remain in, return to, or access employment, i.e. retraining and capacity building, reasonable adjustments and control measures, disability awareness, condition management, and medical treatment

NYHA, New York Heart Association; CCS, Canadian Cardiovascular Society; BP, blood pressure; HR, heart rate; ECG, electrocardiogram; LDL-C, low-density lipoprotein cholesterol; HDL-C, high-density lipoprotein cholesterol; BMI, body mass index

Source data from Piepoli MF, Corrà U, Benzer W, Bjarnason-Wehrens B et al, Cardiac Rehabilitation Section of the European Association of Cardiovascular Prevention and Rehabilitation. Secondary prevention through cardiac rehabilitation: from knowledge to implementation. A position paper from the Cardiac Rehabilitation Section of the European Association of Cardiovascular Prevention and Rehabilitation. *Eur J Cardiovasc Prev Rehabil*. 2010; **17**(1): 1–17.

In terms of the implementation of an individualized intervention for secondary prevention, these core components share aspects which are applicable to all CVD conditions (as outlined in ➲ Table 8.1). However for single clinical conditions, specific components may be identified.

The expected objectives of all these interventions are improved clinical stability and symptom control, reduced overall cardiovascular risk, higher adherence to pharmacological advice, and a better health behaviour profile, all leading to a superior quality of life, social integration, and an improved prognosis.

A CR programme in clinical practice

Several aspects need be addressed in daily clinical practice. ➲ Table 8.2 lists the key items to be considered for implementation in an effective secondary prevention programme, while ➲ Table 8.3 gives the key aspects of lifestyle modification.

Implementation of CR in specific diseases

Acute and chronic coronary disease

➲ Table 8.4 outlines the core components of CR in patients with acute and chronic coronary artery disease. With the availability of myocardial revascularization, CR with risk factor assessment and management is crucial for a patient's prognosis [18]. After an uncomplicated procedure, risk factor management and counselling on physical activity can start the next day, and such patients can be walking on the flat and going up stairs within a few days. After significant and/or complicated myocardial damage, CR should start after clinical stabilization, and physical activity increased slowly,

Table 8.2 Cardiac rehabilitation programme in daily clinical practice (see ➲ Table 8.1)

Individualized plan initiated *prior* to hospital discharge:
- Introduce the concept of risk and the usefulness of individualized targets
- Highlight the importance of cardiovascular risk factors
- Provide results of investigations performed and future investigations required

The programme should address specific areas of concern to the patient and their partners/families:
- Education
  - allaying misconceptions
  - pathophysiology and symptoms
  - exercise, smoking, diet, BP, cholesterol
  - occupation (phased return to work)
  - sexual dysfunction and sexual intercourse
  - psychological
  - medical and surgical interventions
  - cardiopulmonary resuscitation
- Risk factor management
- Lifestyle
  - physical activity
  - diet and weight management
  - smoking cessation
- Psychological status and quality of life
  - valid psychological assessment (anxiety, depression)
  - stress management
  - discussion of social needs (benefits etc.)
- Cardioprotective drug therapy
  - drug titration if needed
- Long-term management strategy
  - ongoing care mainly within primary care with specialist intervention
  - as required; defined pathways
  - exercise groups; community dietetic and weight management services

Table 8.3 Lifestyle modification in daily clinical practice

Eat a healthy, balanced diet ◆ Increase fresh food and reduce processed foods; consider a Mediterranean style diet ◆ Eat less fat—decrease intake of foods high in saturated fat and opt for foods which have unsaturated (polyunsaturated and monounsaturated) fats ◆ Eat more fruit and veg—five portions a day ◆ Increase wholegrain and high-fibre foods ◆ Oily fish—at least two portions a week ◆ Reduce salt intake (<6 g/day). Remember the hidden salt content of foods ◆ Consider foods enriched with plant sterols or stanols, e.g. yoghurt, milk, margarine
Limit alcohol intake ◆ 1–3 units per day
Increase physical activity ◆ Build up gradually over 4–6 weeks ◆ Aim for at least 20–30 min of moderate activity each day to the point of mild breathlessness (walking, jogging, cycling, dancing, or swimming)
Do not smoke ◆ A combination of medication for smoking cessation and behavioural support should be offered (i.e. referred to local stop smoking services)
Manage weight ◆ Education regarding balancing energy intake with energy expenditure ◆ Advise BMI < 25 ◆ To lose around 0.5 kg/1 lb per week

according to the symptoms. After hospital discharge, structured CR should continue, depending upon local facilities. In-hospital CR for 4 weeks can be useful for patients with severe left ventricular dysfunction or relevant comorbidity. All other patients can follow an outpatient CR programme.

The interventional cardiologist can make an important contribution here: he or she should emphasize the importance of these measures directly to the patient, because failure to do so may suggest that secondary prevention therapies are not necessary. The interventional cardiologist should interact with the primary care physician and the physicians in charge of the CR programme to ensure that the necessary secondary prevention therapies initiated during hospitalization are maintained after discharge from hospital.

Uncertainties remain about important aspects such as exercise training programmes or the best way to increase compliance and adherence to a healthy lifestyle. Other general controversies include what to do with Prinzmetal's or microvascular angina pectoris.

Recent cardiovascular surgery and interventions (coronary arteries or structural heart disease including heart valves)

➲ Table 8.5 outlines the core components of CR following recent cardiovascular surgery and interventions. CR programmes should be available for all patients undergoing coronary artery surgery [19,20] and valve surgery [21,22]. For surgical patients,

Table 8.4 Core components of cardiac rehabilitation in patients with acute and chronic coronary artery disease

Components	Method of application
Clinical risk assessment	Evaluation: ◆ Clinical history: review clinical course of ACS ◆ Physical examination: inspect puncture site of PCI, and extremities for presence of arterial pulses
Physical activity counselling	Evaluation: ◆ Exercise capacity and ischaemic threshold: exercise stress testing by bicycle ergometry or treadmill maximal stress test (cardiopulmonary exercise test if available), symptom limited within 4 weeks after the acute event (a sub-maximal test when appropriate, e.g. after extensive MI or complications of MI, while a maximal test afterwards). Exercise or pharmacological imaging technique in patients with an uninterpretable ECG is advisable Intervention: ◆ Exercise stress test guide: in the presence of exercise capacity > 5 METS without symptoms, patients can resume routine physical activity; otherwise, patients should resume physical activity at 50% of maximal exercise capacity and gradually increase ◆ Physical activity: a slow, gradual, and progressive increase of moderate-intensity aerobic activity, such as walking, climbing stairs, and cycling, supplemented by an increase in daily activities (such as gardening or housework)
Exercise training	Intervention: ◆ The programme should include a combination of supervised, medically prescribed aerobic exercise training; and resistance exercise ◆ Aerobic exercise. In *low-risk* patients, at least three sessions of 30–60 min/week aerobic exercise at 55–70% of the maximum work load (in METS) or heart rate at the onset of symptoms; >1500 kcal/week to be spent by low risk patients. In *moderate- to high-risk* patients: similar to low-risk group but starting with <50% of maximum work load. ◆ Resistance exercise: at least 1 hour/week (two sets, with an intensity of 10–15 repetitions maximum) ◆ Medication: prophylactic nitroglycerine can be taken at the start of exercise training session in chronic stable angina
Diet/nutritional counselling	See ➲ Table 8.1
Weight control management	See ➲ Table 8.1

Table 8.4 (*continued*) Core components of cardiac rehabilitation in patients with acute and chronic coronary artery disease

Lipid management	Evaluation: ◆ Assess fasting lipid profile in all patients, preferably within 24 h of an acute event. Initiate lipid-lowering medication as recommended under 'Intervention' as soon as possible Intervention: ◆ Statin therapy for all patients ◆ In case of high triglycerides emphasize weight management and physical activity, abstention from alcohol, and smoking cessation
Blood pressure monitoring	See ➲ Table 8.1
Smoking cessation	See ➲ Table 8.1
Psychosocial management	See ➲ Table 8.1
Vocational management	See ➲ Table 8.1

ACS, acute coronary syndrome; PCI, percutaneous coronary intervention; MI, myocardial infarction; METS, metabolic equivalents.

Source data from Piepoli MF, Corrà U, Benzer W, Bjarnason-Wehrens B et al, Cardiac Rehabilitation Section of the European Association of Cardiovascular Prevention and Rehabilitation Secondary prevention through cardiac rehabilitation: from knowledge to implementation. A position paper from the Cardiac Rehabilitation Section of the European Association of Cardiovascular Prevention and Rehabilitation. *Eur J Cardiovasc Prev Rehabil* 2010; **17**(1): 1–17.

Table 8.5 Core components of cardiac rehabilitation following recent cardiovascular surgery and intervention (coronary arteries or structural heart disease including heart valves)

Components	Method of application
Clinical risk assessment	Evaluation: ◆ Wound (chest and legs) healing, comorbidities, complications, and disabilities ◆ ECG: heart rate, rhythm, repolarization and new Q waves ◆ Chest X-ray: infection, pleural effusion, diaphragm paralysis ◆ Blood testing: anaemia, fasting blood glucose, renal function, and electrolytes ◆ Echocardiography: pleural or pericardial effusion, prosthetic function, and/or valvular heart disease, when appropriate Intervention: ◆ Patient education: about anticoagulation, including drug interactions and self-management if appropriate; in-depth knowledge on endocarditic prophylaxis; secondary prevention medication for CAD; how to progress in order to normalize activities of daily living
Physical activity counselling	Evaluation: ◆ Wound healing and exercise capacity should be considered (see also ➲ Table 8.4)
Exercise training	Intervention: ◆ Individually tailored according to the clinical condition, baseline exercise capacity, ventricular function, and type of valve surgery (see also ➲ Table 8.4) ◆ To be started as early as in the in-hospital phase ◆ Inpatient and/or outpatient programmes immediately after discharge lasting 8–12 weeks are indicated ◆ Upper body training can begin when the chest is stable, i.e. usually after 6 weeks ◆ After mitral valve replacement exercise tolerance is much lower than after aortic valve replacement, particularly if there is residual pulmonary hypertension
Diet/nutritional counselling	◆ Note interaction between anticoagulation and vitamin K-rich food and other drugs, in particularly amiodarone. Special emphasis on the Mediterranean diet
Tobacco cessation	◆ Risk of complications depends on how long before surgery the smoking habit has been changed, and whether smoking was reduced or stopped completely
Psychosocial management	◆ Sleep disturbances, anxiety, depression, and impaired quality of life may occur after surgery
Vocational management	See ➲ Table 8.1

Source data from Piepoli MF, Corrà U, Benzer W, Bjarnason-Wehrens B et al, Cardiac Rehabilitation Section of the European Association of Cardiovascular Prevention and Rehabilitation Secondary prevention through cardiac rehabilitation: from knowledge to implementation. A position paper from the Cardiac Rehabilitation Section of the European Association of Cardiovascular Prevention and Rehabilitation. *Eur J Cardiovasc Prev Rehabil* 2010; **17**(1): 1–17.

the preventive and rehabilitation strategy should also focus on the potential effect of pre-operative rehabilitation. As for other subgroups of patients, CR should be tailored to the individual's risk profile and physical, psychological, and social status assessed as part of the perioperative medical history and examination (➲ Table 8.1). Furthermore, it should be appreciated that the clinical condition and concerns of surgical patients often relate to the surgical procedure itself. Approaching and resolving these issues in addition to understanding the underlying clinical conditions should be part of comprehensive CR.

Table 8.6 Core components of cardiac rehabilitation in chronic heart failure

Components	Method of application
Clinical risk assessment	Evaluation: ◆ Haemodynamic and fluid status: signs of congestion, peripheral and central oedema ◆ Chest X-ray: lung oedema, pleural effusion ◆ Cachexia signs: reduced muscle mass, muscle strength, and endurance ◆ Blood testing: serum electrolytes, creatinine, BUN, and BNP ◆ Other tests: coronary angiography, invasive haemodynamic measurements, endomyocardial biopsy, screening for sleep apnoea is recommended for selected patients or candidates for cardiac transplantation
Physical activity counselling	Intervention: ◆ At least 30 min/day of moderate-intensity physical activity to be gradually increased to 60 min/day
Exercise training	Evaluation: ◆ Exercise capacity: symptom-limited cardiopulmonary exercise test with metabolic gas exchange. For the testing protocol small increments (5–10 W/min) on a bicycle ergometer or modified Bruce or Naughton protocols are indicated. The 6-minute walk test is an acceptable alternative test for assessing exercise tolerance Intervention: ◆ Progression of aerobic exercise for stable patients. *Initial stage*: intensity should be kept at a low level (40–50% of peak VO2), increasing in duration from 15 to 30 min, 2–3 times/week according to perceived symptoms and clinical status for the first 1–2 weeks. *Improvement stage*: a gradual increase of intensity (50, 60, 70 to 80% of peak VO2, if tolerated) is the primary aim. Prolongation of exercise session to 30 min is a secondary goal ◆ Resistance training and inspiratory muscle training are optional training modalities which can be added to endurance training ◆ A supervised, in-hospital training programme may be recommended, especially during the initial phases, to verify individual responses and tolerability, clinical stability, and promptly identify signs and symptoms indicating the need to modify or terminate the programme
Diet/nutritional counselling	Intervention: ◆ Prescribe specific dietary modifications according to fluid intake (<2 L/day) *and* sodium intake (restriction should usually be considered in severe conditions)
Weight control management	Intervention: ◆ Monitoring: patients must be educated to weigh themselves daily. Weight gain is commonly due to fluid retention, which precedes the appearance of symptomatic pulmonary or systemic congestion. A gain > 1.5 kg over 24 hours or >2.0 kg over 2 days suggest developing fluid retention ◆ Reduction: in severe heart failure weight reduction is not recommended since unintentional weight loss and anorexia are common complications. This may be due to loss of appetite, induced by renal and hepatic dysfunction or hepatic congestion, or be a marker of depression
Lipid management	◆ Statins should be considered only in patients with established atherosclerotic disease
Tobacco cessation	See ➲ Table 8.1
Psychosocial management	See ➲ Table 8.1
Vocational management	See ➲ Table 8.1

BUN, blood urea nitrogen; BNP, brain natriuretic peptide; peak VO2, peak oxygen consumption.

Source data from Piepoli MF, Corrà U, Benzer W, Bjarnason-Wehrens B et al, Cardiac Rehabilitation Section of the European Association of Cardiovascular Prevention and Rehabilitation Secondary prevention through cardiac rehabilitation: from knowledge to implementation. A position paper from the Cardiac Rehabilitation Section of the European Association of Cardiovascular Prevention and Rehabilitation. *Eur J Cardiovasc Prev Rehabil* 2010; **17**(1): 1–17.

Chronic heart failure

➲ Table 8.6 lists the core components of CR in CHF. All patients with established CHF, with or without an implantable cardioverter defibrillator and with or without cardiac resynchronization therapy, require a multifactorial approach to CR [8,23–25]. Inpatient rehabilitation should begin as soon as possible after hospital admission. As the length of stay for acute decompensation and intervention procedures continues to decrease, structured outpatient CR is crucial for the development of a lifelong approach to prevention. This may be provided in a wide range of settings, such as CHF clinics, non-clinic settings (community health centres and general medical practices), or a combination of these. Outpatient CR may also be provided on an individual basis at home, including a combination of home visits, telephone support, telemedicine, or specially developed self-education materials.

Cardiac transplantation

It is hard to imagine a group of patients more obviously in need of rehabilitation than heart transplant recipients, because of the multifaceted physical and mental problems encountered pre- and post-operatively [26]. Of the patients who survive the first year after transplant, 50% will live for more than 12 years. As short-term survival is no longer the key issue for heart transplant recipients, a return to a functional lifestyle with a good quality of life becomes the desired outcome [27]. ➲ Table 8.7 lists the core components of CR in cardiac transplantation.

Table 8.7 Core components of cardiac rehabilitation in cardiac transplantation

Components	Method of application
Clinical risk assessment	Evaluation: ◆ Clinical: wound healing, symptoms of rejection ◆ Chest X-ray: infection, pleural effusion, diaphragm paralysis ◆ Echocardiography: right and left ventricular function, pericardial effusion, pulmonary hypertension ◆ Patient education on the risk of acute rejection. Patients should be instructed to practice self-monitoring: unusually low BP, change of HR, unexplained weight gain or fatigue may be early signs of rejection even in the absence of major symptoms. Exercise training should be stopped and prompt intervention is needed ◆ Physician knowledge of the anatomical and physiological reasons for limited exercise tolerance, e.g. the side effects of immune-suppression therapy (impairments of inflammatory response, metabolism, osteoporosis), chronotropic incompetence, diastolic dysfunction ◆ Patients and physiotherapists should be educated to adhere to the recommendations concerning personal hygiene and general measures to reduce the risk of infection
Physical activity counselling	Intervention: ◆ Chronic dynamic and resistance exercises prevent the side effects of immunosuppressive therapy ◆ Exercise intensity relies more on perceived exertion than on a specific HR. Borg scale: achieve scores of 12–14. For example, instruct the patients to start walking 1.5 or 2 km five times a week at a pace resulting in a perceived exertion of 12 to 14 on the Borg scale. The pace should be increased slowly over time
Exercise training	Evaluation: ◆ Exercise capacity: cardiopulmonary exercise stress test 4 weeks after surgery to guide detailed exercise recommendations. For testing protocols, small increments of 10 W/min on a bicycle ergometer, or modified Bruce protocols or Naughton protocols on the treadmill are appropriate Intervention: ◆ Early training programme can be beneficial in the early post-operative period as well as in the long term. Respiratory physiotherapy (to prevent respiratory infection) and kinesiotherapy of the upper and lower limbs are advisable in order to achieve early mobilization ◆ Supervised exercise programme at least during the initial phase may be advisable to verify individual responses (given the chronotropic incompetence in these patients) and tolerability as well as adaptability to exercise and clinical stability ◆ Aerobic exercise may be started in the second or third week after transplant but should be discontinued during corticosteroid bolus therapy for rejection. Resistance exercise should be added after 6 to 8 weeks ◆ Regimen: at least 30–40 min/day of combined aerobic (walking) and resistance (muscle strength) training at a moderate level, slowly progressing warm-up, closed-chain resistive activities (e.g. bridging, half-squats, toe raises, use of therapeutic bands) and walking/Nordic walking/cycling ◆ Resistance training: 2–3 sets with 10–12 repetitions per set at 40–70% 1RM with a full recovery period (>1 min) between each set. The goal is to be able to do 5 sets of 10 repetitions at 70% of 1RM ◆ Aerobic training: the intensity of training should be defined according to peak VO2 [<50% or 10% below the ventilatory anaerobic threshold (VAT) determined by cardiopulmonary exercise testing] or peak workload (<50%)
Diet/ nutritional counselling	Education: ◆ Dietary infection prophylaxis—avoid raw meat, raw seafood, unpasteurized milk, cheese from unpasteurized milk, mouldy cheese, raw eggs, soft ice cream
Weight control management	Education: ◆ Avoidance of overweight is mandatory to balance the side effects of immunosuppressants and to limit the classical cardiovascular risk factors ◆ Obesity increases the risk of CAV. It should be controlled by daily exercise and a healthy diet
Lipid management	Intervention: ◆ Hyperlipidaemia increases the risk of CAV. It should be controlled by statins, daily exercise, and a healthy diet ◆ Statins (pravastatin, simvastatin) not only lower LDL-C levels but also decrease the incidence of CAV and significantly improve survival
Blood pressure monitoring	Education: ◆ Hypertension is linked to immunosuppressive therapy and denervation of cardiac volume receptors Intervention: ◆ BP is sensitive to a low-sodium diet. Treatment with diltiazem and ACE inhibitors is the first choice, usually completed by diuretics. Beta-blockers are contraindicated as they hamper the already delayed chronotropic response of the denervated heart
Tobacco cessation	◆ Cessation of smoking is a prerequisite for transplantation. Psychological support may be needed so the patient does not resume smoking post-transplantation
Psychosocial management	◆ Support for coping strategies (with guilt, high levels of anxiety and apprehensiveness) may be needed
Vocational management	See ➲ Table 8.1

BP, blood pressure; HR, heart rate; RM, repetition maximum (the maximum weight that can be lifted); peak VO2, peak oxygen consumption attained on an incremental exercise test; CAV, cardiac allograft vasculopathy; LDL-C, low-density lipoprotein cholesterol; ACE, angiotensin-converting enzyme.

Source data from Piepoli MF, Corrà U, Benzer W, Bjarnason-Wehrens B et al, Cardiac Rehabilitation Section of the European Association of Cardiovascular Prevention and Rehabilitation Secondary prevention through cardiac rehabilitation: from knowledge to implementation. A position paper from the Cardiac Rehabilitation Section of the European Association of Cardiovascular Prevention and Rehabilitation. *Eur J Cardiovasc Prev Rehabil* 2010; **17**(1): 1–17.

Peripheral arterial disease and surgery/intervention to the great vessels

Peripheral arterial disease (PAD) is one of the multisite presentations of atherosclerosis. At the time of diagnosis of PAD, a history of acute myocardial infarction or stroke or related surgery can be expected in approximately 30% of male and 20% of female patients. Among patients presenting with CAD or cerebrovascular disease, 32% of men and 25% of women also have peripheral arterial involvement, which is two to three times more prevalent than in the respective control groups. Someone with PAD should therefore be regarded as an actual or potential polyvascular patient and an integrated approach to prevention and treatment of atherothrombosis as a whole is called for [28]. ➲ Table 8.8 lists the core components of CR in PAD and vascular surgery/interventions to the great vessels.

Table 8.8 Core components of cardiac rehabilitation in peripheral artery disease and vascular surgery/interventions of the great vessels

Components	Method of application
Clinical risk assessment	Evaluation: ◆ Clinical: any exertional limitation of the lower extremity muscles or any history of walking impairment, i.e. fatigue, aching, numbness, or pain ◆ Primary site(s) of discomfort: buttock, thigh, calf, or foot ◆ Any poorly healing wounds of the legs or feet ◆ Any pain at rest localized to the lower leg or foot and its association with the upright or recumbent positions ◆ Reduced muscle mass, strength, and endurance ◆ Vascular status: bilateral arm BP, palpation of peripheral arteries and abdominal aorta with annotation of any bruits and inspection of feet for trophic defects ◆ Measurement of ankle–brachial index: values 0.5–0.95, claudication range; 0.20–0.49, rest pain; <0.20, tissue necrosis ◆ Difficulty in walking short distances, even at a slow speed, associated with impairment in the performance of activities of daily living ◆ To exclude occult CAD, perform treadmill or bicycle exercise testing to monitor symptoms, ST–T wave changes, arrhythmias, claudication thresholds, HR and BP responses, useful for exercise prescription
Physical activity counselling	◆ Exercise activities, such as walking, lasting >30 min, three or more times a week, until near-maximal pain
Exercise training	Evaluation: ◆ Functional capacity: markedly impaired. Peak VO_2 is <50% of the predicted value Intervention: ◆ Supervised hospital- or clinic-based exercise training programme: to ensure that patients are receiving a standardized exercise stimulus in a safe environment that is effective—recommended as an initial treatment modality for all patients ◆ Exercise–rest–exercise: each training session consists of short periods of treadmill walking interspersed with rest throughout a 60-min exercise session, three times a week ◆ Treadmill exercise: more effective—the initial workload is set to a speed and grade that elicit claudication symptoms within 3 to 5 min. Patients are asked to continue to walk at this workload until they achieve claudication of moderate severity. This is followed by a brief period of rest to permit symptoms to resolve. The exercise–rest–exercise cycle is repeated several times during the hour of supervision (see ➲ Table 8.9) ◆ Resistance training: appropriately prescribed, is generally recommended
Diet/ nutritional counselling	Evaluation: ◆ Serum LDL concentration: <70 mg/dl (1.8 mmol/L) is the target value Intervention: ◆ Treatment with statin to achieve a target LDL ◆ A statin should be given as initial therapy,
Blood pressure monitoring	Evaluation: ◆ <140 mmHg systolic over 90 mmHg diastolic (non-diabetics) or <130 mmHg systolic over 80 mmHg diastolic (diabetics and individuals with chronic renal disease) Intervention: ◆ Antihypertensive therapy to achieve the goal ◆ The use of ACE inhibitors in patients with PAD may confer protection against cardiovascular events beyond that expected from BP lowering
Smoking cessation	◆ Stopping smoking is *exceptionally* important in PAD. Smoking-cessation programmes involving nicotine replacement therapy and the use of medications should be encouraged
Psychosocial management	See ➲ Table 8.1
Vocational management	See ➲ Table 8.1

HR, heart rate; BP, blood pressure; LDL, low-density lipoprotein; ACE, angiotensin-converting enzyme; PAD, peripheral arterial disease; Peak VO_2, peak oxygen consumption.

Source data from Piepoli MF, Corrà U, Benzer W, Bjarnason-Wehrens B et al, Cardiac Rehabilitation Section of the European Association of Cardiovascular Prevention and Rehabilitation Secondary prevention through cardiac rehabilitation: from knowledge to implementation. A position paper from the Cardiac Rehabilitation Section of the European Association of Cardiovascular Prevention and Rehabilitation. *Eur J Cardiovasc Prev Rehabil* 2010; **17**(1): 1–17.

Ventricular-assist device (VAD) recipient

Recently the use of the VADs has revolutionized the treatment of patients with advanced HF. Three categories of patients with VADs have emerged: (1) individuals requiring temporary circulatory support (bridge to recovery); (2) patients awaiting heart transplantation who are unlikely to survive until a suitable organ is available (bridge to transplantation); and (3) individuals who need long-term support but have an absolute or relative contraindication to heart transplantation (destination therapy). This patient group requires the attention of specialized heart failure centres, but a long-term CR approach is also necessary in order to favour the recovery, educate patients and care givers, and manage several components of rehabilitation, such as nutritional status and risk factor control and management. This area of intervention should constitute an important new field for the modern CR specialist [29]. The core components of CR in patients with VADs are summarized in ➲ Table 8.9.

Table 8.9 Core components of cardiac rehabilitation in patients with ventricular assist devices (VAD)

Components	Method of application
Clinical risk assessment	Evaluation: ◆ Anticoagulation and thromboembolism. Close control of anticoagulation is mandatory: daily self-control of anticoagulation by the patient (CoaguChek® device), supplemented by regular laboratory controls. Anticoagulation also has to be checked daily by rehabilitation nurses or physicians. Dose adaption should be done in close communication with the patient ◆ Watch for signs of potential systemic thromboembolism ◆ Avoidance of infections: watch daily wound healing, treat local infections early, screen regularly for systemic infections ◆ Arrhythmias: rapid atrial arrhythmias compromise filling of pulsatile devices. These devices then have to be switched from volume mode to fixed rate. Ventricular tachycardia has to be converted immediately, although it is often haemodynamically well tolerated ◆ Function of assist device and interplay with native heart: watch fluid balance and the function of the native right and left ventricle, watch for aortic valve regurgitation (echocardiogram), control of serum lactate concentration, electrolytes, creatinine, BUN, and BNP ◆ Control of pulsatile assist devices: in the outpatient setting pulsatile devices are usually used in the 'volume mode', and then are strictly dependent on pre-load volume. In the volume mode bradycardia is a consequence of volume depletion (bleeding? excess diuresis? tamponade? RV failure?); tachycardia reflects volume overload (general fluid overload? inflow valve regurgitation? native aortic valve regurgitation? shunting?) ◆ Inadequate filling of an LVAD may be the consequence of right ventricular failure but also of LV recovery ◆ Closely watch the function of inflow and outflow valves (regurgitation? distortions of the conduits?) ◆ Opening of the native aortic valves with 'normal' excursions may be the consequence of either malfunction of LVAD or LV recovery. Decompression of LV is normal in patients with pulsatile LVAD. If decompression does not occur, there may be inadequate LV emptying by LVAD. Intervention: ◆ Medical therapy optimization: anticoagulation with warfarin/phenprocoumon in combination with acetylic salicylic acid in most systems; guideline adjusted medical treatment of HF; close adaption of diuretics to individual needs (especially watch the volume load of pulsatile devices); RV failure—induce inotropic support, call implantation centre; signs of LV recovery, call implantation centre ◆ Patients should not start cardiac rehabilitation before being trained to handle the device independently and securely, and especially to change batteries and controller ◆ The rehabilitation team has to be trained on the specific assist device before starting rehabilitation ◆ The rehabilitation centre should be a short distance from the heart centre, and close cooperation is mandatory ◆ *NOTE: VAD patients are completely dependent on power supply*—batteries may serve as bridging only for some hours and an emergency power supply therefore should be available ◆ Rehabilitation centres should provide an emergency room with beds and monitoring devices ◆ At least two people on the rehabilitation team should be specialized in handling VAD and correctly solving potential functional problems ◆ The rehabilitation team has to be regularly trained in dealing with the systems and potential complications Expected outcomes: ◆ Correct clinical and technical guidance and avoidance of clinical and technical complications ◆ Training of patients in their self-management
Exercise training	Evaluation: ◆ Exercise training may improve the functional status of VAD recipients even at a later time after implantation. It therefore may have additional importance in cases of destination therapy ◆ Determination of peak exercise capacity by peak oxygen consumption (use small increments of 5–10 W/min on a bicycle ergometer or modified Bruce or Naughton protocols) or 6-minute walk test ◆ Continuous ECG monitoring ◆ Control of serum lactate concentration Intervention: ◆ Combination of aerobic endurance and dynamic resistance training with similar restrictions as in other patients after cardiac surgery ◆ Include activities to develop flexibility, coordination, and bodily awareness ◆ *NOTE: Avoid exercise programs that irritate the driveline-outlet. Avoid shaking movements or strong vibrations* Expected outcomes: ◆ Increase fitness and flexibility and rebuild muscular mass and strength ◆ Improved psychosocial wellbeing and social participation

(continued)

Table 8.9 (*continued*) Core components of cardiac rehabilitation in patients with ventricular assist devices (VAD)

Components	Method of application
Diet/ nutritional counselling	◆ Watch fluid regulation and ensure daily weight control by the patient ◆ Reduce salt intake and watch vitamin K intake
Weight control management	See ➲ Table 8.6
Lipid management	See ➲ Table 8.6
Blood pressure management	◆ Systemic blood pressure should be regulated according to the recommendations for the individual assist device
Smoking cessation	See ➲ Table 8.1
Psychosocial management	◆ Patients should be psychologically stable before starting rehabilitation ◆ Include patient's partner and close family members in the rehabilitation process according to the individual needs Expected outcome: ◆ Improved coping

BUN, blood urea nitrogen; BNP, brain natriuretic peptide; LVAD, left ventricular assist device; RV, right ventricular; LV, left ventricular; HF, heart failure.

Source data from Piepoli MF, Corrà U, Benzer W, Bjarnason-Wehrens B et al, Cardiac Rehabilitation Section of the European Association of Cardiovascular Prevention and Rehabilitation Secondary prevention through cardiac rehabilitation: from knowledge to implementation. A position paper from the Cardiac Rehabilitation Section of the European Association of Cardiovascular Prevention and Rehabilitation. *Eur J Cardiovasc Prev Rehabil* 2010; **17**(1): 1–17.

Solution to the case of Mr X

What should be recommended for Mr X in terms of secondary prevention?

Mr X should be referred to an outpatient cardiac rehabilitation/secondary prevention programme. He is not considered to be a high-risk patient. According to the PAMI II criteria (which designate as low risk age < 70 years, with one- or two-vessel disease, successful percutaneous coronary angioplasty and no persistent arrhythmias, and left ventricular ejection fraction < 45%) only the last criterion was not fulfilled since he presented with a left ventricular ejection fraction of 40%.

Nevertheless, a short hospital stay (3 days in the case of Mr X) implies limited time for proper patient education and up-titration of secondary prevention treatments. Advice on lifestyle modification is just the initial step in a secondary prevention intervention (the minimum). This should be done during the acute phase, with the patient still hospitalized or at least at discharge. All patients should receive appropriate information on their clinical status, risk factor control and monitoring, the use of the prescribed therapy, and the targets for an optimal lifestyle. This may not be sufficient to induce optimal and permanent lifestyle changes in many patients: the majority need a more structured and comprehensive secondary prevention intervention through cardiac rehabilitation to effectively achieve their lifestyle targets. Therefore an initial cardiac rehabilitation programme is strongly recommended and this should be followed by adequate long term secondary prevention intervention including follow up monitoring and reinforcement. Consequently, Mr X should be offered planned early post-discharge consultations with a cardiologist or primary care physician and the option of a formal cardiac rehabilitation/secondary prevention programme on an outpatient basis.

However, in some cases (e.g. high-risk patients, patients in an unstable condition, after cardiac surgery, those with multiple risk factors, or in the case of transport difficulties) a personalized in-hospital (residential) cardiac rehabilitation programme with risk factor stratification implemented in a centre-based cardiac rehabilitation setting is more advisable. After an inpatient phase of adequate duration to set up a secondary prevention programme, the intervention should continue in an outpatient setting to check adherence to and the effectiveness of the intervention.

What should be included in Mr X's hospital discharge summary?

The hospital discharge summary should include:

- a confirmed diagnosis
- note of modifiable risk factors
- significant past medical history
- family history
- investigations and results
- procedures and any complications
- medication prescribed and guidance on up-titration
- information on secondary prevention and cardiac rehabilitation (offered/accepted; coordinator), including desirable levels of blood pressure, cholesterol, and lifestyle modifications
- planned follow-up
- recommendations on testing the patient's family.

Acknowledgements

We would like to thank the following: European Association for Cardiovascular Prevention and Rehabilitation members Ugo Corrà, Hugo Saner, and David Wood and Cardiac Rehabilitation Section members Werner Benzer, Birna Bjarnason-Wehrens, Paul Dendale, Dan Gaita, Hannah McGee, Miguel Mendes, Josef Niebauer, Ann-Dorthe Olsen Zwisler, Nana Pogosova, and Jean-Paul Schmid.

Further reading

American Association of Cardiovascular and Pulmonary Rehabilitation. *Guidelines for cardiac rehabilitation and secondary prevention programs*, 3rd edn, 1999. Champaign, IL: Human Kinetics Publishers. [WHO report on the status of implementation of cardiac rehabilitation.]

Balady GJ, Williams MA, Ades PA, et al; American Heart Association Exercise, Cardiac Rehabilitation, and Prevention Committee, the Council on Clinical Cardiology; American Heart Association Council on Cardiovascular Nursing; American Heart Association Council on Epidemiology and Prevention; American Heart Association Council on Nutrition, Physical Activity, and Metabolism; American Association of Cardiovascular and Pulmonary Rehabilitation. Core components of cardiac rehabilitation/secondary prevention programs: 2007 update: a scientific statement from the American Heart Association Exercise, Cardiac Rehabilitation, and Prevention Committee, the Council on Clinical Cardiology; the Councils on Cardiovascular Nursing, Epidemiology and Prevention, and Nutrition, Physical Activity, and Metabolism; and the American Association of Cardiovascular and Pulmonary Rehabilitation. *Circulation* 2007; **115**: 2675–82. [AHA/AACPR scientific statement on the core components in cardiac rehabilitation.]

Bjarnason-Wehrens B, McGee H, Zwisler A-D, et al. on behalf of the Cardiac Rehabilitation Section of the European Association of Cardiovascular Prevention and Rehabilitation. Cardiac rehabilitation in Europe—results from the European Cardiac Rehabilitation Inventory Survey (ECRIS). *Eur J Cardiovasc Prev Rehabil* 2010; **17**: 410–18. [The first European survey on the implementation of cardiac rehabilitation.]

British Association for Cardiac Rehabilitation. *Standards and core components for cardiac rehabilitation*, 2007. URL; <http://www.bcs.com/documents/affiliates/bacr/BACR%20Standards%202007.pdf> [British scientific statement on the core components in cardiac rehabilitation.]

Leon AS, Franklin BA, Costa F, et al; American Heart Association; Council on Clinical Cardiology (Subcommittee on Exercise, Cardiac Rehabilitation, and Prevention); Council on Nutrition, Physical Activity, and Metabolism (Subcommittee on Physical Activity); American Association of Cardiovascular and Pulmonary Rehabilitation. Cardiac rehabilitation and secondary prevention of coronary heart disease: an American Heart Association scientific statement from the Council on Clinical Cardiology (Subcommittee on Exercise, Cardiac Rehabilitation, and Prevention) and the Council on Nutrition, Physical Activity, and Metabolism (Subcommittee on Physical Activity), in collaboration with the American Association of Cardiovascular and Pulmonary Rehabilitation. *Circulation* 2005; **111**: 369–76. [AHA/AACPR scientific statement on the core components in cardiac rehabilitation and secondary prevention in coronary artery disease.]

Fernandez RS, Davidson P, Griffiths R, et al. Overcoming barriers to guideline implementation: the case of cardiac rehabilitation. *Qual Saf Healthcare* 2010; **19**: e15. [A report on the barriers to implementation of cardiac rehabilitation in practice.]

Piepoli MF, Corrà U, Benzer W, et al; Cardiac Rehabilitation Section of the European Association of Cardiovascular Prevention and Rehabilitation. Secondary prevention through cardiac rehabilitation: from knowledge to implementation. A position paper from the Cardiac Rehabilitation Section of the European Association of Cardiovascular Prevention and Rehabilitation. *Eur J Cardiovasc Prev Rehabil* 2010; **17**: 1–17. [A review of the outcome measures in secondary prevention in clinical practice.]

Piepoli MF, Corrà U, Adamopoulos S, et al. Secondary prevention in the clinical management of patients with cardiovascular diseases. Core components, standards and outcome measures for referral and delivery. *Eur J Prev Cardiol* 2012; **21**: 664–81. [EACPR scientific statement on the core components in cardiac rehabilitation.]

Rehabilitation after cardiovascular diseases, with special emphasis on developing countries. Report of a WHO Expert Committee. *World Health Organ Tech Rep Ser* 1993; **831**; 1–122.

References

1 The European Heart Health Charter. URL: <http://www.heartcharter.eu/>

2 Piepoli MF, Corrà U, Benzer et al; Cardiac Rehabilitation Section of the European Association of Cardiovascular Prevention and Rehabilitation. Secondary prevention through cardiac rehabilitation: from knowledge to implementation. A position paper from the Cardiac Rehabilitation Section of the European Association of Cardiovascular Prevention and Rehabilitation. *Eur J Cardiovasc Prev Rehabil* 2010; **17**: 1–17.

3 Steg PG, James SK, Atar D, et al. ESC guidelines for the management of acute myocardial infarction in patients presenting with ST-segment elevation. The Task Force on the Management of Acute Myocardial Infarction of the European Society of Cardiology. *Eur Heart J* 2012; **33**: 2569–619.

4 Hamm CW, Bassand JP, Agewall S, et al. ESC Guidelines for the management of acute coronary syndromes in patients presenting without persistent ST-segment elevation: The Task Force for the management of acute coronary syndromes (ACS) in patients presenting without persistent ST-segment elevation of the European Society of Cardiology (ESC). *Eur Heart J* 2011; **32**: 2999–3054.

5 Antman EM, Hand M, Armstrong PW, et al. 2007 focused update of the ACC/AHA 2004 guidelines for the management of patients with ST-elevation myocardial infarction. *J Am Coll Cardiol* 2008; **51**: 210–47.

6 Anderson JL, Adams CD, Antman EM, et al. ACC/AHA 2007 guidelines for the management of patients with unstable angina/non-ST-elevation myocardial infarction: a report of the American College of Cardiology/American Heart Association Task Force on Practice Guidelines (Writing Committee to Revise the 2002 Guidelines for the management of patients with unstable angina/non-ST-elevation myocardial infarction): developed in collaboration with the American College of Emergency Physicians, American College of Physicians, Society for Academic Emergency Medicine, Society for Cardiovascular Angiography and Interventions, and Society of Thoracic Surgeons. *J Am Coll Cardiol* 2007; **50**: 1–157.

7 Gibbons RJ, Abrams J, Chatterjee K, et al. ACC/AHA 2002 guideline update for the management of patients with chronic stable angina. *J Am Coll Cardiol* 2003; **41**: 159–68.

8 The Task Force for the Diagnosis and Treatment of Acute and Chronic Heart Failure 2012 of the European Society of Cardiology. Developed in collaboration with the Heart Failure Association (HFA) of the ESC. ESC Guidelines for the diagnosis and treatment of acute and chronic heart failure 2012. *Eur Heart J* 2012; **33**: 1787–847.

9 Hunt SA, Abraham WT, Chin MH, et al; American College of Cardiology; American Heart Association Task Force on Practice Guidelines; American College of Chest Physicians; International Society for Heart and Lung Transplantation; Heart Rhythm Society. ACC/AHA guideline update for the diagnosis and management of chronic heart failure in the adult: summary article: a report of the American College of Cardiology/American Heart Association Task Force on Practice Guidelines. *Circulation* 2005; **112**: 1825–52.

10 Rehabilitation after cardiovascular diseases, with special emphasis on developing countries. Report of a WHO Expert Committee. *World Health Organ Tech Rep Ser* 1993; **831**; 1–122.

11 Papadakis S, Oldridge NB, Coyle D, et al. Economic evaluation of cardiac rehabilitation: a systematic review. *Eur J Cardiovasc Prev Rehabil* 2005; **12**: 513–20.

12 Piepoli MF, Davos C, Francis DP, et al. ExTraMATCH Collaborative Exercise training meta-analysis of trials in patients with chronic heart failure (ExTraMATCH). *Br Med J* 2004; **328**: 189–93.

13 Kotseva K, Wood D, De Backer G, et al. EUROASPIRE III: a survey on the lifestyle, risk factors and use of cardioprotective drug therapies in coronary patients from twenty-two European countries. EUROASPIRE Study Group. *Eur J Cardiovasc Prev Rehabil* 2009; **16**: 121–37.

14 Bjarnason-Wehrens B, McGee H, Zwisler A-D., et al. on behalf of the Cardiac Rehabilitation Section of the European Association of Cardiovascular Prevention and Rehabilitation. Cardiac rehabilitation in Europe—results from the European Cardiac Rehabilitation Inventory Survey (ECRIS). *Eur J Cardiovasc Prev Rehabil* 2010; **17**: 410–18.

15 Kotseva K, Wood D, De Backer G, et al. Cardiovascular prevention guidelines in daily practice: a comparison of EUROASPIRE I, II and III surveys in 8 European countries. EUROASPIRE Study Group. *Lancet* 2009; **373**: 929–40.

16 Wood DA, Kotseva K, Connolly S, et al., on behalf of the EUROACTION Study Group. Nurse-coordinated multidisciplinary, family-based cardiovascular disease prevention programme (EUROACTION) for patients with coronary heart disease and asymptomatic individuals at high risk of cardiovascular disease: a paired, cluster-randomised controlled trial. *Lancet* 2008; **371**: 1999–2012.

17 Giannuzzi P, Temporelli PL, Marchioli R, et al. Global secondary prevention strategies to limit event recurrence after myocardial infarction: results of the GOSPEL study, a multicenter, randomized controlled trial from the Italian Cardiac Rehabilitation Network. *Arch Intern Med* 2008; **168**: 2194–204.

18 Task Force on Myocardial Revascularization of the European Society of Cardiology (ESC) and the European Association for Cardio-Thoracic Surgery (EACTS); European Association for Percutaneous Cardiovascular Interventions (EAPCI); Wijns W, Kolh P, Danchin N, et al. Guidelines on myocardial revascularization. *Eur Heart J*. 2010; **31**: 2501–55.

19 Eagle KA, Guyton RA, Davidoff R, et al. ACC/AHA guidelines for coronary artery bypass graft surgery: a report of the American College of Cardiology/American Heart Association Task Force on Practice Guidelines (committee to revise the 1991 guidelines for coronary artery bypass graft surgery). American College of Cardiology/American Heart Association. *J Am Coll Cardiol* 1999; **34**: 1262–347.

20 Eagle KA, Guyton RA, Davidoff R, et al. ACC/AHA 2004 guideline update for coronary artery bypass graft surgery: a report of the American College of Cardiology/American Heart Association Task Force on Practice Guidelines (committee to update the 1999 guidelines for coronary artery bypass graft surgery). *Circulation* 2004; **110**: e340–e437.

21 Vahanian A, Baumgartner H, Bax J, et al. Guidelines on the management of valvular heart disease: the Task Force on the Management of Valvular Heart Disease of the European Society of Cardiology. *Eur Heart J* 2007; **28**: 230–68.

22 Butchart EG, Gohlke-Barwolf C, Antunes MJ, et al. Recommendations for the management of patients after heart valve surgery. *Eur Heart J* 2005; **26**: 2463–71.

23 Hunt SA, Baker DW, Chin MH, et al. ACC/AHA guidelines for the evaluations and management of chronic heart failure in the adult: a report of the American College of Cardiology/American Heart Association Task Force on Practice Guidelines. *J Am Coll Cardiol* 2001; **38**: 2101–13.

24 Arnold JMO, Howlett JG, Ducharme A, et al. The 2001 Canadian Cardiovascular Society consensus guidelines update for the management and prevention of heart failure. *Can J Cardiol* 2001; **17**(Suppl. E): 5E–25E.

25 Krum H. Guidelines for management of patients with chronic heart failure in Australia. *Med J Aust* 2001; **174**: 459–66.

26 Taylor DO, Edwards LB, Boucek MM, et al. Registry of the International Society for Heart and Lung Transplantation: twenty-first official adult heart transplant report—2005. *J Heart Lung Transplant* 2005; **24**: 945–55.

27 Niset G, Vachiery JL, Lamotte M, et al. Rehabilitation after heart transplantation. In: M. Rieu (ed.) *Physical work capacity in organ transplantation*, pp. 67–84, 1998. Basel: Karger.

28 Hirsch AT, Haskal ZJ, Hertzer NR, et al. ACC/AHA 2005 practice guidelines for the management of patients with peripheral arterial disease (lower extremity, renal, mesenteric, and abdominal aortic): a collaborative report from the American Association for Vascular Surgery/Society for Vascular Surgery, Society for Cardiovascular Angiography and Interventions, Society for Vascular Medicine and Biology, Society of Interventional Radiology, and the ACC/AHA Task Force on Practice Guidelines. *Circulation* 2006; **113**: e463–e654.

29 Corrà U, Pistono M, Piepoli MF, et al. Ventricular assist device patients on the horizon of cardiovascular prevention and rehabilitation. *Eur J Prevent Cardiol* 2012; **19**: 490–3.

CHAPTER 9

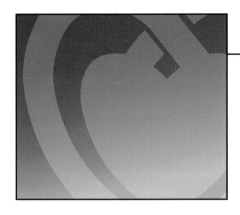

Behaviour and motivation

Christian Albus and Christoph Herrmann-Lingen

Contents

Summary

Caregivers need to be aware that lifestyle change is difficult and that adherence to medication in people at high cardiovascular risk and established cardiovascular disease (CVD) is low. Lifestyle is usually based on long-standing patterns and is highly determined by someone's social environment and socioeconomic status. Additional factors such as chronic stress, cognitive impairment, and negative emotions (e.g. depression, anxiety) further impede the ability to adopt a healthy lifestyle, as does complex or confusing advice from medical caregivers. Reasons for poor adherence to medication and lifestyle recommendations can be multifactorial, ranging from factors related to the health system (e.g. poor communication) to complexity of the therapeutic regimen and the condition of the patient (e.g. asymptomatic disease, disabilities, lack of motivation). In clinical practice, increased awareness of these factors by caregivers is important, as it facilitates empathetic counselling and the provision of simple and explicit advice. Established cognitive–behavioural strategies, such as motivational interviewing, goal setting, repetitive monitoring, and feedback, are important tools to help with behaviour change and adherence to medication. Specialized healthcare professionals (e.g. nurses, dieticians, psychologists, etc.) should be involved wherever necessary and feasible. In addition, reducing dosage demands to the lowest applicable level is the single most effective means for enhancing adherence to medication. In individuals at very high risk or with clinically manifest CVD, multimodal interventions, integrating education on healthy lifestyle and medical resources, exercise training, stress management, and counselling on psychosocial risk factors, are recommended.

Clinical case

Mr A is a 48-year-old man who comes to the surgery once in a while to receive a new prescription for his antihypertensive drugs. The intervals between consultations suggest that he is not taking his prescribed drugs regularly. Mr A is obese (BMI 34 kg/m^2) and has poorly controlled type 2 diabetes [glycated haemoglobin (HbA1c) 8.5% with metformin] and dyslipidaemia (low-density lipoprotein cholesterol 183 mg/dl). His current office blood pressure is 155/95 mmHg and he currently smokes 20 cigarettes a day (32 pack-years). Some years ago his father, who was also a smoker, died from his first myocardial infarction at the age of 68. After his father's death Mr A had made an attempt to quit smoking but relapsed after a few weeks. Mr A himself has not suffered a cardiac event so far and has no typical symptoms of angina.

(*continued*)

Clinical case *(continued)*

Mr A has a poorly paid and insecure sedentary job as a clerk and lives in a lower-class neighbourhood. In his leisure time he has no physically active hobbies. He is married to a smoker, who works as a cleaner for a few hours per week. Their 25-year-old daughter lives with her husband. Their 21-year-old son still lives at home and has a poorly paid trainee job. The couple are in chronic conflict about how to deal with the permanent scarcity of money. Mr A tends to react to conflicts with high levels of anger and uses overeating and increased smoking to calm down in such situations.

Why do individuals find it hard to change their lifestyle?

A person's lifestyle is usually based on long-standing behavioural patterns. These patterns are framed during childhood and adolescence by the interaction of environmental and genetic factors, and are maintained or even promoted by one's social environment as an adult. Consequently, marked differences in health behaviours can be observed among individuals and social groups. In particular, individuals with a low level of education or low income, social isolation, chronic stress at work and at home, and negative emotions such as depression, anxiety, and hostility are more likely to have an unhealthy lifestyle [1–4]. In addition, these factors impede someone's ability to adopt a healthy lifestyle and to maintain health-promoting behaviours, as does complex or confusing advice from medical caregivers. In clinical practice, increased awareness of these factors by caregivers is important. It facilitates empathetic counselling and the provision of simple and explicit advice. Psychosocial risk factors that interfere with health behaviours should be assessed by clinical interview or standardized questionnaires, and tailored clinical management should be considered in order to enhance quality of life and cardiac prognosis [5].

Attempts to facilitate behavioural change typically start by increasing the motivation for change. However, they also have to consider the so-called 'intention–behaviour gap' [6]. People at risk might feel motivated to change their behaviour, but barriers like dysfunctional beliefs, perceived lack of time, or situations where people give in to temptations might occur. Thus, just focusing on 'motivation' or 'intention' often does not necessarily translate into action. In addition, while many people start to engage in healthy behaviours after a significant event (e.g. myocardial infarction), maintenance of lifestyle change is typically low [7]. Even in the context of structured programmes, low adherence and maintenance are among the main factors limiting the effects of behavioural interventions (such as exercise training) and require special attention [8].

A recent model for predicting and modifying the adoption and maintenance of health behaviours is the 'health action process approach' (HAPA) [6]. In addition to the assumption of other social-cognitive theories that the individual's intention to change is the best predictor for action, the HAPA model suggests a distinction between (1) pre-intentional motivational processes that lead to a behavioural intention and (2) post-intentional volitional processes that lead to the actual health behaviour [6].

According to the HAPA model, factors important for building an intention, for example risk perception, outcome expectancies, and action self-efficacy (the motivational phase), have necessarily to be followed by post-intentional factors like maintenance and recovery self-efficacy and strategic planning, resulting in a repetitive, cyclic process of action, involving initiative, maintenance, and recovery after a relapse (volitional phase) [6].

The HAPA model is shown in ➲ Fig. 9.1. In the initial, motivational phase, risk perception (e.g. 'I could get a heart attack') sets the stage for a contemplative process, in which the person balances the pros and cons of certain behaviours (outcome expectancies; e.g. 'Smoking cessation might be good for my heart' versus 'I do not know how to cope with inner tension without smoking', or 'I might get fat when I quit smoking'). However, even if the pros outweigh the cons, a stable intention can only be established if the person feels capable of performing the desired action (action self-efficacy). In the case of low perceived action self-efficacy (e.g. 'I will never be able to quit smoking'), patients will not even intend to change their behaviour although they 'know' that they should. Hence, positive outcome expectancies together with high action self-efficacy comprise the most important factors in the motivational phase.

Of the processes that are important for the volitional phase, perceived self-efficacy has been found to be important at all stages in the process of changing health behaviour [9]. However, there are distinct differences in the exact meaning of 'self-efficacy' depending on the stage of the health action process. In the motivational phase, 'action self-efficacy' means a strong, optimistic belief that an action will be successful with respect to its outcome (e.g. 'I will be able to quit smoking') and is more likely to initiate a new behaviour. The terms 'maintenance self-efficacy' and 'recovery self-efficacy' are instrumental to the subsequent volitional phase. People with high maintenance self-efficacy feel optimistic that they will be able to cope with barriers that could or will occur during the maintenance period of the new behaviour (e.g. 'I will overcome inner tension without smoking'). 'Recovery self-efficacy', finally, is

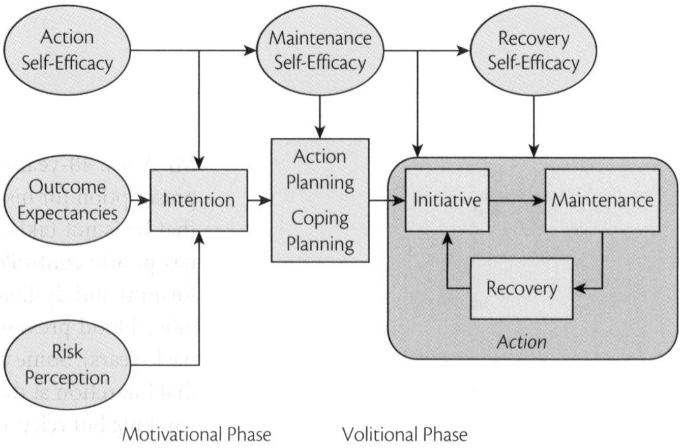

Fig. 9.1 Generic diagram of the health action process approach [6].
Source: 'Modeling health behavior change: how to predict and modify the adoption and maintenance of health behaviors', Schwarzer R, 2008, *Applied Psychology*, John Wiley & Sons.

an important factor if someone faces a relapse. Relapses are common in all kinds of health behaviours, but are only deleterious to maintenance if the individual dramatises the event as due to overwhelming, stable internal or external reasons (e.g. 'I cannot cope with my job without smoking'). People with high 'recovery self-efficacy' are able to recover hope and find ways to restore their required behaviour [6].

A firm intention, together with high 'maintenance self-efficacy', enables the individual to undertake concrete 'action planning' (e.g. 'I will quit smoking on June 1st, at noon') as well as 'coping planning' (e.g. 'I will cope with inner tension by breathing techniques'). Prepared like this, the individual will go for action (e.g. initiate a new health behaviour). A high 'recovery self-efficacy' will help to maintain the desired behaviour, even if there are short relapses [6]. Thus, intervention aimed at achieving an enduring healthy lifestyle change should always take the two phases or 'stages' of behaviour change into account, i.e. the motivational and the volitional phase, and address these stages specifically.

In addition to individual psychological processes, there are several other dimensions with potential relevance for behaviour change. Michie et al. [10] have categorized seven policy categories (e.g. environmental/social planning, service provision, legislation, fiscal) and nine intervention functions (e.g. education, training, restrictions, incentivization) that might have an impact on tobacco control and obesity by enhancing an individual's motivation, capability, and opportunity for lifestyle change. Because this chapter focuses on individual health processes, further details on policies relevant to the general public are given in Chapter 24.

Why is adherence to medication so low?

Numerous studies have shown that adherence to medication in individuals at high risk and patients with cardiovascular disease (CVD) is low, resulting in poor cardiac prognosis [11,12]. For example, 1 month after an acute myocardial infarction, almost 25–30% of patients stop at least one medication, with a progressive decline in adherence over time. After 1 year, less than 50% report persistent use of either statins, beta-blockers, or antihypertensive therapy [13].

The reasons for poor adherence are complex and can be categorized into five broad groupings that include factors related to the patient, the condition, therapy, socioeconomics, and the health system [14] (➲ Table 9.1). In addition, low adherence may be the result of cognitive processes, such as implicit cost–benefit analyses in which (correct or incorrect) beliefs about the need of a specific drug are weighed against concerns about its potential adverse effects, and more or less conscious decisions are made not to take it [15].

In clinical practice, reasons for non-adherence tend to cluster together, for example complex medication regimens may occur in individuals with chronic, asymptomatic disease or multiple risk factors who lack motivation and a clear understanding of the therapeutic regimen [12]. This situation makes high demands on the physician, who needs to give explicit and clear advice and continuous care. However, physicians often fail to communicate critical elements of medication use, such as possible adverse effects, how long to take the medication for, and the exact timing and dosage [16].

Table 9.1 Potential reasons for non-adherence to medication [14]

Categories of reasons for non-adherence	Examples
Health system	Poor quality of provider–patient relationship; poor communication (e.g. limited, complex, or confusing advice); lack of access to healthcare; lack of continuity of care
Condition	Asymptomatic chronic disease (lack of physical cues); comorbid mental health disorders (e.g. depression)
Patient	Physical impairments (e.g. vision problems or impaired dexterity); cognitive impairment; psychological/behavioural factors (e.g. lack of motivation, low self-efficacy); younger age
Therapy	Complexity of regimen; side effects
Socioeconomic	Low literacy; high medication costs; poor social support

Source: World Health Organization. Adherence to long term therapies: evidence for action, 2003.

Physicians should assess adherence to medication, and identify reasons for non-adherence in order to tailor further interventions to the individual needs of the patient or person at risk. In addition, physicians should be aware that low adherence to medication may reflect generally poor health behaviour. Therefore, measures should always be taken to improve adherence and health behaviour in general [5].

Effective communication and cognitive–behavioural strategies as a means towards lifestyle change and better adherence to medication

A friendly and positive interaction with caregivers is a powerful tool for enhancing an individual's ability to cope with illness and adhere to recommended lifestyle changes and medication use. The social support provided by caregivers may be of primary importance in helping patients maintain healthy habits and follow medical advice. It is particularly important to explore each individual patient's experiences, thoughts and worries, previous knowledge, and circumstances of their everyday life. Individualized counselling is the basis for gaining the patient's motivation and commitment. Decision-making should be shared between the caregiver and patient (also including the patient's spouse and family) to the greatest extent possible, thus ensuring the active involvement of both the individual and his or her family in lifestyle change and adherence to medication [5,17,18].

The way in which advice is given, or rather the offering of relevant information and support, must be sensitive to the particular patient's thoughts (including, among others, beliefs about the illness and its treatment) and feelings [15]. This is a specific clinical skill; therefore, communication training is important for health

Table 9.2 Principles of effective communication for facilitating behavioural change [5]

◆ Spend enough time with the individual to create a therapeutic relationship—even a few more minutes can make a difference
◆ Acknowledge the individual's personal view of his/her disease and contributing factors
◆ Encourage expression of worries and anxieties, concerns, and self-evaluation of motivation for behaviour change and chances of success
◆ Speak to the individual in his/her own language and be supportive of every improvement in lifestyle
◆ Ask questions to check that the individual has understood the advice and has any support they require to follow it
◆ Acknowledge that changing lifelong habits can be difficult and that gradual change that is sustained is often more permanent than a rapid change
◆ Accept that individuals may need support for a long time and that repeated efforts to encourage and maintain lifestyle change may be necessary in many individuals
◆ Make sure that all health professionals involved provide consistent information

Source: Perk J, De Backer G, Gohlke H, Graham I, Reiner Z, Verschuren M, Albus C, Benlian P, Boysen G, Cifkova R, Deaton C, Ebrahim S, Fisher M, Germano G, Hobbs R, Hoes A, Karadeniz S, Mezzani A, Prescott E, Ryden L, Scherer M, Syvänne M, Scholte op Reimer WJ, Vrints C, Wood D, Zamorano JL, Zannad F. European guidelines on cardiovascular disease prevention in clinical practice (version 2012). *Eur Heart J* 2012; **33**: 1635–1701.

professionals. ➲ Table 9.2 sets out the principles of effective communication needed to facilitate successful treatment and prevention of CVD [5].

Regarding specific interventions for behavioural change, caregivers can build on established cognitive–behavioural strategies to assess an individual's thoughts, attitudes, and beliefs concerning their willingness and perceived ability to change behaviour, as well as the environmental context in which attempts to change are made, and subsequently maintain the lifestyle change.

Michie et al. [19] have performed a meta-regression analysis on 26 behavioural and/or cognitive techniques for increasing physical activity and healthy eating in adults in order to identify effective individual techniques and theoretically derived combinations of techniques. After extracting outcome data from 101 papers reporting 122 interventional studies ($n = 44\,747$ participants), the random-effects model produced a small but significant overall effect size of 0.31 (95% CI 0.26–0.36). In view of the moderate level of heterogeneity ($I^2 = 69\%$, $Q = 393$, $P < 0.001$), meta-regression identified five techniques that explained the greatest amount of variance: self-monitoring of behaviour, in combination with at least one other behavioural technique—prompting intention formation, prompting the setting of specific goals, providing feedback on performance, and prompting a review of behavioural goals [19]. Thus, promoting sustained lifestyle change requires not only interventions to improve motivation but also repetitive monitoring and feedback over a long period of time.

Another crucial step in behaviour change is to help the individual set realistic goals; goal-setting combined with self-monitoring of the chosen behaviour are important tools needed to achieve a positive outcome [18]. This will in turn increase self-efficacy for the chosen behaviour, and thereafter new goals can be set. Moving forward in small, consecutive steps is one of the key points in changing long-term behaviour [18]. Translated into implications for clinical practice, the 'ten strategic steps' listed in ➲ Table 9.3 are recommended to enhance counselling on behavioural change [5].

Table 9.3 Ten strategic steps for enhancing counselling on behavioural change [5]

1. Develop a therapeutic alliance
2. Counsel all individuals at risk of or with manifest CVD
3. Assist individuals to understand the relationship between their behaviour and health
4. Help individuals assess the barriers to behaviour change
5. Gain commitments from individuals to own their behaviour change
6. Involve individuals in identifying and selecting the risk factors to change
7. Use a combination of strategies including reinforcement of the individual's capacity for change
8. Design a lifestyle modification plan
9. Involve other healthcare staff whenever possible
10. Monitor progress through follow-up contact

Source: Perk J, De Backer G, Gohlke H, Graham I, Reiner Z, Verschuren M, Albus C, Benlian P, Boysen G, Cifkova R, Deaton C, Ebrahim S, Fisher M, Germano G, Hobbs R, Hoes A, Karadeniz S, Mezzani A, Prescott E, Ryden L, Scherer M, Syvänne M, Scholte op Reimer WJ, Vrints C, Wood D, Zamorano JL, Zannad F. European guidelines on cardiovascular disease prevention in clinical practice (version 2012). *Eur Heart J* 2012; **33**: 1635–1701.

One established behavioural intervention that can help with lifestyle change is motivational interviewing [20]. In a systematic review and meta-analysis of 73 randomized controlled trials, motivational interviewing was shown to significantly induce favourable changes in body mass index, total blood cholesterol, systolic blood pressure, and alcohol use [21]. Rollnik et al. [20] provide a set of 'top ten useful questions' that can be used in a 15-minute clinical interview (see ➲ Table 9.4).

Many efforts have been made to replace personal contact with caregivers by e-learning approaches. However, current clinical and economic evidence does not suggest that e-learning devices designed to promote change in dietary behaviour will produce clinically

Table 9.4 The top ten most useful questions for motivational interviewing [20]

1. What changes would you most like to talk about?
2. What have you noticed about ...?
3. How important is it for you to change ...?
4. How confident do you feel about changing ...?
5. How do you see the benefits of ...?
6. How do you see the drawbacks of ...?
7. What will make the most sense to you ...?
8. How might things be different if you ...?
9. In what way ...?
10. Where does that leave you now?

Source: Rollnik S, Butler CC, Kinnersley P, Gregory J Mash B. Motivational interviewing. *BMJ* 2010; **340**: c1900.

Table 9.5 Recommendations for promoting adherence to medication [5]

◆ Provide clear (written) advice regarding the benefits and possible adverse effects of the medication, and the duration and timing of dosage
◆ Consider patients' habits and preferences
◆ Reduce dosage demands to the lowest feasible level
◆ Ask patients in a non-judgemental way how the medication works for them, and discuss possible reasons for non-adherence (e.g. side effects, worries)
◆ Implement repetitive monitoring and feedback
◆ In case of lack of time, introduce physician's assistants and/or trained nurses whenever it is necessary and feasible
◆ In case of persistent non-adherence, offer multisession or combined behavioural interventions

Source: Perk J, De Backer G, Gohlke H, Graham I, Reiner Z, Verschuren M, Albus C, Benlian P, Boysen G, Cifkova R, Deaton C, Ebrahim S, Fisher M, Germano G, Hobbs R, Hoes A, Karadeniz S, Mezzani A, Prescott E, Ryden L, Scherer M, Syvänne M, Scholte op Reimer WJ, Vrints C, Wood D, Zamorano JL, Zannad F. European guidelines on cardiovascular disease prevention in clinical practice (version 2012). *Eur Heart J* 2012; **33**: 1635–1701.

significant changes [22]. Furthermore, at a population level, e-learning interventions are at least as expensive as other interventions for changing individuals' behaviour [22]. Hence, a personal intervention, delivered by physicians or other healthcare professionals, can currently be considered the 'gold standard' for behaviour change.

In clinical practice, physicians should identify reasons for possible non-adherence to medication, and promote adherence according to the principles outlined in ➲ Table 9.5 [5].

In addition to these measures, some specific pragmatic steps may help to improve adherence to medication. A recent meta-analysis of interventions among older adults (age at least 60 years; $n = 11\,287$ participants) emphasized that, in addition to repetitive monitoring and reducing dosage demands, special medication packaging and succinct written instructions are significantly associated with improved adherence to medication (ES 0.33), knowledge (ES 0.48), diastolic blood pressure (ES 0.21), and healthcare utilization (ES 0.16) [23].

Multimodal, behavioural interventions as further tools to help lifestyle change and promote adherence to medication

According to a recent systematic review and meta-analysis involving 13 RCTs ($n = 68\,556$ subjects), patient education alone can improve health-related quality of life and decrease healthcare costs in patients with coronary heart disease. However, there is no strong evidence for an effect on cardiac morbidity and hospitalization [24].

Therefore, in individuals at very high risk and those with clinically manifest CVD, 'multimodal, behavioural interventions' are recommended [5,25]. These interventions combine the skills of multiple healthcare professionals, such as physicians, nurses, psychologists, and experts in nutrition and sports medicine, into a complex intervention. Specifically, multimodal, behavioural interventions integrate education on a healthy lifestyle and medical resources, exercise training, and smoking cessation programmes for resistant smokers [25]. Psychosocial risk factors (stress, social isolation, and negative emotions) that may act as barriers to behavioural change are addressed in individual or group counselling sessions, according to the specific needs of the participants [25].

In patients with hypertension and diabetes, but no evidence for CVD, complex behavioural interventions significantly reduce total mortality and cardiac events [odds ratio (OR) 0.78 and 0.61, respectively] [26]. In patients with coronary heart disease, exercise-based rehabilitation alone or in combination with psychosocial or educational interventions could significantly reduce overall and cardiovascular mortality (OR 0.87 and 0.74, respectively) and hospital readmissions (OR 0.69). However, there was no clear evidence for a favourable impact on rates of myocardial infarction, coronary artery bypass graft, or percutaneous coronary intervention, and no differential effect of types and dosages of the interventions [27].

In a recent randomized trial, depressed patients with poorly controlled diabetes and/or coronary artery disease were assigned to either usual care or collaborative care, simultaneously addressing depression and control of risk factors with regular monitoring and shared decision making on step-by-step improvements. The intervention led to an overall improvement in depressive symptoms and risk factor burden [28] as well as reduced healthcare costs and an improved quality of life [29].

There is evidence that more extensive/longer interventions (i.e. longer than 6 months) lead to better long-term results with respect to behaviour change and somatic outcome [18]. Individuals with a low socioeconomic status, older age, or female gender may need tailored programmes in order to meet their specific needs for information and emotional support [18,30]. More detailed information on the content and structure of current preventive care is given in ➲ Chapters 22 and 23.

Solution to the case of Mr A

To increase his willingness and ability to cooperate in reducing his cardiovascular risk, Mr A needs a stable and continuous relationship with his physician, who can provide regular guidance and support. He has some perception of his cardiac risk (as can be seen from his earlier attempt to quit smoking) but needs more information on the increased risk conferred by obesity, diabetes, and lack of exercise. He also has some misconceptions about the need to take his antihypertensive drugs regularly, and he feels uncomfortable about changing too much at a time.

(continued)

Solution to the case of Mr A *(continued)*

After Mr A has been educated about his current risk and the advantages of good adherence to medication and behavioural change, he will benefit from advice on single steps that may be helpful in his current situation. Since he had indirectly indicated that he might be willing to quit smoking, one of the first steps to be recommended will be another attempt to quit. However, as he often uses smoking as a method to cope with anger, alternative means for anger regulation should be discussed. Physical activity could be introduced here (e.g. he could go out for a walk instead of smoking cigarettes after angry conflicts with his wife). Further suggestions will include healthier food choices and better adherence to medication, with self-monitoring of blood pressure and glucose. Weight reduction might be a goal for the future, but to gain no more weight might be an adequate aim in the short term.

Patient education is followed by shared decision making on a clear and explicit (possibly written and commonly signed) stepped lifestyle change plan with a defined time schedule. After general agreement has been reached, each step needs to be operationalized.

It would be valuable to involve Mrs A as a partner, getting her commitment to stop smoking together with her husband and to collaborate in choosing healthier food. Exercising together might also be an attractive option for the couple—unless in situations of conflict, where the wife could support her husband by letting him leave the situation for a walk as a chance for de-escalation. They are both offered nicotine replacement and referral to a cognitive–behavioural smoking cessation programme and receive dietary advice with a specific focus on the dietary needs of diabetics, and information about healthy amounts of exercise, existing walking groups, sports clubs etc.

Asking for patients' (and spouses') views and preferences helps to identify types of food and exercise that are likely to be adopted and maintained. Mr and Mrs A would enjoy joining a dancing group once a week and each partner wants to take up some additional individual endurance exercise once a week.

Finally, the medication plan is reviewed with the patient and simplified, if possible. Misconceptions (e.g. 'I only need to take my blood pressure pills, if my blood pressure is high') are corrected and details of regular self-monitoring as well as practical means to increase medication adherence (e.g. pill boxes) are agreed upon.

Regular monthly follow-up appointments are scheduled over the next year. During follow-up appointments, achieved changes are documented and valued. Feedback about improved parameters (e.g. reduced risk SCORE) is used to encourage maintenance. Unforeseen barriers and failures to adhere to the initial agreement sometimes occur and are discussed. A new agreement on the next or modified steps is made each time. If Mr A remains behind initial targets during several follow-up visits, referral to specialist care or a multimodal prevention programme might be needed.

After 6 months the monthly appointments have become important to Mr and Mrs A and they have managed to quit smoking with the help of the smoking cessation programme and nicotine replacement. Due to dancing classes and weekly walking, Mr A has maintained his body weight despite smoking cessation. Both partners have understood the need for a healthier lifestyle and better self-control of high blood pressure and diabetes. Mr A is now taking his medication almost regularly and home measurements of blood pressure usually lie around 130/90 mmHg. Mrs A pays more attention to healthy cooking. The money saved by smoking cessation and the recommendations for conflict de-escalation help alleviate the regular discussions about finances. Mr A's HbA1c has improved to 7.5%. Both partners can be commended for their achievements and a new agreement is made to increase the frequency of weekly exercise from this week on.

Further reading

Artinian NT, Fletcher GF, Mozaffarian D, et al. Interventions to promote physical activity and dietary lifestyle changes for cardiovascular risk reduction in adults. AHA scientific statement. *Circulation* 2010; **122**: 406–41.

Balady GJ, Williams MA, Ades PA, et al. Core components of cardiac rehabilitation/secondary prevention programs: 2007 update. *Circulation* 2007; **115**: 2675–82.

Burell G, Granlund B. Women's hearts need special treatment. *Int J Behav Med* 2002; **9**: 228–42.

General Medical Council. *Consent: patients and doctors making decisions together*, 2008. London: General Medical Council. URL: <http://www.gmc-uk.org/static/documents/content/Consent_-_English_0911.pdf>

Ho PM, Bryson CL, Rumsfeld JS. Medication adherence. Its importance in cardiovascular outcomes. *Circulation* 2009; **119**: 3028–35.

National Institute for Health and Care Excellence. *Behaviour change at population, community and individual level.* NICE Public Health Guidance **6**, 2007. London: National Institute for Health and Care Excellence.

Perk J, De Backer G, Gohlke H, et al. European guidelines on cardiovascular disease prevention in clinical practice (version 2012). *Eur Heart J* 2012; **33**: 1635–701.

Rollnik S, Butler CC, Kinnersley P, et al. Motivational interviewing. *Br Med J* 2010; **340**: c1900.

Schwarzer R. Modeling health behaviour change: how to predict and modify the adoption and maintenance of health behaviours. *Appl Psychol* 2008; **57**: 1–29.

World Health Organization. *Adherence to long term therapies: evidence for action*, 2003. Geneva: World Health Organization. URL: <http://whqlibdoc.who.int/publications/2003/9241545992.pdf>

References

1 Stringhini S, Sabia S, Shipley M, et al. Association of socioeconomic position with health behaviors and mortality. *J Am Med Assoc* 2010; **303**: 1159–66.

2 Albert MA, Glynn RJ, Buring J, et al. Impact of traditional and novel risk factors on the relationship between socioeconomic status and incident cardiovascular events. *Circulation* 2006; **114**: 2619–26.

3 Whooley MA, de Jonge O, Vittinghoff E, et al. Depressive symptoms, health behaviours and the risk of cardiovascular events in patients with coronary heart disease. *J Am Med Assoc* 2008; **300**: 2379–88.

4 Chandola T, Britton A, Brunner E, et al. Work stress and coronary heart disease: what are the mechanisms? *Eur Heart J* 2008; **29**: 640–8.

5 Perk J, De Backer G, Gohlke H, et al. European guidelines on cardiovascular disease prevention in clinical practice (version 2012). *Eur Heart J* 2012; **33**: 1635–701.

6 Schwarzer R. Modeling health behaviour change: how to predict and modify the adoption and maintenance of health behaviours. *Appl Psychol* 2008; **57**: 1–29.

7 National Institute for Health and Care Excellence. *Behaviour change at population, community and individual level.* NICE Public Health Guidance **6**, 2007. London: National Institute for Health and Care Excellence.

8 Conraads VM, Deaton C, Piotrowicz E, et al. Adherence of heart failure patients to exercise: barriers and possible solutions: a position statement of the Study Group on Exercise Training in Heart Failure of the Heart Failure Association of the European Society of Cardiology. *Eur J Heart Fail* 2012; **14**: 451–8.

9 Bandura A. *Self-efficacy: the exercise of control*, 1997. New York: Freeman.

10 Michie S, van Stralen MM, West R. The behaviour change wheel: a new method for characterising and designing behaviour change interventions. *Implement Sci* 2011; **6**: 42.

11 Ho PM, Bryson CL, Rumsfeld JS. Medication adherence. Its importance in cardiovascular outcomes. *Circulation* 2009; **119**: 3028–35.

12 Osterberg L, Blaschke T. Adherence to medication. *N Engl J Med* 2005; **353**: 487–97.

13 Ho PM, Spertus JA, Masoudi FA, et al. Impact of medication therapy discontinuation on mortality after myocardial infarction. *Arch Intern Med* 2006; **166**: 1842–7.

14 World Health Organization. *Adherence to long term therapies: evidence for action*, 2003. Geneva: World Health Organization. URL: <http://whqlibdoc.who.int/publications/2003/9241545992.pdf>

15 Horne R, Weinman J. Patients' beliefs about prescribed medicines and their role in adherence to treatment in chronic physical illness. *J Psychosom Res* 1999; **47**: 555–67.

16 Tarn DM, Heritage J, Peterniti DA, et al. Physician communication when prescribing medication. *Arch Intern Med* 2006; **166**: 1855–62.

17 General Medical Council. *Consent: patients and doctors making decisions together*, 2008. London: General Medical Council. URL: <http://www.gmc-uk.org/static/documents/content/Consent_-_English_0911.pdf>

18 Artinian NT, Fletcher GF, Mozaffarian D, et al. Interventions to promote physical activity and dietary lifestyle changes for cardiovascular risk reduction in adults. AHA scientific statement. *Circulation* 2010; **122**: 406–41.

19 Michie S, Abraham C, Whittington C, et al. Effective techniques in healthy eating and physical activity interventions: a meta-regression. *Health Psychol* 2009; **28**: 690–701.

20 Rollnik S, Butler CC, Kinnersley P, et al. Motivational interviewing. *Br Med J* 2010; **340**: c1900.

21 Rubak S, Sandbaek A, Lauritzen T, et al. Motivational interviewing: systematic review and meta-analysis. *Br J Gen Pract* 2005; **55**: 305–12.

22 Harris J, Felix L, Miners A, et al. Adaptive e-learning to improve dietary behaviour: a systematic review and cost-effectiveness analysis. *Health Technol Assess* 2011; **15**: 1–160.

23 Conn VS, Hafdahl AR, Cooper PS, et al. Interventions to improve medication adherence among older adults: meta-analysis of adherence outcomes among randomized controlled trials. *The Gerontologist* 2009; **49**: 447–62.

24 Brown JP, Clark AM, Dalal H, et al. Effect of patient education in the management of coronary heart disease: a systematic review and meta-analysis of randomised controlled trials. *Eur J Prev Cardiol* 2013; **20**: 701–14.

25 Balady GJ, Williams MA, Ades PA, et al. Core components of cardiac rehabilitation/secondary prevention programs: 2007 update. *Circulation* 2007; **115**: 2675–82.

26 Ebrahim S, Taylor F, Ward K, et al. Multiple risk factor interventions for primary prevention of coronary heart disease. *Cochrane Database Syst Rev* 2011; (1): CD001561.

27 Heran BS, Ebrahim S, Moxham T, et al. Exercise-based cardiac rehabilitation for coronary heart disease. *Cochrane Database Syst Rev* 2011; (7): CD001800.

28 Katon WJ, Lin EH, Von Korff M, et al. Collaborative care for patients with depression and chronic illnesses. *N Engl J Med* 2010; **363**: 2611–20.

29 Katon W, Russo J, Lin EH, et al. Cost-effectiveness of a multicondition collaborative care intervention: a randomized controlled trial. *Arch Gen Psychiatry* 2012; **69**: 506–14.

30 Burell G, Granlund B. Women's hearts need special treatment. *Int J Behav Med* 2002; **9**: 228–42.

CHAPTER 10

Smoking

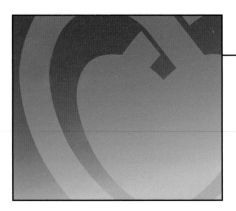

Charlotta Pisinger and Serena Tonstad

Contents

Summary

Smoking causes all forms of atherosclerotic cardiovascular disease. Smokers are about 10 years younger than never smokers at the time of their first myocardial infarction. Even occasional, light, and passive smoking are harmful; there is no safe level. The health benefits of quitting smoking are immediate. In patients with coronary heart disease, smoking cessation results in a dramatic decline in future cardiovascular events and reduces cardiovascular death. Tobacco dependence produces structural and functional changes in the central nervous system and should be regarded as a chronic disease with a lifelong risk of relapse. The addictive nature of nicotine and craving for cigarettes make continued abstinence difficult to maintain. The majority of serious attempts to quit smoking will fail within a year, as seen with other addictions. Making treatment readily available and reducing barriers to treatment increase the likelihood that smokers will accept treatment. Treatment starts with very brief advice: asking about smoking, advising on quitting, and offering/referring to assistance—a combination of supportive counselling and smoking cessation pharmacotherapy. Medication and supportive follow-up should be arranged for all smokers upon discharge from hospital and in outpatient settings. Abbreviated motivational interviewing can be used to help ambivalent smokers become willing to make an attempt to quit. Three types of pharmacotherapy have evidence-based effects in promoting cessation. These include nicotine-replacement therapy, bupropion, and varenicline. All three are clinically appropriate for patients with stable cardiovascular disease. Less evidence is available regarding their use in patients with acute disease. Nicotine-replacement therapy may be started up to 2 weeks prior to or on the target quit day. Bupropion and varenicline should be titrated up for 1–2 weeks in order to reach a therapeutic level before the target quit day. In every cardiovascular setting high priority should be given to identification and documentation of the smoking status of all patients and systematic provision of cessation support. Furthermore, clinicians should ask about exposure to second-hand smoke and recommend avoidance. Even though relapse rates are high, efforts to help smokers must not cease. Smoking cessation is the most effective, and certainly the cheapest, treatment for preventing new or recurrent cardiovascular disease. Furthermore, clinicians must play a more active role than ever before in advocating for stronger tobacco control.

What is in a cigarette?

> A cigarette is the only consumer product which, when used as directed, kills its consumer (Gro Harlem Brundtland, World Health Organization).

Nicotine is the best known component of cigarettes but tobacco smoke contains more than 7000 chemicals and compounds. Hundreds of these chemicals are toxic and at least 69 are carcinogenic [1]. Previously it was believed that nicotine played the most important role in cardiovascular disease, but that does not now appear to be the case. Carbon monoxide, benzopyrenes, glycoproteins, and other substances in tobacco smoke seem to play the major part.

The risks of smoking and the benefits of quitting

Smoking cigarettes is the single greatest preventable cause of death; it is estimated to have caused around 100 million deaths during the twentieth century [1]. Smoking harms the heart and results in premature ageing, causes serious damage to most organs, and costs the smoker about 10 years of life [2–4]. Helping patients quit smoking improves cardiovascular health and significantly reduces the risk of numerous other serious conditions. There is no lower safe level of smoking. There is no other intervention as effective as quitting smoking for improving health and longevity.

In patients with coronary heart disease (CHD) smoking cessation results in a dramatic decline in the risk of future cardiovascular disease (CVD) and reduces the risk of cardiovascular death markedly [5,6]. The reduction in risk of a non-fatal cardiac event is about 36% [7] and of premature death about 50% or more. The decrease in smoking prevalence in the last decades has accounted for the same reduction in cardiovascular mortality as all the combined medical treatments for CVD [8].

The benefits of quitting are rapid. The excess risk of CHD caused by smoking is halved after 1 year of smoking cessation, after controlling for all possible relevant confounders. After 15 years of abstinence, the risk of CHD is as low as in people who have never smoked. Quitting smoking also reduces the risk of ischaemic stroke and subarachnoid haemorrhage. In patients with left ventricular dysfunction after MI, who are at particularly high risk for recurrent adverse outcomes, smoking cessation is associated with a 40% lower hazard of death and a 30% lower hazard of recurrent myocardial infarction (MI). Among patients with peripheral artery disease, smoking cessation improves exercise tolerance, reduces the risk of amputation after surgery, and increases overall survival.

Smoking cessation is not only the cheapest treatment for the patient with CVD and the one with fewest adverse events, it is also one of the most effective. A review found that mortality risk was reduced by 36% in quitters [7], compared with much lower risk reductions due to use of aspirin [9], angiotensin-converting enzyme (ACE) inhibitors [10], beta-blockers [11], or lipid-lowering therapy [12] (➲ Fig. 10.1).

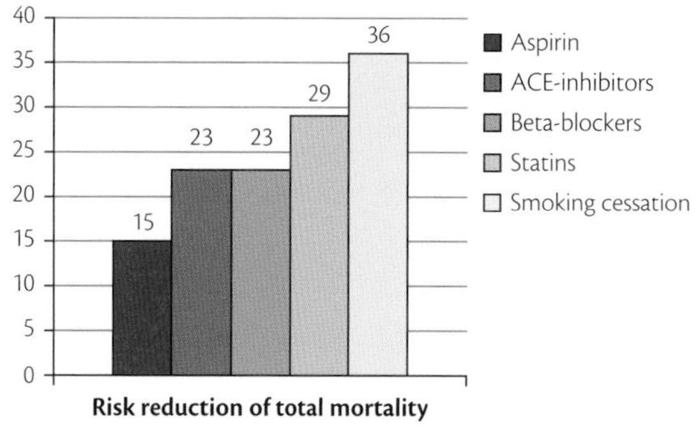

Fig. 10.1 Reduction in mortality risk associated with smoking cessation or use of pharmacotherapy in patients with coronary heart disease.

- The health benefits of quitting smoking are immediate.
- The excess risk of CHD caused by smoking is halved after 1 year of cessation.
- Smoking cessation is more effective than other secondary preventive measures.

How smoking harms the cardiovascular system

Some of the acute effects of smoking include decreased myocardial oxygen supply and increased demand, acute haemodynamic alterations with increases in heart rate, systemic and coronary vascular resistance and myocardial contractility, and reduced artery compliance (➲ Fig. 10.2). Smoking is associated with an acute increase in the endothelial cell count in circulating blood; smoking only two cigarettes a day more than doubles the number of damaged endothelial cells [13].

Some of the long-term effects of smoking include endothelial dysfunction, increased oxidative modification of low-density lipoprotein (LDL), decreased high-density lipoprotein (HDL) cholesterol levels, induced systemic inflammatory response, increased leucocyte count, elevation of the level of C-reactive protein, increased platelet activity and aggregation, imbalance of antithrombotic versus pro-thrombotic factors, decrease of fibrinolytic activity, and increased thickness and stiffness of the arterial wall.

Smoking produces insulin resistance and is associated with an increased risk of type 2 diabetes [14]. A review based on more than a million participants and over 45 000 incident cases of diabetes found an almost 50% increased risk, as well as a dose–response relationship [15]. Beyond being an independent risk factor, smoking appears to have a multiplicative interaction with the other major risk factors for CVD (➲ Fig. 10.3).

- Smoking is a major cause of CVD.
- Even very low tobacco consumption is harmful; there is no safe level.
- Smoking produces insulin resistance and chronic inflammation.
- Smoking has a multiplicative interaction with other risk factors for CVD.

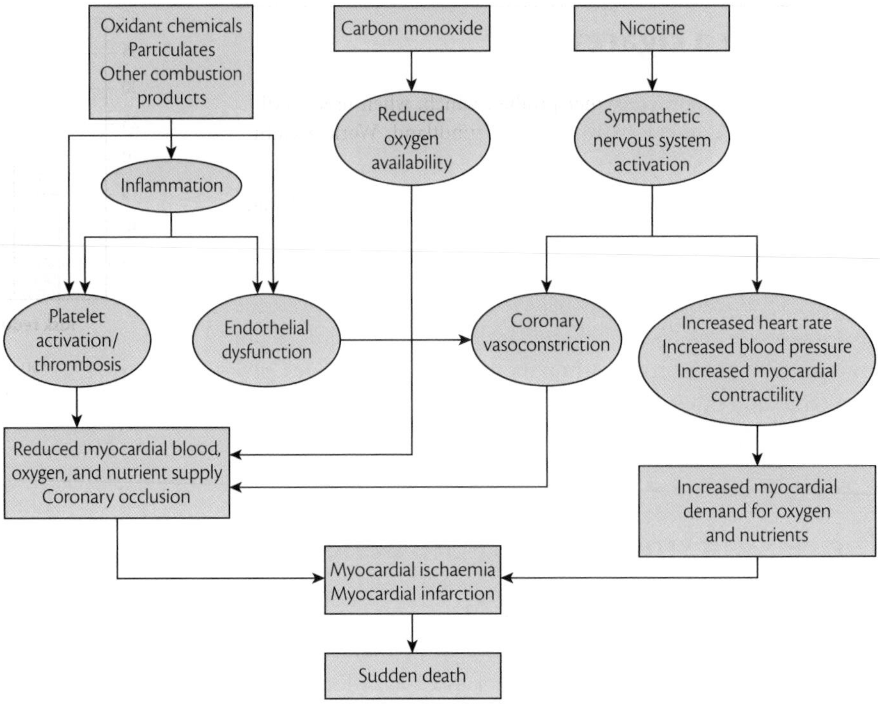

Fig. 10.2 Overview of the mechanisms by which smoking causes an acute cardiovascular event.
Reproduced from 'Cigarette smoking and cardiovascular disease: pathophysiology and implications for treatment', Neal L Benowitz, *Progress in Cardiovascular Diseases*, Vol. 46, No. 1, (July/August) 2003: pp. 91–111.

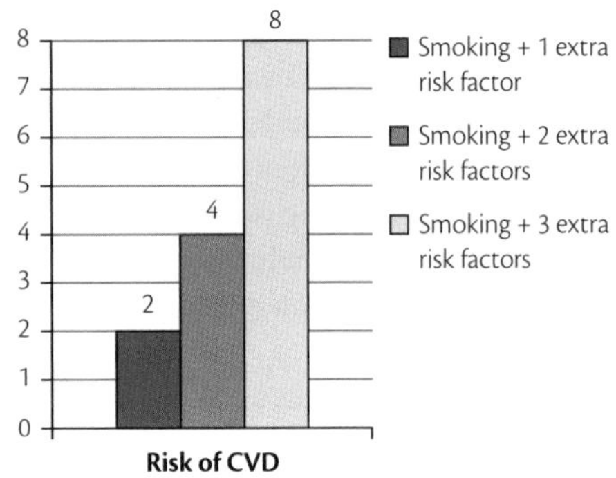

Fig. 10.3 Smoking has a multiplicative interaction with the other major risk factors for CVD.

Light and occasional smoking

Intermittent smoking, smoking just few cigarettes a day, or not inhaling are all shown to carry a significantly increased risk of developing MI and of premature mortality, with higher relative risk being found in women than in men [16–18]. In contrast to the dose–response relationship between smoking and cancer there is a non-linear dose–response relationship between the number of cigarettes smoked per day and CVD. Platelet aggregation is suggested to be the most important harm of low tobacco consumption (➲ Fig. 10.4). Risk increases sharply with only a few cigarettes per day, then tends to plateau at higher levels of consumption. One explanation could be that lighter smokers compensate by inhaling cigarettes more deeply and intensively.

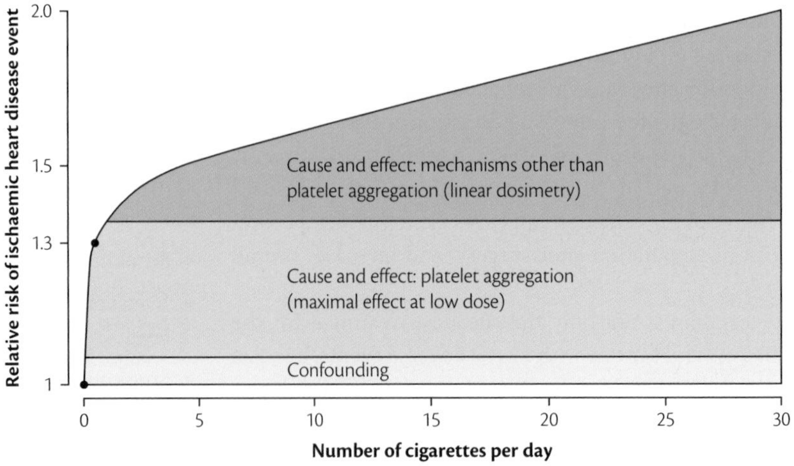

Fig. 10.4 Dose–response relationship between tobacco smoke and ischaemic heart disease events.
Source: Law M, Wald N. Environmental tobacco smoke and ischemic heart disease. *Progress in Cardiovascular Diseases*, Vol 46, Issue 1, 2003, 31–38.

Smoking and CVD

Smoking causes the following conditions:

- asymptomatic atherosclerosis
- CHD (including sudden death, acute coronary syndrome, stable angina, and congestive heart failure)
- stroke
- aortic abdominal aneurysm
- peripheral arterial disease

Smoking appears to have a greater impact on acute coronary events than on atherogenesis. The relative risk is highest for aortic aneurysm and peripheral vascular disease, and lowest for stroke. Smoking increases the risk of sudden death more than acute MI.

Subclinical atherosclerosis

Studies have shown a remarkably consistent significant positive association between smoking and markers of subclinical atherosclerosis. Furthermore, studies have established evidence of a dose–response relationship—the more cigarettes smoked the more pronounced the early changes.

CHD (including MI, sudden death, and congestive heart failure)

In a worldwide case–control study (INTERHEART), current smoking was associated with an almost tripled risk of non-fatal MI compared with never smoking [19]. Also, risk of MI increased by 6% for every additional cigarette smoked. Young male current smokers had the highest population-attributable risk (about 60%). Even though the relative risk of smoking is highest at younger ages, the magnitude of the CHD burden produced by smoking increases with advancing age [20]. Smoking is one of the major risk factors for more severe MI. In a large study of 100 000 consecutive patients with a first MI, smoking was a major determinant for ST-elevation MI (STEMI), compared with non-STEMI [21]. The largest impact of smoking was seen among younger patients and among women.

The 'smokers' paradox' stated that smokers with acute MI have better short-term survival than non-smokers; this was explained by their younger age and lower risk in general. A recent review concluded that this paradox was only observed in some older studies in the pre-thrombolytic era. Studies of present-day populations have not observed this paradox [22].

Cigarette smoking is associated with sudden cardiac death of all types [5]. Smokers have a double to triple increased risk of sudden death compared with non-smokers. The risk of congestive heart failure from smoking is probably mediated through atherosclerosis. The estimated population attributable risk has been found to be higher than for any other risk factor, with the exception of pre-existing CHD [5].

- The risk of CHD is increased two- to four-fold among current smokers of 20 cigarettes/day.
- Smokers are about 10 years younger than never smokers at the time of their first MI.

Stroke

Only hypertension appears to be as consistently related to risk of stroke as smoking [5]. The risk for a current smoker is about two- to four-fold higher than for lifetime non-smokers. Smoking increases the risk of both ischaemic stroke and subarachnoid haemorrhage and the relative risk is highest in younger people.

Abdominal aortic aneurysm

Smoking is the most important avoidable cause of abdominal aortic aneurysm [5]. The risk increases with number of years of smoking and amount smoked. Smoking less than 20 pack-years increases risk of abdominal aorta aneurysm abut three-fold whereas smoking 50 pack-years or more increases the risk up to ten-fold.

Peripheral arterial disease

There is a strong dose–response relationship between smoking and peripheral arterial disease. Prospective studies have shown that in patients with intermittent claudication, current smokers had worse 6-minute walk performance and more severe ischaemic leg symptoms. A higher rate of late arterial occlusion is found in continuing smokers after peripheral vascular surgery than in quitters.

Other effects on the heart

Smoking increases the risk of supraventricular and ventricular arrhythmias. In a large prospective study the risk of atrial fibrillation was more than doubled in smokers [23].

Even though smoking acutely increases blood pressure, mainly through stimulation of the sympathetic nervous system, there does not appear to be a causal relationship between chronic smoking and hypertension [24]. Furthermore, long-term smoking cessation does not result in lower blood pressure. However, smoking increases central blood pressure as it impairs arterial stiffness and wave reflection, which are more closely related to target organ damage than brachial blood pressure. Also, hypertensive smokers have a higher risk of developing severe forms of hypertension, including malignant and renovascular hypertension, most likely due to accelerated atherosclerosis.

In patients with CHD, smoking is associated with an acute decrease in systolic ventricular function and development of widespread hypokinesis [25]. Patients who smoke or have smoked until shortly before heart transplantation have a poorer prognosis and longer recovery time [26].

Differences in susceptibility

Genes, gender, and smoking

About half of the phenotypic variance in smoking is attributable to genetic influences.

Some clinicians believe that smoking is more harmful to men, but there is compelling evidence that the opposite is true. A meta-analysis including data from 2.4 million participants concluded that female smokers have a 25% higher relative risk for CHD than male smokers [27]. Whether the mechanisms underlying the sex difference are biological or related to differences in smoking behaviour is not known. As women in general are smaller they might be exposed to a higher quantity of toxic agents from the same number of cigarettes.

Female smokers taking oral contraceptives have an increased risk of coronary and peripheral artery diseases, MI, and stroke, compared with non-smoking women who use oral contraceptives.

Drug interactions with smoking

Many interactions have been identified between tobacco smoke and medications. These are mostly important for drugs metabolized by the hepatic cytochrome P450 enzymes (primarily CYP1A2), especially antipsychotic drugs [28]. Smokers may need increased doses of beta-blockers, acetyl salicylic acid, propranolol, and opioids.

Types of tobacco other than cigarettes

Cigars, water pipes, and smokeless tobacco

Smokers of pipes and cigars absorb nicotine orally, inhaling their own environmental smoke in the same way that non-smokers inhale other people's smoke. Their risk of CHD is lower relative to that of cigarette smokers.

Water-pipe smoke contains very much the same harmful substances as cigarette smoke and results in substantial increases in plasma nicotine concentrations, while increases in carbon monoxide are higher than from cigarette smoking. Water-pipe smoke is associated with metabolic syndrome, induces increases in heart rate and blood pressure, and markedly impairs baroreflex sensitivity [29]. A high incidence of stroke has been observed in countries where water-pipe smoking is prevalent, but overall there is little research in this field.

Due to the lack of smoke production, harm associated with smokeless tobacco is thought to be lower than with cigarettes. Some kinds of smokeless tobacco contain health-damaging chemicals in addition to producing high nicotine levels, while snus seems to be less toxic. Systematic reviews have concluded that that smokeless tobacco increases the risk of some cancers and of CVD mortality [30,31]. A recent pooled analysis of prospective studies found no association between snus and development of MI; however, case fatality seemed to be increased [32]. In a Swedish study, no relation was found between Swedish snuff and incident CVD [33].

Low-tar, filter, and low-nicotine cigarettes

Switching to low-tar, filter, or low-nicotine cigarettes has very little, or no effect, on reducing the risk for CHD [20].

Electronic cigarettes

Electronic cigarettes, or e-cigarettes, are battery operated, and can deliver high concentrations of nicotine as a vapour. Small experimental studies have found that heart rate increased significantly and remained elevated throughout the puffing period and that there were immediate adverse physiological pulmonary effects after short-term use similar to the effects seen with tobacco smoking [34,35]. However, other studies found no elevation in complete blood count markers, or heart rate. Recent evidence indicate they are not harmless and more research is needed before we can recommend e-cigarettes as a harm reduction strategy for the smoker unable to stop. However, if no other method seems to help, or the smoker insists trying e-cigarettes rather than proven methods of stopping, the harm of short-term use of e-cigarettes is likely to be lower than the harm of continued smoking. The same applies to short-term use of smokeless tobacco for cessation.

Exposure to second-hand smoke

Exposure to second-hand smoke (SHS), or passive smoking, describes inhalation of sidestream smoke that comes from the end of a lighted cigarette, pipe, or cigar. Pooled relative risks from meta-analyses indicate a 25–30% increase in the risk of CHD from exposure to SHS [36]. The risk increases with increased exposure, but there is no safe level of exposure to SHS. Constituents other than nicotine probably play a more important role in the damaging effects of SHS. Platelet aggregation and endothelial dysfunction seem to be important biological mechanisms. Experimental studies have shown that only 30 minutes of exposure to SHS compromised the endothelial function in the coronary arteries in healthy non-smokers to an extent that was indistinguishable from habitual smokers [37].

Avoidance of SHS swiftly reduces this risk, which declines with time after exposure. Therefore, physicians should always ask about exposure to SHS and strongly recommend avoidance.

Understanding addiction

Smoking cessation is the most cost-effective of all interventions to prevent the development or progression of CVD [38]. In every cardiovascular setting high priority should be given to identification and documentation of the smoking status of all patients and provision of cessation assistance. Understanding addiction underpins all interventions for smoking cessation.

Why don't smokers quit?

Most smokers do not quit even though they understand that smoking is a major cause of their disease, and quitting smoking can save their life. There may be many reasons why smokers do not quit.

Tobacco dependence

The most important reason for not quitting is tobacco dependence. Smoking is extremely addictive, and relapse rates in smokers are similar to relapse rates in cocaine or heroin users (➲ Fig. 10.5).

Tobacco dependence is often physical, mental, and social:

- Physical dependence is caused by the highly addictive substance nicotine and other substances in tobacco smoke.
- Mental dependence: nicotine has a rapid relaxing effect and smokers get used to handling difficult or stressful situations in life by lighting up. Many smokers feel anxious without this mental 'lifebelt'.

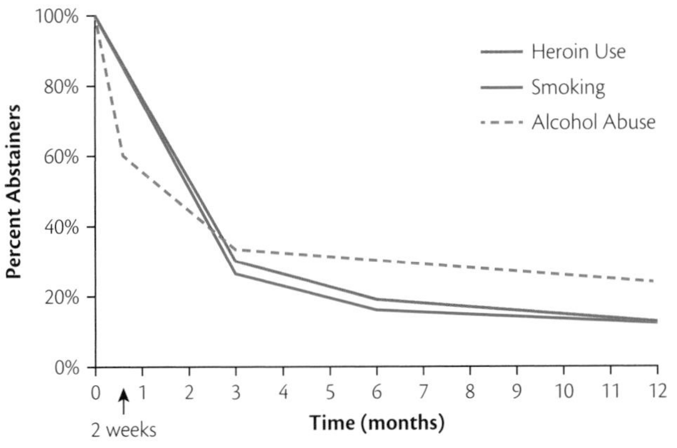

Fig. 10.5 Relapse rate over time for heroin use, smoking, and alcohol abuse.
Source: The Department of Health and Human Services, 'The Health Consequences of Smoking, Nicotine Addiction: A Report by the Surgeon General', DHHS Publication No. CDC 88-8406, 1988.

- Social dependence: many smokers or ex-smokers have an urge to light up a cigarette when somebody else starts smoking. Quitting smoking can be experienced as loss of identity and/or social network.

A 20 pack-day smoker has probably lit up nearly 900 000 times in the course of 10 years. Smoking becomes more ingrained and overlearned than almost any other behaviour.

Defensiveness

Thinking about smoking can lead to feelings of guilt or shame, which puts the smoker on the defensive and raises levels of anxiety.

Lack of self-efficacy

Self-blame, guilt, previous frustrating attempts to quit, and withdrawal symptoms may result in hopelessness. Many smokers believe they are unable to quit—even though they wish they did not smoke.

Mental vulnerability

People with mental vulnerability/disease have a high prevalence of smoking. As the smoking prevalence in the general population decreases, a higher percentage of smokers will be mentally vulnerable. These are the smokers who may have the greatest difficulty in quitting. It is a myth that mentally ill people are unable or unwilling to quit, or that their disease will worsen when they quit smoking. However, they need more assistance to succeed.

Lack of knowledge

Studies have shown that patients do not understand all the medical information they are given and that doctors presume that smokers know much more than they actually do about the health hazards of smoking. Many patients do not believe that smoking is the cause of their disease. They find that health professionals are 'obsessed' with blaming cigarettes. Bad luck, pollution, heredity, and other factors the smoker cannot be blamed for are often believed to be the causes of disease.

Table 10.1 Nicotine abstinence symptoms (diagnosis DSM IV 292.0)

Craving plus:
◆ bad mood or depressive symptoms
◆ insomnia
◆ irritability
◆ frustration or anger
◆ anxiety
◆ difficulties concentrating
◆ restlessness
◆ increased appetite or/and weight gain

Table 10.2 A simple test of nicotine dependence (the Heavy Smoking Index). A score of 4 or more indicates a high level of nicotine dependence, 2–3 moderate dependence, and 0–1 light dependence

How many cigarettes, on average, do you smoke per day?
◆ 1–10 (score 0)
◆ 11–20 (score 1)
◆ 21–30 (score 2)
◆ 31+ (score 3)
How soon after waking do you smoke your first cigarette?
◆ within 5 minutes (score 3)
◆ 6–30 minutes (score 2)
◆ 31–60 minutes (score 1)
◆ 61+ minutes (score 0)

Nicotine dependence and withdrawal symptoms

Nicotine binds to a particular type of acetylcholine receptor in the brain, known as the nicotinic receptor. Binding leads to release of the neuromediator dopamine. Chronic smokers maintain a high enough concentration of nicotine to deactivate the receptors and slow down their recovery, thus developing a tolerance to nicotine. When a smoker does not smoke for some time the receptors become functional again and cholinergic neurotransmission is raised to an abnormally high level. The smoker will experience this as discomfort (i.e. withdrawal symptoms) that drives lighting up.

Many smokers wrongly believe that this discomfort will last for the rest of their life. In some people withdrawal symptoms can be rather severe and the individual feels unable to function in their daily life for weeks (➲ Table 10.1). The smoker may feel that they have had a personality change and need to start smoking again to feel normal. However, most symptoms, excepting for craving and increased appetite, wane after about 2 weeks.

A simple test for nicotine dependence, useful in a busy clinical setting, is the Heavy Smoking Index [39] (➲ Table 10.2). A very dependent smoker, for example one who starts smoking within 30 minutes after waking up and smokes 20 or more cigarettes a day will probably experience more severe withdrawal and have a very high relapse rate. Such smokers require more intensive support.

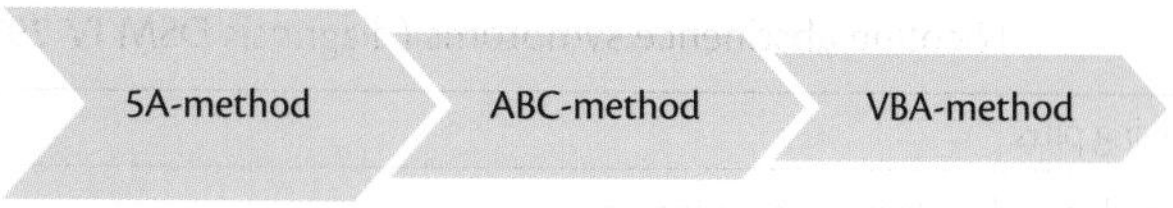

Fig. 10.6 Smoking cessation counselling methods. The main elements of the 5 As are: Ask (smoking status), Advise (to quit smoking), Assess (the motivation to quit), Assist (offer help), Arrange (follow-up). The ABC method is a shorter version of counselling. The main elements are: Ask (smoking status), Brief counselling (advise to quit), Cessation support (offer help). The VBA method is even shorter (30 seconds): Ask (smoking status), Advise (advising on *how* to quit) and Act (offer help).

Smoking cessation treatment

Evidence-based counselling

Several evidence-based approaches have been developed for smoking cessation counselling and have been proven to increase abstinence rate effectively. In general the higher the intensity of counselling, the higher the quit rate. All methods require that the clinician offers help or refers the patient to help.

The 'Very Brief Advice' (VBA) method is the shortest: Ask (smoking status), Advise (advising on how to quit), and Act (offer help) (➲ Fig. 10.6) (see also <http://www.ncsct.co.uk/publication_very-brief-advice.php>). VBA is probably the best choice for the doctor who is not a smoking cessation specialist and has very limited time. The method takes only 30 seconds and does not require any specific skills. However, the doctor must have options and knowledge of referral to trained smoking cessation specialists/centres. In a systematic review and meta-analysis, advice to quit on medical grounds increased quit attempts, but not as much as giving behavioural support or offering medication [40]. These results indicate that offering assistance to all smokers is probably more effective than advising and only offering help to smokers who are interested.

Smokers who are not motivated

Even though a majority of smokers state they wish to quit, most do not have any serious plans to quit within the next 6 months or so. However, new evidence shows that smokers not ready to quit can change their mind very quickly, and accept an assisted quit attempt without longer contemplation. Furthermore, a quit attempt without long preparation can be as successful as one that has been in preparation for a long time [41]. This means that even smokers who are not contemplating quitting deserve an offer of help to quit.

On the other hand, if the reluctant smoker says 'no thanks' they should not be left with a feeling of guilt or defensiveness. As tobacco dependence is a chronic disease, smoking should be addressed at every contact with the patient, and assistance to quit should be offered repeatedly. A 'no thanks' to smoking cessation is not a life-long rejection—it is, hopefully, a step on the way to another chance. However, another chance may not come because of premature morbidity and mortality. A further option is to encourage smokers to reduce their smoking while using nicotine-replacement therapy. A meta-analysis of smokers unwilling to quit showed that starting nicotine-replacement therapy was associated with higher quit rates than no therapy [42]. This approach appears safe—only nausea was increased in the nicotine-replacement group.

Abbreviated motivational interviewing

Motivational interviewing involves the use of counselling to resolve ambivalence about quitting and encourage choices that are consistent with the smoker's long-term goals. A meta-analysis showed that motivational interviewing increased 6-month cessation rates by about 30% [43]. To help the patient explore and resolve ambivalence, the clinician may ask the smoker to rate their motivation to quit on a scale from 1 to 10. This can be followed by the question 'Why are you a __ and not a 10 (or 1) on the scale?'. This is followed by eliciting suggestions from the patient on how to overcome barriers. For example, if the patient says, 'My motivation to quit is only a 5, because I got so irritable last time that my wife asked me to start again' the clinician can respond, 'I understand that quitting may make you difficult to get along with. But these symptoms usually last only two weeks or so. Is there anything you can do during those two weeks that may help?'. Be sure to add, 'Medication that I can offer you can help'.

Expressing empathy and avoiding arguments is another important tenet of motivational interviewing. The clinician may say: 'Many doctors have probably asked you to quit smoking, and you are getting fed up with the subject. I would like to understand how you really feel about your smoking these days. Does your smoking give you some pleasures? Do you have some concerns?'. This could lead to a discussion of what it would take for the smoker to be ready to quit.

Also, developing discrepancies is part of motivational interviewing. The clinician helps the patient understand the difference between behaviour and goals and ties the advantages and disadvantages of quitting to the patient's core values and life goals. The clinician may state: 'I think you know that stopping smoking will help you avoid another MI, or a new stent. What are your roadblocks to stopping smoking? What can you do to overcome these difficulties?'. This may lead to a discussion of the long-term goals and short-term difficulties.

Reasons not to quit should be met with understanding and not opposing arguments. This technique is often called 'rolling with resistance'. When smokers express reasons for not making change they can be helped to find ways to succeed. But the clinician needs to ensure that the atmosphere is relaxed, and information and help are offered, rather than counterarguments.

Smoking cessation pharmacotherapy

Three types of pharmacotherapy are recommended for smoking cessation, based on efficacy and safety [44–49]:

- nicotine-replacement therapy
- bupropion
- varenicline

The advantages, disadvantages, and clinically important parameters of these are summarized in ➲ Table 10.3. A meta-analysis

Table 10.3 Evidence-based recommendations for pharmacotherapy for smoking cessation

Nicotine-replacement therapy	Advantages	Many years of experience. High safety. Dose and combination of several different products can be adapted individually
	Disadvantages	High risk of under-dosing (i.e. no effect)
	Long-term abstinence rates	17% (approx.)
	Special recommendations	Start 1–2 weeks before stop date. Use patches combined with, e.g., inhaler, spray, or gum p.r.n. Let the patient try different types
	Side effects	Common: heart palpitations and chest pains, nausea and vomiting, gastrointestinal complaints, insomnia, skin irritation, mouth and throat soreness, mouth ulcers, hiccups and coughing
	Contraindications	Patch: allergic reactions (caution). Gum: temporomandibular joint disease, ulcers
	NNT	14
Bupropion	Advantages	Easy to dose. Well-known safety profile as the drug has previously been used in psychiatric patients for decades
	Disadvantages	Many interactions with other types of medicine, e.g. antidepressants, antipsychotics, and type 1c anti-arrhythmics
	Long-term abstinence rates	19% (approx.)
	Special recommendations	Start 1–2 weeks before stop date. Dose reduction advised in patients taking propafenone or flecainide. All patients should be observed for neuropsychiatric symptoms
	Side effects	Insomnia, headache, dry mouth, dizziness, and nausea are common. Risk exists for serious adverse effects such as seizures
	Contraindications	History of hypersensitivity to bupropion. Concurrent use of MAO inhibitors. Current or past epilepsy, bulimia, or anorexia nervosa. Alcohol withdrawal or withdrawal from benzodiazepines. Bipolar disorder. Severe liver cirrhosis. Known CNS tumour. Pregnancy
	NNT	11
Varenicline	Advantages	Highest quit rates. Easy to dose
	Disadvantages	Neuropsychiatric cautions. Expensive
	Long-term abstinence rates	21% (approx.)
	Special recommendations	Start 1–2 weeks or up to 35 days before stop date. Titration recommended and is part of packaging. All patients should be observed for neuropsychiatric symptoms including changes in behaviour, hostility, agitation, depressed mood, and suicide-related events, including ideation. Due to possible drowsiness patients should not drive, use machinery etc. until they can perform such activity safely. Avoid use of alcohol
	Side effects	Common: nausea, insomnia, headache, abnormal dreams, constipation, flatulence, and abdominal pain. Severe: neuropsychiatric and cardiac adverse events have been reported
	Contraindications	History of serious hypersensitivity or skin reactions to varenicline. Pregnancy
	NNT	8

NNT, number needed to treat; p.r.n., as needed; MAO, monoamine oxidase.

concluded that both behavioural therapy and pharmacotherapy are more efficacious than usual care for smoking cessation in patients with CVD [50]. Overall, the benefits of cessation in patients with stable CVD far exceed any risks of pharmacotherapy delivered over the short term, i.e. up to 6 months. The smoker should be informed about the importance of compliance with treatment during the whole period, as many experience relapse if they stop treatment too fast. Although these therapies have demonstrated efficacy in the acute stages of quitting, the duration of treatment that is currently recommended may not be sufficient for smokers to maintain abstinence from smoking [51]. Less evidence is available on the efficacy of medications in patients with acute CVD.

- Smoking cessation pharmacotherapy may double or triple quit rates.
- Combining pharmacotherapy with counselling improves quit rates further.
- The use of pharmacotherapy is far safer than continued smoking.

Nicotine-replacement therapy

Nicotine-replacement therapy ameliorates withdrawal symptoms and craving and, with the exception of the transdermal patch, can be used ad libitum throughout the day. The various forms of nicotine-replacement therapy (gums, patches, sprays, inhalers, lozenges, and sublingual tablets) seem to have similar efficacy. Combining a nicotine patch with fast-acting nicotine-replacement therapies like gums, lozenges, or tablets is significantly more effective than use of a single form [52]. Starting nicotine-replacement therapy 1–2 weeks before the quit date may be another way to boost quit rates [53].

Absorption of nicotine from all these nicotine products is slower and the increase in nicotine blood levels more gradual than from smoking. This slow increase in blood and especially brain levels of nicotine results in low likelihood of abuse [54]. The mouth spray reaches maximum blood concentrations significantly faster than the other oral products. Use of nicotine-replacement therapy in patients with stable coronary disease does not increase cardiovascular risk [55]. An angiographic study found no enhancement of sympathetic stimulation or coronary vasoconstriction in subjects using nicotine gum [56]. Adverse events are local (skin reactions to the patch, irritation of the throat and stomach with oral forms, and jaw tenderness and hiccups with gum). Because nicotine-replacement therapies do not lead to the same instantaneous rises and rapid falls in nicotine blood levels as cigarette smoking, only a minority of users become dependent on them.

There is no direct evidence regarding how soon after a cardiac event nicotine-replacement therapy may be administered. An observational study of smokers admitted to hospital after acute coronary syndrome found no difference in mortality in smokers receiving patches or not [57]. It is recommended to discontinue nicotine-replacement therapy during acute cardiac events; however, short-acting nicotine-replacement therapies can be used for haemodynamically stable smokers with withdrawal symptoms. Smokers who quit during hospitalization may be prescribed nicotine-replacement therapies upon discharge.

Bupropion

Bupropion has been used for over two decades as an antidepressant. Bupropion reduces cravings and withdrawal symptoms during smoking cessation and limits weight gain during the treatment period only. Bupropion has proven effectiveness in a wide range of populations including smokers with stable CVD [58]. However, studies in smokers with acute CVD have not shown any efficacy [59].

Bupropion is started 1–2 weeks before the target quit date. During this period of time smokers may experience a decrease in the pleasure or taste derived from smoking, sensations that may pre-condition the smoker to quit. Bupropion does not produce dependence.

Bupropion is associated with an increased risk of seizure (about 1/1000) and serious allergic reactions. More common adverse events are dry mouth and insomnia. Other adverse events are tremor, taste or visual disturbance, and neuropsychiatric disorders (e.g. activation of mania, extreme irritability and restlessness, hyperactivity). Bupropion has several contraindications (hypersensitivity, epileptic disorder, anorexia or bulimia, a history of bipolar depression, severe hepatic cirrhosis, and use of monoamine oxidase inhibitors) and cautions (mainly conditions that may lower the risk of seizure). Bupropion interacts with drugs metabolized via various cytochrome P450 isoenzymes.

Varenicline

Varenicline activates neuronal $\alpha 4\beta 2$ and other nicotinic acetylcholine receptors, particularly in the ventral tegmental area, causing the release of dopamine. The time course of dopamine release has been shown to be more gradual and flattened compared with that induced by nicotine in cigarette smoke. Varenicline attenuates craving for cigarettes and other withdrawal symptoms. As a partial agonist that binds tightly to the nicotinic receptors, varenicline limits the binding of nicotine to the receptors and thus acts as a nicotine antagonist. Satisfaction with a smoke, the psychological reward of smoking, and respiratory tract sensations are all attenuated with varenicline.

Varenicline requires 4 days to reach steady state, and is started 1–2 weeks prior to the target quit date. Extended treatment with varenicline for 12 weeks in smokers who quit following an initial 12-week course of treatment increased quit rates compared with placebo 6 months after the cessation of therapy [60]. Varenicline's only contraindication is hypersensitivity. No interactions of clinical significance have been reported.

The most common adverse event associated with varenicline is dose-dependent nausea that occurs in about a third of users. Nausea diminishes with continued treatment and when varenicline is taken after the ingestion of food or fluids. Titrating the dose during the first week of treatment has been shown to increase tolerability. Other gastrointestinal adverse events that have been observed with frequencies of 2–5% in individuals taking varenicline versus placebo are constipation, abdominal pain, flatulence, dyspepsia, and vomiting. Insomnia, headache, and abnormal dreams are the most frequent neuropsychiatric adverse events. Patients need to be observed for changes in behaviour, hostility, agitation, depressed mood, and suicide-related events. However, increases in neuropsychiatric events were not observed in a review of placebo-controlled studies [61]. Furthermore, a study of varenicline in patients with stably treated current, or past major, depression found that varenicline increases smoking cessation rates without exacerbating anxiety or depression [62].

In a randomized controlled trial of 696 persistent high-risk smokers with established CVD, or at high multifactorial risk of developing CVD, and all willing to make a quit attempt, the combination of a nurse-led preventive cardiology programme (EUROACTION) using a behavioural approach together with the option of varenicline achieved more than a four-fold increase in abstinence (self-report plus breath CO $<$ 10 p.p.m.) at 16 weeks compared with usual care. In addition this comprehensive approach to reducing total cardiovascular risk also achieved healthier eating habits (Mediterranean diet score), increased levels of physical activity, and better blood pressure control with no increase in the use of antihypertensive drugs compared with usual care [63].

In another randomized controlled clinical trial of 714 patients the focus was smokers with stable CVD. They were given smoking cessation counselling and either varenicline or matching placebo. Varenicline was over three times more effective than placebo in promoting continuous abstinence from smoking, validated by breath CO, after 1 year [64]. Though the study was not powered to examine event rates, an analysis of adjudicated events was done. This revealed that the varenicline- and placebo-treated groups did not differ significantly with regard to serious adverse events, cardiovascular events, CVD mortality, or all-cause mortality.

However, the Federal Drug Administration (FDA) in the United States noted a potential increased risk of certain cardiovascular events in smokers with stable CVD—this was subsequently added to the label. A meta-analysis reported that ischaemic or arrhythmic cardiovascular events including MI, unstable angina, coronary revascularization, coronary artery disease, arrhythmias, transient ischaemic attacks, stroke, sudden death, cardiovascular-related death, or congestive heart failure occurred in slightly more varenicline- than placebo-treated subjects [65]. The number of deaths was considered too small for separate analysis. Two subsequent meta-analyses which used other statistical methods, included all trials published, and focused on events occurring during drug exposure found no significant increase in serious adverse cardiovascular events associated with varenicline use [66,67]. A cohort study from Denmark found no increased risk of major cardiovascular events associated with use of varenicline versus bupropion for smoking cessation [68]. A recent meta-analysis by Pfizer, performed at the request of the FDA, showed no significant increase in serious adverse cardiovascular events, but all analyses consistently showed a numerically higher occurrence of events in patients using varenicline. However, as the serious adverse events are very rare and the risk of new cardiac events in a CVD patient is very high in continuous smokers, and given the high quit rates achieved with varenicline, treatment is likely to result in net benefits.

Weight gain after smoking cessation

Unfortunately, some clinicians still believe that weight gain after smoking cessation is more harmful than continued smoking. Most of the post-cessation weight gain occurs quickly, during the first months and decelerates afterwards. The average gain in weight after smoking cessation is approximately 5 kg after 1 year. Studies show that the risk of death from CHD is not reduced sufficiently by lower body weight to justify smoking. A gain in body mass index of 15.9 units (kg/m^2) for men and 15.8 units for women would be required to offset the harmful effects of smoking [69]!

Alternative therapies and vaccines and other future treatment options

There is no evidence that hypnosis, acupuncture, acupressure, laser therapy, electrostimulation, or anxiolytics are effective for long-term smoking cessation. Smokers who deeply believe in alternative therapy should not be discouraged from trying it, but inform that there are effective alternatives and that you will provide evidence-based treatment if they fail to succeed or relapse.

No easy miracle cures for smokers are under development. Three antinicotine vaccines are today in an advanced stage of clinical evaluation, but clinical effects have not so far been established. Other smoking cessation strategies are under various stages of development [70].

The ex-smoker

Tobacco dependence is a chronic disease, and an ex-smoker has a lifelong risk of relapse to smoking. Most relapses occur within the first 2 weeks and absolute abstinence is essential in this period. Long-term abstinence is defined as 1 year or more, and at this time relapse rates are low. Many ex-smokers will sabotage their abstinence after some months, finding excuses to smoke such as: smoking a single cigarette will do no harm, or it is better to smoke one cigarette now than be stressed. The ex-smoker may benefit from discussion of this tobacco dependence-driven self-sabotage mechanism and the need to stay 100% smoke free. Assistance with smoking cessation should not stop when the smoker has smoked the 'last cigarette' after an MI or a cardiac intervention.

Smoking cessation in the hospital

Treatments initiated in hospital following a CHD-related event or procedure are more effective than those initiated outside hospital. A recent Cochrane review based on 50 randomized trials concluded that high-intensity behavioural interventions that begin during a hospital stay and include at least 1 month of supportive contact after discharge promote smoking cessation among hospitalized patients [71]. The effect of these interventions was independent of the patient's diagnosis at admission and was found in rehabilitation settings as well as acute care hospitals. There was no evidence of effect for interventions of lower intensity or shorter duration. It was found that adding nicotine-replacement therapy to intensive counselling significantly increased cessation rates over counselling alone. There is insufficient direct evidence to conclude that adding bupropion or varenicline to intensive counselling increases cessation rates over what is achieved by counselling alone; however, studies of varenicline in this setting have not yet been done.

Cost-effectiveness of smoking cessation in CVD prevention

A study investigated 11 CVD prevention activities and found that the only cost-saving activity was smoking cessation, even if $600 was spent annually helping a smoker quit. When looking at cost per quality-adjusted life year only smoking cessation could be expected to save money over a 30-year follow-up period [38].

Smoking and public health

There is evidence that banning smoking in public places reduces the risk of MI in the general population. However, the reductions vary very much across nations/states and some recent publications report no significant effect. These differences can be explained by differences in how strict the law is and how many local restrictions there were before implementation of a national ban, together with different methodologies (e.g. inclusion of confounders, year of study, change of social norm) and other factors.

Physicians should be acquainted with the Framework Convention on Tobacco Control (FCTC), which was signed by 173 nations in 2012. The FCTC gives evidence-based and detailed recommendations on tobacco control at all levels [72,73]. Most countries aim to achieve smoking prevalences of below 5%. To achieve optimal tobacco control, physicians, at the top of the pyramid in ➲ Fig. 10.7, should also work at influencing all levels.

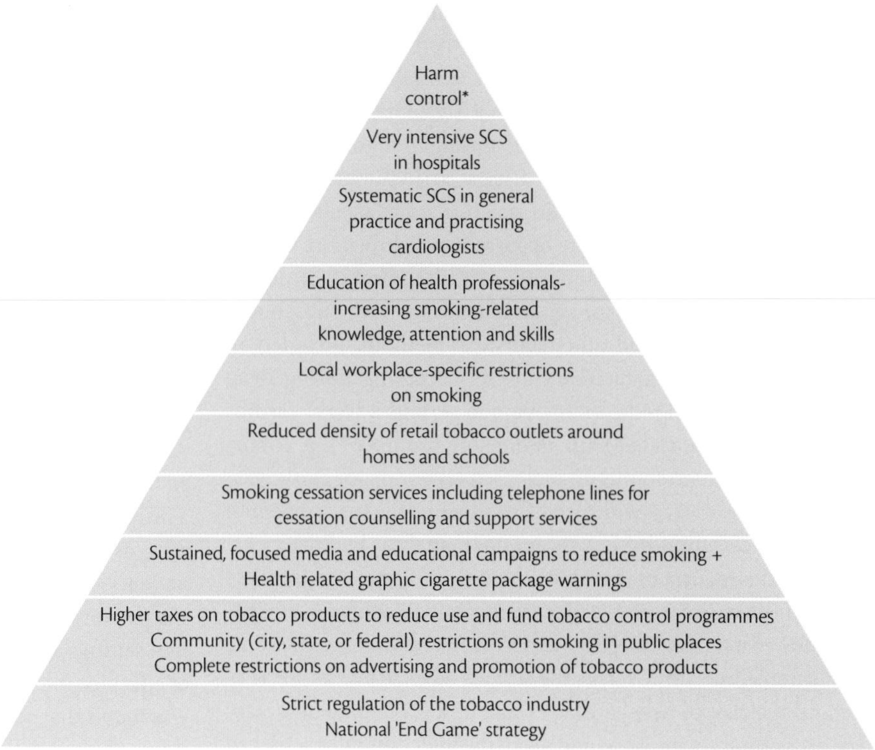
Harm
control*
Very intensive SCS
in hospitals
Systematic SCS in general
practice and practising
cardiologists
Education of health professionals-
increasing smoking-related
knowledge, attention and skills
Local workplace-specific restrictions
on smoking
Reduced density of retail tobacco outlets around
homes and schools
Smoking cessation services including telephone lines for
cessation counselling and support services
Sustained, focused media and educational campaigns to reduce smoking +
Health related graphic cigarette package warnings
Higher taxes on tobacco products to reduce use and fund tobacco control programmes
Community (city, state, or federal) restrictions on smoking in public places
Complete restrictions on advertising and promotion of tobacco products
Strict regulation of the tobacco industry
National 'End Game' strategy

Fig. 10.7 Overview of tobacco control on several levels. Even though doctors/cardiologists act at the top of the pyramid they can and should influence all levels. SCS, smoking cessation support. *Harm control for reluctant smokers (e.g. substantial smoking reduction, long-term nicotine-replacement therapy).

Conclusion

Helping smokers quit should be the highest priority for all doctors, especially cardiovascular specialists. The health benefits of quitting smoking are immediate and cessation markedly reduces the risk of cardiovascular events and death. Evidence-based smoking cessation methods are available, and cessation is one of the most effective and cheapest treatments for cardiac patients. Very high priority should be given to the identification and documentation of the smoking status of all patients, systematic provision of cessation, and recommendation of avoidance of exposure to tobacco smoke.

Further reading

Doll R, Peto R, Boreham J, et al. Mortality in relation to smoking: 50 years' observations on male British doctors. *Br Med J* 2004; **328**: 1519.

Eriksen M, Mackay J, Ross H. *The tobacco atlas*, 4th edn, 2012. Atlanta, GA: American Cancer Society.

Department of Health and Human Services. *The 2004 United States Surgeon General's Report: the health consequences of smoking*, 2004. Atlanta, GA: Department of Health and Human Services. Centers for Disease Control and Prevention.

The Surgeon General's 1990 Report on the health benefits of smoking cessation. Executive Summary. *MMWR Recomm Rep* 1990; **39** (RR-12): i-xv, 1–12.

A clinical practice guideline for treating tobacco use and dependence: 2008 update.: A US Public Health Service report. *Am J Prev Med* 2008; **35**: 158–76.

See also [20], [36], [50], [71–77], and <http://www.ncsct.co.uk/publication_very-brief-advice.php>

References

1 Eriksen M, Mackay J, Ross H. *The tobacco atlas*, 4th edn, 2012. Atlanta, GA: American Cancer Society.

2 Valdes AM, Andrew T, Gardner JP, et al. Obesity, cigarette smoking, and telomere length in women. *Lancet* 2005; **366**: 662–4.

3 Doll R, Peto R, Wheatley K, et al. Mortality in relation to smoking: 40 years' observations on male British doctors [see comments]. *Br Med J* 1994; **309**: 901–11.

4 Doll R, Peto R, Boreham J, et al. Mortality in relation to smoking: 50 years' observations on male British doctors. *Br Med J* 2004; **328**: 1519.

5 Department of Health and Human Services. *The 2004 United States Surgeon General's Report: the health consequences of smoking*, 2004. Atlanta, GA: Department of Health and Human Services. Centers for Disease Control and Prevention.

6 The Surgeon General's 1990 Report on the health benefits of smoking cessation. Executive Summary. *MMWR Recomm Rep* 1990; **39** (RR-12): i-xv, 1–12.

7 Critchley JA, Capewell S. Mortality risk reduction associated with smoking cessation in patients with coronary heart disease: a systematic review. *J Am Med Assoc* 2003; **290**: 86–97.

8 Aspelund T, Gudnason V, Magnusdottir BT, et al. Analysing the large decline in coronary heart disease mortality in the Icelandic population aged 25-74 between the years 1981 and 2006. *PLoS One* 2010; **5**: e13957.

9 Antithrombotic Trialists' Collaboration. Collaborative meta-analysis of randomised trials of antiplatelet therapy for prevention of death, myocardial infarction, and stroke in high risk patients. *Br Med J* 2002; **324**: 71–86.

10 Flather MD, Yusuf S, Kober L, et al. Long-term ACE-inhibitor therapy in patients with heart failure or left-ventricular dysfunction: a systematic overview of data from individual patients. ACE-Inhibitor Myocardial Infarction Collaborative Group. *Lancet* 2000; **355**: 1575–81.

11 Freemantle N, Cleland J, Young P, et al. Beta blockade after myocardial infarction: systematic review and meta regression analysis. *Br Med J* 1999; **318**: 1730–7.

12 Pignone M, Phillips C, Mulrow C. Use of lipid lowering drugs for primary prevention of coronary heart disease: meta-analysis of randomised trials. *Br Med J* 2000; **321**: 983–6.

13 Puranik R, Celermajer DS. Smoking and endothelial function. *Prog Cardiovasc Dis* 2003; **45**: 443–58.

14 Wannamethee SG, Shaper AG, Perry IJ. Smoking as a modifiable risk factor for type 2 diabetes in middle-aged men. *Diabetes Care* 2001; **24**: 1590–5.

15 Willi C, Bodenmann P, Ghali WA, et al. Active smoking and the risk of type 2 diabetes: a systematic review and meta-analysis. *J Am Med Assoc* 2007; **298**: 2654–64.

16 Schane RE, Ling PM, Glantz SA. Health effects of light and intermittent smoking: a review. *Circulation* 2010; **121**: 1518–22.

17 Prescott E, Scharling H, Osler M, Schnohr P. Importance of light smoking and inhalation habits on risk of myocardial infarction and all cause mortality. A 22 year follow up of 12 149 men and women in The Copenhagen City Heart Study. *J Epidemiol Commun Health* 2002; **56**: 702–6.

18 Luoto R, Uutela A, Puska P. Occasional smoking increases total and cardiovascular mortality among men. *Nicotine Tob Res* 2000; **2**: 133–9.

19 Teo KK, Ounpuu S, Hawken S, et al. Tobacco use and risk of myocardial infarction in 52 countries in the INTERHEART study: a case-control study. *Lancet* 2006; **368**: 647–58.

20 Centers for Disease Control and Prevention (US); National Center for Chronic Disease Prevention and Health Promotion (US); Office on Smoking and Health (US). *2010 Surgeon General's report—how tobacco smoke causes disease: the biology and behavioral basis for smoking-attributable disease*, 2010. Atlanta, GA: Centers for Disease Control and Prevention.

21 Bjorck L, Rosengren A, Wallentin L, et al. Smoking in relation to ST-segment elevation acute myocardial infarction: findings from the Register of Information and Knowledge about Swedish Heart Intensive Care Admissions. *Heart* 2009; **95**: 1006–11.

22 Aune E, Roislien J, Mathisen M, et al. The 'smoker's paradox' in patients with acute coronary syndrome: a systematic review. *BMC Med* 2011; **9**: 97.

23 Chamberlain AM, Agarwal SK, Folsom AR, et al. Smoking and incidence of atrial fibrillation: results from the Atherosclerosis Risk in Communities (ARIC) study. *Heart Rhythm* 2011; **8**: 1160–6.

24 Virdis A, Giannarelli C, Neves MF, et al. Cigarette smoking and hypertension. *Curr Pharm Des* 2010; **16**: 2518–25.

25 Hoilund-Carlsen PF, Marving J, Gadsboll N, et al. Acute effects of smoking on left ventricular function and neuro-humoral responses in patients with known or suspected ischaemic heart disease. *Clin Physiol Funct Imaging* 2004; **24**: 216–23.

26 Sanchez-Lazaro IJ, Almenar L, Martinez-Dolz L, et al. Impact of smoking on survival after heart transplantation. *Transplant Proc* 2007; **39**: 2377–8.

27 Huxley RR, Woodward M. Cigarette smoking as a risk factor for coronary heart disease in women compared with men: a systematic review and meta-analysis of prospective cohort studies. *Lancet* 2011; **378**: 1297–305.

28 Li WJ, Zhang HY, Miao CL, et al. Cigarette smoking inhibits the anti-platelet activity of aspirin in patients with coronary heart disease. *Chin Med J (Engl)* 2011; **124**: 1569–72.

29 Al-Kubati M, Al-Kubati AS, al'Absi M, et al. The short-term effect of water-pipe smoking on the baroreflex control of heart rate in normotensives. *Auton Neurosci* 2006; **126-7**: 146–9.

30 Boffetta P, Hecht S, Gray N, et al. Smokeless tobacco and cancer. *Lancet Oncol* 2008; **9**: 667–75.

31 Boffetta P, Straif K. Use of smokeless tobacco and risk of myocardial infarction and stroke: systematic review with meta-analysis. *Br Med J* 2009; **339**: b3060.

32 Hansson J, Galanti MR, Hergens MP, et al. Use of snus and acute myocardial infarction: pooled analysis of eight prospective observational studies. *Eur J Epidemiol* 2012; **27**: 771–9.

33 Janzon E, Hedblad B. Swedish snuff and incidence of cardiovascular disease. A population-based cohort study. *BMC Cardiovasc Disord* 2009; **9**: 21.

34 Vansickel AR, Eissenberg T. Electronic cigarettes: effective nicotine delivery after acute administration. *Nicotine Tob Res* 2013; **15**: 267–70.

35 Vardavas CI, Anagnostopoulos N, Kougias M, et al. Short-term pulmonary effects of using an electronic cigarette: impact on respiratory flow resistance, impedance, and exhaled nitric oxide. *Chest* 2012; **141**: 1400–6.

36 US Department of Health and Human Services. *The health consequences of involuntary exposure to tobacco smoke: a report of the Surgeon General*, 2006. Atlanta, GA: US Department of Health and Human Services, Centers for Disease Control and Prevention, Coordinating Center for Health Promotion, National Center for Chronic Disease Prevention and Health Promotion, Office on Smoking and Health.

37 Davis JW, Shelton L, Watanabe IS, et al. Passive smoking affects endothelium and platelets. *Arch Intern Med* 1989; **149**: 386–9.

38 Kahn R, Robertson RM, Smith R, et al. The impact of prevention on reducing the burden of cardiovascular disease. *Circulation* 2008; **118**: 576–85.

39 Chabrol H, Niezborala M, Chastan E, et al. Comparison of the Heavy Smoking Index and of the Fagerstrom test for nicotine dependence in a sample of 749 cigarette smokers. *Addict Behav* 2005; **30**: 1474–7.

40 Aveyard P, Begh R, Parsons A, et al. Brief opportunistic smoking cessation interventions: a systematic review and meta-analysis to compare advice to quit and offer of assistance. *Addiction* 2012; **107**: 1066–73.

41 Pisinger C, Vestbo J, Borch-Johnsen K, et al. It is possible to help smokers in early motivational stages to quit. The Inter99 study. *Prev Med* 2005; **40**: 278–84.

42 Moore D, Aveyard P, Connock M, et al. Effectiveness and safety of nicotine replacement therapy assisted reduction to stop smoking: systematic review and meta-analysis. *Br Med J* 2009; **338**: b1024.

43 Lai DT, Cahill K, Qin Y, et al. Motivational interviewing for smoking cessation. *Cochrane Database Syst Rev* 2010; (1): CD006936.

44 National Institute for Health and Care Excellence. *Brief interventions and referral for smoking cessation in primary care and other settings*, 2006. NICE Public Health Intervention Guidance 1. London: National Institute for Health and Care Excellence.

45 Ministry of Health. *New Zealand smoking cessation guidelines*, 2007. Wellington, New Zealand: Ministry of Health.

46 Stead LF, Perera R, Bullen C, et al. Nicotine replacement therapy for smoking cessation. *Cochrane Database Syst Rev* 2008; (1): CD000146.

47 Department of Family and Community Medicine, University of Toronto. *Smoking cessation guidelines. How to treat your patient's tobacco addiction*, 2000. Toronto: Department of Family and Community Medicine; Pegasus Healthcare International.
48 Zwar N, Richmond R, Borland R, et al. *Smoking cessation guidelines for Australian general practice. Practice handbook*, 2004. Canberra: Australian Government Department of Health and Ageing.
49 A clinical practice guideline for treating tobacco use and dependence: 2008 update. A US Public Health Service report. *Am J Prev Med* 2008; **35**: 158–76.
50 Eisenberg MJ, Blum LM, Filion KB, et al. The efficacy of smoking cessation therapies in cardiac patients: a meta-analysis of randomized controlled trials. *Can J Cardiol* 2010; **26**: 73–9.
51 Sims TH, Fiore MC. Pharmacotherapy for treating tobacco dependence: what is the ideal duration of therapy? *CNS Drugs* 2002; **16**: 653–62.
52 Stead LF, Perera R, Bullen C, et al. Nicotine replacement therapy for smoking cessation. *Cochrane Database Syst Rev* 2012; 11: CD000146.
53 Lindson N, Aveyard P. An updated meta-analysis of nicotine preloading for smoking cessation: investigating mediators of the effect. *Psychopharmacology (Berl)* 2011; **214**: 579–92.
54 Hukkanen J, Jacob P, III, Benowitz NL. Metabolism and disposition kinetics of nicotine. *Pharmacol Rev* 2005; **57**: 79–115.
55 McRobbie H, Hajek P. Nicotine replacement therapy in patients with cardiovascular disease: guidelines for health professionals. *Addiction* 2001; **96**: 1547–51.
56 Nitenberg A, Antony I. Effects of nicotine gum on coronary vasomotor responses during sympathetic stimulation in patients with coronary artery stenosis. *J Cardiovasc Pharmacol* 1999; **34**: 694–9.
57 Meine TJ, Patel MR, Washam JB, et al. Safety and effectiveness of transdermal nicotine patch in smokers admitted with acute coronary syndromes. *Am J Cardiol* 2005; **95**: 976–8.
58 Tonstad S, Farsang C, Klaene G, et al. Bupropion SR for smoking cessation in smokers with cardiovascular disease: a multicentre, randomised study. *Eur Heart J* 2003; **24**: 946–55.
59 Rigotti NA, Thorndike AN, Regan S, et al. Bupropion for smokers hospitalized with acute cardiovascular disease. *Am J Med* 2006; **119**: 1080–7.
60 Hajek P, Tonnesen P, Arteaga C, et al. Varenicline in prevention of relapse to smoking: effect of quit pattern on response to extended treatment. *Addiction* 2009; **104**: 1597–602.
61 Tonstad S, Davies S, Flammer M, et al. Psychiatric adverse events in randomized, double-blind, placebo-controlled clinical trials of varenicline: a pooled analysis. *Drug Saf* 2010; **33**: 289–301.
62 Anthenelli RM, Morris C, Ramey TS, et al. Effects of varenicline on smoking cessation in adults with stably treated current or past major depression. A randomized trial. *Ann Intern Med* 2013; **159**: 390–400.
63 Jennings CS, Kotseva K, De Bacquer D, et al. Effectiveness of a preventive cardiology programme for high risk persistent smokers: the EUROACTION plus Varenicline trial. *Eur Heart J* 2014; **35**: 1411–20.
64 Rigotti NA, Pipe AL, Benowitz NL, et al. Efficacy and safety of varenicline for smoking cessation in patients with cardiovascular disease: a randomized trial. *Circulation* 2010; **121**: 221–9.
65 Singh S, Loke YK, Spangler JG, et al. Risk of serious adverse cardiovascular events associated with varenicline: a systematic review and meta-analysis. *Can Med Assoc J* 2011; **183**: 1359–66.
66 Prochaska JJ, Hilton JF. Risk of cardiovascular serious adverse events associated with varenicline use for tobacco cessation: systematic review and meta-analysis. *Br Med J* 2012; **344**: e2856.
67 Krebs P, Sherman SE. Review: varenicline for tobacco cessation does not increase CV serious adverse events. *Ann Intern Med* 2012; **157**: JC2.
68 Svanstrom H, Pasternak B, Hviid A. Use of varenicline for smoking cessation and risk of serious cardiovascular events: nationwide cohort study. *Br Med J* 2012; **345**: e7176.
69 Diverse Populations Collaboration. Smoking body weight, and CHD mortality in diverse populations. *Prev Med* 2004; **38**: 834–40.
70 D'Souza MS, Markou A. Neuronal mechanisms underlying development of nicotine dependence: implications for novel smoking-cessation treatments. *Addict Sci Clin Pract* 2011; **6**: 4–16.
71 Rigotti NA, Clair C, Munafo MR, et al. Interventions for smoking cessation in hospitalised patients. *Cochrane Database Syst Rev* 2012; 5: CD001837.
72 Nikogosian H. WHO Framework Convention on Tobacco Control: a key milestone. *Bull World Health Organ* 2010; **88**: 83.
73 Shibuya K, Ciecierski C, Guindon E, et al. WHO Framework Convention on Tobacco Control: development of an evidence based global public health treaty. *Br Med J* 2003; **327**: 154–7.
74 Beaglehole R, Bonita R, Horton R, et al. Priority actions for the non-communicable disease crisis. *Lancet* 2011; **377**: 1438–47.
75 Ambrose JA, Barua RS. The pathophysiology of cigarette smoking and cardiovascular disease: an update. *J Am Coll Cardiol* 2004; **43**: 1731–7.
76 Raupach T, Brown J. Treatment of tobacco addiction and the cardiovascular specialist. *Curr Opin Cardiol* 2012; **27**: 525–32.
77 Mozaffarian D, Afshin A, Benowitz NL, et al. Population approaches to improve diet, physical activity, and smoking habits: a scientific statement from the American Heart Association. *Circulation* 2012; **126**: 1514–63.

CHAPTER 11

Nutrition

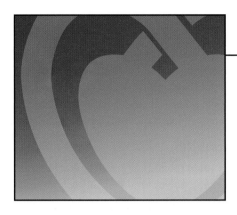

Jean Dallongeville, Deborah Lycett, and Monique Verschuren

Contents

Summary

Different aspects of the human diet are causally related to atherosclerosis and its clinical consequences, therefore a balanced and healthy diet is the cornerstone of the prevention of cardiovascular disease (CVD). This chapter gives an overview of the medical evidence supporting the importance of nutrition in the prevention of CVD. Practical ways to cultivate cardioprotective dietary habits are summarized not only in terms of macro- and micronutrients but also in relation to foods, functional foods, and portfolio diets.

Case study

The following describes a man, Mr X, with a medium to high risk of a cardiovascular event in the next 10 years (a SCORE risk of 4%/10 years), his dietary history, and the support he should be offered to help him improve his diet.

Mr X is a 58-year-old white European man. He is a non-smoker with a family history of heart disease in a first-degree relative before the age of 60, he is being treated for hypertension but does not have diabetes or any other comorbidities. His weight is 74 kg, height 1.8 m, and BMI 22.8 kg/m^2. He has a total serum cholesterol of 7.1 mmol/L (274 mg/dl), low-density lipoprotein (LDL) cholesterol of 5.2 mmol/L (201 mg/dl), high-density lipoprotein (HDL) cholesterol of 1.0 mmol/L (39 mg/dl), triglycerides of 2.2 mmol/L (195 mg/dl), and his blood pressure reading is 140/90 mm/Hg.

The rationale for dietary intervention

Mr X's BMI is desirable and his triglycerides are slightly elevated. His total cholesterol to HDL cholesterol ratio is high and his LDL cholesterol is significantly elevated, so the key targets for dietary intervention are to reduce his risk of cardiovascular events and reduce his LDL cholesterol (in combination with statin therapy). Further reduction in blood pressure through dietary means may also need to be addressed. What should the strategy be and what recommendations should he be given regarding his dietary habits?

Effects of common dietary components on CVD risk

Fats

Total fat intake

Fats have an important role in the development and prevention of atherosclerosis—mainly by influencing cardiovascular risk factors.

Triglycerides are the main constituent of nutritional fat. The mean daily intake ranges from 50 to 100 g, depending on age and gender. Unlike carbohydrates, fat intake increases total cholesterol, low-density lipoprotein (LDL) cholesterol and high-density lipoprotein (HDL) cholesterol [1–4]. Fats constitute an important source of energy. Hence, a high fat intake may be associated with an excessive energy intake, which in turn may result in excess body weight, obesity, and its complications (such as insulin resistance and diabetes). However, epidemiological studies have failed to provide clear evidence of a relationship between fat intake on the one hand and the risk of cardiovascular disease (CVD) and diabetes on the other. However, clinical trials have shown that a low-fat diet promotes weight loss [5] and long-term weight reduction may be explained by the fact that low-energy-density diets tend to increase feelings of satiety [6–11].

Several clinical trials have assessed the effect of reducing fat intake prevention of CVD. Although the earliest studies failed to observe a statistically significant relationship between a low fat intake and cardiovascular events this was probably due to low statistical power [12,13]. In the Women's Health Initiative Randomized Controlled Dietary Modification Trial [14], 48 000 American women were randomly assigned to a low-fat diet (20% of total energy intake) to assess whether this would reduce the incidence of cardiovascular events. However, after 6 years of follow-up, the mean fat intake was only 8.3% lower in the intervention group than in the control group; the difference in serum cholesterol between intervention and control groups was also minor and there was no intergroup difference with respect to cardiovascular events. Taken as a whole, these data suggest that lowering fat intake does not have a clear impact on cardiovascular risk. However, reducing excessive fat intake is recommended in overweight and obese subjects because of its effect on body weight.

Fat composition

Fatty acids differ with respect to the length of the carbon chain, the presence and number of double bonds, and the spatial configuration of the double bond (*cis* or *trans*). The n-3 and n-6 families of fatty acids are defined by the location of the first double bond in the chain (at the third and sixth carbon from the methyl end, respectively). The effects of fatty acids on cardiovascular risk are closely related to their chemical structure.

Saturated fatty acids

In clinical trials, saturated fatty acids were found to raise LDL cholesterol, when compared with mono- and polyunsaturated fatty acids [15]. More precisely, intake of lauric (C12:0) and myristic (C14:0) fatty acids was associated with a greater plasma LDL cholesterol level than seen with palmitic acid (C16:0) [16–18]. In contrast, the saturated fatty acid stearic acid (C:18) had much the same effect as oleic acid (C18:1) on levels of LDL cholesterol. Epidemiological investigations of saturated fat intake have yielded contradictory findings regarding cardiovascular risk [19–21]. Intakes of C-12 and C-18 fatty acids were associated with an elevated cardiovascular risk, whereas shorter fatty acids were not [16].

Monounsaturated fatty acids

Oleic acid is the most common monounsaturated fatty acid. Compared with carbohydrates and polyunsaturated fatty acids, the intake of monounsaturated fatty acids is associated with an elevated HDL/LDL ratio [21] and lower triglyceride levels [22]—suggesting a favourable impact on the lipoprotein profile. Cohort studies have reported similar results. In general, cardiovascular event rates are lower in people who consume a high proportion of monounsaturated fatty acids than in those who consume saturated fatty acids [23–25]. However, these observations have not yet been validated in randomized, prevention-focused trials.

Trans unsaturated fatty acids

The principal dietary sources of trans fatty acids are meat, hard margarines, and hydrogenated oils. Trans fatty acids result from the hydrogenation of vegetable oils, but are also produced during the digestion of animal-based food products [26]. In the past decade, significant efforts by industry have decreased the trans fatty acid content of margarine in Europe. Compared with oleic acid, trans fatty acids raise LDL cholesterol levels and tend to decrease HDL cholesterol levels [27].

For similar intakes, the effects of trans fatty acids on LDL cholesterol are more pronounced than those of saturated fatty acids [28]. Epidemiological studies in Europe and North America have shown a clear association between the intake of trans fatty acids and elevated cardiovascular morbidity/mortality [19,25,29–36]. As with levels of LDL cholesterol, the effects of trans fatty acids on the risk of coronary heart disease (CHD) are more pronounced than those of saturated fatty acids. Recent studies have compared the respective effects of animal-derived and plant-derived trans fatty acids, but failed to draw clear conclusions [37,38]. Taken as a whole, these data suggest that a high intake of trans fatty acids is associated with an elevated cardiovascular risk.

Polyunsaturated fatty acids

Polyunsaturated fatty acids (PUFAs) lower LDL-cholesterol levels and, to a lesser extent, HDL-cholesterol levels when they replace saturated fatty acids [21]. PUFAs can be largely divided into two subgroups: n-6 fatty acids and n-3 fatty acids, which will be discussed in this subsection.

n-6 PUFAs

n-6 PUFAs are the main type of PUFA in the diet, accounting for about 85–90% of the total intake of PUFAs [39]. Linoleic acid is the most abundant n-6 PUFA in the diet, and is mainly obtained from vegetable oils, such as sunflower and soybean oil. Linoleic acid is an essential PUFA, which means that it cannot be synthesized by humans and has to be provided by the diet. The protective effect of n-6 PUFAs on CHD is assumed to be mediated largely by their impact on serum cholesterol levels. Two meta-analyses on the relation between PUFAs and CHD in prospective cohort studies have reported conflicting results. Jakobsen et al. [40] reported a 13% lower CHD risk when 5% of the energy from saturated fat was replaced by PUFAs, while Siri-Tarino et al. [41] concluded that there was no evidence that replacement of saturated fat by PUFAs reduced CHD. A meta-analysis of randomized trials, however, supported the protective effect of PUFA intake, showing that replacement of 5% of the energy from saturated fat by PUFAs would reduce coronary events by 10% [42].

n-3 PUFAs

The most important n-3 fatty acids are alpha-linolenic acid (ALA), ecosapentaenoic acid (EPA), and docosahexanoic acid (DHA). ALA is an essential fatty acid of vegetable origin, present in, for example, soybeans and sunflower oil. Fish is the main source of EPA and DHA.

The impact of ALA on CHD and stroke is still inconclusive, as is the possible mechanism by which ALA could exert a protective effect. Suggested mechanisms include anti-inflammatory, antithrombotic, and anti-arrhythmic effects, but these have not been conclusively demonstrated [43]. Several prospective cohort studies have shown inverse associations of ALA with CHD, but others observed no protective effect of ALA intake. A meta-analysis of five prospective cohort studies reported that ALA intakes of around 2 g/day were associated with a borderline significant 21% lower risk of fatal CHD compared with an intake of 0.8 g/day [44]. However, the overall conclusion to date is that the role of ALA in prevention of CHD is inconclusive, and even more so with respect to prevention of stroke.

EPA and DHA do not have an impact on serum cholesterol levels, but in various epidemiological studies they are associated with a lower risk of fatal CHD but not of non-fatal CHD, even at a low level of intake (compared with no intake). A hypothesis for this differential effect on fatal compared with non-fatal events is that EPA/DHA could prevent fatal cardiac arrhythmia [45].To a lesser extent, EPA and DHA are also associated with a lower stroke mortality [46].

As EPA and DHA are of marine origin, EPA and DHA intake equates to fish intake. Most evidence on fish consumption comes from epidemiological observational studies (see the section Fish). The protective effects of EPA and DHA have been tested in randomized controlled trials (RCTs). Several meta-analyses of trials have been published, and in some of them the patient groups and end-points that were studied were quite heterogeneous. Leon et al. [47] restricted their meta-analysis to patients after myocardial infarction (MI) or with coronary artery disease (CAD), and observed a 20% risk reduction for cardiac death when an additional amount of 0.9–2.8 g/day EPA/DHA was taken. In 2010, the results of three secondary prevention RCTs were published, and the results were quite disappointing [48–50]. None of the three trials, in post-MI or CHD patients, observed a reduction in cardiovascular events in the intervention group, who received an extra 400–800 mg of EPA/DHA daily. The explanation for these results, compared with the more positive results from cohort studies and older trials, could be that the current evidence-based treatment that CHD patients receive is so good that no additional effect of fish oils is observed. Further, the question remains whether fish oil supplements are equivalent to consumption of actual fish.

Dietary cholesterol

The impact of dietary cholesterol on serum cholesterol levels is weak compared with that of dietary fatty acids. When recommendations to reduce the intake of saturated fat are implemented, this will also usually lead to a reduction in dietary cholesterol. Therefore, some healthy diet recommendations do not give specific guidelines on dietary cholesterol; others recommend a limited intake of <300 mg/day.

Carbohydrates

When a reduction in fat intake is replaced by an increase in carbohydrate intake no reduction in cardiovascular risk is apparent. Although total LDL cholesterol levels may be reduced [51], HDL cholesterol levels may also be reduced, increasing the total/HDL cholesterol ratio, small dense atherogenic LDL particles may be produced, and triglyceride levels may be increased [52]. These effects may depend on the type of carbohydrate consumed. Our understanding of this process has improved in recent years with a move away from biochemical classifications of carbohydrates as simple (sugars) and complex (starches) to classifications based on physiological responses.

Sweetened beverages

Large prospective studies do not support an association between a high intake of total sugar and cardiovascular risk [53,54]. However, there is increasing evidence to suggest that consuming sugar in liquid form in sweetened beverages may be detrimental. First, this may be because it contributes to obesity because liquid sugar may have a minimal impact on satiety [55]. Secondly, evidence from cohort studies suggests an independent association of sweetened beverages with cardiovascular disease. In women a 35% higher risk of developing CHD has been associated with drinking two sweetened beverages a day compared with one a month [56]. In men a 20% higher relative risk of CHD has been associated with daily consumption of sweetened drinks compared with never consuming them [57]. Increased risk of hypertension, increased levels of triglycerides, and lower levels of HDL cholesterol have also been demonstrated with higher consumption [58,59].

In studies by Fung et al. [56] and de Koning et al. [57] the same effects were not seen for artificially sweetened beverages. However, there has been one prospective cohort study to date which found an association between higher consumption of diet drinks and vascular events [60]. There is some evidence from cohort studies that diet drinks raise the risk of weight gain and metabolic syndrome but residual confounding of diabetes may explain such associations [61].

Most of the studies investigating sweetened beverages are from the United States where drinks are typically sweetened with high-fructose corn syrup (HFCS), an ingredient not commonly used in Europe. However, there is evidence from laboratory studies that drinks sweetened just with fructose (but not glucose) have a similar effect on raising triglycerides and LDL cholesterol as those sweetened with HFCS [62]. Therefore it seems prudent to encourage sugar-free beverages, such as water, over those with added sugars. The ingredients list of beverages should be checked for HFCS, fructose, and sucrose in particular.

The effect of added fructose on blood pressure (BP) has also been investigated, but a recent meta-analysis of isoenergetic exchange studies found no adverse effects [63].

The glycaemic index (GI)

Carbohydrates are classified according to their glycaemic response:

- carbohydrates with a high GI, or in large enough quantity to exert a high glycaemic response
- carbohydrates with a low GI, or in a small enough quantity to exert a low glycaemic response.

➲ Table 11.1 gives examples of high-carbohydrate foods with a low GI. Meta-analysis from eight cohort studies shows a 32% increased risk of CHD [relative risk (RR) 1.32, 95% CI 1.10–1.54)] with a high intake of high-GI foods. This analysis meets the Bradford Hill causality criteria of strength, consistency, temporality, and coherence [64]. However, meta-analyses of RCTs comparing diets with a high or low GI have detected only a slight reduction in total cholesterol with a low-GI diet, and no effect on LDL cholesterol, HDL cholesterol, or triglycerides—but the studies included were of short duration and poorly powered [65]. Nonetheless the benefit of low-GI diets on glycated haemoglobin (HbA1c) in those with diabetes was apparent [65,66] (see ➲ Chapter 16).

Fibre

Soluble fibre

Fibre has traditionally been classified as soluble and insoluble. Until fairly recently it was soluble fibre, found predominantly in fruit and vegetables, legumes, pulses, and oats, which was highly promoted for its glucose- and cholesterol-lowering effect. In 1999 Brown et al. [67] showed in a meta-analysis of RCTs that for each gram increase in soluble fibre, LDL cholesterol was lowered by about 2 mg/dl (0.052 mmol/L). Beta-glucan from oats has received particular attention; a meta-analysis of RCTs has shown that 3 g/day (approximately three servings of oat breakfast cereal or bread made with oat flour) can reduce total cholesterol by 6 mg/dl (0.16 mmol/l) [68]. However, any superior effect of oat beta-glucan over other fibre has been recently challenged with RCT evidence [69].

Table 11.1 Low-GI examples of high-carbohydrate foods

Bread	Seeded, granary, rye, wholegrain pitta, chapatti, oat bread
Pasta	All pasta (al dente), noodles
Rice	Basmati rice or long grain
Breakfast cereals	Bran and oat based cereals e.g. bran flakes, porridge, muesli. Rye flakes
Potatoes	New potatoes (unpeeled), sweet potato, yam
Other grains	Bulgur wheat, barley, couscous, quinoa
Most fruit and vegetables, legumes, pulses, and dairy foods (i.e yoghurt and milk) also have a low glycaemic index	

Wholegrains

Insoluble fibre, often considered as the bran of cereals, is more congruent with the term wholegrain, which refers to the unrefined, intact grain containing the bran, germ, and endosperm. Wholegrains include whole oats. Meta-analytic evidence from 11 prospective cohort studies has shown a 19% reduction in the risk of developing CHD (RR 0.81, 95% CI 0.75–0.86) with higher wholegrain consumption [64]. At least three servings a day of wholegrain foods to replace refined grain varieties is recommended.

Total fibre

There is considerable overlap between definitions of soluble and insoluble fibres, and evidence from EPIC cohort data shows no difference in benefit between fibre type. A 10 g/day increase in total fibre is associated with a 15% reduced risk in CHD mortality [70]. A meta-analysis of RCT data for fibre supplementation found that an increase of 11.5 g/day reduced diastolic and systolic BP by 1 mmHg [71].

Dietary strategies should focus on increasing all types of fibre. This can be achieved in the following ways:

- Replacing refined flours and cereal products such as white breads, white rice, and white pastas with wholegrain varieties, i.e. wholegrain breads, wholegrain pastas, and brown rice.
- Checking food labels for a minimum fibre content of 3 g/100 g.
- Replacing breakfast cereals such as crisped rice cereals and cornflakes with wholegrain cereals such as porridge oats, muesli, and bran-based cereals. Wholegrain cereals like Shredded Wheat and Weetabix, although high in fibre have a high GI. Products which are both wholegrain and have a low GI potentially offer the maximum benefit (see ➲ Table 11.2).
- Increase fruit and vegetables consumption, including beans and pulses.

Table 11.2 Low-fibre, high-fibre and high-fibre/low-GI foods

	Low fibre	High fibre (but not low GI)	High fibre/low GI
Bread	White bread, white rolls, white baguettes, ciabatta, white pitta bread, bagels	Wholemeal bread, wholemeal rolls, wholemeal baguettes, other breads made with wholemeal flour	Seeded wholemeal and wholemeal granary breads, wholegrain pitta, rye (pumpernickel), oat bread
Pasta	Pastas made with white flour		Pastas made with wholemeal flour and cooked *al dente*
Rice	White rice	Brown/wholegrain rice	Wholegrain basmati rice
Breakfast cereals	Cornflakes, crisped rice cereals	Shredded Wheat, Weetabix, mini wheat squares, multigrain hoops	Bran- and oat-based cereals, e.g. bran flakes, porridge, muesli, rye flakes

Alcoholic beverages

Results from observational cohort studies show a protective effect of moderate alcohol consumption on the occurrence of CVD. The relation is J-shaped, meaning that non-drinkers are at higher risk than moderate drinkers, and at higher levels of consumption cardiovascular risk is increased. A recent comprehensive meta-analysis showed that the level of alcohol consumption giving the greatest protection differed for the different cardiovascular endpoints [72]. For CHD incidence, the lowest risk occurred with an alcohol intake of 15–30 g/day (34% lower risk than non-drinkers), and even at higher levels of intake (> 60 g/day) risk was still reduced by 25%. One drink can be considered equivalent to 10 g of alcohol. For stroke incidence, risk was reduced by 20% for up to 1.5 drinks per day; for intakes between 1.5 and 6 drinks per day no statistically significant protective effect was observed, while at intake levels of 6 drinks per day or more a 62% increased risk was observed. It has to be kept in mind that for cancer incidence the associations are different. Still, the meta-analysis [72] showed that the lowest risk of all-cause mortality was observed for alcohol intake of 2.5–14.9 g/day, which is equivalent to up to 1.5 glasses/day. For a long time it has been debated whether the J-shape was explained by special characteristics of the non-drinkers. It was suggested, for example, that people may stop drinking because of illness, which would lead to the observation in epidemiological studies that non-drinkers are at higher risk than drinkers. The meta-analysis [72] concluded that it was very unlikely that this was the case. Apart from alcohol intake itself, it has been studied whether the type of alcoholic beverage is of importance. There seems to be an especially favourable effect of red wine, which may be due to its polyphenol content. Evidence for the protective effects of alcohol must be applied with caution in public health and clinical practice. The public health message can easily be misinterpreted or misused, leading to alcohol abuse. The current recommendation, from a broad public health perspective, is that drinkers should limit their alcohol intake to a maximum of one glass a day for women (10 g of alcohol) or two glasses a day for men (20 g of alcohol) to obtain the lowest level of risk for chronic disease.

Micronutrients

Sodium

The effect of sodium intake on BP is well established. A meta-analysis estimated that even a modest reduction in sodium intake of 1 g/day reduces systolic BP by 3.1 mmHg in hypertensive patients and 1.6 mmHg in normotensive patients [73]. The DASH trial showed a dose–response relation between reduction in sodium intake and BP reduction [74]. In most western countries salt intake is high (around 9–10 g/day), whereas the recommended maximum intake is 5 g/day. Optimal intake levels might be as low as around 3 g/day. Processed foods are an important source of sodium. A recent simulation study estimated that for the United States a reduction in salt intake of 3 g/day would result in a reduction of 5.9–9.6% in the incidence of CHD (low and high estimates based on different assumptions), a reduction of 5.0–7.8% in the incidence of stroke, and a reduction of 2.6–4.1% in death from any cause [75].

Potassium

Potassium is another mineral that affects BP. The main sources of potassium are fruits and vegetables. A higher potassium intake has been shown to reduce BP. Risk of stroke varies largely with potassium intake: the relative risk of stroke in the highest quintile of potassium intake (average of 110 mmol/day) is almost 40% lower than that in the lowest quintile (average intake of 61 mmol/day) [76].

Vitamins and the prevention of CVD

Vitamins with antioxidant properties

In the last few decades, the potentially preventive effects of vitamin and mineral supplements for CVD and cancer have come under intense scrutiny from scientists and health authorities.

The scientific basis for today's guidelines consists of experiments that have identified bioactive molecules in cell systems and laboratory animals. It is known that oxidative processes are involved in the development of atherosclerosis. Accordingly, antioxidant treatment of cell cultures and laboratory animals exposed to oxidative stress has been shown to reduce inflammatory processes. These results have been underpinned by epidemiological, population-level observations of an inverse correlation between antioxidant intake and CVD [77].

However, many rigorous, placebo-controlled, interventional trials with antioxidant vitamins have failed to confirm the laboratory-based and epidemiological observations.

Vitamin E

The term vitamin E refers to several different isomers of the same compound, the most active, and most active in the plasma, being α-tocopherol. In Europe and North America, vegetable oils and vegetables are the most abundant sources of vitamin E. The mean daily intake is 10–15 mg. Vitamin E is a potent, liposoluble antioxidant that inhibits the peroxidation of cell membrane lipids and LDLs and tumour angiogenesis [78,79]. Several meta-analyses of prevention-focused trials have addressed the relationship of vitamin E to cardiovascular mortality [80–84]. In one meta-analysis of 19 trials with a total of 130 000 participants, follow-up periods of between 1.8 and 8.2 years, and a mean daily dose of between 16.5 and 2000 IU, high-dose vitamin E supplementation was associated with increased all-cause mortality [81]. These results were confirmed in another trial [85].

Vitamin A: beta-carotene and retinol

The term 'vitamin A' refers to a group of molecules, including carotenoids (pro-vitamin A) and retinoids. Many epidemiological studies have found an inverse correlation between dietary or plasma vitamin A levels and cardiovascular events [86]. A meta-analysis of clinical trials revealed excess mortality in patients receiving active vitamin A supplements [84]. These results were confirmed in another meta-analysis [85].

Vitamin C: ascorbic acid

Vitamin C is a potent, water-soluble antioxidant [87]. Fruits and vegetables are the main sources of dietary vitamin C. There is a large body of evidence to suggest that vitamin C prevents oxidation of LDLs and improves endothelial function. However, there is no adequate evidence from randomized clinical trials to suggest that vitamin C supplements prevent cardiovascular events [88].

There are several possible explanations for the harmful effects of antioxidant vitamins evidenced in clinical trials. However, the presence of various methodological issues means that the trial data should be interpreted with caution: these include inappropriate dosing and insufficient duration of intake, both of which may influence the efficacy of intervention [89]. The most effective isomers and the most effective combinations of vitamins for the prevention of CVD may not yet have been identified. Lastly, the CVD prevention trials might have been performed in subjects who were unlikely to benefit from treatment, such as patients with advanced lesions or a satisfactory vitamin status.

Vitamin D

Vitamin D deficiency is highly prevalent worldwide [90]. The best characterized consequences of vitamin D deficiency involve the musculoskeletal system, with rickets in children and osteomalacia and osteoporosis in adults. However, it is now acknowledged that vitamin D receptors are present on a large variety of cell types, including osteoblasts, immune system cells, neurones, pancreatic beta cells, vascular endothelial cells, and (possibly) myocytes and cardiomyocytes [90]. A growing body of evidence indicates that low levels of vitamin D have a role in determining the risk of cardiometabolic outcomes in general and metabolic syndrome, type 2 diabetes mellitus, and systemic hypertension in particular [91,92]. However, most of the recent clinical trials of supplementation with various forms and dosages of vitamin D have failed to provide clear evidence of a beneficial effect on cardiovascular risk.

Folic acid, B vitamins (B_6, folic acid, and B_{12}), and homocysteine

The B vitamins B_6, B_{12}, and folic acid have been studied for their potential to lower homocysteine levels. Homocysteine has been postulated as a risk factor for CVD [93]. Many epidemiological studies have reported on the association between homocysteine levels and CVD. A meta-analysis of observational and case–control studies published in 2008 estimated that each 5 μmol/L increase in homocysteine was associated with a 18% increase in coronary events [94]. However, the question remained whether homocysteine was merely a marker of risk (an innocent bystander) or a causally related factor. Several RCTs have been set up to answer this question. In a recent meta-analysis of eight RCTs [95] the Cochrane collaboration concluded that homocysteine-lowering interventions did not reduce the risk of fatal/non-fatal myocardial infarction (RR 1.03, 95% CI 0.94–1.13), stroke (RR 0.89, 95% CI 0.73–1.08) or death by any cause (RR 1.00, 95% CI 0.92–1.09). Since publication of the Cochrane review, three large secondary prevention trials [Study of the Effectiveness of Additional Reductions in Cholesterol and Homocysteine (SEARCH), VITAmins TO Prevent Stroke (VITATOPS), and Supplementation with Folate, vitamin B_6 and B_{12} and/or OMega-3 fatty acids (SU.FOL.OM3)] have been completed and published [48,96]. All trials concluded that supplementation with folic acid and vitamin B_6 and/or B_{12} offers no protection against the development of CVD. Therefore, the evidence is quite consistent that supplementation with B vitamins to lower homocysteine levels does not lower cardiovascular risk.

Food types

Fruits, vegetables, and CVD

The putative relationship between fruit and vegetable consumption and cardiovascular risk is based largely on observational, epidemiological studies [97–106]. The epidemiological studies have varied considerably in terms of their subject recruitment methods and inclusion criteria. Most were performed in North America and Northern Europe. The inclusion dates cover a 50-year period (i.e. the latter half of the twentieth century) during which lifestyles and dietary habits have changed considerably. The various dietary assessment methods include dietary history, 24-hour recall, food (frequency) questionnaires and 3- or 7-day food diaries. Interstudy comparisons are further complicated by the considerable heterogeneity of sample size, duration of follow-up, definition of events, adjustment factors, and presentation of the results. However, meta-analyses of observational studies of fruit and vegetable intake have shown a clear negative association with CVD.

The results of biological experiments are controversial. Of the many nutrients in fruits and vegetables, vitamins occupy a special position because they have been tested in prevention-focused clinical trials. Despite abundant biological evidence [107] and observational, epidemiological data [77,86,108] that emphasize the role of vitamins in atherosclerosis, the meta-analyses of interventional trials have not shown a clear, beneficial effect of fruits and vegetables on the risk of CVD [84,109–112]. In contrast, a recent randomized clinical trial has underpinned epidemiological observations by showing that fruit and vegetable intake was associated with a dose-dependent improvement in endothelium-dependent forearm blood flow responses—an integrated marker of vascular health with known prognostic value [113].

Very few randomized trials have evaluated the effect of high fruit and vegetable consumption on the incidence or recurrence of CHD [14,114,115] and those that have done so do not provide conclusive evidence to show that fruit and vegetable consumption is cardioprotective in secondary prevention. However, the difficulties in modifying long-term fruit and vegetable intake by the provision of nutritional advice alone should be borne in mind when considering these disappointing results.

Lastly, fruit and vegetable intake can affect established CVD risk factors. Numerous findings in observational, population-based studies [116–121] support the hypothesis that fruit and vegetable consumption has an effect on BP regulation. Under the strictly controlled experimental conditions of the DASH study, fruit and vegetable consumption decreased BP over an 8-week period (with changes in systolic and diastolic BP of –2.8 and –1.1 mmHg, respectively). Other researchers have reported similar results [122]. The effect on cholesterol is less well documented. Fruit and vegetables may act through an effect of their fibre content [107]. Several studies have reported effects of fruit and vegetable consumption on lipid profiles [123,124]. Given that these trials were generally not specifically designed to test the effects of fruits and vegetables in hypercholesterolaemic patients, the majority found either only a modest effect or no effect [14,125–131]. Lastly, in cohort studies, components of fruits and vegetables (such as antioxidants, fibre, and magnesium) appeared to protect against the onset of diabetes [132,133]. In contrast, studies of the relationship between fruit and vegetable intake alone and the risk of diabetes have yielded contradictory results [134–136]. Although randomized trials have proved the efficacy of complex lifestyle interventions (including promotion of fruit and vegetable intake, physical activity, and reduction of body weight) in reducing the risk of diabetes [137,138] the contribution of fruits and vegetables per se in these studies is difficult to estimate. On the contrary, nutritional intervention trials have failed to show that fruit and vegetable intake affects either the risk of diabetes [139] or glycaemia and insulin sensitivity [127,140–142]. Thus, the studies published to date do not provide evidence to suggest that fruits and vegetables affect the occurrence of diabetes. The observed discrepancies between studies may be due to confounding factors and possibly antagonistic effects of the sugars, fibres, and antioxidants in fruits and vegetables.

Fish

The protective effect of fish on CVD is attributed to their n-3 fatty acid content. These essential fatty acids have a number of physiological effects, such as anti-inflammatory effects, inhibition of platelet aggregation, lowering of triglycerides, improvement of endothelial function, and anti-arrhythmic effects.

Observations from the 1950s, comparing Inuit from Greenland who consumed about 14 g of n-3 fatty acids per day and Danes eating about 3 g of fatty acids per day showed a ten-fold lower incidence of MI in the Inuit. In 1985, Kromhout et al. [143] showed that even a small amount of fish in the diet was associated with a lower risk of CHD mortality in a cohort of men from the general population. A similar protective effect was shown in a secondary prevention trial that was published a few years later [144]. Since then a lot of research has been done, and knowledge about the mechanism of action of n-3 fatty acids has increased. On the other hand, recently completed secondary prevention trials have not been able to show the positive effects that were expected based on the epidemiological findings and mechanistic properties attributed to n-3 fatty acids (see section 'n-3 PUFAs').

Pooled risk estimates show that eating fish at least once a week results in a 15% reduction in risk of CHD (RR 0.85, 95% CI 0.76–0.96) [45]. Another meta-analysis showed that eating fish two to four times a week reduced the risk of stroke by 18% (RR 0.82, 95% CI 0.72–0.94) compared with eating fish less than once a month [46].The relation between fish intake and cardiovascular risk is not linear. Compared with eating no fish, cardiovascular risk decreases rapidly when eating small to moderate amounts of fish. The public health impact of a small increase in fish consumption in the general population is therefore potentially large. It is estimated that a modest increase in fish consumption of one to two servings a week would reduce CHD mortality by 36% and all-cause mortality by 17% [145]. The recommendation therefore is to eat fish at least twice a week, of which one serving should be oily fish.

Nuts

Meta-analysis of data from six cohort studies shows a 30% reduction in developing CHD (RR 0.70, 95% CI 0.57–0.82); these associations meet the Bradford Hill causality criteria of strength, consistency, temporality, and coherence [64]. Meta-analysis of 25 RCTs found that a daily serving of about 70 g of nuts, significantly reduced total cholesterol [–10.9 mg/dl (–0.28 mmol/L)], LDL cholesterol [–10.2 mg/dl (–0.26 mmol/L)], and total/HDL cholesterol ratio (–0.24). Triglyceride levels were reduced by 20.6 mg/dl (0.23 mmol/L) in those with blood triglyceride levels above 150 mg/dl (1.7 mmol/L). The effects of nut consumption were dose related, and different types of nuts had similar effects on blood lipid levels. The effects were greatest in those with a high LDL cholesterol and low body mass index [146].

Despite the high energy density of nuts, evidence does not suggest increased consumption leads to an increase in body weight. It is estimated that 55–75% of the energy from nuts is offset by dietary compensation, 10–15% by faecal loss, and 10% via increased energy expenditure (although this is less well established) [147]. However, in those with less competent appetite regulation dietary compensation may be ineffective. In such cases it would be prudent to account for the energy content from nuts within a calorie-controlled diet, where they can be used as a replacement for other high-protein foods such as meat. A 60 g serving of nuts contains approximately 200 kcal. Daily consumption can be recommended and can include a variety of nuts such as almonds, walnuts, hazelnuts, pecans, pistachios, macadamia, and peanuts. Nuts should be unsalted (see section 'Salt').

Soy

The lipid-lowering effects of soy have been investigated, but whether the active constituent is soy protein or soy isoflavones is unclear. Meta-analysis of 11 RCTs have shown both soy isoflavones and soy protein to significantly reduce total [–3.9 mg/dl (–0.1 mmol/L)] and LDL [–5.3 mg/dl (–0.13 mmol/L)] cholesterol, but not HDL cholesterol or triglycerides. The greatest effects are seen in those with raised cholesterol levels [148].

Another meta-analysis of 30 RCTs has shown that around 25 g (15–40 g) of soy protein a day lowers LDL cholesterol by 0.23 mmol/L (95% CI –0.160 to –0.306), total cholesterol by 0.22 mmol/L (95% CI –0.142 to –0.291), and triglycerides by 0.08 mmol/L (95% CI –0.004 to –0.158) [149]. Meta-analysis of RCTs have shown isoflavones to exert a modest but significant improvement on endothelial function [150].

There have been a small number of cohort studies showing that soy consumption is associated with lower rates of heart disease. A weak association with heart disease mortality has been shown in one study [151]. Another, the Shanghai women's health study, found a dose–response relationship between soy intake and CHD. This was strongest for non-fatal MI (RR 0.14; 95% CI 0.04–0.48) for the highest (11 g a day soy protein) compared with the lowest (<4.5 g/day) quartile of intake [152].

Table 11.3 Servings of foods high in soy protein

Soy food	Serving size
Soy milk (should be fortified with calcium)	200 ml
Soy yoghurt or dessert (should be fortified with calcium)	150 g
Soy beans	80 g
Soy mince	80 g
Tofu	80 g

Meeting a target to consume 25 g soy protein each day requires eating about three or four servings of soy-rich foods daily (see ➲ Table 11.3). Achieving this requires a drastic dietary change with at least one soy product at each meal, and this may not be achievable for many. A complete switch in the European population from dairy products to soy alternatives has not been investigated with respect to long-term outcomes for bone health and iodine status.

Dairy

Since the results of the DASH trial there has been an interest in the part played by dairy products in cardiovascular risks and outcomes. Meta-analysis of eight cohort studies did not find a significant reduction in CVD risk with high versus low intakes of milk (RR 0.94, 95% CI 0.75–1.13) [64]; however, the effect could be masked by higher levels of saturated fat from consumption of full-fat milk as differentiation could not be made between full-fat and low-fat milk. RCT evidence of the effects of constituents in milk, such as calcium and conjugated linoleic acid, on cardiovascular risk factors have been inconsistent [64]. However, low-fat dairy food is a source of many essential nutrients and is an important part of a balanced diet.

Functional foods

Phytosterols

Phytosterols (including both plant sterols and stanols) are plant compounds that are structurally related to cholesterol. Milk, yoghurt, yoghurt drinks, and margarines enriched in phytosterol ester are available and can be used to supplement natural dietary sources. Many clinical trials have investigated the effect of phytosterol consumption on plasma lipoprotein levels and have consistently found that phytosterol consumption lowers overall plasma lipoprotein levels (and especially concentrations of LDL cholesterol) without affecting levels of HDL cholesterol. A recent meta-analysis showed that a daily phytosterol intake of 2 g lowers levels of LDL cholesterol by about 10% [153, 154, 155, 156]. The cholesterol-lowering effect of phytosterols appears to plateau at intakes above 2.0–3.0 g/day, although in a recent study additional reduction in LDL cholesterol with increasing plant sterol intake was observed [157].

Over the past decade, the results of several epidemiological studies [158, 159, 160, 161, 162] have suggested that slightly elevated plasma plant sterol concentrations are associated with an increased risk of cardiovascular events, independently of the serum total plasma cholesterol; this was already known to be the case for pathologically elevated plasma levels, such as those seen in sitosterolaemia [163]. Recent observational studies have failed to confirm these findings and hence do not support the presence of this type of association in non-sitosterolaemic subjects [155,164–170]. However, the hypothesis whereby phytosterols decrease the incidence of cardiovascular events has not yet been tested in a randomized clinical trial.

Miscellaneous topics

Chocolate

The cardioprotective effects of chocolate consumption have gained a lot of attention recently. A meta-analysis of six cohort studies and one cross-sectional study concluded that the highest level of chocolate intake (which was quite heterogeneous between studies) was associated with a 37% reduction in CVD and a 29% reduction in stroke compared with the lowest levels [171]. It was suggested that the high polyphenol content of chocolate could be one of the mechanisms underlying this association. However, experimental studies are needed to confirm the protective effect of chocolate. For clinical practice, it must be kept in mind that chocolate contains a lot of energy (kilocalories) and is high in sugar and fat.

Cardioprotective diets

Portfolio diet

Several cardioprotective diets which contain a blend of nutrients and foods in the proportions associated with cardioprotection have been investigated. One such diet is the portfolio diet which is low in saturated fat and combines an increase in soy protein (50 g/day), soluble fibre (20 g/day), plant sterols (2g/day), and nuts (almonds, 30 g/day) (each of these elements has already been described). In a randomized controlled laboratory study the effect of the portfolio diet was comparable to the 30% reduction in LDL cholesterol achieved with lovastatin [172]. Longer-term effects under free-living conditions in compliant and motivated individuals has shown a 20% reduction in LDL cholesterol at 1 year [173]. However, while we know that lowering cholesterol through statin use reduces clinical end-points of cardiovascular events [174] we do not have the same evidence from long-term studies that reduction in cholesterol using this combination of specific dietary components translates into reduced cardiovascular events. In view of this, we should perhaps focus on the combination of dietary components which have both RCT evidence for reducing risk factors such as cholesterol and also long-term evidence from cohort studies of an association with reduced cardiovascular events (see ➲ Table 11.4 where a summary is given of the effects of food and nutrients on cardiovascular risk factors and the consequent recommendations).

The Mediterranean diet

Because interactions and correlations among nutrients will influence their bioavailability and absorption, investigating the relationship of single nutrients to CVD is not sufficient. More and more research is focusing on dietary patterns instead of single nutrients. The impact of a total dietary pattern theoretically shows the full preventive potential of diet, yielding a combined estimate of the impact of several favourable dietary habits.

Table 11.4 Summary of evidence for associations of food and nutrients with CHD risk factors

Food or nutrient	Association with cardiovascular events	Association with cardiovascular risk factors	Dietary recommendations
Carbohydrate: glycaemic index	+++ HGI increases CHD risk (MA PC)	+++ Slight reduction in total cholesterol with LGI +++ Reduced HbA1c in diabetes with LGI (MA RCT)	Encourage LGI carbohydrate choices
High intake of sweetened beverages	++ Increased CHD incidence (PC)	+ Increased hypertension, triglycerides, lower HDL concentrations (PC) + Increased weight (PC) ++ Increased C-reactive protein (RCT) – Increased weight gain and metabolic syndrome risk (PC)	Avoid sweetened beverages. Diet beverages remain a reasonable alternative but water should be the cold drink of choice
High intake of diet beverages	+ Increased risk of cardiovascular events (PC)		
High fibre intake	+++ Reduced risk of CHD (MA PC)	+++ Reduction in cholesterol (soluble fibre) (MA RCT) +++ Very small reduction in BP (MA RCT)	Increase total fibre both soluble fibre and wholegrains (three servings a day). Maximum benefit from those which are also low GI
High intake of nuts	+++ Reduced risk of CHD (MA PC)	+++ Cholesterol lowering (MA RCT)	A daily 60 g serving of unsalted nuts can be recommended
Soy products	++ Reduced risk of CHD (PC)	+++ Cholesterol lowering (MA RCT)	Advice to increase intakes should be made on a case by case basis
Dairy foods	+++ No association of intake with CHD (MA PC)	Inconsistent results	Neither increase nor decrease of dairy products is recommended but low-fat choices should be made
Portfolio diet	Not investigated	++ Cholesterol lowering (RCT)	Those aspects of the portfolio diet (reducing saturated fat, increasing fibre and nuts) for which there is strong evidence of reducing cardiovascular events should be prioritized

PC, prospective cohort; MA, meta-analysis; LGI/HGI, low/high glycaemic index.
–,+,++,+++: strength of evidence, based on number of studies and study type.

The Seven Countries study that started in the late 1950s showed striking differences in cardiovascular mortality rates between northern and southern Europe. Even at similar cholesterol levels, and after adjusting for BP and smoking, the large difference in cardiovascular risk remained (➲ Fig. 11.1) [175]. The diet consumed in the Mediterranean cohorts of the Seven Countries study is probably an important factor underlying the large difference in CVD rates between southern and northern Europe.

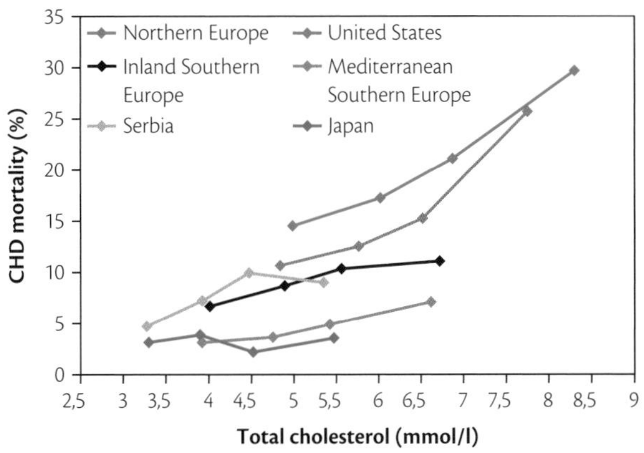

Fig. 11.1 Cumulative 25-year CHD mortality rates in different cohorts of the Seven Countries study, according to baseline quartiles of total cholesterol level, adjusted for age, smoking, and blood pressure [175].

The concept of the Mediterranean diet comprises many of the nutrients and foods that have already been discussed: a high intake of fruits, vegetables, legumes, wholegrain products, fish, and unsaturated fatty acids (especially olive oil), a moderate consumption of alcohol (mostly wine, preferably consumed with meals), and a low consumption of (red) meat, dairy products, and saturated fatty acids.

A number of studies have demonstrated the protective effect of this diet, and recently a meta-analysis was performed in 2010 [176]. Adherence to the Mediterranean diet was operationalized by a scoring system (the Mediterranean diet score), in which one point was obtained for each component of the diet where the intake is above the median intake level for the study population (fruits, vegetables, legumes, cereals, fish, moderate consumption of red wine) or below the median (red and processed meats, dairy products). Depending on the number of food items for which information was obtained, the score could range from 0 to 7–9. The meta-analysis showed that greater adherence to the Mediterranean diet (by a score two points higher) was associated with a 10% reduction in cardiovascular incidence or mortality (pooled RR 0.90, 95% CI 0.87–0.93) and also with an 8% reduction in all-cause mortality (pooled RR 0.92, 95% CI 0.90–0.94).

The effect of adhering to a Mediterranean diet was also tested in the PREDIMED study, an RCT with primary prevention of CVD as the outcome; the results were clearly positive [177].

Solution to the case study

Dietary assessment

Relevant dietary advice cannot be given without understanding an individual's eating patterns and food choice. In a brief consultation a 24-hour dietary recall is a good way to achieve this (e.g. 'Can you tell me everything you ate and drank yesterday, beginning from when you woke up?'). Prompt questions may be necessary to get a complete picture (e.g. 'Did you have any snacks between meals?'). Asking about food type will provide an indication of specific nutrient levels, for example whether low-fat choices are made (e.g. 'What type of milk do you use?').

It is difficult to get an accurate idea of the quantity of food consumed and food pictures or models for comparison can help with this. It is also important to ascertain whether the last 24 hours are considered by the patient to be a typical reflection of their eating.

Supporting dietary change

Mr X's 24-hour dietary recall showed specific foods contributing to a high intake of saturated fat and a low intake of fibre. Food suggestions can be made to reverse this and incorporate other elements having good evidence for preventing cardiovascular events (see ➲ Table 11.5). Other dietary components for which the evidence on clinical end-points is less certain should take lesser priority and be addressed in subsequent consultations, for example increasing plant stanols and increasing soy products.

Particular consideration should be given to the way in which dietary change is supported. While it is necessary to impart correct dietary information and consolidate this with literature on which foods to eat less of and which to eat more of, this alone is unlikely to lead to dietary change. Rather, a patient-led discussion with negotiated achievable goals for dietary change is much more likely to be effective (see ➲ Chapter 9). Helping patients to find their own solutions is much more likely to lead to change than simply telling them what to do. For example, having explained that it is important to eat less saturated fat, rather than give prescriptive advice such as 'so don't eat cheese sandwiches' you could say: 'Your sandwich is high in saturated fat, what do you feel you can do to change that?'.

Table 11.5 Mr X's diet and cardioprotective alternatives

	Mr X's diet	**Cardioprotective alternatives**
Breakfast	Black americano coffee (unsweetened) and two croissants[a,b]	Two seeded wholegrain rolls[c] spread with sunflower soft margarine[d] OR muesli[c] with low-fat natural yoghurt OR branflakes[c] with berries[c] and skimmed milk
Mid-morning	Coffee and two biscuits[a,b]	A piece of fruit, e.g. apple[c]
Lunch	Sandwich containing two pieces of white bread[b], butter[a], cheese[a] (sometimes salami[a]), and salad. Potato crisps[a] (one 40 g packet)	Two pieces of seeded wholegrain bread[c], sunflower spread[d], sliced chicken breast OR canned fish (salmon, mackerel, sardines), and salad. Unsalted nuts[c] (one 50 g packet)
Mid-afternoon	One glass of iced peach tea	Iced mineral water and a piece of fruit, e.g. peach[c]
Evening meal	Three glasses of red wine (125 ml each). Spaghetti bolognaise containing white spaghetti[b] (350 g), minced beef[a] in a bolognaise sauce (300 g), green salad drizzled with olive oil and balsamic vinegar. Fruit salad with Greek yoghurt[a] (200 g)	Two glasses of red wine. Wholegrain spaghetti[c]. Lean minced beef (replace half with cooked red lentils[c]) in a bolognaise sauce. Green salad, with half an avocado[d], sprinkled with sunflower seeds[c,d], and drizzled with olive oil[d] and balsamic vinegar. Fruit salad with low-fat natural yoghurt
		Diet is now low in saturated fat, higher in unsaturated fat and fibre, contains an additional three portions of fruit and vegetables, a portion of oily fish, and three servings of low-GI wholegrain foods

[a]High in saturated or trans-fat.
[b]Low in fibre.
[c]High in fibre and low GI.
[d]High in unsaturated fat.

Further reading

European Heart Network. *Diet, physical activity and cardiovascular disease prevention in Europe*, 2011. Brussels: EHN.

Hooper L, Summerbell CD, Thompson R, et al. Reduced or modified dietary fat for preventing cardiovascular disease. *Cochrane Database Syst Rev* 2012; 5: CD002137.

Mente A, de Koning L, Shannon HS, et al. A systematic review of the evidence supporting a causal link between dietary factors and coronary heart disease. *Arch Intern Med* 2009; **169**: 659–69.

Mozaffarian D, Appel LJ, Horn LV. Recent advances in preventive cardiology and lifestyle medicine: components of a cardioprotective diet: new insights. *Circulation* 2011; **123**: 2870–91.

84 Vivekananthan DP, Penn MS, Sapp SK, et al. Use of antioxidant vitamins for the prevention of cardiovascular disease: meta-analysis of randomised trials. *Lancet* 2003; **361**: 2017–23.

85 Bjelakovic G, Nikolova D, Gluud LL, et al. Mortality in randomized trials of antioxidant supplements for primary and secondary prevention: systematic review and meta-analysis. *J Am Med Assoc* 2007; **297**: 842–57.

86 Marchioli R, Schweiger C, Levantesi G, et al. Antioxidant vitamins and prevention of cardiovascular disease: epidemiological and clinical trial data. *Lipids* 2001; **36** (Suppl.): S53–S63.

87 Sauberlich HE. Pharmacology of vitamin C. *Ann Rev Nutr* 1994; **14**: 371–91.

88 Frei B. To C or not to C, that is the question! *J Am Coll Cardiol* 2003; **42**: 253–5.

89 Steinhubl SR. Why have antioxidants failed in clinical trials? *Am J Cardiol* 2008; **101**: 14D–19D.

90 Holick MF. Vitamin D deficiency. *N Engl J Med* 2007; **357**: 266–81.

91 Lavie CJ, Lee JH, Milani RV. Vitamin D and cardiovascular disease will it live up to its hype? *J Am Coll Cardiol* 2011; **58**: 1547–56.

92 Pittas AG, Dawson-Hughes B. Vitamin D and diabetes. *J Steroid Biochem Mol Biol* 2010; **121**: 425–9.

93 Boushey CJ, Beresford SA, Omenn GS, et al. A quantitative assessment of plasma homocysteine as a risk factor for vascular disease. Probable benefits of increasing folic acid intakes. *J Am Med Assoc* 1995; **274**: 1049–57.

94 Humphrey LL, Fu R, Rogers K, et al. Homocysteine level and coronary heart disease incidence: a systematic review and meta-analysis. *Mayo Clin Proc* 2008; **83**: 1203–12.

95 Marti-Carvajal AJ, Sola I, Lathyris D, et al. Homocysteine lowering interventions for preventing cardiovascular events. *Cochrane Database Syst Rev* 2009; (4): CD006612.

96 Armitage JM, Bowman L, Clarke RJ, et al. Effects of homocysteine-lowering with folic acid plus vitamin B12 vs placebo on mortality and major morbidity in myocardial infarction survivors: a randomized trial. *J Am Med Assoc* 2010; **303**: 2486–94.

97 Bazzano LA, Serdula MK, Liu S. Dietary intake of fruits and vegetables and risk of cardiovascular disease. *Curr Atheroscler Rep* 2003; **5**: 492–9.

98 Bazzano LA. *Dietary intake of fruit and vegetables and risk of diabetes mellitus and cardiovascular diseases*, 2005. URL: <http://www.who.int/dietphysicalactivity/publications/f%26v_cvd_diabetes.pdf>

99 Dauchet L, Amouyel P, Dallongeville J. Fruit and vegetable consumption and risk of stroke: a meta-analysis of cohort studies. *Neurology* 2005; **65**: 1193–7.

100 Dauchet L, Amouyel P, Hercberg S, et al. Fruit and vegetable consumption and risk of coronary heart disease: a meta-analysis of cohort studies. *J Nutr* 2006; **136**: 2588–93.

101 He FJ, Nowson CA, MacGregor GA. Fruit and vegetable consumption and stroke: meta-analysis of cohort studies. *Lancet* 2006; **367**: 320–6.

102 He FJ, Nowson CA, Lucas M, MacGregor GA. Increased consumption of fruit and vegetables is related to a reduced risk of coronary heart disease: meta-analysis of cohort studies. *J Hum Hypertens* 2007; **21**: 717–28.

103 Hu FB. Plant-based foods and prevention of cardiovascular disease: an overview. *Am J Clin Nutr* 2003; **78**: 544S–551S.

104 Law MR, Morris JK. By how much does fruit and vegetable consumption reduce the risk of ischaemic heart disease? *Eur J Clin Nutr* 1998; **52**: 549–56.

105 Law MR, Morris JK. By how much does fruit and vegetable consumption reduce the risk of ischaemic heart disease: response to commentary. *Eur J Clin Nutr* 1999; **53**: 903–4.

106 Ness AR, Egger M, Powles J. Fruit and vegetables and ischaemic heart disease: systematic review or misleading meta-analysis? *Eur J Clin Nutr* 1999; **53**: 900–4.

107 Lampe JW. Health effects of vegetables and fruit: assessing mechanisms of action in human experimental studies. *Am J Clin Nutr* 1999; **70**: 475S–490S.

108 Ye Z, Song H. Antioxidant vitamins intake and the risk of coronary heart disease: meta-analysis of cohort studies. *Eur J Cardiovasc Prev Rehabil* 2008; **15**: 26–34.

109 Albert CM, Cook NR, Gaziano JM, et al. Effect of folic acid and B vitamins on risk of cardiovascular events and total mortality among women at high risk for cardiovascular disease: a randomized trial. *J Am Med Assoc* 2008; **299**: 2027–36.

110 Bazzano LA, Reynolds K, Holder KN. Effect of folic acid supplementation on risk of cardiovascular diseases: a meta-analysis of randomized controlled trials. *J Am Med Assoc* 2006; **296**: 2720–6.

111 Cook NR, Albert CM, Gaziano JM, et al. A randomized factorial trial of vitamins C and E and beta carotene in the secondary prevention of cardiovascular events in women: results from the Women's Antioxidant Cardiovascular Study. *Arch Intern Med* 2007; **167**: 1610–18.

112 Sesso HD, Buring JE, Christen WG, et al. Vitamins E and C in the prevention of cardiovascular disease in men: the Physicians' Health Study II randomized controlled trial. *J Am Med Assoc* 2008; **300**: 2123–33.

113 McCall DO, McGartland CP, McKinley MC, et al. Dietary intake of fruits and vegetables improves microvascular function in hypertensive subjects in a dose-dependent manner. *Circulation* 2009; **119**: 2153–60.

114 Burr ML, Ashfield-Watt PA, Dunstan FD, et al. Lack of benefit of dietary advice to men with angina: results of a controlled trial. *Eur J Clin Nutr* 2003; **57**: 193–200.

115 Ness AR, Ashfield-Watt PA, Whiting JM, et al. The long-term effect of dietary advice on the diet of men with angina: the diet and angina randomized trial. *J Hum Nutr Diet* 2004; **17**: 117–19.

116 Ascherio A, Rimm EB, Giovannucci EL, et al. A prospective study of nutritional factors and hypertension among US men. *Circulation* 1992; **86**: 1475–84.

117 Dauchet L, Kesse-Guyot E, Czernichow S, et al. Dietary patterns and blood pressure change over 5-y follow-up in the SU.VI.MAX cohort. *Am J Clin Nutr* 2007; **85**: 1650–6.

118 Sacks FM, Rosner B, Kass EH. Blood pressure in vegetarians. *Am J Epidemiol* 1974; **100**: 390–8.

119 Shah M, Jeffery RW, Laing B, et al. Hypertension Prevention Trial (HPT): food pattern changes resulting from intervention on sodium, potassium, and energy intake. Hypertension Prevention Trial Research Group. *J Am Diet Assoc* 1990; **90**: 69–76.

120 Hypertension Prevention Trial Research Group. The Hypertension Prevention Trial: three-year effects of dietary changes on blood pressure. *Arch Intern Med* 1990; **150**: 153–62.

121 Margetts BM, Beilin LJ, Vandongen R, et al. Vegetarian diet in mild hypertension: a randomised controlled trial. *Br Med J* 1986; **293**: 1468–71.

122 John JH, Ziebland S, Yudkin P, et al. Effects of fruit and vegetable consumption on plasma antioxidant concentrations and blood pressure: a randomised controlled trial. *Lancet* 2002; **359**: 1969–74.

123 Zino S, Skeaff M, Williams S, et al. Randomised controlled trial of effect of fruit and vegetable consumption on plasma concentrations of lipids and antioxidants. *Br Med J* 1997; **314**: 1787–91.

124 Smith-Warner SA, Elmer PJ, Tharp TM, et al. Increasing vegetable and fruit intake: randomized intervention and monitoring in an at-risk population. *Cancer Epidemiol Biomarkers Prev* 2000; **9**: 307–17.

125 Broekmans WM, Klopping-Ketelaars WA, Kluft C, et al. Fruit and vegetables and cardiovascular risk profile: a diet controlled intervention study. *Eur J Clin Nutr* 2001; **55**: 636–42.

126 Djuric Z, Ren J, Mekhovich O, et al. Effects of high fruit-vegetable and/or low-fat intervention on plasma micronutrient levels. *J Am Coll Nutr* 2006; **25**: 178–87.

127 Lanza E, Schatzkin A, Daston C, et al. Implementation of a 4-y, high-fiber, high-fruit-and-vegetable, low-fat dietary intervention: results of dietary changes in the Polyp Prevention Trial. *Am J Clin Nutr* 2001; **74**: 387–401.

128 Maskarinec G, Chan CL, Meng L, et al. Exploring the feasibility and effects of a high-fruit and -vegetable diet in healthy women. *Cancer Epidemiol Biomarkers Prev* 1999; **8**: 919–24.

129 Obarzanek E, Sacks FM, Vollmer WM, et al. Effects on blood lipids of a blood pressure-lowering diet: the Dietary Approaches to Stop Hypertension (DASH) Trial. *Am J Clin Nutr* 2001; **74**: 80–9.

130 Pierce JP, Newman VA, Flatt SW, et al. Telephone counseling intervention increases intakes of micronutrient- and phytochemical-rich vegetables, fruit and fiber in breast cancer survivors. *J Nutr* 2004; **134**: 452–8.

131 Rock CL, Flatt SW, Thomson CA, et al. Plasma triacylglycerol and HDL cholesterol concentrations confirm self-reported changes in carbohydrate and fat intakes in women in a diet intervention trial. *J Nutr* 2004; **134**: 342–7.

132 Hu FB, van Dam RM, Liu S. Diet and risk of type II diabetes: the role of types of fat and carbohydrate. *Diabetologia* 2001; **44**: 805–17.

133 Lopez-Ridaura R, Willett WC, Rimm EB, et al. Magnesium intake and risk of type 2 diabetes in men and women. *Diabetes Care* 2004; **27**: 134–40.

134 Hamer M, Chida Y. Intake of fruit, vegetables, and antioxidants and risk of type 2 diabetes: systematic review and meta-analysis. *J Hypertens* 2007; **25**: 2361–9.

135 Bazzano LA, Li TY, Joshipura KJ, et al. Intake of fruit, vegetables, and fruit juices and risk of diabetes in women. *Diabetes Care* 2008; **31**: 1311–17.

136 Villegas R, Shu XO, Gao YT, et al. Vegetable but not fruit consumption reduces the risk of type 2 diabetes in Chinese women. *J Nutr* 2008; **138**: 574–80.

137 Tuomilehto J, Lindstrom J, Eriksson JG, et al. Prevention of type 2 diabetes mellitus by changes in lifestyle among subjects with impaired glucose tolerance. *N Engl J Med* 2001; **344**: 1343–50.

138 Pan XR, Li GW, Hu YH, et al. Effects of diet and exercise in preventing NIDDM in people with impaired glucose tolerance. The Da Qing IGT and Diabetes Study. *Diabetes Care* 1997; **20**: 537–44.

139 Tinker LF, Bonds DE, Margolis KL, et al. Low-fat dietary pattern and risk of treated diabetes mellitus in postmenopausal women: the Women's Health Initiative randomized controlled dietary modification trial. *Arch Intern Med* 2008; **168**: 1500–11.

140 Ard JD, Grambow SC, Liu D, et al. The effect of the PREMIER interventions on insulin sensitivity. *Diabetes Care* 2004; **27**: 340–7.

141 Beresford SA, Johnson KC, Ritenbaugh C, et al. Low-fat dietary pattern and risk of colorectal cancer: the Women's Health Initiative randomized controlled dietary modification trial. *J Am Med Assoc* 2006; **295**: 643–65.

142 Pierce JP, Natarajan L, Caan BJ, et al. Influence of a diet very high in vegetables, fruit, and fiber and low in fat on prognosis following treatment for breast cancer: the Women's Healthy Eating and Living (WHEL) randomized trial. *J Am Med Assoc* 2007; **298**: 289–98.

143 Kromhout D, Bosschieter EB, de Lezenne CC. The inverse relation between fish consumption and 20-year mortality from coronary heart disease. *N Engl J Med* 1985; **312**: 1205–9.

144 Burr ML. Lessons from the story of n-3 fatty acids. *Am J Clin Nutr* 2000; **71**: 397S–398S.

145 Mozaffarian D, Rimm EB. Fish intake, contaminants, and human health: evaluating the risks and the benefits. *J Am Med Assoc* 2006; **296**: 1885–99.

146 Sabate J, Oda K, Ros E. Nut consumption and blood lipid levels: a pooled analysis of 25 intervention trials. *Arch Intern Med* 2010; **170**: 821–7.

147 Mattes RD, Dreher ML. Nuts and healthy body weight maintenance mechanisms. *Asia Pac J Clin Nutr* 2010; **19**: 137–41.

148 Taku K, Umegaki K, Sato Y, et al. Soy isoflavones lower serum total and LDL cholesterol in humans: a meta-analysis of 11 randomized controlled trials. *Am J Clin Nutr* 2007; **85**: 1148–56.

149 Harland JI, Haffner TA. Systematic review, meta-analysis and regression of randomised controlled trials reporting an association between an intake of circa 25 g soya protein per day and blood cholesterol. *Atherosclerosis* 2008; **200**: 13–27.

150 Li SH, Liu XX, Bai YY, et al. Effect of oral isoflavone supplementation on vascular endothelial function in postmenopausal women: a meta-analysis of randomized placebo-controlled trials. *Am J Clin Nutr* 2010; **91**: 480–6.

151 Nagata C. Ecological study of the association between soy product intake and mortality from cancer and heart disease in Japan. *Int J Epidemiol* 2000; **29**: 832–6.

152 Zhang X, Shu XO, Gao YT, et al. Soy food consumption is associated with lower risk of coronary heart disease in Chinese women. *J Nutr* 2003; **133**: 2874–8.

153 Abumweis SS, Barake R, Jones PJ. Plant sterols/stanols as cholesterol lowering agents: a meta-analysis of randomized controlled trials. *Food Nutr Res* 2008; **52**: doi: 10.3402/fnr.v52i0.1811

154 Demonty I, Ras RT, van der Knaap HC, et al. Continuous dose-response relationship of the LDL-cholesterol-lowering effect of phytosterol intake. *J Nutr* 2009; **139**: 271–84.

155 Genser B, Silbernagel G, De Backer G, et al. Plant sterols and cardiovascular disease: a systematic review and meta-analysis. *Eur Heart J* 2012; **33**: 444–51.

156 Katan MB, Grundy SM, Jones P, et al. Efficacy and safety of plant stanols and sterols in the management of blood cholesterol levels. *Mayo Clin Proc* 2003; **78**: 965–78.

157 Musa-Veloso K, Poon TH, Elliot JA, et al. A comparison of the LDL-cholesterol lowering efficacy of plant stanols and plant sterols over a continuous dose range: results of a meta-analysis of randomized, placebo-controlled trials. *Prostaglandins Leukot Essent Fatty Acids* 2011; **85**: 9–28.

158 Assmann G, Cullen P, Erbey J, et al. Plasma sitosterol elevations are associated with an increased incidence of coronary events in men: results of a nested case-control analysis of the Prospective Cardiovascular Munster (PROCAM) study. *Nutr Metab Cardiovasc Dis* 2006; **16**: 13–21.

159 Glueck CJ, Speirs J, Tracy T, et al. Relationships of serum plant sterols (phytosterols) and cholesterol in 595 hypercholesterolemic subjects, and familial aggregation of phytosterols, cholesterol, and premature coronary heart disease in hyperphytosterolemic probands and their first-degree relatives. *Metabolism* 1991; **40**: 842–8.

160 Rajaratnam RA, Gylling H, Miettinen TA. Independent association of serum squalene and noncholesterol sterols with coronary artery disease in postmenopausal women. *J Am Coll Cardiol* 2000; **35**: 1185–91.

161 Sehayek E, Fung YY, Yu HJ, et al. A complex plasma plant sterol locus on mouse chromosome 14 has at least two genes regulating intestinal sterol absorption. *J Lipid Res* 2006; **47**: 2291–6.

162 Sudhop T, Gottwald BM, von Bergmann K. Serum plant sterols as a potential risk factor for coronary heart disease. *Metabolism* 2002; **51**: 1519–21.

163 Weingartner O, Bohm M, Laufs U. Controversial role of plant sterol esters in the management of hypercholesterolaemia. *Eur Heart J* 2009; **30**: 404–9.

164 Fassbender K, Lutjohann D, Dik MG, et al. Moderately elevated plant sterol levels are associated with reduced cardiovascular risk—the LASA study. *Atherosclerosis* 2008; **196**: 283–8.
165 Pinedo S, Vissers MN, von Bergmann K, et al. Plasma levels of plant sterols and the risk of coronary artery disease: the prospective EPIC-Norfolk Population Study. *J Lipid Res* 2007; **48**: 139–44.
166 Pinedo S, Vissers MN, von Bergmann K, et al. Plasma levels of plant sterols and the risk of coronary artery disease: the prospective EPIC-Norfolk Population Study. *J Lipid Res* 2007; **48**: 139–44.
167 Silbernagel G, Fauler G, Renner W, et al. The relationships of cholesterol metabolism and plasma plant sterols with the severity of coronary artery disease. *J Lipid Res* 2009; **50**: 334–41.
168 Wilund KR, Yu L, Xu F, et al. No association between plasma levels of plant sterols and atherosclerosis in mice and men. *Arterioscler Thromb Vasc Biol* 2004; **24**: 2326–32.
169 Windler E, Zyriax BC, Kuipers F, et al. Association of plasma phytosterol concentrations with incident coronary heart disease. Data from the CORA study, a case-control study of coronary artery disease in women. *Atherosclerosis* 2009; **203**: 284–90.
170 Gylling H, Plat J, Turley S, et al. Plant sterols and plant stanols in the management of dyslipidaemia and prevention of cardiovascular disease. *Atherosclerosis* 2014; **232**: 346–60.
171 Buitrago-Lopez A, Sanderson J, Johnson L, et al. Chocolate consumption and cardiometabolic disorders: systematic review and meta-analysis. *Br Med J* 2011; **343**: d4488.
172 Jenkins DJ, Kendall CW, Marchie A, et al. Effects of a dietary portfolio of cholesterol-lowering foods vs lovastatin on serum lipids and C-reactive protein. *J Am Med Assoc* 2003; **290**: 502–10.
173 Jenkins DJ, Kendall CW, Faulkner DA, et al. Assessment of the longer-term effects of a dietary portfolio of cholesterol-lowering foods in hypercholesterolemia. *Am J Clin Nutr* 2006; **83**: 582–91.
174 LaRosa JC, Grundy SM, Waters DD, et al. Intensive lipid lowering with atorvastatin in patients with stable coronary disease. *N Engl J Med* 2005; **352**: 1425–35.
175 Verschuren WM, Jacobs DR, Bloemberg BP, et al. Serum total cholesterol and long-term coronary heart disease mortality in different cultures. Twenty-five-year follow-up of the seven countries study. *J Am Med Assoc* 1995; **274**: 131–6.
176 Sofi F, Abbate R, Gensini GF, et al. Accruing evidence on benefits of adherence to the Mediterranean diet on health: an updated systematic review and meta-analysis. *Am J Clin Nutr* 2010; **92**: 1189–96.
177 Estruch R, Ros E, Salas-Salvadó J, et al., for the PREDIMED Study Investigators. Primary prevention of cardiovascular disease with a Mediterranean diet. *N Engl J Med* 2013; **368**: 1279–90.

CHAPTER 12

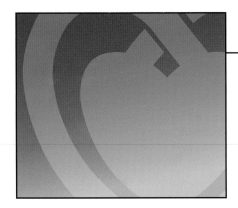

Physical activity and inactivity

Stephan Gielen, Alessandro Mezzani, Paola Pontremoli, Simone Binno, Giovanni Q. Villani, Massimo F. Piepoli, Josef Niebauer, and Daniel Forman

Contents

Summary

Physical activity plays a central role in the prevention and treatment of cardiovascular diseases. In this chapter the current evidence for regular aerobic exercise in primary prevention is discussed and recommendations for exercise interventions in the general population are given. Regular physical exercise is an established therapeutic strategy in a number of cardiovascular diseases, most notably for patients after an acute myocardial infarction, with stable coronary artery disease (CAD), and with stable chronic heart failure. In these disease entities moderate-intensity aerobic endurance training is the basis of most training programmes. However, high-intensity interval training has been found to be more effective in improving cardiovascular exercise capacity without any measurable additional risks. Resistance training can be used as an optional training component in patients with pronounced loss of lean muscle mass (i.e. patients with chronic heart failure and geriatric patients). In recent years new areas for application of exercise-based intervention have been explored: training interventions proved to be safe and effective in pulmonary hypertension, heart failure with preserved ejection fraction, and compensated subcritical valvular heart disease. However, in contrast to training in CAD and in heart failure, the prognostic benefit is not yet established.

Case study—the clinical problem

A 78-year-old patient is referred to your institution for in-hospital cardiac rehabilitation. He has survived two myocardial infarctions (anterior and inferior) 2 and 10 years ago, has type 2 diabetes, orthopaedic problems in his lower back, and chronic heart failure with a severely reduced left ventricular ejection fraction of 23%. He received an implantable cardioverter defibrillator with biventricular pacing for cardiac resynchronization therapy a year ago.

His last unscheduled hospitalization was just 3 weeks ago because of worsening dyspnoea and fluid overload. That episode occurred after the patient went on a bus trip with his local church community and discontinued his diuretics for 2 days. He leads an independent life with his wife, who is 72 years old, and has complained of increasing exercise intolerance over the last 6–8 months. He is able to climb just one flight of stairs and has problems carrying the shopping bags from the car to his apartment.

After recompensation and reinstitution of the diuretic therapy, he is sent to your institution because the cardiologist in the tertiary care hospital heard a talk at the last ESC Congress that exercise training can improve exercise capacity and quality of life in heart failure patients.

On examination, you find a slim patient of 70 kg, height 1.78 m (BMI 22.1 kg/m^2). His temperature is 37.6 °C. He explains that he lost about 5 kg unintentionally over the last 6 months but says that he was never a big man. His blood pressure is 110/86 mm Hg and pulse rate 92 beats/minute (irregular). Auscultation of the lungs is normal and his respiration rate is 25/minute. He has a holosystolic murmur at the apex with propagation into the left axilla. The abdomen is normal, non-tender and the liver slightly enlarged on palpation. Despite the diuretic therapy he still has ++ pitting oedema at both ankles extending way up to the knees.

You need to consider the following questions:

- Which diagnostic blood tests would you like to have on admission to your institution?
- What kind of apparative diagnostic tests do you need/not need to assess the patient's ability to start an exercise programme, to determine the initial target heart rate, and to assess the risk of adverse events?
- Which medications would you check and possibly increase in dose before starting the training programme?
- What kind of exercise programme would you prescribe to increase exercise capacity and improve prognosis?

Introduction

Over 2000 years ago the Greek philosopher Plato wrote that 'Lack of activity destroys the good condition of every human being, while movement and methodical physical exercise save it and preserve it'. That ancient wisdom has now been documented in large-scale observational trials which confirmed a clear dose-dependent reduction of all-cause and cardiovascular mortality with regard to time spent on leisure-time physical activity. According to the largest of these studies, involving over 400 000 individuals, even 15 minutes of exercise per day confer a 14% reduction in mortality [1]. A 4% reduction can be added for each additional 15 minutes of daily exercise [1].

The effects on mortality and morbidity are even greater in patient populations with manifest coronary artery disease (CAD), survivors of myocardial infarction (MI), and those with stable chronic heart failure (CHF). In patients with CAD a consistent reduction of 18–20% in all-cause mortality was confirmed in a meta-analysis [2,3]. After acute coronary syndrome the effects seem to be even more pronounced, leading to a 40% decline in 6-month mortality [4].

In heart failure with reduced ejection fraction (HFREF) a European meta-analysis of pooled patient data from randomized studies found a significant reduction of 35% in total mortality and 28% in hospitalization [5]. However, this was not confirmed in a prospective large-scale multicentre study, probably because of lower than expected adherence to the prescribed training programme [6]. It is clear, however, that training programmes result in a 15–25% increase in exercise capacity, a concomitant improvement in the New York Heart Association (NYHA) functional class, and a reverse left ventricular remodelling with reduction of cardiomegaly.

Recently, in the ExDHF study [7], the beneficial effects of training on symptoms, exercise capacity, and left ventricular diastolic function were also confirmed in heart failure with preserved ejection fraction (HFPEF). Training as a therapeutic concept is also being extended to groups of patients who were formerly advised not to engage in sporting activities—patients with pulmonary hypertension [8] and valvular and congenital heart disease. Clinical research in these areas is just beginning, and although first proof-of-concept studies have confirmed safety and efficacy it is too early to extrapolate the findings to prognostic improvements.

Exercise training has multiple physiological effects on the cardiovascular system, most notably a reduction in resting heart rate as a result of increased parasympathetic tone, improved vascular endothelial function with augmented flow-mediated vasodilation during exercise, increased vasculogenesis through endothelial progenitor cells, and multiple metabolic changes in the myocardium resulting in improved tolerance for ischaemia and reperfusion injury (➲ Fig. 12.1; for review see [9,10]).

The evolutionary perspective on physical activity and inactivity

According to Neel's hypothesis [11], during the human hunter–gatherer phase there was genetic selection for endurance performance and 'thrifty genes' that permit effective storage of energy in fuel depots during times when food is abundant. The regular alternation of periods of famine and physical activity (i.e. during hunting) and periods of rest with replenishment of the fuel stores after successful hunts represents the human physiological lifestyle (➲ Fig. 12.2) [11,12].

The abundance of food and lack of physical activity in the modern technical world have shifted this balance between energy intake and energy expenditure through physical activity towards a continuous stalling process, leading to central obesity, constantly low beta-oxidation in skeletal muscles, high insulin levels, and insulin resistance—finally leading to the development of metabolic syndrome (➲ Fig. 12.3). In animal experiments only 4 weeks of forced physical inactivity (by housing mice in smaller cages) lead to a significant reduction of normal flow-mediated arterial vasodilatation [13]. This so-called endothelial dysfunction is regarded as the initial step in atherogenesis.

Should we measure physical activity levels or physical fitness?

Physical activity and physical fitness are not two sides of the same coin: while physical activity indicates the time and energy an

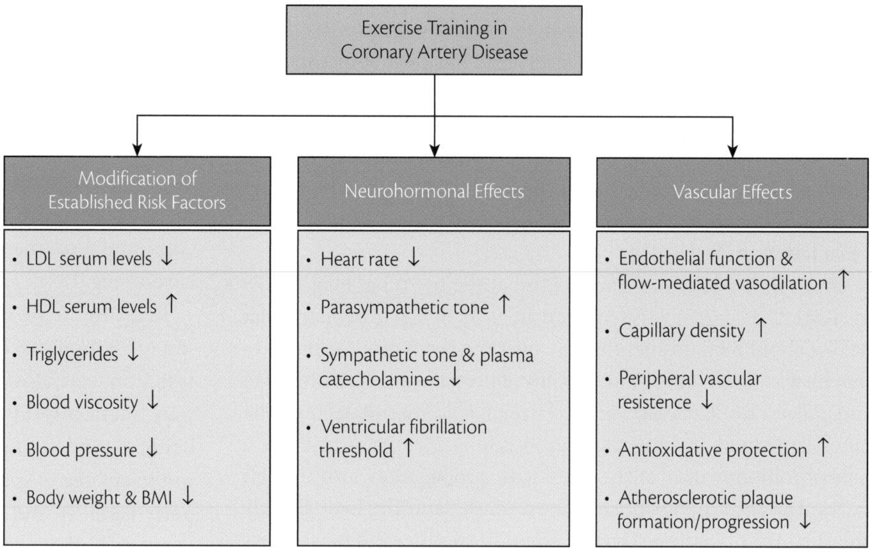

Fig. 12.1 In patients with cardiovascular disease exercise training positively modifies the risk factor profile, normalizes the neurohormonal balance, and improves vascular function resulting in prevention of plaque development/plaque progression. LDL, low-density lipoprotein; HDL, high-density lipoprotein; BMI, body mass index.

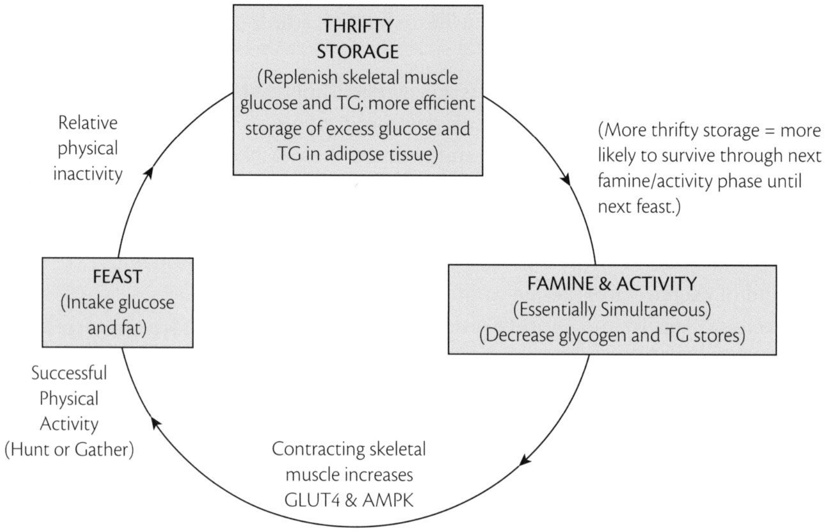

Fig. 12.2 In Palaeolithic times the life of hunter–gatherers was characterized by regular cycles of famine and physical activity and feasting with ample food supply after successful hunting. Evolutionary selection favoured 'thrifty genes' which enhance efficient energy storage to survive the next famine/activity phase. TG, total glycogen; GLUT4, Glucose transporter type 4; AMPK, AMP-activated protein kinase.

Reproduced with permission from Chakravarthy MV, Booth FW. Eating, exercise, and 'thrifty' genotypes: connecting the dots toward an evolutionary understanding of modern chronic diseases. *J Appl Physiol Bethesda Md 1985* 2004; **96**: 3–10.

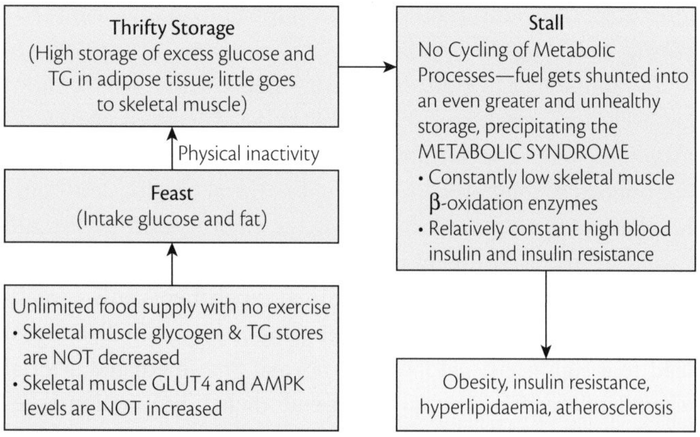

Fig. 12.3 Today, unlimited food supply and absence of famine/activity phases lead to continuous high storage of glucose and triglycerides with the known consequences of obesity, insulin resistance, hyperlipidaemia, and finally atherosclerosis.

Reproduced with permission from Chakravarthy MV, Booth FW. Eating, exercise, and 'thrifty' genotypes: connecting the dots toward an evolutionary understanding of modern chronic diseases. *J Appl Physiol Bethesda Md 1985* 2004; **96**: 3–10.

individual invests in exercise and is mainly influenced by motivation and perseverance, physical fitness carries an important genetic component. If two different people invest the same time and energy in the same type of training programme their resulting fitness levels will be different. In consequence, it has been debated whether fitness predicts mortality independent of the level of physical activity [14].

Indeed, fitness and physical activity have different dose–response relations with cardiovascular events. In a large meta-analysis Williams [15] described that: (1) the risk reduction per 10% increment in physical fitness showed a sharp drop in cardiovascular event rates between the 15th and 25th percentiles, while there was a steady decline over the entire range of physical activity levels; and (2) for all percentiles greater than the 25th the relative risk reduction is greater for fitness than for physical activity (➲ Fig. 12.4). These data indicate that the least fit individuals derive the greatest prognostic benefit from training interventions.

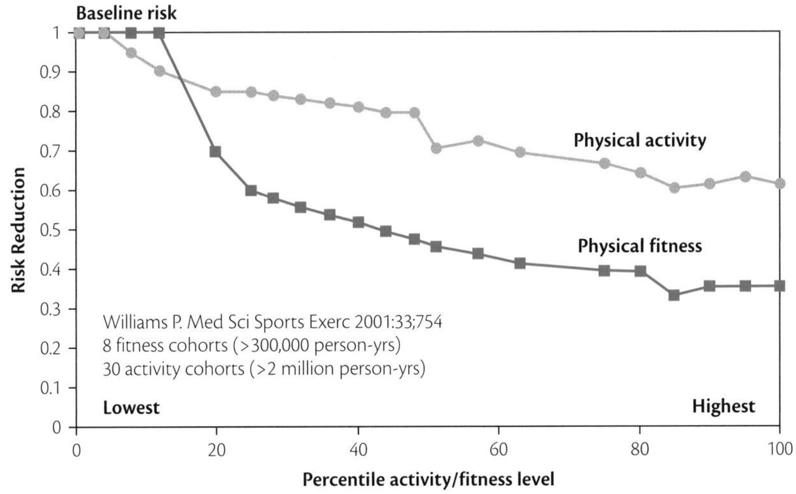

Fig. 12.4 In a recent meta-analysis comparing the dose–response relationships between leisure-time physical activity and fitness and their association with cardiovascular events, Williams [15] found that the risk reduction per 10% increment in physical fitness showed a sharp drop for fitness between the 15th and 25th percentiles of fitness while there was a steady decline over the entire range of physical activity levels. This indicates the potential for a 'threshold effect', i.e. a minimal physical fitness to reduce one's cardiovascular risk. The meta-analysis included a total of eight fitness cohorts with over 300 000 person-years and 30 physical activity cohorts with over 2 000 000 person-years of data.

Reproduced from Williams, P, Physical fitness and activity as separate heart disease risk factors: a meta-analysis, *Medicine & Science in Sports & Exercise*, **33**:5 2001, with permission from Wolters Kluwer.

The advantage of using physical fitness rather than physical activity for assessing the association between individual lifestyle and incidence of cardiovascular events lies in the fact that fitness can be objectively measured by a maximal exercise test (ideally ergospirometry) while physical activity is usually measured by recall questionnaires. In questionnaires patients usually overestimate the time devoted to physical activity and the calculation of leisure-time-related energy expenditure for different activities is very unreliable. Thus fitness probably gives a more objective assessment of a lifestyle with regular exercise.

Prognostic implications of physical activity and physical fitness

In the last three decades long-term observational studies have shown a significant relationship between above average levels of leisure-time physical activity and reduced cardiac and all-cause mortality [16, 17, 18]. In relative terms mortality was 30–40% lower in moderately active people (leisure-time energy expenditure 1000 kcal/week) compared with inactive individuals (➲ Fig. 12.5) [19].

The results of these questionnaire-based physical activity studies were corroborated by longitudinal studies that objectively measured physical fitness at baseline and compared fitness levels with mortality rates [14,20]. An increase in exercise capacity of just 1 metabolic equivalent (MET; in an average 70-kg man an exercise intensity of 25 W is equal to 1.6 METs) is associated with a mortality reduction of 12% [21]. Although it has traditionally been recommended that a minimum energy expenditure of 1000 kcal/week during leisure-time physical activity should be achieved to obtain a prognostic benefit, newer studies suggest that the greatest reduction in morbidity and mortality is attained when formerly inactive people begin to exercise regularly. Recommendations may therefore need to consider individual fitness levels instead of globally prescribing activities of ≥3 METs [22].

Basic components of exercise

In principle, exercise activities can be either endurance or resistance training activities. The primary purpose of endurance training is to improve a person's aerobic exercise capacity, which permits prolonged submaximal activities typically associated with locomotion (e.g. walking, long-distance running, cycling, rowing, and swimming). Resistance exercise aims to improve a person's maximal muscular strength and hence his or her ability to perform activities where maximal strength is important (e.g. weightlifting, boxing, short-distance sprints). The corresponding terminology in muscle physiology is isotonic contraction, in which the muscle contracts with a constant minor load, and isometric contraction, in which the muscle length is kept constant with maximal load.

In recent years resistance exercise has entered the field of cardiac rehabilitation (CR) and its effectiveness has been much debated. However, the debate is to a certain degree artificial because in training interventions there is no strict endurance or resistance training just as there is no pure isotonic or isometric muscle

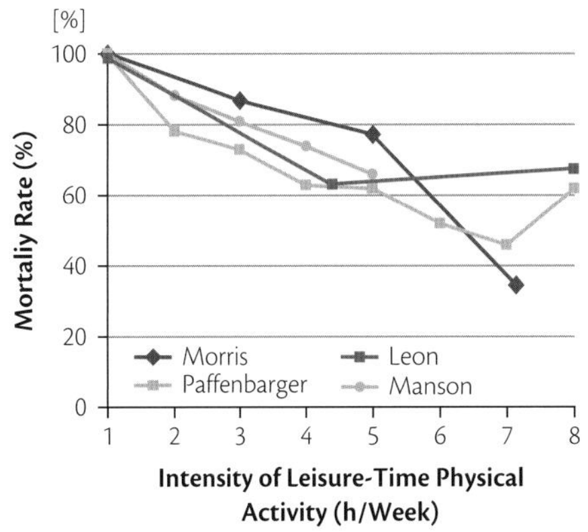

Fig. 12.5 Relationship between the intensity of leisure-time physical activity in hours per week and all-cause mortality in the seminal publications by Morris et al. [16], Paffenbarger et al. [17], Leon et al. [173], and Manson et al. [174].

Source: data from [173] Leon AS, Connett J, Jacobs DR Jr, Rauramaa R. Leisure-time physical activity levels and risk of coronary heart disease and death. The Multiple Risk Factor Intervention Trial. *JAMA J Am Med Assoc*. 1987; **258**: 2388–2395. [174] Manson JE, Greenland P, LaCroix AZ, Stefanick ML, Mouton CP, Oberman A, Perri MG, Sheps DS, Pettinger MB, Siscovick DS. Walking compared with vigorous exercise for the prevention of cardiovascular events in women. *N Engl J Med*. 2002; **347**: 716–725.

contraction. The physiological reality is auxotonic contraction, which is contraction occurring against increasing load (e.g. in cycling). Pure endurance and resistance training represent theoretical concepts which mark the extreme forms of training. In reality there is a continuum between both extremes, and the level of exercise intensity/percentage of one repetition maximum (RM) determines whether a given training intervention has more endurance or resistance components.

Whole body exercise testing in cardiovascular health and disease

The role of exercise testing

Exercise testing is used extensively in both healthy subjects and cardiac patients [1,2] because the measurements obtained during exercise describe the functional reserve of the cardiopulmonary system.

Protocols adopted for exercise testing distinguish between incremental and constant work rate, according whether there is progressive increase in work rate or constancy during the test, respectively [23,24]. Incremental tests aim at maximally stressing the cardiovascular system and are routinely used in the clinical setting, whereas constant work-rate tests are usually performed at submaximal effort intensities and are mainly used for research purposes. In step incremental protocols the work rate is increased by a uniform amount every 1, 2, or 3 minutes (➲ Fig. 12.6). In ramp incremental protocols work rate is increased continuously during each minute of exercise (➲ Fig. 12.6), allowing better adaptation to the increasing workload on the part of the subject/patient and a more linear trend over time of physiological parameters compared with non-ramp incremental protocols [25,26].

When a thorough evaluation of the efficiency of the O_2 transport and/or utilization system is required for clinical or research purposes [25,27,28], measurement of ventilation (VE), oxygen consumption (VO_2), and carbon dioxide production (VCO_2) can be added to standard exercise testing measurements in cardiopulmonary exercise testing (CPET). ➲ Table 12.1 defines the abbreviations used in cardiopulmonary exercise testing.

Table 12.1 Glossary of abbreviations used in cardiopulmonary exercise testing

Abbreviation	Explanation	Unit
VE	Ventilation	L/min
VO_2	Oxygen uptake	L/min
VCO_2	Carbon dioxide output	L/min
PO_2	Oxygen partial pressure	mmHg
PCO_2	Carbon dioxide partial pressure	mmHg
V_T	Tidal volume	L
V_D	Dead space volume	L
EELV	End-expiratory lung volume	L
$PETO_2$	End-tidal oxygen partial pressure (i.e. at the end of the expiratory phase)	mmHg
$PETCO_2$	End-tidal carbon dioxide partial pressure (frequently used as an approximation of arterial PCO_2)	mmHg
VAT	Ventilatory anaerobic threshold	ml/min (or ml/kg min if adjusted for body weight)
Peak VO_2	Maximal oxygen uptake as a measure of individual maximal exercise capacity	ml/min (or ml/kg min if adjusted for body weight)

Indications for exercise testing

This section discusses the main indications for incremental exercise testing. For a complete summary of exercise test indications see ➲ Table 12.2.

Risk stratification

Several parameters obtained by exercise testing are powerful predictors of all-cause and cardiac death in normal subjects and/or cardiac patients [21,29–32] (➲ Box 12.1). It must be noted,

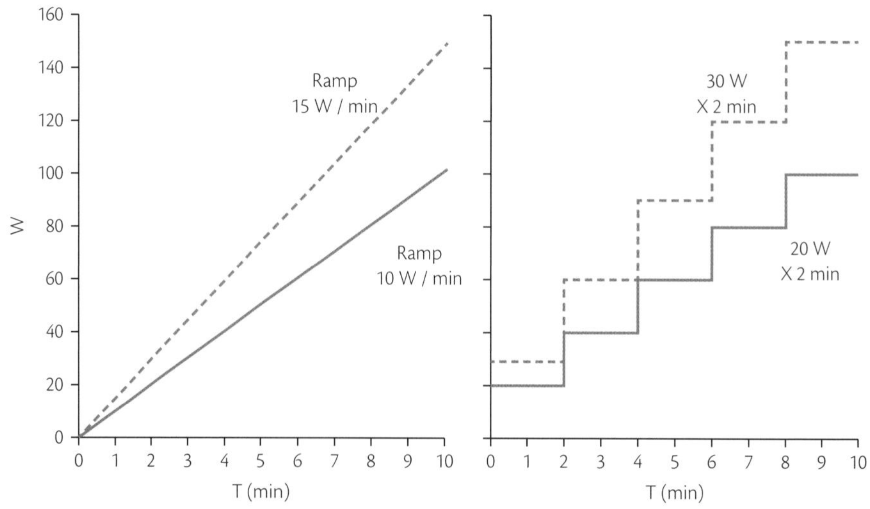

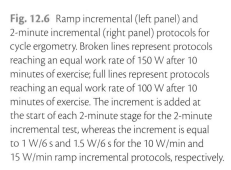

Fig. 12.6 Ramp incremental (left panel) and 2-minute incremental (right panel) protocols for cycle ergometry. Broken lines represent protocols reaching an equal work rate of 150 W after 10 minutes of exercise; full lines represent protocols reaching an equal work rate of 100 W after 10 minutes of exercise. The increment is added at the start of each 2-minute stage for the 2-minute incremental test, whereas the increment is equal to 1 W/6 s and 1.5 W/6 s for the 10 W/min and 15 W/min ramp incremental protocols, respectively.

Table 12.2 Indications for the use of exercise testing in cardiovascular medicine

◆ CAD diagnosis in subjects with no history of ischaemic heart disease, especially in adults with intermediate pre-test CAD probability and interpretable ECG
◆ New-onset CAD diagnosis in patients with history of ischaemic heart disease, previous revascularization procedures, and interpretable ECG
◆ Differentiation of cardiac versus pulmonary causes of exercise-induced dyspnoea and/or impaired exercise capacity
◆ Prognostic stratification of patients with: suspected or known CAD recent acute myocardial infarction chronic heart failure
◆ Functional evaluation of patients with: suspected or known CAD recent acute myocardial infarction previous revascularization procedures valvular heart disease chronic heart failure previous heart transplantation
◆ Exercise prescription for patients with: suspected or known CAD recent acute myocardial infarction previous revascularization procedures valvular heart disease chronic heart failure previous heart transplantation
◆ Evaluation of therapy efficacy in patients with: suspected or known CAD recent acute myocardial infarction previous revascularization procedures exercise-induced arrhythmias chronic heart failure
◆ Evaluation of heart rhythm response/disorders in patients with: rate-responsive pacemakers known or suspected exercise-induced arrhythmias
◆ Evaluation of normal subjects: functional evaluation prognostic stratification exercise prescription

CAD, coronary artery disease

Source: data from The ESC Textbook of Cardiovascular Medicine 2nd Edition edited by Camm, Luscher, and Serruys (2009) Tab.25.1 by permission of Oxford University Press.

Box 12.1 Prognostic descriptors obtainable from exercise testing

- Exercise capacity, expressed as estimated metabolic equivalents (METs)
- ST segment depression
- Chronotropic response
- Blood pressure response
- Heart rate recovery
- Right bundle branch block and multiple morphology exercise-induced ventricular arrhythmias
- Exercise test-derived multiparametric scores (Duke treadmill score, Athens score, etc.)

Box 12.2 Descriptors of exercise capacity

Physiological parameters:
- peak VO_2
- peak estimated METs (treadmill)

Performance parameters:
- peak work rate (cycle ergometer)
- exercise time

however, that parameters provided by CPET (i.e. peak VO2 and the VE/VCO2 slope) are superior predictors of prognosis to those reported in ➲ Box 12.1, not only in patients with CHF but also in several other groups of cardiac and non-cardiac patients. [28,32]

Determination of capacity for physical exercise

By definition, exercise testing is the gold standard method for assessing the capacity for physical exercise [27]. Exercise capacity can be described by using physiological and/or performance parameters, as indicated in ➲ Box 12.2.

Determination of target exercise levels

Exercise testing can be used to determine target exercise levels for prescription of exercise training in both cardiac patients and healthy subjects [33]. To this end, both a direct and an indirect approach can be used according to whether or not data from CPET are available.

Detection of myocardial ischaemia

Exercise testing has traditionally been used as a screening tool for myocardial ischaemia. The possible electrocardiogram (ECG) changes with exercise-induced myocardial ischaemia are illustrated in ➲ Fig. 12.7, the most common of which is a downsloping ST segment. This ECG change is considered diagnostic when reaching at least 1 mm with respect to baseline at 80 ms from the J-point of the QRS complex [23].

Detection of exercise-induced arrhythmia

Exercise testing can be used to detect exercise-induced tachy- or bradyarrhythmias which may put subjects/patients at risk of cardiac events when performing exercise and/or in the long term [34,35].

Physiology of exercise testing

Cardiovascular response to incremental exercise

In the early phases of incremental exercise, up to around 50% of maximal effort, cardiac output rises thanks to an increase in both heart rate and stroke volume, whereas at higher work intensities the increase in cardiac output depends largely on increases in heart rate [25] (➲ Table 12.3). Systolic and mean blood pressures increase in parallel during incremental exercise, while diastolic blood pressure remains unchanged or decreases (➲ Table 12.3). In addition, when a large skeletal muscle mass is involved in exercise, a significant decrease in systemic vascular resistance is observed at both submaximal and maximal effort (➲ Table 12.3).

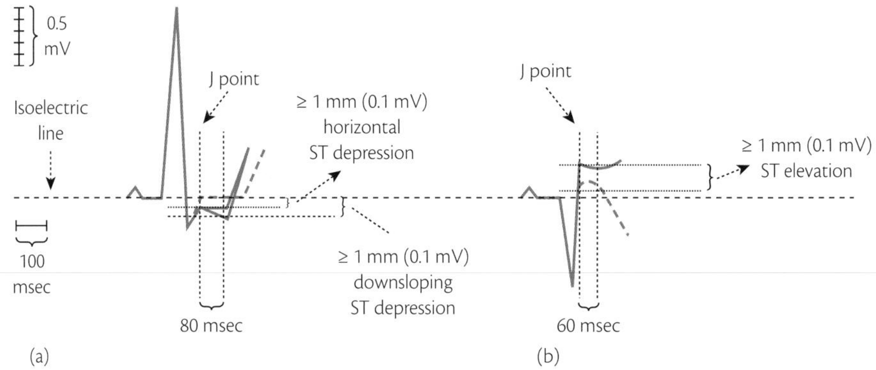

Fig. 12.7 A downsloping of the ST segment is the most common ECG sign of exercise-induced myocardial ischaemia, and is considered diagnostic when reaching at least 1 mm with respect to baseline at 80 ms from the J-point of the QRS complex in peripheral leads (I, II, III, aVF, aVL) (a). ST-elevations >= 0.1 mV also indicate significant myocardial ischemia (b).

Table 12.3 Physiological response to incremental exercise

	Rest	Peak exercise*
HR (beats/min)	70	180 (2.6)
SV (ml)	80	140 (1.7)
CO (L/min)	5.6	25 (4.5)
SBP (mmHg)	120	180 (1.5)
DBP (mmHg)	80	80 (1)
MAP (mmHg)	93	113 (1.2)
TPR (mmHg/L/min)	16.6	4.5 (0.27)
Δa-vO_2 (ml/dl)	5	16 (3.2)
VO_2 (ml/min)	280	4000 (14.3)
V_T (ml)	500	1800 (3.6)
BF (breaths/min)	12	40 (3.3)
VE (L/min)	6	72 (12)

*The figures in brackets are the fold increases versus rest values.
HR, heart rate; SV, stroke volume; CO, cardiac output; SBP, systolic blood pressure; DBP, diastolic blood pressure; MAP, mean arterial pressure; TPR, total peripheral resistance; Δa-vO_2, arterio-mixed venous oxygen concentration difference; VO_2, oxygen consumption; V_T, tidal volume; BF, breathing frequency; VE, ventilation.

Metabolic response of skeletal muscle to incremental exercise

During incremental exercise an energy requirement is reached, termed the 'lactate threshold', above which blood lactate concentration begins to increase at a progressively steeper rate [25,27,33]. This is due to the activation of anaerobic glycolysis, which occurs because the rate of supply of oxygen is not rapid enough to reoxidize cytosolic NADH + H^+. Almost all of the H^+ generated in the cell by the dissociation of lactic acid is buffered by intracellular bicarbonate. Such buffering generates CO_2 in excess of that produced by aerobic metabolism (excess CO_2), causing the VCO_2 versus VO_2 relationship, as evaluated at the mouth by CPET, to become steeper [25,27,33]. The 'first ventilatory threshold' can thus be determined as the point of transition of the VCO_2 versus VO_2 slope from less than 1 to greater than 1 (➲ Fig. 12.8) [25,27,33]. The first ventilatory threshold occurs at around 50–60% of peak VO_2 in most normal subjects and cardiac patients, with a trend towards higher percentages of peak VO_2 in patients with CHF [27,33].

Ventilatory response to incremental exercise

The ventilatory response during incremental exercise increases at the rate required to remove the CO_2 produced by energetic metabolism [25,27,33]. The excess CO_2 produced by intracellular lactate buffering (see section 'Metabolic response of skeletal muscle to incremental exercise') increases ventilatory drive, keeping the VE versus VCO_2 relationship linear and the value of the end-tidal CO_2 pressure ($PETCO_2$) constant. In the final phase of incremental exercise, a 'second ventilatory threshold' is identifiable when hyperventilation occurs with respect to CO_2 as respiratory compensation for exercise-induced metabolic acidosis (➲ Fig. 12.9), causing VE/VCO_2 to increase and $PETCO_2$ to decrease [25,27,33].

Maximal effort attainment criteria

Achievement of maximal or near-maximal effort during incremental exercise testing can be assumed in the presence of one or more of the criteria reported in ➲ Box 12.3 [36].

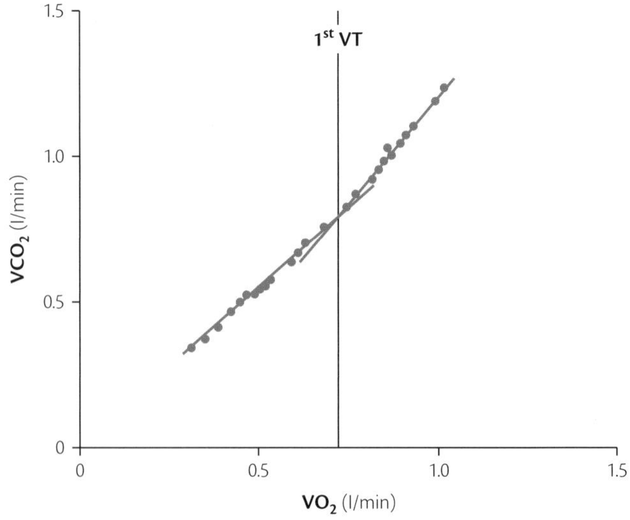

Fig. 12.8 VCO_2 as a function of VO_2 during ramp incremental exercise (V-slope plot). The point where the VCO_2 versus VO_2 slope increases in steepness is the first ventilatory threshold (1st VT).

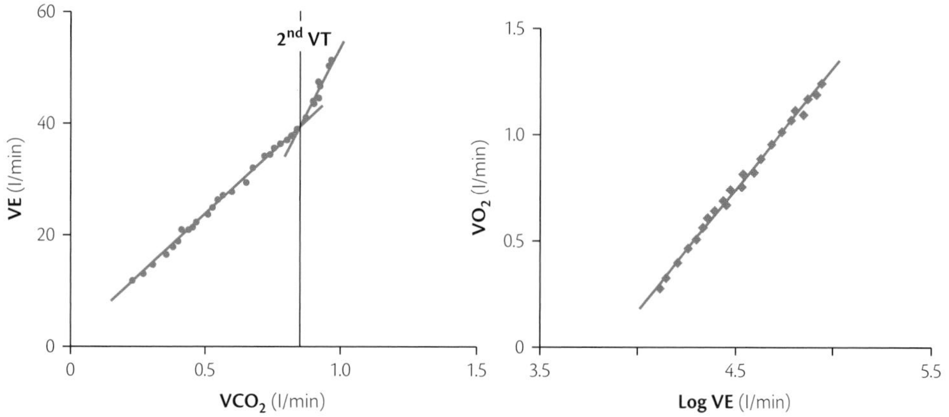

Fig. 12.9 Left panel: Ventilation as a function of VCO_2 during ramp incremental exercise. In the final phase of exercise, hyperventilation occurs after the second ventilatory threshold (2nd VT) to compensate for exercise-induced acidosis, making the ventilation (VE)/VCO_2 slope increase. Given the linearity of the VE/VCO_2 relationship below the 2nd VT, the VE/VCO_2 slope can be assessed even in case of non-maximal effort. Right panel: VO_2 as a function of the logarithm of ventilation during ramp incremental exercise. The slope of the relationship is the oxygen uptake efficiency slope. The logarithmic transformation of ventilation is aimed at linearizing the otherwise curvilinear relation of VO_2 versus VE, so making the oxygen uptake efficiency slope theoretically independent of the patient-achieved effort level.

Box 12.3 Criteria for maximal effort attainment

- Failure of VO_2 and/or heart rate to increase with further increases in work rate
- Peak respiratory exchange ratio (VCO_2/VO_2) ≥ 1.10–1.15
- Post-exercise blood lactate concentration ≥ 8 mmol/L
- Rating of perceived exertion ≥ 8 (on the 10-point Borg scale)
- Subject/patient appears exhausted

Source: data from Howley ET, Bassett DR Jr, Welch HG. Criteria for maximal oxygen uptake: review and commentary. *Med Sci Sports Exerc* 1995; **27**: 1292–1301.

Safety aspects of exercise testing

Contraindications to exercise testing

Absolute and relative contraindications to exercise testing are listed in ➲ Box 12.4. It is essential to implement these criteria in clinical practice because their neglect may have legal consequences in case of an adverse event.

Statistical risk of adverse events during incremental exercise testing

Despite its undisputed clinical value, incremental exercise testing confers a certain risk of adverse events. In an unselected patient population referred for exercise testing, mortality and morbidity are reported to be below 0.01% and 0.05%, respectively [21]. When performed in patients within 4 weeks of an acute MI, mortality rises to 0.03% and the rate of non-fatal MI or the need for cardiac resuscitation reaches 0.09% [37]. No additional risk of incremental exercise testing has been reported in patients with stable compensated CHF [38]. Intuitively, the risk of complications can be minimized by strictly adhering to established standards with regard to the conduction of exercise testing provided in the available guidelines [39].

Formal requirements for exercise testing facilities

Even if rare, the possible occurrence of adverse events during exercise tests makes the presence of instrumentation for cardiopulmonary resuscitation mandatory in all exercise testing laboratories. Emergency drugs, defibrillators, and endotracheal intubation

Box 12.4 Contraindications to exercise testing

Absolute:
- ongoing or recent acute myocardial infarction
- decompensated heart failure
- unstable angina
- acute myocarditis, pericarditis, or endocarditis
- complex atrial or ventricular arrhythmias
- severe aortic stenosis
- severe systemic or pulmonary hypertension
- severely dilated aortic aneurysm
- acute extracardiac disease
- severe anaemia
- severe orthopaedic limitations

Relative:
- moderate aortic stenosis
- severe proximal stenosis of left coronary branches
- severe subaortic hypertrophic stenosis
- advanced atrioventricular block
- electrolytic disorders
- cognitive and/or psychiatric disorders

Box 12.5 Criteria for interrupting the exercise testing

- Muscle fatigue
- Severe dyspnoea, especially when disproportionate to effort intensity
- Moderate to severe angina pectoris
- Horizontal/descending ST segment downsloping > 3 mm with respect to baseline
- ST segment upsloping > 1 mm with respect to baseline in leads different from V1 and aVR, in the absence of Q waves
- Exercise-induced complex arrhythmias (2nd and 3rd degree atrioventricular block, atrial fibrillation, paroxysmal supraventricular tachycardia, ventricular tachycardia)
- Exercise-induced complete bundle branch block, especially when indistinguishable from ventricular tachycardia
- Systolic and/or diastolic blood pressure > 240 and > 120 mmHg, respectively
- Systolic blood pressure fall > 10 mmHg with respect to baseline, especially when associated with other signs/symptoms of myocardial ischaemia
- Increasing atypical chest pain
- Signs of peripheral hypoperfusion (pallor, cyanosis, cool sweating, etc.)
- Neurological signs/symptoms (ataxia, vertigo, lightheadness, phosphenes, etc.)
- Lower limb(s) claudication
- Orthopaedic limitation
- Technical impossibility of ECG monitoring
- Patient request

equipment must be available, and regular checks regarding the expiry date of drugs and the functioning of instrumentation must be carried out. Exercise tests must be supervised by a physician or by non-physician assistant personnel with a physician present within calling distance. In addition, periodical drills on cardiopulmonary resuscitation procedures should be performed by all personnel. It must be ensured that additional assistance can readily be summoned from inside and/or outside the facility by the presence of easy-to-reach telephones and/or alarms in the exercise testing laboratory.

Criteria for interrupting exercise testing

The criteria for interrupting exercise tests that are commonly adopted in the clinical setting are reported in ➲ Box 12.5.

Methodological aspects of exercise testing in particular disease and patient groups

Exercise testing in coronary artery disease

Exercise testing with step incremental protocols is extensively used for the diagnosis of obstructive CAD: this applies to diagnosis of both previously unknown CAD and progression of CAD in native coronary vessels or coronary bypass grafts in patients with previous coronary events and/or revascularization procedures. However, several causes of both false positive and false negative exercise tests have been described (see ➲ Box 12.6).

In addition, the predictive accuracy of the exercise test is known to increase with increasing pre-test probability of CAD in the patient under examination. As a consequence, sensitivity and specificity values ranging between 50 and 90% and predictive accuracy values ranging from 65 to 75% can occur when performing exercise testing in different patient populations [23].

Exercise testing in chronic heart failure

Ramp incremental CPET is increasingly used in patients with CHF as it provides not only a precise and repeatable evaluation of functional capacity but also powerful exercise-derived prognostic indicators currently used in heart transplantation work-up. In this regard, peak VO_2 values ≤ 10 ml/kg/min are used as a decisional cut-off for indication to heart transplantation in CHF patients both on and off beta-blockers [40]. In patients with a peak

Box 12.6 Causes of false positive and false negative exercise tests

False positive:

- left ventricular hypertrophy
- resting repolarization abnormalities (left bundle branch block, Wolff–Parkinson–White pre-excitation, etc.)
- non-ischaemic cardiomyopathy
- digoxin
- systemic hypertension
- mitral valve prolapse
- pericardial disease
- hypokalaemia
- anaemia
- female gender
- interpretative error

False negative:

- lack of ischaemic threshold attainment
- lack of appreciation of symptoms or non-ECG signs possibly associated with CAD
- significant obstructive CAD well compensated by collateral circulation
- interpretative error

VO_2 >10 ml/kg/min, ventilation-related indices, such as slopes of VE versus VCO_2 and VO_2 versus VE (➲ Fig. 12.9), seem to be the most powerful prognostic predictors, with the advantage of also being assessable at submaximal levels of effort if the exercise test is prematurely interrupted [28]. Finally, CPET is a valuable tool in the rehabilitative setting for prescription of the intensity of aerobic training and evaluation of its effects [33].

Exercise testing in peripheral artery occlusive disease

Exercise testing can be used in patients with known lower limb peripheral artery disease (PAD) and claudication to objectively document the magnitude of functional limitation and its improvement in response to therapeutic interventions and exercise training. Exercise testing should be performed on treadmill, walking at 3.2 km/h with a 10% slope or introducing a steady increase in elevation of the treadmill every 3 min while keeping the speed constant [40]. In patients with suspected lower extremity PAD, exercise-induced vasodilation in the claudicating limb(s) is associated with the development of a significant blood pressure gradient across the arterial stenosis, and the post-exercise ankle–brachial index, i.e. the ratio of the systolic blood pressure from the dorsalis pedis and/or the posterior tibial arteries and that from the brachial artery, will fall by more than 20% from its baseline value [40].

Exercise testing in the elderly

Exercise testing has been demonstrated to be usable for functional evaluation, prognostic stratification, and exercise prescription in elderly subjects and patients [8,22,23]. In this population, exercise protocols will have to be carefully matched to exercise capacity, using less aggressive ramp incremental protocols (i.e. 5–10 W/min) with low starting workloads in most functionally compromised individuals [22]. A cycle ergometer may be preferable to a treadmill in elderly subjects/patients due to possible poor balance, impaired neuromuscular coordination, and impaired vision and/or gait pattern.

Exercise testing in patients with orthopaedic comorbidities

The exercise capacity of patients with orthopaedic comorbidities (e.g. osteoarthritis and osteoporosis) may be limited by joint pain, which may lead to interruption of the exercise test (see ➲ Box 12.5) and prevent maximal effort being attained [41,42]. The choice of the exercise modality to minimize such a risk (e.g. treadmill versus cycle ergometer) is thus very important in this population. When maximal effort is not attained and CPET is not available, lactate measurements may be useful to detect if the lactate threshold has been reached and provide a reference for prescription of exercise training [42].

Exercise testing in patients with cognitive or psychiatric comorbidities

Patients with cognitive (e.g. Alzheimer's) or psychiatric (e.g. depression, schizophrenia, personality disorders) diseases often have a low fitness level and may not be accustomed to the instrumentation and procedures involved in exercise testing [42,43]. However, the presence of a cognitive or psychiatric disease is not an absolute formal contraindication to exercise testing (see ➲ Box 12.4). In these patient groups cycle ergometry may be preferable to treadmills due to drug- and/or disease-induced gait disturbance. Note that the face mask or mouthpiece needed for CPET may not be tolerated, and may even induce panic attacks in patients with panic disorders [43]. The need for these patients to undergo CPET should thus be carefully evaluated on an individual basis.

Local muscle strength testing in cardiovascular health and disease

The role of strength testing

Strength testing (i.e. measuring the maximal contractile force of a muscle) has received increasing clinical attention in recent years, for several reasons:

1. Muscle strength is an independent predictor of mortality in healthy men [44–46] and women [47]. Low handgrip strength is a better predictor of cardiovascular mortality than body mass index (➲ Fig. 12.10) [48].
2. In patients aged 80 or more handgrip strength predicts all-cause mortality, and the older patients are the larger the mortality

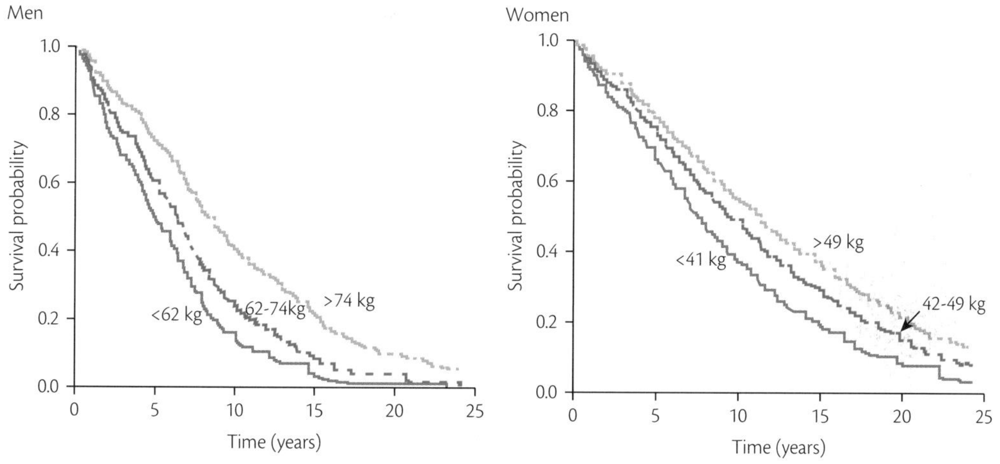

Fig. 12.10 Kaplan–Meier survival curves for all-cause mortality according to tertiles of handgrip strength in men and women.
Reproduced from Gale CR, Martyn CN, Cooper C, Sayer AA. Grip strength, body composition, and mortality. *Int J Epidemiol.* 2007; **36**: 228–235, by permission of Oxford University Press.

differences between patients in the highest versus the lowest tertile of handgrip strength [49]. Low handgrip strength is part of the definition of operational frailty (see [50]).

3. In patients with heart failure, muscle wasting has been identified as a key component of the disease process [51–54]. Cachectic patients have a significantly reduced quadriceps muscle strength [55] and it has therefore been hypothesized that resistance training may be particularly beneficial in halting the wasting process in patients with heart failure [56].

In practical terms strength testing occurs in three settings: (1) measurement of muscle strength as part of a test battery to assess individual fitness and estimate prognosis, (2) measurement of muscle strength to determine the optimal dosing of resistance training programmes, and (3) measurement of respiratory muscle strength (especially in patients with heart failure) for prognostic or therapeutic reasons.

Measurement of muscle strength to assess individual fitness

Strength tests as part of a battery of fitness tests should be simple, fast, reliable, and reproducible without the need for expensive equipment. The majority of epidemiological studies assessing the relation between muscle strength and mortality use the maximal handgrip strength test.

The classical device for measurement of maximal handgrip force is the Jamar dynamometer (➲ Fig. 12.11), for which the intra- and inter-test reliability is ≥0.97 and reference values are available for different age groups [57]. This dynamometer has an adjustable top-workbench to fit different hand sizes and is a hydraulic isometric hand dynamometer with readings in kilograms (kg) with 2-kg gradations.

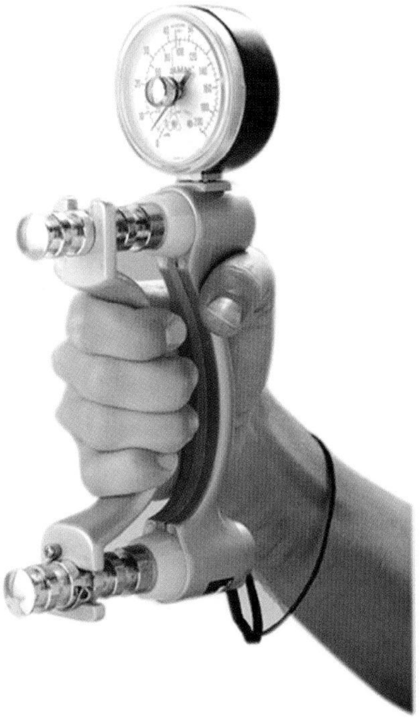

Fig. 12.11 The Jamar dynamometer is the classical tool for measuring handgrip force. This dynamometer has an adjustable top-workbench to fit different hand sizes and is a hydraulic isometric hand dynamometer with readings in kilograms (kg) with 2 kg gradation.

The handgrip test is performed in: (1) a standing position with straight back; (2) the shoulder adducted and in neutral rotation; (3) the elbow flexed 90°; (4) the lower arm in neutral position; and (5) the wrist in neutral position [58–60]. Patients are instructed to 'squeeze the handle as hard as possible'. The peak value is registered after a maximal squeeze for about 5 seconds. If the test needs to be repeated because of an error, for example rotation of the wrist, the test should be repeated after a 5-minute rest. According to Peolsson et al. [57] women should normally use grip breadth 2 and men grip breadth 3 (the smallest possible grip breadth is 1, and the largest is 5).

Advantages of handgrip measurement are the use of a small, inexpensive, and portable measuring device, excellent intra- and inter-test reproducibility, the availability of age-related normal values, and good relative predictive value for mortality. The disadvantages include that individuals with manual occupations may have better hand strength than expected, that handgrip strength is not useful for follow-up in rehabilitation programmes that are highly focused on lower-limb aerobic exercise, and that orthopaedic problems may invalidate the measurements in individuals with rheumatoid disease or arthritis.

Measurement of muscle strength to optimize strength training

In strength/resistance training it is essential to measure the 'one repetition maximum' (1RM) as the upper limit in order to determine the desired load for the training programme. The 1RM needs to be measured for each of the planned training sessions (i.e. leg press, curl) individually—usually on the training device itself.

Classically, the 1RM is defined as the maximum amount of weight one can lift in a single repetition for a given exercise. It is usually determined by stepwise increase of weight until the individual can no longer perform the exercise adequately. However, actually testing the maximal load carries a certain risk of injury due to overload of the musculoskeletal system. Therefore, a number of formulae have been developed to extrapolate the 1RM from multiple repetitions with submaximal loads (e.g. Epley, Brzycki, Lander, Lombardi, Mayhew, O'Connor, Wathan).

In the clinical context the 1RM is measured after a warm-up with ten repetitions of a light weight followed by a resting period and five repetitions with a medium weight. The testing includes single attempts at progressively heavier weights until the 1RM is identified. A successful attempt is defined by lifting the weight by 90% or more of the patient's unloaded range of motion [61]. A minimum of 2 minutes rest should be observed between the tests because that is the time needed for replenishment phosphocreatine [62]. Elderly patients need more testing sessions than young healthy subjects to obtain stable measurements of 1RM (eight or nine rather than three or four).

The 1RM should not be used to assess the effect of strength training on muscle strength. To objectively measure muscle isometric strength, dynamometers that measure muscle contractile force (usually in newtons, N) for different limbs should be used. These dynamometers ensure that strength measurements are made at reproducible positions and angles of the joints and allow continuous measurement of changes, while measurements of the 1RM are always discrete (at 0.5 or 1.0 kg intervals).

In cardiovascular patients the general recommendation for the initiation of a resistance training programme is to start rehabilitation with aerobic endurance training for about 2 weeks, then use a three-step approach to start a muscle build-up exercise programme (for details see [63]):

- Step I, pre-training: <30% 1RM, five to ten repetitions, two or three sessions/week, one to three circuits per session.
- Step II, resistance–endurance training: 30-50% 1RM, two or three sessions/week, one circuit per session.
- Step III, muscle build-up training: 40–60% 1RM, two or three sessions/week, one circuit per session.

Measurement of respiratory muscle strength

In the early 1990s observational studies reported a marked reduction of respiratory muscle strength in CHF [64,65]. In long-term follow-up studies peak inspiratory muscle strength (Pi_{max}) emerged as an independent predictor of survival in patients with heart failure [66]. It is therefore hoped that respiratory training programmes that aim to improve Pi_{max} will ultimately improve patient prognosis.

For the measurement of Pi_{max} patients wear a flanged mouthpiece and first undergo a normal ventilator function test. The purpose of this test is to determine functional residual capacity and total lung capacity. In deep inspiration from functional residual capacity against a shutter with a minor air leak to prevent undesirable glottis closure Pi_{max} is measured in triplicate [66]. A minimum period of 2 minutes should be observed between two consecutive measurements.

Maximal expiratory pressure (Pe_{max}) can be measured at total lung capacity during maximal expiratory effort. Again, measurements should be done in triplicate [66].

Respiratory muscle training is usually done with the help of a device to permit an individually adapted resistive breathing exercise (e.g. the Threshold inspiratory muscle trainer). The Threshold trainer is set at approximately 30% of Pi_{max} and patients exercise under supervision for 20 min three times a week (➲ Fig. 12.12) [67].

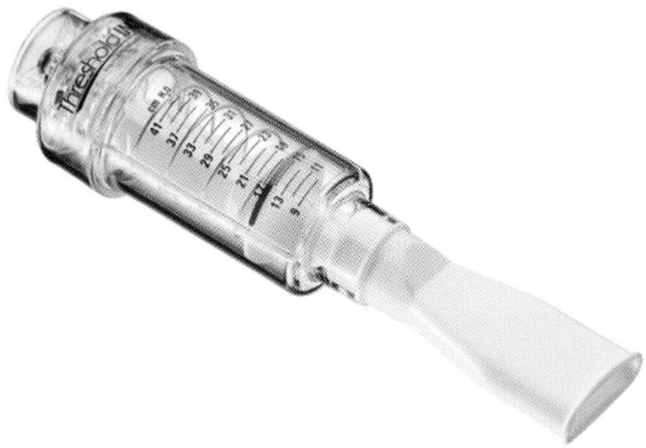

Fig. 12.12 The Threshold inspiratory muscle trainer (IMT) incorporates a flow-independent one-way valve to ensure consistent resistance and features an adjustable pressure threshold setting in cmH_2O. When the patient breathes through the Threshold IMT, a spring-loaded valve provides a resistance that exercises respiratory muscles through conditioning.

Physical exercise in primary prevention

Physical activity: health effects beyond the cardiovascular system

Guidelines suggest that physical activity and aerobic exercise training are very important non-pharmacological tools for primary and secondary cardiovascular prevention (class I, level A recommendation) [68].

In healthy subjects, growing levels of both physical activity and cardiorespiratory fitness are associated with a significant reduction (around 20–30%) in the risk of all-cause and cardiovascular mortality, in a dose–response fashion. The evidence suggests that the risk of dying during a given period continues to decline with increasing levels of physical activity and cardiorespiratory fitness [69].

Although much of the evidence to date is cross-sectional and the evidence base is still being developed, we have sufficient information to warrant public health actions that support physical activity.

The epidemic of physical inactivity: evidence and causes

The levels of physical activity in the general population have been decreasing, with more than 60% of the world's population not being active enough [70]. Technology and economic incentives tend to discourage activity: technology by reducing the energy needed for activities of daily living and economics by better wages for sedentary than active work. Moreover in a number of areas our daily living environments are simply less conducive to physical activity [71]:

- transport: for example, increased use of cars and perceived or real danger of walking or cycling
- urban planning: for example, lack of public parks and athletic fields, work places and shopping centres becoming more distant from homes
- technical advances: for example, elevators and escalators rather than stairs
- occupational changes: for example, increasing service sector instead of manual work seen in agricultural/industrial settings
- institutionalization of childhood: for example, longer school hours with increasing academic demands and changing leisure-time activities (e.g. computer-related activities).

With this in mind, three strategies for the prevention of cardiovascular diseases (CVD) by promotion of PA can be distinguished: population (primary), high-risk (primary), and secondary prevention. The population strategy in particular is critical—this involves environmental and lifestyle changes that affect the whole population without necessarily requiring medical examination.

The challenge of building environments which are activity-friendly

The built environment has been defined as 'the neighbourhoods, roads, buildings, food sources and recreational facilities in which people live, work, are educated, eat and play' [72] and it impacts on physical activity, particularly walking. Adults are more likely to walk for transport in compact, pedestrian-friendly neighbourhoods characterized by connected street networks with access to mixed-use areas, the presence of places to walk to (such as public transport hubs, delicatessens, and newsagents), and in neighbourhoods with higher population densities. Greater attention needs to be given to designing attractive and convivial neighbourhoods and facilities. Neighbourhood design is also a powerful determinant of physical activity in young people.

Lifestyle approaches for increasing physical activity in the general population

There are two main target areas for population interventions to increase physical activity in the population [73]:

- children and adolescents, at school and during leisure time
- adults, at work and during leisure time.

Children and adolescents

School interventions

Schools should be a prime target for interventions to increase physical activity, for a number of reasons [74]:

- school-based physical education increases physical activity to the recommended levels
- test results in core academic subjects are not reduced by increasing the time spent on physical education
- increasing physical education increases children's health
- superior cognitive functioning, including better concentration in class, has been described in children and adolescents with higher levels of physical activity.

Schools should therefore be mandated to provide recommended amounts of physical activity every day. Schools and parents should also be encouraged to promote walking or cycling as the main mode of transport when travelling to school. A variety of organized or unorganized physical activities need to be promoted throughout the school day.

Leisure-time interventions

Non-school-based variables that have been associated with lower levels of physical activity are as follows: low levels of physical activity by a child's father, less time spent outdoors, less social support, lower educational level of a child's mother, lower family income, and higher rates of crime. Consideration of such factors may suggest promising opportunities for effective interventions. Indeed, multifactorial interventions are the best way to increase physical activity in adolescents. Screen-based methods may also be looked on as an opportunity for promoting physical activity. Recent reviews have demonstrated that interventions on physical activity delivered via the internet appear to achieve a similar response to more established interventions. There is also a suggestion from the literature that exergaming may provide increased levels of moderate-intensity PA—although not as much as doing the actual activity [75].

Adults

Interventions to increase PA need to be targeted at the work environment and leisure-time activities.

Interventions for increasing physical activity at work

A recent meta-analysis of studies of interventions regarding physical activity in the workplace showed significant increases in the following: general physical activity, fitness, lipids, and anthropometric measures, with positive benefits for work attendance and job-related stress. Evidence-based guidance on promoting physical activity in the workplace is widely available [76].

Exercise and corporate wellness

Many corporations have included exercise facilities and/or programmes as a part of their worksite health promotion, fitness, wellness, and CR programmes. The Johnson and Johnson 'Live for Life' programme [77] compared the effectiveness of selected cardiovascular/lifestyle risk reduction interventions through a randomized controlled study. It showed significant improvements in weight reduction, exercise tolerance, and blood pressure control within the treatment population with healthcare savings of $225 per employee. Burton et al. [78] examined the effect of participation in a worksite fitness programme on productivity. Non-participants in the study were twice as likely as participants to report health-related work limitations in the areas of time management and physical work. They also recorded more days absent from work when compared with their more active counterparts. This trial promoted 15–45 minutes of exercise every other day.

Active commuting to work

Walking has been shown to be protective of incident CVD, with those engaging in high levels of walking having a 31% reduced risk of developing CVD compared with those in the lowest walking category [79]. The benefits of walking or cycling to work have been also demonstrated [80].

Leisure-time physical activity

Levels of leisure-time physical activity seem to be increasing for adults while work-related activity is decreasing, and these reductions actually outweigh the increases seen for leisure-time activity [81]. A meta-analysis of 26 studies showed that, compared with those reporting low levels of physical activity (or none), those who reported high levels of activity were 27% less likely to develop CHD, and those who reported moderate levels were 12% less likely to develop CHD.

There is evidence that interventions delivered without face-to-face contact do provide increases in physical activity, at least in the short term [82], and effective results may be achieved relatively inexpensively. Point-of-decision prompts (e.g. signs encouraging the use of stairs instead of lifts/elevators) are also effective for increasing physical activity. A median increase of 54% in the use of stairs with the use of such prompts has been demonstrated. Enhancing access to locations for activity (e.g. providing walking routes and access to exercise facilities) was reported to be especially effective: the frequency of activity increased by 48%, energy expenditure by 8%, and aerobic capacity by 5%. Furthermore cost–benefit analysis has shown that active transport, comprehensive worksite approaches, individually adapted behaviour change, and the creation of places for physical activity along with information services are all cost-effective interventions [83].

Recommendations for physical exercise in primary prevention

Aerobic dynamic exercise: intensity and volume

The European Prevention Guidelines recommend that healthy people in all age groups should choose enjoyable physical activities which fit into their daily routine [68]. Moderate-intensity activities such as walking and cycling have a considerable impact on cardiovascular events and therefore undertaking such activities for a few hours per week should be recommended to all adults. The additional benefit of intensive aerobic activity can be deduced from the dose–response curve for physical activity, and the addition of 2 hours a week of high-intensity activities can be recommended (➲ Table 12.4).

The effect of exercise on cardiovascular risk reduction already appears at low or moderate intensities. The amount of *moderate-intensity* physical activity or aerobic exercise training that can provide a reduction in all-cause and cardiovascular mortality ranges from 2.5 to 5 hours a week—the longer the duration of physical activity/aerobic exercise training performed over the week the greater the observed benefits (➲ Box 12.7).

Table 12.4 Definitions of exercise intensity

Intensity	Peak VO_2 or HRR	Borg scale	METs in young	METs in old
Moderate	40–59%	5–6	4.8–7.1	3.2–4.7
e.g. brisk walk with a noticeable acceleration of heart rate				
Vigorous	60–85%	7–8	7.2–10.1	4.8–6.7
e.g. jogging, causes rapid breathing and a substantial increase in heart rate				

HRR, heart rate reserve; MET, metabolic equivalent, equal to the consumption of 3.5 ml of O_2 per kg of body weight, per minute; Peak VO_2, peak oxygen consumption by cardiopulmonary exercise testing (the ideal physiological marker of intensity): practical surrogate intensity markers are presented here.

Source: data from the European Association of Cardiovascular Prevention and Rehabilitation Committee for Science Guidelines, EACPR, Corrà U, Piepoli MF, Carré F, Heuschmann P, Hoffmann U, Verschuren M, Halcox J, Document Reviewers, Giannuzzi P, Saner H, Wood D, Piepoli MF, Corrà U, Benzer W, Bjarnason-Wehrens B, Dendale P, Gaita D, McGee H, Mendes M, Niebauer J, Zwisler A-DO, Schmid J-P. Secondary prevention through cardiac rehabilitation: physical activity counselling and exercise training: key components of the position paper from the Cardiac Rehabilitation Section of the European Association of Cardiovascular Prevention and Rehabilitation. *Eur Heart J* 2010; **31**: 1967–1974.

Box 12.7 General recommendations for physical activity at the population level

1. To perform enjoyable physical activities (PA) which fit into daily routine on most days of the week, and consist of the following:
   - Aerobic training:
     - moderate-intensity aerobic PA for a minimum of 30 minutes on 5 days a week

     or

     - vigorous-intensity aerobic PA for a minimum of 20 minutes on 3 days a week

     or

     - a combination of the above, to meet the global weekly amount of PA
   - Muscular strength training: twice weekly on major muscle groups
2. Evaluation of the risk for performing PA varies according to the intended level of physical activity and of the individual's cardiac risk profile:
   - Self-assessment of the habitual PA level and of the risk factors is recommended for screening of large populations
   - Individuals deemed to be at risk require further evaluation by a qualified physician
   - In senior/adult individuals with an increased risk for coronary events, maximal exercise testing (and possibly further evaluations) is advocated

Source: data from Vanhees L, Sutter J De, GeladaS N, Doyle F, Prescott E, Cornelissen V, Kouidi E, Dugmore D, Vanuzzo D, Börjesson M, Doherty P, EACPR. Importance of characteristics and modalities of physical activity and exercise in defining the benefits to cardiovascular health within the general population: recommendations from the EACPR (Part I). *Eur J Prev Cardiol* 2012; **19**: 670–686.

Similar results can be obtained by performing 1 to 1.5 hours a week of *vigorous-intensity* physical activity/aerobic exercise training or an equivalent combination of moderate-intensity and vigorous-intensity training. Moreover, the available evidence suggests that the total weekly amount of activity/aerobic training can be obtained by summing multiple daily bouts of exercise, each lasting for 10 minutes or longer, and that such activity/training should be distributed over most days of the week. Examples of suitable activities include not only sport-related activities such as hiking, running or jogging, skating, cycling, rowing, swimming, cross-country skiing, and aerobic classes, but also common daily activities such as climbing stairs at a speed of 20 steps in 20 seconds, walking briskly, doing housework and gardening, and engaging in active recreational pursuits.

Strength and resistance exercise

These activities should be backed up by exercises to maintain muscle strength and improve joint function: they include daily gymnastic exercises with bodyweight and/or light weights, involving the major joints and major muscle groups of the limbs and trunk. Stretching exercises, used in the warm-up and cool-down phases, serve to maintain the flexibility of the muscles and promote the transition from inactivity to challenging activity. They are very useful in elderly and middle-aged sedentary individuals as they facilitate coordination and the execution of movements.

Therefore, eight to ten exercises should be performed on two or more non-consecutive days each week using the major muscle groups. To maximize strength development, a resistance (weight) should be used that allows 8 to 12 repetitions of each exercise resulting in volitional fatigue. Muscle-strengthening activities include a progressive weight-training programme, weight-bearing calisthenics, stair climbing, and similar resistance exercises that use the major muscle groups.

Is medical monitoring necessary when moving from being sedentary to being active?

The exercise-related risk of major cardiovascular events in ostensibly healthy people is exceedingly low, ranging from 1 in 500 000 to 1 in 2 600 000 patient-hours of exercise [84].

As recently proposed for leisure-time sport activities in middle-aged/elderly subjects, the accuracy of risk assessment should be tailored to the individual's cardiac risk profile, the current level of habitual physical activity, and the intended level of physical activity/aerobic exercise training, with more aggressive screening (i.e. exercise testing) possibly being reserved for people who are sedentary and/or have cardiovascular risk factors and/or are proposing to engage in vigorous-intensity activities.

Vigorous physical exertion is associated with an increased risk for cardiac events, including sudden cardiac death in individuals harbouring CVD. Moreover, individuals who exercise only occasionally seem to have an increased risk of acute coronary events and sudden cardiac death during or after exercise.

It is recommended that sedentary subjects and those with cardiovascular risk factors start with a low-intensity activity. An appropriate evaluation of middle-aged and older individuals should take place before they engage in regular physical activities. Such evaluation should vary according to the individual's cardiac risk profile and the intended level of activity. Different screening modalities have been proposed according to the person's habits (sedentary versus active) and level of activity (low versus high intensity) (➲ Figs 12.13 and 12.14) [85].

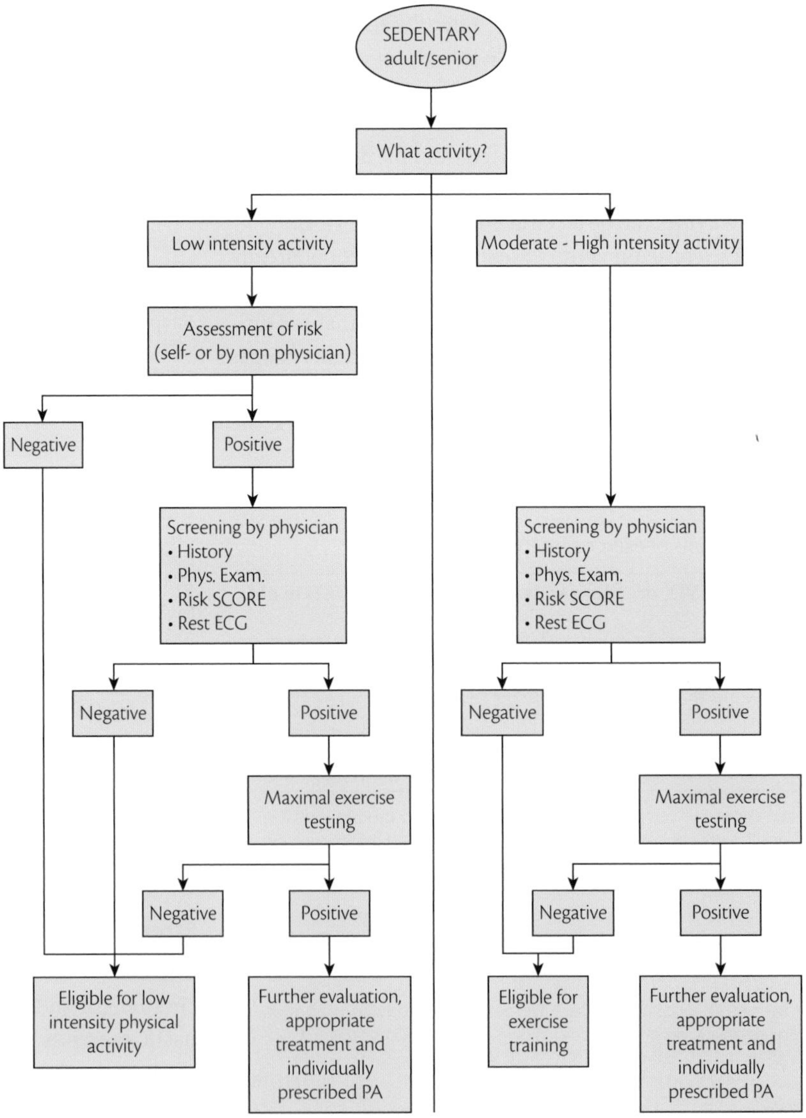

Fig. 12.13 Proposed pre-participation cardiovascular evaluation protocol for asymptomatic sedentary adult/senior individuals. PA, physical activity.

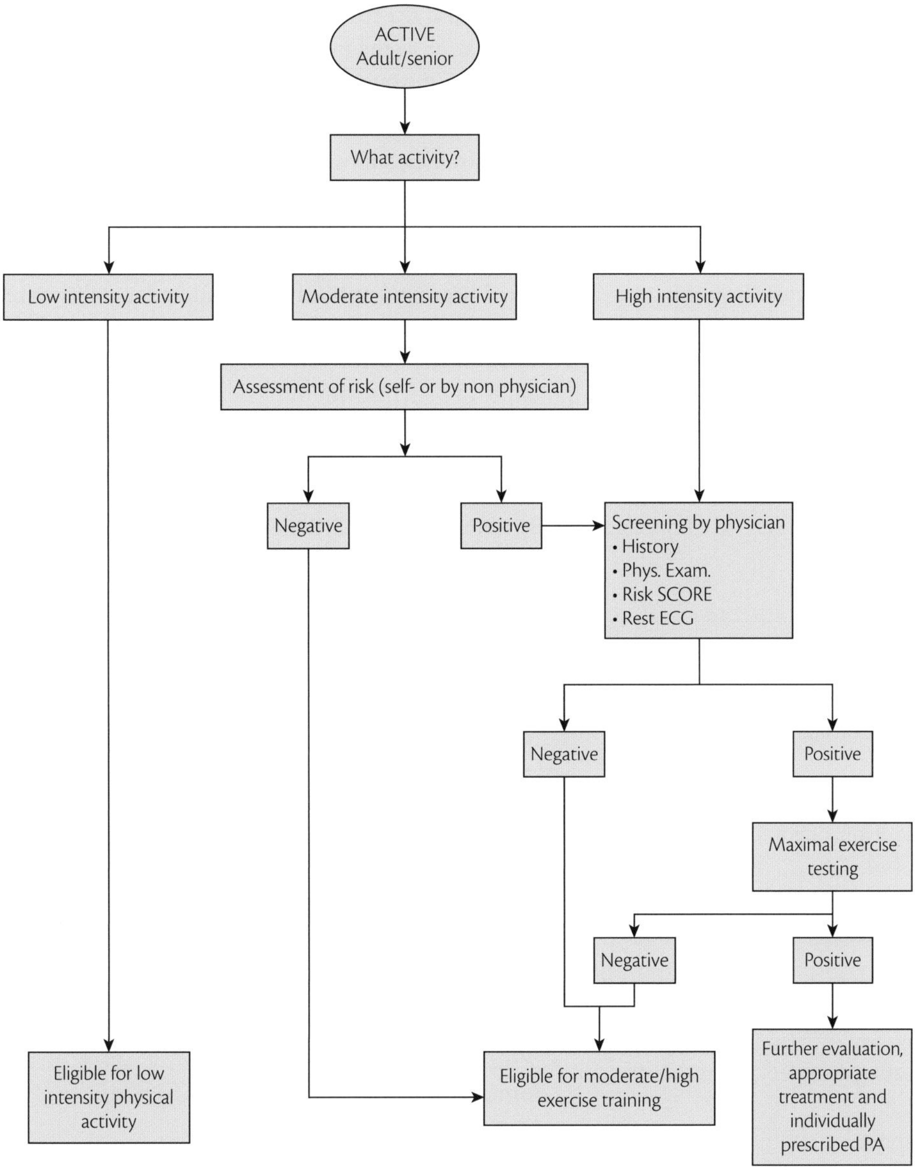

Fig. 12.14 Proposed pre-participation evaluation protocol for asymptomatic active adult/senior individuals. PA, physical activity.

Exercise interventions in cardiovascular diseases

Health effects of exercise in cardiovascular diseases

There are many sophisticated symptomatic therapies among the interventional techniques used in modern cardiovascular medicine, but exercise-based CR offers effective treatment of the causes of atherosclerotic coronary and peripheral disease. The lifestyle and risk factor modifications achieved by CR have been shown to halt disease progression and to reduce cardiovascular mortality and the rate of non-fatal MI in patients with stable CAD. In CHF exercise intolerance is primarily related to the degree of peripheral change (such as muscle atrophy, reduced peripheral perfusion due to endothelial dysfunction, abnormalities in ventilation, etc.) and pharmacological treatment alone sometimes fails to significantly improve exercise capacity. Regular aerobic endurance training in stable CHF has been shown to improve peak oxygen uptake by 15–25%, to reduce peripheral vascular resistance, to retard or reverse muscle wasting, and to reduce morbidity and mortality.

Despite its documented clinical effectiveness, rehabilitation/prevention interventions are still widely under-utilized in the clinical context. However, it is becoming increasingly clear that the use of interventional procedures without simultaneous lifestyle modification, including regular physical exercise and aggressive treatment of cardiovascular risk factors, is suboptimal therapy.

Contraindications for exercise training and risk stratification

Exercise training in patients with established CVD is not risk free. Based on large clinical databases the risk for a cardiac arrest during exercise sessions is 1 per 112 000 patient training hours (PTH), the risk for an acute MI is 1 per 294 000 PTH, and the risk for a cardiac death is 1 per 784 000 PTH.

The challenge is to identify those patients with clear contraindications and exclude them (at least temporarily) from training, and to identify patients at very high risk who can be trained but may need special supervision (i.e. continuous ECG monitoring or in-hospital training).

Medical evaluation before exercise training

The primary purpose of medical evaluation before beginning exercise-based CR is (1) to establish the likelihood of medical conditions which put the patient at an increased risk for adverse events during physical exertion and (2) to assess the patient's baseline physical fitness/exercise capacity. ➲ Box 12.8 gives an overview of the relevant components of such a baseline medical assessment. The main goal of the baseline assessment is to identify the individual level of risk for CVD complications during exercise. However, it is not clear if the risk for an exercise-induced event is related to the exercise or to the overall risk of morbidity and mortality associated with the presence of CVD [87].

Clear contraindications for exercise training

Clear contraindications for training are similar to those for any exercise testing procedure (➲ Box 12.9). In addition to the list in ➲ Box 12.8 an assessment of sensory and cognitive function may be warranted, especially in geriatric patients. Issues such as impaired hearing, impaired vision, and poor ability to remember important safety issues such as the targeted training pulse should be noted and addressed before engaging in a formal training programme. In patients with overt dementia supervised exercise interventions may be the only safe option.

Prior to enrolling a patient with CAD in a training programme the ischaemic threshold needs to be determined in a maximal exercise test with 12-lead ECG monitoring. A maximal exercise test is recommended for all other patients to determine the heart rate reserve and the targeted training pulse.

Box 12.8 Components of a medical history assessment

1. Collect the patient's medical diagnoses, focusing on:
   - CHD (previous MI, angioplasty, coronary bypass surgery, angina pectoris)
   - known heart rhythm disorders (atrial fibrillation, ventricular arrhythmias, sudden cardiac death, ongoing beta-blocker therapy)
   - cerebrovascular and peripheral vascular disease (stroke, claudication, carotid artery stenosis, thromboembolic diseases)
   - pulmonary disease (asthma, emphysema, bronchitis)
   - major illnesses limiting exercise capacity (weight loss, cancer, musculoskeletal diseases, eating disorders, gastrointestinal disorders)
2. Look for exercise-induced symptoms:
   - angina pectoris
   - dyspnoea
   - dizziness/lightheadedness
   - syncope
3. Risk factors for progression of atherosclerotic disease (hypertension, diabetes, obesity, dyslipidaemia, smoking, physical inactivity)
4. Recent illness, hospitalization, or surgical procedure
5. Medication dose and schedule, drug allergies
6. Other habits (alcohol and drug abuse)
7. Exercise history (habitual level of physical activity, including frequency, duration and type of exercise)
8. Work history (emphasis on current or expected physical and mental demands, upper and lower extremity requirements, estimated time to return to work)
9. Psychosocial history (family support, domestic and emotional problems, depression, anxiety)

Source: data from AACVPR Guidelines for Cardiac Rehabilitation and Secondary Prevention, 5th edition, 2013, p. 58.

Box 12.9 Contraindications for exercise training

Absolute contraindications:

- recent change in resting ECG suggesting significant ischaemia, recent MI, or other acute cardiac event
- unstable angina
- uncontrolled cardiac arrhythmia
- symptomatic severe aortic stenosis or other valvular disease
- decompensated symptomatic heart failure
- acute pulmonary embolus or pulmonary infarction
- acute non-cardiac disorder that may affect exercise performance or may be aggravated by exercise (e.g. infection, thyrotoxicosis)
- acute myocarditis or pericarditis
- acute thrombophlebitis
- physical disability that would preclude safe and adequate exercise performance

Relative contraindications (can be superseded if benefits outweigh the risks of exercise):

- electrolyte abnormalities
- tachyarrhythmias or bradyarrhythmias
- high-degree atrioventricular block
- atrial fibrillation with uncontrolled ventricular rate
- hypertrophic obstructive cardiomyopathy with peak resting left ventricular outflow gradient of > 25 mmHg
- known aortic dissection
- severe resting arterial hypertension (systolic BP > 200 mmHg and diastolic BP > 110 mmHg)
- mental impairment leading to inability to cooperate with testing

Source: data from AACVPR Guidelines for Cardiac Rehabilitation and Secondary Prevention, 5th edition, 2013, p. 58.

Stratification of risk for cardiac events during exercise participation according to the AACVPR guidelines

The risk stratification scheme proposed by the American Association of Cardiovascular and Pulmonary Rehabilitation (AACVPR) in their fifth guideline is mainly based on a diagnostic maximal ergometer test to assess the likelihood of exercise-induced myocardial ischaemia or arrhythmias. Consequently patients who do not have a diagnostic maximal exercise test cannot be adequately classified according to the risk stratification scheme. This patient group includes [87]:

- patients with abnormal resting ECG, including left bundle branch block, left ventricular hypertrophy, non-specific intraventricular conduction delays, Wolff–Parkinson–White ECG pattern, and ventricular-paced rhythms
- patients on digitalis therapy
- patients who fail to achieve 85% of the predicted maximal heart rate
- patients who are unable to perform a maximal exercise test due to significant non-cardiac comorbidities that limit exercise capacity

(and see ➲ Chapter 8). In these patients precise classification of risk may be challenging and a reasonable approach would be to treat them as high risk during the initiation of exercise therapy. All other patients can be stratified as low, moderate, or high risk as shown in ➲ Fig. 12.15.

Strategies to minimize the risk of adverse events during exercise participation

The risk for adverse cardiovascular events is highest in unaccustomed activity and at the beginning of an exercise training programme [88] but will be outweighed by the significant reduction in exercise-induced cardiovascular events after completion of an exercise-based CR programme [89,90].

To reduce the risk of adverse cardiovascular events at the start of the training programme the following actions are recommended:

- start with low to moderate exercise levels during the first days of the new training programme
- regularly ask the patients about symptoms suggestive of myocardial ischaemia and/or arrhythmias
- perform regular training of personnel involved in CR and exercise training in emergency response and advanced cardiopulmonary resuscitation
- consider continuous ECG monitoring in high-risk patients (note that ECG monitoring has not been shown to be related to the event rate during exercise-based cardiac rehabilitation) [91]
- monitor blood pressure at regular intervals
- monitor pulse, heart rate, or both by palpation
- rate perceived exertion (Borg scale).

Low Risk

Exercise Test Findings:
- Absence of complex ventricular dysrhythmias during exercise testing and recovery
- Absence of angina or other significant symptoms (e.g. unusual shortness of breath, light-headedness, or dizziness during exercise testing or recovery
- Presence of normal haemodynamics during exercise testing and recovery (i.e.. Appropriate increases and decreases in heart rate and systolic blood pressure with increasing workloads and recovery)
- Functional capacity ≥7 metabolic equivalents (METs)

Nonexercise Testing Findings:
- Rest ejection fraction ≥50%
- Uncomplicated myocardial infarction (MI) or revascularization procedure
- Absence of complicated ventricular arrhythmias at rest
- Absence of congestive heart failure (CHF)
- Absence of signs or symptoms of postevent or postprocedure ischaemia
- Absence of clinical depression

Moderate Risk

Exercise Test Findings:
- Presence of angina or other significant symptoms (e.g., unusual shortness of breath, light-headedness, or dizziness occurring only at high levels of exertion [≥7 METs])
- Mild to moderate level of silent ischaemia during exercise testing or recovery (ST-segment depression ≤2 mm from baseline)
- Functional capacity ≤5 METs

Nonexercise Testing Findings:
- Rest ejection fraction 40 to 49%

High Risk

Exercise Test Findings:
- Presence of complex ventricular arrhythmias during exercise testing or recovery
- Presence of angina or other significant symptoms (e.g, unusual shortness of breath, light-headedness, or dizziness at low levels of exertion [≤5 METs] or during recovery)
- High level of silent ischaemia (ST-segment depression ≥0.2 mm from baseline) during exercise testing or recovery
- Presence of abnormal haemodynamics with exercise testing (i.e., chronotropic incompetence or flat or decreasing systolic SP with increasing workloads) or recovery (i.e, severe postexercise hypotension)

Nonexercise Testing Findings:
- Rest ejection fraction ≤40
- History of cardiac arrest, or sudden death
- Complex dysrhythmias at rest
- Complicated MI or revascularization procedure
- Presence of CHF
- Presence of signs or symptoms of postevent or postprocedure ischaemia
- Presence of clinical depression

Fig. 12.15 Risk stratification for cardiac events during exercise participation according to Williams [175].

Reproduced from Williams MA. Exercise testing in cardiac rehabilitation. Exercise prescription and beyond. *Cardiol Clin*. 2001; **19**: 415–431, with permission from Elsevier.

Low Risk

Recommendations for Supervision and Monitoring:

- Direct medical supervision of exercise should occur for a minimum of 6 to 18 exercise sessions or 30 days postevent or postprocedure, beginning with continuous electrocardiogram (ECG) monitoring and decreasing as appropriate (e.g., at 6-12 sessions).
- For the patient to remain at lowest risk, the ECG and haemodynamic findings must remain normal; there should be no development or progression of abnormal signs and symptoms or intolerance to exercise within or outside the supervised programme. Progression of the exercise regimen should be appropriate.

Moderate Risk

Recommendations for Supervision and Monitoring:

- Direct staff supervision of exercise should occur for a minimum of 12 to 24 exercise sessions or 60 days postevent or postprocedure; begin with continuous ECG monitoring and decrease to intermittent or no ECG monitoring as appropriate (e.g., at 12-18 sessions).
- To move the patient to the lowest risk category, ECG and haemodynamic findings during exercise must be normal; there should be no development or progression of abnormal signs and symptoms or intolerance to exercise within or outside the supervised programme. Progression of the exercise regimen should be appropriate.
- Abnormal ECG or haemodynamic findings during exercise or the development or progression of abnormal signs and symptoms or intolerance to exercise within or outside the supervised programme, or the need to severely decrease exercise levels, may result in the patient's remaining in the moderate risk category or even moving to the high risk category.

High Risk

Recommendations for Supervision and Monitoring:

- Direct staff supervision of exercise should occur for a minimum of 18 to 36 exercise sessions or 90 days postevent or postprocedure, beginning with continuous ECG monitoring and decreasing to intermittent ECG monitoring as appropriate.
- For a patient to move to the moderate risk category, ECG and haemodynamic findings during exercise should be normal; there should be no development or progression of abnormal signs and symptoms or intolerance to exercise within or outside the supervised programme. Progression of the exercise regimen should be appropriate.
- Findings of the development or progression of abnormal ECG or haemodynamic findings during exercise including intolerance to exercise within or outside the supervised programme should be evaluated immediately. Significant limitations in the ability to participate may result in discontinuation of the exercise programme until appropriate evaluation, and intervention where necessary, can take place.

Fig. 12.16 Recommendations for the intensity of supervision and monitoring related to the risk of participation in an exercise programme according to Williams [175].

Reproduced from Williams MA. Exercise testing in cardiac rehabilitation. Exercise prescription and beyond. *Cardiol Clin*. 2001; **19**: 415–431, with permission from Elsevier.

Recommendations for the intensity of supervision and monitoring related to the stratification of risk (i.e. low, moderate, or high risk) are given in ➲ Fig. 12.16.

Exercise therapy in stable coronary artery disease

Evidence supporting the clinical use of exercise in this patient population

Regular aerobic exercise attenuates the progression of coronary lesions [92–96] and can even induce regression at an average energy expenditure during exercise of 2200 kcal/week, which translates to 5–6 hours/week of moderate-intensity exercise training [97]. Epidemiological [21,98–100] and interventional [101] studies indicate that aerobic exercise training reduces cardiovascular morbidity and mortality both in the general population [21,98–100] and in patients with CAD [21,95,101]. A sedentary lifestyle increases the risk of developing and dying from CAD [100,102]. While exercise may trigger MI and sudden cardiac death in patients with a sedentary lifestyle [103,104] training reduces these risks. Consequently, exercise training is recommended by the American Heart Association (AHA), American College of Cardiology (ACC), European Society of Cardiology (ESC), and American College of Sports Medicine (ACSM) guidelines as a class I, level A recommendation [68,105,106].

Indications, contraindications, and clinical examination

Exercise training is a class I indication in patients with stable CAD and one or more of the following diagnoses [18–20]:

- acute coronary syndrome (ST-segment elevation MI and non-ST-segment elevation MI)
- percutaneous coronary intervention (PCI)
- aortocoronary bypass surgery.

Exercise training is temporarily contraindicated as long as one or more of the following diagnoses are present and cannot be stabilized [107]:

- unstable angina pectoris
- acute endomyocarditis or other acute infections
- recent pulmonary artery embolism or phlebothrombosis
- haemodynamically relevant arrhythmia
- critical obstruction of the left ventricular outflow tract.

The clinical examinations necessary for the determination of individual risk and baseline exercise capacity prior to starting a training programme are given in ➲ Table 12.5.

Recommendations for exercise training

At the beginning of an exercise programme patients should be supervised by trained staff (an exercise physiologist, physiotherapists,

Table 12.5 Clinical examinations necessary for determination of individual risk and baseline exercise capacity prior to starting a training programme for patients with CAD

Components	Established/agreed issues
Patient risk assessment	◆ **Clinical history**: review clinical course of CAD ◆ **Physical examination**: inspect puncture site of PCI, and extremities for presence of arterial pulses, sternal wound inspection post-aortocoronary bypass surgery ◆ **Resting ECG** ◆ **Exercise capacity and ischaemic threshold**: symptom-limited, maximal exercise stress test by cycle ergometry or treadmill (cardiopulmonary exercise test if available) within 4 weeks after acute event; a submaximal test might be warranted, e.g. after an extensive MI or complications of a MI. Exercise or pharmacological imaging technique in patients with uninterpretable ECG ◆ Other tests as indicated (e.g. echocardiography, cardiac CT or MRI)

Source: data from European Association of Cardiovascular Prevention and Rehabilitation Committee for Science Guidelines, EACPR, Corrà U, Piepoli MF, Carré F, Heuschmann P, Hoffmann U, Verschuren M, Halcox J, Document Reviewers, Giannuzzi P, Saner H, Wood D, Piepoli MF, Corrà U, Benzer W, Bjarnason-Wehrens B, Dendale P, Gaita D, McGee H, Mendes M, Niebauer J, Zwisler A-DO, Schmid J-P. Secondary prevention through cardiac rehabilitation: physical activity counselling and exercise training: key components of the position paper from the Cardiac Rehabilitation Section of the European Association of Cardiovascular Prevention and Rehabilitation. *Eur Heart J* 2010; **31**: 1967–1974.

or nurses in addition to a cardiologist or an internist trained in rehabilitation medicine) in order to assess individual responses to exercise training and to identify signs and symptoms of angina pectoris. Heart rate and rhythm have to be monitored continuously throughout the training session, blood pressure should be measured before, during, and after training. ➲ Table 12.6 presents the duration and number of sessions as well as dose adjustment during the training course and ➲ Table 12.7 the recommendations for muscle hypertrophy training.

Exercise therapy in chronic heart failure

Evidence supporting the clinical use of exercise in this patient population

Traditionally, strenuous exercise was discouraged in patients with CHF because of concerns that any extra haemodynamic workload during physical exertion could lead to a further deterioration of cardiac function. In the early 1990s it became clear that there is no correlation between left ventricular function and exercise capacity in patients with CHF but a clear relation between muscle mass and exercise capacity, highlighting the relevance of peripheral factors for exercise intolerance [109]—peripheral hypoperfusion due to impaired endothelium-dependent vasodilation, reduced

Table 12.6 Duration and number of sessions as well as dose adjustment during the training course for patients with CAD

Physical activity	◆ **Exercise intensity**: patients with an exercise capacity > 5 METs without symptoms can resume physical activity at their previous intensity; otherwise, patients should resume physical activity at 50% of maximal work load or VO_2max and gradually increase intensity according to the subjective feeling of exertion, symptoms but also objective criteria like heart rate and/or lactate ◆ **Energy expenditure > 2000 kcal/week:** • Every day 30 minutes of a slow, gradual, and progressively increasing moderate intensity aerobic activity, e.g. occupational physical activity, walking, climbing stairs, bicycling to work or to run errands, gardening, etc.; approximately 1000 kcal in total • 2 hours/week of structured endurance training (3 × 40 min), approximately 800 kcal in total with the additional goal of increasing the maximum oxygen uptake by >20% and/or the performance on the bicycle ergometer to 100–120% of the age-adjusted index value • 1 hour resistance training per week (2 × 30 min), 200 kcal in total to increase muscle mass and muscle force
Exercise training	**Medically prescribed supervised aerobic exercise training:** ◆ **Low-risk patients:** at least three sessions of 30–60 minutes/week aerobic exercise at 55–70% of the maximum work load or heart rate at the onset of symptoms • >1500 kcal/week to be spent by low-risk patients ◆ **Moderate- to high-risk patients:** similar to low-risk group but starting with <50% maximum work load ◆ **Resistance exercise:** at least 1 hour/week: all major muscle groups; two sets each, with an intensity of 10–15 RM ◆ **Medication:** prophylactic nitroglycerine can be taken at the start of an exercise training session in chronic stable angina

Source: data from European Association of Cardiovascular Prevention and Rehabilitation Committee for Science Guidelines, EACPR, Corrà U, Piepoli MF, Carré F, Heuschmann P, Hoffmann U, Verschuren M, Halcox J, Document Reviewers, Giannuzzi P, Saner H, Wood D, Piepoli MF, Corrà U, Benzer W, Bjarnason-Wehrens B, Dendale P, Gaita D, McGee H, Mendes M, Niebauer J, Zwisler A-DO, Schmid J-P. Secondary prevention through cardiac rehabilitation: physical activity counselling and exercise training: key components of the position paper from the Cardiac Rehabilitation Section of the European Association of Cardiovascular Prevention and Rehabilitation. *Eur Heart J*. 2010;**31**:1967–1974. and Niebauer J, Mayr K, Tschentscher M, Pokan R, Benzer W. Outpatient cardiac rehabilitation: the Austrian model. *Eur J Prev Cardiol* 2013; **20**: 468–479.

Table 12.7 Recommendations for muscle hypertrophy training in patients with CAD

Design	Goals	Mode	Intensity	Repetitions	Frequency
Step I: preliminary training (3–4 weeks)	Learning and practising correct exercises; improvement of intermuscular coordination	Dynamic	< 50% RM*	8–15	Two units/week; six to eight muscle groups; one to two sets/muscle group
Step II: hypertrophy strength training	Muscle hypertrophy; improvement of intramuscular coordination	Dynamic	60–80% RM*	8–15	Two units/week; six to eight muscle groups; two sets/muscle group

The intensity has to be chosen so that the chosen number of repetitions can be performed.

*RM (repetition maximum) = load (kg)/(1 repetition × 0.025).

Source: data from Niebauer J, Mayr K, Tschentscher M, Pokan R, Benzer W. Outpatient cardiac rehabilitation: the Austrian model. *Eur J Prev Cardiol*. 2013;**20**:468–479. and Piepoli MF, Corrà U, Benzer W, Bjarnason-Wehrens B, Dendale P, Gaita D, McGee H, Mendes M, Niebauer J, Zwisler A-DO, Schmid J-P, Cardiac Rehabilitation Section of the European Association of Cardiovascular Prevention and Rehabilitation. Secondary prevention through cardiac rehabilitation: from knowledge to implementation. A position paper from the Cardiac Rehabilitation Section of the European Association of Cardiovascular Prevention and Rehabilitation. *Eur J Cardiovasc Prev Rehabil* Off J Eur Soc Cardiol Work Groups Epidemiol Prev Card Rehabil Exerc Physiol. 2010; **17**: 1–17.

strength of the respiratory muscles, and profound morphological, metabolic, and functional alterations in the skeletal muscles [53,55,109–112].

Randomized training studies in patients with systolic heart failure (i.e. HFREF) established the safety and efficacy of aerobic endurance training interventions [5,113–115] and documented that endurance training reduced cardiomegaly and heart failure-related hospitalization [116] and improved systolic and diastolic function [115,117,118], exercise capacity [117,119], and quality of life.

Training effects on all-cause and cardiac mortality continue to be disputed. In the EXTRA-MATCH case-based meta-analysis including a total of 395 exercise-trained patients with HFREF and 406 control patients a significant 35% reduction in all-cause mortality and a 28% reduction in the combined end-point of death or hospital admission were described [5]. The consecutive multicentre HF-ACTION study, however, showed no significant reduction in all-cause mortality or hospitalization in the protocol-specified analysis—most likely due to low rates of compliance with the prescribed training protocol (approximately 60%). However, after adjustment exercise training was associated with modest significant reductions in both all-cause mortality or hospitalization and cardiovascular mortality or hospitalization with heart failure [6]. Due to the large number of participants (2331 patients) this result was also carried over into the 2010 Cochrane systematic meta-analysis, which described no significant training effect on all-cause mortality and all-cause hospitalizations [116]. Subsequent sub-analysis confirmed a dose–response relationship between training intensity (as measured by MET-h per week) and outcome improvement, indicating significant reductions in adjusted hazard ratios for all-cause/cardiac mortality or all-cause/cardiac hospitalization between 3 and 7 MET-h per week (➲ Figs 12.17 and 12.18) [120]. Taken together, available data are consistent with a dose-related improvement in clinical outcomes that reaches significant levels above 3 MET-h per week of aerobic continuous exercise training.

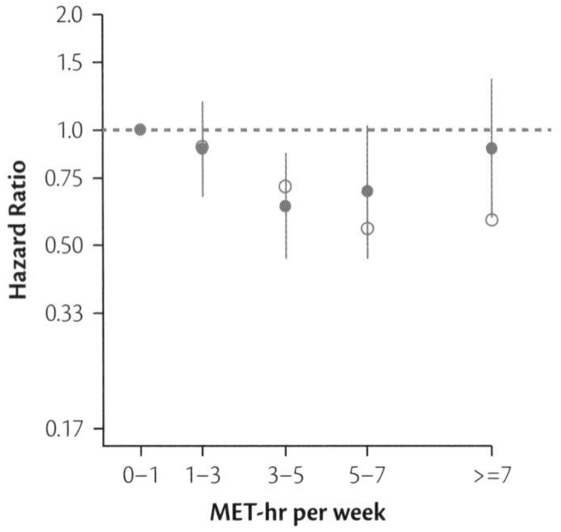

Fig. 12.17 Hazard ratios for all-cause mortality or hospitalization. Among patients who were event-free for at least 3 months the figure shows adjusted hazard ratios (filled circles, log scale) for all-cause mortality or hospitalization with 95% confidence intervals. The reference category is 0–1 MET-h per week. Unadjusted hazard ratios are plotted with open circles.

Reproduced from Keteyian SJ, Leifer ES, Houston-Miller N, Kraus WE, Brawner CA, O'Connor CM, Whellan DJ, Cooper LS, Fleg JL, Kitzman DW, Cohen-Solal A, Blumenthal JA, Rendall DS, Piña IL, HF-ACTION Investigators. Relation between volume of exercise and clinical outcomes in patients with heart failure. *J Am Coll Cardiol* 2012; **60**: 1899–1905, with permission from Elsevier.

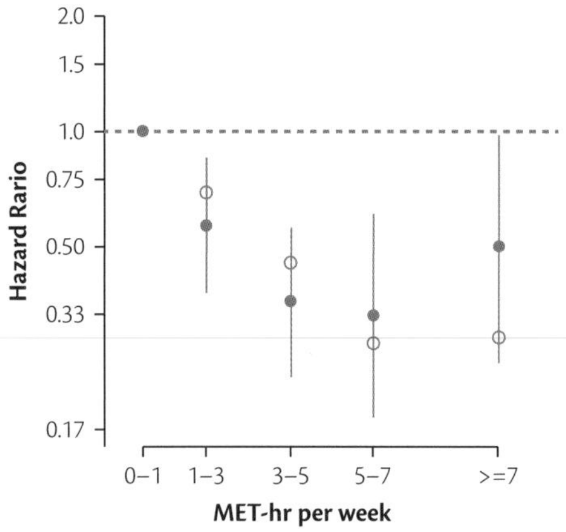

Fig. 12.18 Hazard ratios for cardiovascular mortality or heart failure hospitalization. Among patients event-free for at least 3 months the figure shows adjusted hazard ratios (filled circles, log scale) for cardiovascular mortality or heart failure hospitalization with 95% confidence intervals. The reference category is 0–1 MET-h per week. Unadjusted hazard ratios are plotted with open circles.

Reproduced from Keteyian SJ, Leifer ES, Houston-Miller N, Kraus WE, Brawner CA, O'Connor CM, Whellan DJ, Cooper LS, Fleg JL, Kitzman DW, Cohen-Solal A, Blumenthal JA, Rendall DS, Piña IL, HF-ACTION Investigators. Relation between volume of exercise and clinical outcomes in patients with heart failure. *J Am Coll Cardiol* 2012; **60**: 1899–1905, with permission from Elsevier

Recently, interval training and strength training have been introduced in HFREF patients. Clearly, interval training with exercise peaks at 90% of VO_2 max for 2–3 minutes leads to superior improvements in exercise capacity and quality of life, with no apparent difference in the improvement in left ventricular remodelling [121,122]. Training can be recommended for stable, motivated patients with no significant comorbidities limiting exercise capacity. Pure strength training without any dynamic/aerobic component does not improve exercise capacity [56] while combined strength–endurance training seems to lead to greater improvements in muscle strength and muscle mass compared with steady-state endurance training [123–125]. However, the beneficial effects on vascular function and reverse remodelling seem to depend on the aerobic component of the training programme.

About half of all patients with heart failure have HFPEF. Recently, pilot studies indicated that improved exercise capacity and diastolic function can be achieved by aerobic training in HFPEF patients [7]. Outcome studies are planned.

Indications, contraindications, and clinical examination

Based on current ESC Heart Failure Guidelines 'It is recommended that regular aerobic exercise is encouraged in patients with heart failure to improve functional capacity and symptoms' (class I, level A) [126]. Detailed recommendations on patient selection are given in ➲ Fig. 12.19 and by Piepoli et al. [127]. Indications for training are as follows:

- Patients with stable compensated HFREF in NYHA functional class I–III.
- Patients with stable compensated HFPEF may be considered for aerobic endurance training interventions based on pilot study data.

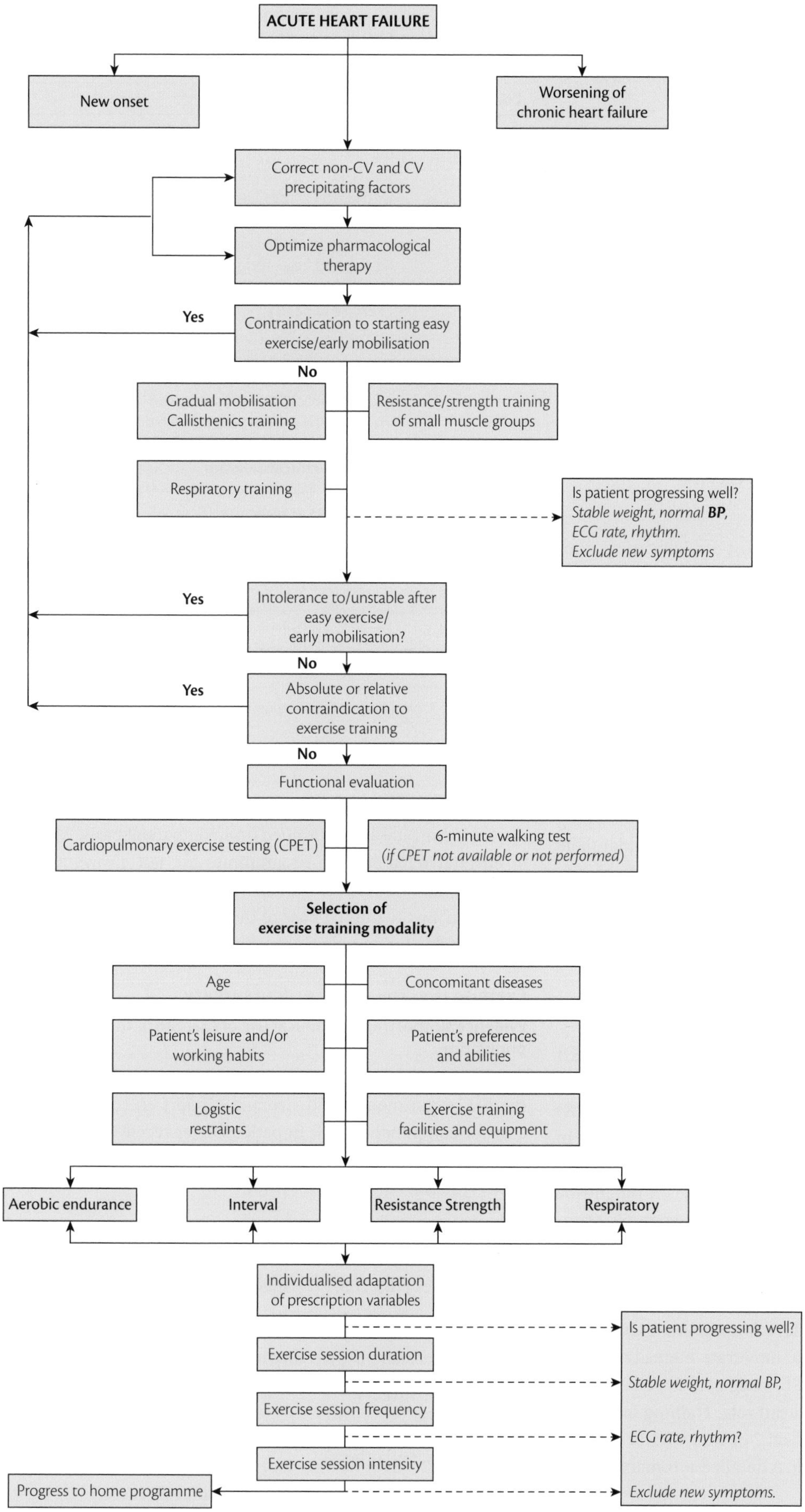

Fig. 12.19 Flow-chart to guide the tailoring of an exercise training programme according to the individual clinical conditions and needs of the patient.
From Piepoli MF, Conraads V, Corrà U, Dickstein K, Francis DP, Jaarsma T, McMurray J, Pieske B, Piotrowicz E, Schmid J-P, Anker SD, Solal AC, Filippatos GS, Hoes AW, Gielen S, Giannuzzi P, Ponikowski PP. Exercise training in heart failure: from theory to practice. A consensus document of the Heart Failure Association and the European Association for Cardiovascular Prevention and Rehabilitation. *Eur J Heart Fail* 2011; **13**: 347–357, with permission from Wiley.

In patients with HFREF, exercise training is contraindicated in the following circumstances [127]:

- progressive worsening of exercise tolerance or dyspnoea at rest over the previous 3–5 days
- significant ischaemia during low-intensity exercise (2 METs, 50 W)
- uncontrolled diabetes
- recent embolism
- thrombophlebitis
- new-onset atrial fibrillation/atrial flutter.

In patients with HFREF the risk of exercise training is increased in the following circumstances [127]:

- 1.8 kg increase in body mass over the previous 1–3 days
- concurrent, continuous, or intermittent dobutamine therapy
- decrease in systolic blood pressure with exercise
- NYHA functional class IV
- complex ventricular arrhythmia at rest or appearing with exertion
- supine resting heart rate > 100 beats/minute
- pre-existing comorbidities limiting exercise tolerance.

These patients need clinical stabilization prior to being enrolled in a structured exercise programme and should be monitored during the initial training phase. In exercise training studies in stable CHF patients, however, adverse events are surprisingly low with post-exercise hypotension, atrial or ventricular arrhythmias, and worsening heart failure symptoms being the most common complications. Training after implantable cardioverter defibrillator (ICD) implantation appears to be safe and feasible [128,129].

The clinical examinations necessary for determination of individual risk and baseline exercise capacity prior to starting the training programme are shown in ➲ Table 12.8.

Recommendations for exercise training

As highlighted in the 2011 consensus document of the Heart Failure Association (HFA) and the European Association for Cardiovascular Prevention and Rehabilitation (EACPR) there is no universal agreement on exercise prescription in CHF [127].

The classical approach with the largest database on prognostic and symptomatic efficacy is based on steady-state aerobic training starting at 40–50% of the maximal exercise capacity, aiming for 70–80% during the course of the training programme [127]. This approach is also favoured in the 2013 update of the Canadian Cardiovascular Society's Heart Failure Management Guidelines [130] which recommends continuous moderate-intensity training at a rating of perceived exertion (RPE) scale of 3–5, or 50–75% of peak VO_2, or at 65–85% of maximal heart rate. Training sessions of 15–30 minutes should be performed on 2 or 3 days a week aiming for 30 minutes a day on 5 days a week. A detailed summary is given in ➲ Tables 12.9 and 12.10.

Table 12.8 Clinical examinations necessary for determination of individual risk and baseline exercise capacity prior to starting a training programme in patients with CHF

Components	Established/agreed issues
Patient risk assessment	◆ **Clinical history**: review clinical course of past or recent history of heart failure including assessment of functional status (NYHA) and quality of life (e.g. Minnesota Living with Heart Failure Questionnaire) ◆ **Physical examination**: inspect for peripheral oedema, auscultation of the lungs for rales, auscultation of the heart (third heart sound, mitral regurgitation) ◆ **Resting ECG** ◆ **Exercise capacity**: symptom limited, maximal exercise stress test by cycle ergometry or treadmill (cardiopulmonary exercise test if available); a submaximal test might be warranted, e.g. after an extensive MI or complications of an MI. Exercise or pharmacological imaging technique in patients with uninterpretable ECG and known CAD ◆ **Baseline echocardiogram** with determination of left ventricular ejection fraction and mitral regurgitation ◆ **Other tests as indicated** (BNP, MRI, etc.)

BNP, brain natriuretic peptide.

Source: data from European Association of Cardiovascular Prevention and Rehabilitation Committee for Science Guidelines, EACPR, Corrà U, Piepoli MF, Carré F, Heuschmann P, Hoffmann U, Verschuren M, Halcox J, Document Reviewers, Giannuzzi P, Saner H, Wood D, Piepoli MF, Corrà U, Benzer W, Bjarnason-Wehrens B, Dendale P, Gaita D, McGee H, Mendes M, Niebauer J, Zwisler A-DO, Schmid J-P. Secondary prevention through cardiac rehabilitation: physical activity counselling and exercise training: key components of the position paper from the Cardiac Rehabilitation Section of the European Association of Cardiovascular Prevention and Rehabilitation. *Eur Heart J* 2010; **31**: 1967–1974.

Traditionally, training programmes in heart failure patients are started in hospital and continued on an outpatient basis. Although in-hospital rehabilitation programmes are not always available and are cost- and resource-intensive they provide optimal supervision during the initial phase of the training programme and are indispensable for complex interventions such as interval training.

Exercise therapy after cardiac surgery

Evidence supporting the clinical use of exercise in this patient population

Guidelines and recommendations from the AHA, ACC, and the ESC unanimously and strongly support exercise training as a major component of CR in patients after recent surgical revascularization [133,134], valvular surgery, or surgery due to other structural heart diseases [135,136].

Indications, contraindications, and clinical examination

Exercise training is a class I indication in patients with the following diagnoses [107,108,137] or after a previous event:

- all indications listed for stable CAD and in particular:
  - aortocoronary bypass surgery
  - valvular surgery
  - surgery of major vessels (aorta, carotids and/or subclavian arteries, and others)
  - surgery due to other structural cardiac diseases.

Table 12.9 Duration and number of sessions as well as dose adjustment during the training course for patients with CHF

Physical activity	◆ Patients should be encouraged to engage in moderate aerobic activities
Exercise training	**Endurance aerobic training (continuous and interval):** ◆ Start at low intensity (i.e. 40–50% of peak VO_2) and short session durations (i.e. 5–10 minutes) twice a week ◆ Bicycle ergometers are first choice for ECG monitoring if needed ◆ If well-tolerated first increase the training duration per session to 30, then 45 min, then the number of training sessions (i.e. up to five a week) ◆ Aim for 20–60 min at moderate-to-high intensity (i.e. 70–80% of peak VO_2) on 3–5 days a week ◆ If cardiopulmonary exercise testing is not available heart rate-based or RPE-based monitoring of training intensity is recommended: ◆ 40–70% of heart rate reserve (defined as peak heart rate during maximal exercise testing—basal heart rate) ◆ 10/20–14/20 Borg RPE rating ◆ **Interval training** provides an even more effective method for aerobic training interventions but needs more sophisticated exercise equipment (usually electronically steered bicycle ergometers): • Short high-intensity exercise bouts (10–30 s at 90–95% of peak VO_2) are interspersed with 1–3 min recovery periods at no or low intensity [121,131] • 5–10 min warm-up and cool-down periods are recommended • Typically, the intensity of the first three hard segments is reduced to allow for warm-up • 10–12 work phases can be performed per 15–30 minute training session **Resistance/strength training** [63]: see ➲ Table 12.9 **Respiratory training:** ◆ Screen for inspiratory muscle weakness in every HFREF patient ◆ Start respiratory training at 30% of the maximal inspiratory mouth pressure (Pi_{max}) and readjust the intensity every 7–10 days up to a maximum of 60% [132] ◆ 20–30 min per day ◆ Three to five sessions a week ◆ Minimum duration of exercise programme of 8 weeks ◆ Methodologies with documented efficacy include the use of the Threshold inspiratory muscle trainer (Respironics Health Scan Inc., Cedar Grove, NJ, USA) and Power-Breathe (HaB International Ltd, Southam, Warwickshire, UK).

Source: data from Piepoli MF, Conraads V, Corrà U, Dickstein K, Francis DP, Jaarsma T, McMurray J, Pieske B, Piotrowicz E, Schmid J-P, Anker SD, Solal AC, Filippatos GS, Hoes AW, Gielen S, Giannuzzi P, Ponikowski PP. Exercise training in heart failure: from theory to practice. A consensus document of the Heart Failure Association and the European Association for Cardiovascular Prevention and Rehabilitation. *Eur J Heart Fail* 2011; **13**: 347–357.

Box 12.10 Clinical examinations needed to determine individual risk and baseline exercise capacity prior to starting a training programme after cardiac surgery

◆ All examinations listed in ➲ Table 12.5 plus assessment of:
  • wound healing of the chest and, where applicable, legs
  • comorbidities
  • complications
  • disabilities
◆ ECG: heart rate, rhythm, repolarization and new Q waves
◆ X-ray: infection, pleural effusion, diaphragm paralysis
◆ Blood testing: anaemia, fasting blood glucose, ($HbA1_C$ if fasting blood glucose is elevated), renal function, and electrolytes
◆ Echocardiography: pleural or pericardial effusion, prosthetic function, and/or valvular heart disease, when appropriate
◆ Exercise capacity to guide exercise prescription
◆ Patient education:
  • anticoagulation, including drug interactions and self-management
  • in-depth knowledge on endocarditic prophylaxis
  • secondary prevention medication for CAD
  • how to progress in order to normalize activities of daily living

Exercise training is temporarily contraindicated as long as one or more of the following diagnoses are present and cannot be stabilized [107]:

◆ all contraindications listed for stable CAD and in addition:

  wound infection after sternotomy, harvesting of saphenous veins, and/or radial arteries

  respiratory infection, for example secondary to sternotomy.

The clinical examinations necessary for the determination of individual risk and baseline exercise capacity prior to starting a training programme in patients after cardiac surgery are shown in ➲ Box 12.10.

Recommendations for exercise training

All the recommendations given in ➲ Tables 12.6 and 12.7 are relevant plus [107,108]:

◆ Exercise training has to be started early in the acute care hospital.

Table 12.10 Minimum recommendations for the implementation of a resistance/strength training programme in CHF patients

Training programme	Training objectives	Stress form	Intensity	Repetitions	Training volume
Step I: pre-training	To learn and practise the correct implementation, to learn perception, to improve intermuscular coordination	Dynamic	<30% 1RM, RPE < 12	5–10	Two to three training sessions a week, one to three circuits during each session
Step II: resistance/endurance training	To improve local aerobic endurance and intermuscular coordination	Dynamic	30–40% 1RM, RPE 12–13	12–55	Two to three sessions a week, one circuit per session
Step III: strength training, muscle build-up training	To increase muscle mass (hypertrophy), to improve intramuscular coordination	Dynamic	40–60% 1RM, RPE < 15	8–15	Two to three sessions a week, one circuit per session

1RM, one repetition maximum; RPE, rating of perceived exertion.
Modified according to Bjarnson-Wehrens et al. [63].

- Thereafter, inpatient and/or outpatient CR programmes need to be initiated immediately after discharge.
- A minimum of 8–12 weeks of CR is indicated.
- Upper-body training can begin when the chest is stable, i.e. usually after 6 weeks.
- Exercise training has to be individually tailored according to the patient's clinical condition, baseline exercise capacity, ventricular function, and kind of surgery. Generally speaking, after mitral valve replacement exercise tolerance is much lower than after aortic valve replacement, particularly if there is residual pulmonary hypertension.

Further recommendations with regard to type of physical activity, duration per session, number of sessions per day, need for supervision/monitoring, and dose adjustment during the training course can found be in ➲ Table 12.10.

Exercise therapy in valvular heart disease

Only a few studies have specifically evaluated training interventions in patients with valvular heart disease. Therefore, recommendations are necessarily less reliable and are based on pathophysiological considerations rather than on hard clinical evidence.

Indications, contraindications, and clinical examination

In patients with stable asymptomatic moderate-degree valvular heart disease (up to grade II) moderate-intensity exercise is possible. There is, however, no evidence to suggest that regular exercise interventions influence the progression of valvular heart disease.

Clear contraindications to exercise training include:

- All critical and highly symptomatic valvular lesions on the edge to cardiac decompensation.
- Stable aortic stenosis with a valvular orifice area < 0.75 cm^2 and a peak pressure gradient > 50 mmHg.
- In general, patients with valvular heart disease and a clear (class I and IIa) indication for cardiac surgery should abstain from exercise training until after valve surgery.

There are specific risks for special valvular lesions, namely:

- Mitral valve prolapse. Although considered a benign abnormality occurring in up to 5% in the general population sudden death has been reported as a rare complication. Exercise is considered safe in patients without significant arrhythmias at rest and during exercise, without a family history of sudden cardiac death, and without any previous thromboembolic event or syncope.
- Mitral regurgitation. Relative mitral regurgitation is frequent in patients with CHF and does not preclude the initiation of training therapy provided the patient is in stable condition (NYHA grades II–III).
- Mitral stenosis. Patients with a mitral valve orifice > 1.5 cm^2 may safely participate in normal exercise training sessions. Those with moderate to severe mitral stenosis (< 1.5 cm^2) are usually limited by exercise-induced dyspnoea and can only tolerate low levels of physical exertion. In these symptomatic patients treatment of mitral stenosis by balloon valvuloplasty or valve replacement should be performed prior to starting a training programme.
- Aortic regurgitation. Patients with mild to moderate aortic regurgitation may engage in training without problems. However, left ventricular diameters need to be reassessed every 3–6 months to watch for worsening of the valve disease.

Table 12.11 Clinical examinations necessary for the determination of individual risk and baseline exercise capacity prior to starting the training programme in patients with valvular heart disease

Components	Established/agreed issues
Patient risk assessment	◆ **Clinical history**: review clinical course of valvular heart disease including assessment of functional status (NYHA), history of syncope or angina pectoris, and quality of life (e.g. Minnesota Living with Heart Failure Questionnaire) ◆ **Physical examination**: inspect for peripheral oedema, auscultation of the lungs for rales, auscultation of the heart ◆ **Resting ECG** ◆ **Exercise capacity**: submaximal exercise testing is generally recommended except in asymptomatic patients with valvular heart disease ≤ NYHA grade II ◆ **Baseline echocardiogram** with determination of left ventricular ejection fraction and assessment of valvular function ◆ **Invasive assessment of valvular heart disease** in symptomatic patients and whenever indicated

The clinical examinations necessary for the determination of individual risk and baseline exercise capacity prior to starting a training programme in patients with valvular heart disease are given in ➲ Table 12.11.

Recommendations for exercise training

In valvular heart disease changes in afterload or pre-load associated with changes in peripheral resistance may greatly affect cardiac output. Therefore, resistance training of large muscle groups is generally discouraged in valvular heart disease. Endurance training sessions—preferably with ECG and blood pressure monitoring during the initial phase—are more reproducible with regard to haemodynamic load and should be at moderate intensity (i.e. 50–70% of VO_2 max).

Exercise therapy in patients with arrhythmias, pacemakers, and ICDs

Evidence supporting the clinical use of exercise in this patient population

Despite the fact that physical exertion might serve as a trigger for arrhythmias and sudden cardiac death [103,104], deconditioning secondary to a sedentary lifestyle will expose the patient to increasing levels of stress during daily activities, so that daily routines will become exhausting and thus pro-arrhythmic. As a consequence, submaximal exercise training has also been recommended in patients with arrhythmias, pacemakers, and ICDs [107,108,137].

Indications, contraindications, and clinical examinations

Exercise training is indicated in patients with arrhythmias [107,108,137], especially after

- implantation of a pacemaker or an ICD
- electrophysiological intervention
- haemodynamically stable arrhythmia
- sustained ventricular tachycardia or cardiac arrest.

Exercise training is temporarily contraindicated in the following situations or as long as one or more of the following diagnoses is present and cannot be stabilized [107]:

- all contraindications shown for stable CAD
- local infections of lower extremities
- systemic infection
- pain at rest.

The following clinical examinations are necessary to determine individual risk and baseline exercise capacity prior to starting a training programme:

- Perform wound inspection; gain knowledge about wire and device placement.
- Echocardiography: left ventricular function is a crucial prognosticator.
- Note details of device sensing, pacing, and shock thresholds as well as pacing mode.
- Staff have to be aware of the fact that lead failure might result in inappropriate or missing shocks. Therefore external defibrillators have to be in the training room at all times and staff have to be trained how to use them.
- Perform a maximal symptom-limited stress test. Note that rate-responsive devices are preferable since they do not limit the patient during exercise. Rate-limited devices will only permit exercise training at submaximal intensity.

Recommendations for exercise training

Type of physical activity

- Continuous endurance training as well as resistance training are encouraged. For details see ➲ Tables 12.6 and 12.7.
- To avoid unwarranted shocks the training heart rate should be set to 10–20 beats below the therapy threshold.
- Avoid excessive arm movement so as to not risk lead dislocation or breakage.

Duration of session/number of sessions per day

- As in all patients, training intensity has to be defined according to peak VO_2 or maximal heart rate achieved during maximal ergometry or ergospirometry.
- Basing exercise prescription on an estimated training heart rate is unacceptable, since incorrect training heart rates might be above the detection threshold of the ICD and could lead to inappropriate ICD therapy.
- Continuous physical activity of 30 minutes or more, or multiple activity sessions of 10 to 15 minutes on the same day, on most days of the week.
- Avoid contact sports as bruising or breaking of the skin over the site of the device may lead to infections.
- Swimming can be undertaken after wound healing. During swimming patients should be accompanied at all times by someone able to rescue the patient.
- SCUBA diving is discouraged.

Dose adjustment during the training course

- Depending on the underlying diagnosis, initial training intensity will have to be determined for each individual. In patients with ICD/cardiac resynchronization therapy due to heart failure the initial exercise intensity could, for example, be set to 40–60% of the maximal work capacity reached during maximal ergometry.

Need for supervision/monitoring

- Supervised training programmes have been shown to be beneficial if they last between 12 weeks and up to 1 year. Patients should initially train under ECG monitoring, which can later on be replaced by heart rate monitors.

Exercise therapy in special patient groups

Older adults

Elements of ageing (e.g. inflammation, oxidative stress, telomere shortening) accumulate over a lifetime, as do the mounting effects of CV risk factors, predisposing to CVD as well as other chronic diseases [138–140]. These diseases often occur in combination, making management more complex [141]. Amidst these risks, and the related tendencies for pain, deconditioning, and fatigue, many older adults lapse into sedentary behaviours. Paradoxically, inactivity generally worsens medical instability, accelerates morbidity and mortality, increases weakness and falls, diminishes independence, and reduces quality of life [50,142].

Exercise moderates many of the basic mechanisms of ageing and age-related vulnerability to disease [143,144]. Training can thereby moderate morbidity and even prevent the manifestation of disease in the elderly [145]. It also plays a key role in secondary prevention in those with established CVD [146]. In addition, exercise improves cognition, respiration, bone strength, gastrointestinal motility, sleep, and mood [147,148]. While the life-prolonging benefits of exercise remain relevant for seniors, an even greater value is often ascribed to the ability of exercise to maintain or even improve quality of life, independence, and self-efficacy.

Physical activity

In the 2007 ACSM/AHA recommendations on physical activity in older adults [106] the importance of regular physical activity, including aerobic, strength, and balance activities, as part of healthy ageing is emphasized. Even the accumulation of light activities throughout the day can have a significant effect on total energy expenditure and overall health outcomes. Self-transportation (i.e. walking or cycling), housework, and gardening are potential opportunities to structure active, healthy lifestyles. Participation in activities that provide positive social and intellectual stimulation (e.g. dancing) reduces cognitive decline [149].

Box 12.11 Recommendations for exercise training in older adults

Caveats for older adults:

- For frail elders, priorities often centre on building strength, stability, and balance, before progressing to aerobic modalities
- For some infirm adults, exercises may be restricted to arm movements, seated machines, or water activities
- Warm-up and cool-down activities are particularly important for elderly individuals, counterbalancing risks and limitations from reduced autonomic responsiveness, peripheral flow and joint instability

General exercise training recommendations:

- Exercise training 5 days a week for 30 minutes at moderate intensity

or

- Exercise training vigorous intensity on 3 days a week for 20 minutes
- For adults who are frail, starting with exercises to build strength, stability, and balance must often precede aerobic exercise training

Aerobic training recommendations:

- Indoors: walking (treadmill or indoor track), bicycle ergometer, or recumbent steppers
- Outdoors: walking, cycling, gardening, swimming (laps or water aerobics), and golfing (especially if walking with a pull cart)
- Moderate-training effect, older adults are typically advised to exercise at a level that feels 'somewhat hard'
- High-intensity interval training (HIT) may be especially well-suited to older adults since it maximizes cardiovascular stimulation with preserved stability overall [121]; however, HIT is more complex than continuous training, necessitating more supervision for implementation and safety

Strength training recommendations:

- Eight to 12 repetitions of moderate to heavy intensity. Regimens will vary relative to comorbidity, baseline conditioning, and training goals
- Two to three sets of repetitions, two to three times a week on non-consecutive days, is generally recommended, but even one set is beneficial

Stretching and balance training:

- Stretching on 2 days a week for at least 10 minutes each time, but can also be completed more frequently
- Balance training with walking activities (backward, sideways, heel-to-toe), Bosu ball activities, clockwise sway, standing on one foot, and tai chi exercises

Source: data from Nelson ME, Rejeski WJ, Blair SN, Duncan PW, Judge JO, King AC, Macera CA, Castaneda-Sceppa C, American College of Sports Medicine, American Heart Association. Physical activity and public health in older adults: recommendation from the American College of Sports Medicine and the American Heart Association. *Circulation* 2007; **116**: 1094–1105.

Exercise prescription

Exercise goals need to be tailored to the broad range of seniors, including those who are frail and those who are robust. Strength training is often particularly important in the elderly since the natural susceptibility to sarcopenia and osteoporosis often limits the capacities of frail older adults to initiate aerobic-type training. Strength-training programmes increase muscle strength and mass through muscle hypertrophy and neuromuscular adaptation, facilitating improvements in gait, balance, and overall functional capacity and resistance to falls [150,151]. Strength training also increases bone mineral density and content, increases metabolic rate [152], and assists with maintenance of body weight by increasing lean mass, thereby improving muscle metabolism [153]. ➲ Box 12.11 summarizes the recommendations for exercise training in older adults.

Women

In the 2008 United States physical activity guidelines [154] a meta-analysis included more women (>200 000) than men (>120 000) in epidemiological studies of physical activity and CHD risk published after 1995, and documented a median risk reduction of 38% in the most active women compared with the least active. Physiological differences in exercise training dynamics in women compared with men include a smaller average body size in women with shorter stride length and greater stride frequency, leading to higher exercise intensity for an equivalent exercise workload. Peak oxygen consumption (VO_2) is also 5–15% lower in women than in men [41] due to differences in body fat per kilogram of body weight, smaller lung volumes, and lower stroke volume. Exercise-induced cardiac remodelling may be different in women due to their ability to increase end-diastolic volume as a means to augment stroke volume and cardiac output [155].

Exercise training may benefit women disproportionately in relation to gender-specific pathophysiological vulnerabilities. Microvascular myocardial ischaemia entails clinical signs and symptoms of ischaemia, primarily due to endothelial dysfunction. Women are particularly predisposed to this, and exercise training can moderate the pathophysiological mechanisms [156]. HFPEF also occurs more commonly in women: exercise can help restore lusitropy [7] and also moderate hypertension, diabetes, and other predisposing risks. Still other literature points to the gender-specific advantages of exercise training in relation to affect, anxiety, and self-efficacy [157].

Due to the generally lower intrinsic strength and aerobic capacities of women exercise training may best start at low to moderate intensities. However, as training proceeds, women can often advance to high-intensity regimens similar to men. Strength training may provide particular benefit to counteract the relatively lower muscle mass and strength in many women. Exercise training among post-menopausal women is an important strategy for mitigating osteoporosis and frailty in old age [158].

Exercise is also considered safe for healthy women with an uncomplicated pregnancy [159]. While there are few randomized, controlled data regarding exercise training during pregnancy, multiple observational studies [160–162] suggest the safety of continued exercise routines. Moreover, reductions in gestational diabetes [163,164] and post-partum depression have been demonstrated [165].

Obesity

Obese patients need a higher volume of exercise to achieve weight reduction compared with non-obese patients, who aim to improve their exercise capacity [166,167]. Furthermore, initial exercise can be challenging: not only are many obese adults deconditioned, but the physiological burden associated with carrying extra weight during exercise implies greater workload and exercise intensity. Walking is the preferred exercise modality for maximizing caloric expenditure rather than weight-supported exercises (cycling or rowing) which burn fewer calories [168]. Longer-duration training at a lower intensity is based on the premise that glycogen is the predominant fuel source during the first 20 minutes of exercise, followed by a shift to fat stores after 30 minutes [169]. The following training recommendations can be made for obese patients:

- 150 minutes of aerobic activity per week as a minimum for the treatment of obesity.
- For weight loss exercise duration should progress to 200–300 minutes a week.
- A training frequency of 5 to 7 days a week, with sessions lasting from 45 to 60 minutes is recommended.

Obese people may benefit from a resistance training programme which improves muscular strength and favourably affects functional tasks. Resistance training may also stimulate an increase in fat-free mass and intrinsic energy expenditure [170].

The risk of hyperthermia is another concern as the proportion of surface area relative to body size is lower in obese adults compared with those of normal weight. The exercise environment should be appropriately adapted to avoid overheating and the associated cardiovascular risks. ➲ Table 12.12 details the clinical examinations necessary for the determination of individual risk and baseline exercise capacity prior to starting a training programme in obese patients.

Type 2 diabetes mellitus

A Joint Position Stand by ACSM and the American Diabetes Association [171] recommends the combination of aerobic and strength training to maximize glucose control in patients with type 2 diabetes mellitus with benefits attributable to improved glucose metabolism as well as to changes in body composition and improvements in the cardiovascular risk profile.

Hyperglycaemia can be worsened by exercise, particularly in those with type 1 diabetes who are insulin deficient. In contrast, patients with type 2 diabetes rarely develop similar insulin deficiency. However, concerns regarding hypoglycaemia in patients with type 2 diabetes are relatively greater, particularly in those using insulin or sulfonylureas, nateglinide, or repaglinide. These risks may also be influenced by the time of day at which exercise is initiated and the relative influences of meals. Patients with a pre-exercise blood glucose < 100 mg/dl should ingest carbohydrate prior to exercise. Hypoglycaemia is also a concern during high-intensity or prolonged exercise. In such circumstances, consumption of carbohydrate during or soon after exercise can help lower the risk of hypoglycaemia. Glucose monitoring and the availability of carbohydrate supplements are important safeguards.

Diabetes also predisposes to other intrinsic complications. CVD, peripheral neuropathy, autonomic neuropathy, and retinopathy are all more likely in people with diabetes, and each compounds the complexity of exercise training. Patients with CVD and diabetes are generally at higher risk and may benefit from CR or a supervised setting in which cardiac parameters can be assessed and monitored to best facilitate the safe progression of therapeutic exercise. In general these patients benefit from careful pre-exercise assessment for unstable atherosclerotic heart disease, especially since symptoms provide a less reliable indication of concern. Older age and increased weight add to these concerns.

Peripheral neuropathy may be manifest as burning, tingling, and numbness in the feet, or even foot ulcers. Weight-bearing exercises should be minimized or avoided, relying more on seated modalities. Routine monitoring of foot health and optimal shock-absorbing footwear are also indicated. Autonomic neuropathy is manifest in changes in heart rate, blood pressure, arrhythmia, and ischaemia, as well as postural hypotension and falls. Exercise-related risks are increased. Thorough pre-screening is indicated and patients may benefit from supervised exercise training. Diabetic retinopathy is also a concern. In patients with uncontrolled proliferative disease, activities that increase intraocular pressure and haemorrhagic risks are best avoided. These include

Table 12.12 Clinical examinations necessary for the determination of individual risk and baseline exercise capacity prior to starting the training programme in obese patients

Components	Established/agreed issues
Patient risk assessment	◆ **Clinical history**: look for a history of hypertension, insulin resistance, and lipid abnormalities ◆ **Physical examination**: weight, height, BMI, body fat. Signs/symptoms of arthritis. Assess coordination/mobility ◆ **Resting ECG** ◆ **Exercise capacity**: symptom limited, maximal exercise stress test by cycle ergometry or treadmill (cardiopulmonary exercise test if available); a submaximal test might be warranted e.g. after an extensive myocardial infarction or complications of an MI. Exercise or pharmacological imaging technique in patients with uninterpretable ECG and known CAD ◆ **Baseline echocardiogram** with determination of left ventricular ejection fraction ◆ **Other tests as indicated**: BNP, HbA1c, oral glucose tolerance test Holter R–R measurement etc.

BMI, body mass index; BNP, brain natriuretic peptide.

Box 12.12 Recommendations for exercise training in diabetes mellitus

Established/agreed components:

- 150 minutes (or more) a week of moderate-intensity aerobic physical activity (≥ 4.5 METs) and/or 90 minutes a week of vigorous aerobic exercise (≥ 7.5 METs)
- The physical activity should be for at least 30 minutes on at least 5 days a week
- Resistance training three times a week, targeting all major muscle groups, two to four sets of 7–40 repetitions

Components requiring further evidence:

- Relative benefits of *resistance training* (e.g. eight muscle groups, two sets per muscle group, 8–12 repetitions, 70–80% of RM) versus *endurance training* (e.g. eight muscle groups, two sets per muscle group, 25–30 repetitions, 40–55% of RM)

high-intensity aerobic or resistance training, head-down activities, and jumping/jarring activities.

The recommendations for exercise training in diabetes mellitus are summarized in ➲ Box 12.12.

Future challenges in exercise therapy

We now have well-established scientific evidence for the clinical and prognostic benefits of exercise training in the majority of CVD. More importantly, we are beginning to understand the complex mechanisms by which exercise positively modifies the disease process [10]. Are there any further research challenges left for exercise training in CVD? It is the view of the authors that the following areas will become a focus of research as a result of the changes we are seeing in the patient population:

- Although an increasing number of studies are being published on exercise interventions for geriatric patients we still lack studies comparing different training programmes and types of interventions in regard to their clinical efficacy.
- Women are still underrepresented in exercise programmes in relation to their share of CVD. One reason is that they are affected by CVD at more advanced ages, another is related to social role perceptions that have not yet been adequately targeted.
- Increasing numbers of patients with valvular and congenital heart disease before or after surgical correction live to older ages. We lack larger-scale multicentre studies on appropriate training interventions to prevent CVD in this heterogeneous patient cohort.
- In primary prevention, childhood obesity will be the major challenge for societal exercise programmes at school and in the community. The evidence is there, we need more data on implementation strategies that work and on motivation strategies that catch children's attention.

Solution to the case study

Diagnostic blood tests

Renal function is important for determination of the underlying cause of the patient's oedema (cardiac decompensation versus renal failure) and for potential dose adjustments of the medications. Electrolytes are necessary to monitor for hypokalaemia as a side effect of diuretic therapy and hyperkalaemia resulting from ACE inhibition and aldosterone-antagonist treatment. The full blood count should be part of the routine to rule out anaemia as a negative prognostic indicator and a factor that is exercise limiting.

Apparative diagnostic tests

Echocardiography is needed to measure the left ventricular ejection fraction and look for concomitant functional/structural valvular heart disease. A bicycle ergometer test, if possible with gas exchange measurement, should be done. Chest X-ray is routine. An ICD programming report should be produced indicating detection and intervention thresholds for ventricular arrhythmias. A cardiac MRI is not routinely needed.

Medication/dosage checks

Because of this patient's tachyarrhythmia and pitting oedema it is most important to check digitoxin, beta-blockers, and diuretics.

Prescription of an exercise programme

Although jogging would be possible, this patient needs heart rate monitoring at least when starting the training programme. Interval training is more effective than steady-state endurance training in improving exercise capacity and has similar effects on reverse cardiac remodelling and improved vascular function.

Further reading

Introduction

Gielen S, Schuler G, Adams V. Cardiovascular effects of exercise training: molecular mechanisms. *Circulation* 2010; **122**: 1221–38.

Heran BS, Chen JM, Ebrahim S, et al. Exercise-based cardiac rehabilitation for coronary heart disease. *Cochrane Database Syst Rev* 2011; (7): CD001800.

Wen CP, Wai JPM, Tsai MK, et al. Minimum amount of physical activity for reduced mortality and extended life expectancy: a prospective cohort study. *Lancet* 2011; **378**: 1244–53.

Williams PT. Physical fitness and activity as separate heart disease risk factors: a meta-analysis. *Med Sci Sports Exerc* 2001; **33**: 754–61.

Whole body exercise testing in cardiovascular health and disease

ACSM's resource manual for guidelines for exercise testing and prescription, 2009. Philadelphia, PA: Lippincott Williams & Wilkins.

Farrell PA, Joyner MJ, Caiozzo VJ. *ACSM's advanced exercise physiology*, 2011. Philadelphia, PA: Lippincott Williams & Wilkins.

Mezzani A, Hamm LF, Jones AM, et al. Aerobic exercise intensity assessment and prescription in cardiac rehabilitation: a joint position statement of the European Association for Cardiovascular Prevention and Rehabilitation, the American Association of Cardiovascular and Pulmonary Rehabilitation and the Canadian Association of Cardiac Rehabilitation. *Eur J Prev Cardiol.* 2013; **20**: 442–67.

Local muscle strength testing in cardiovascular health and disease

Bjarnason-Wehrens B, Mayer-Berger W, Meister ER, et al. Recommendations for resistance exercise in cardiac rehabilitation. Recommendations of the German Federation for Cardiovascular Prevention and Rehabilitation. *Eur J Cardiovasc Prev Rehabil* 2004; **11**: 352–61.

Peolsson A, Hedlund R, Oberg B. Intra- and inter-tester reliability and reference values for hand strength. *J Rehabil Med* 2001; **33**: 36–41.

Ruiz JR, Sui X, Lobelo F, et al. Association between muscular strength and mortality in men: prospective cohort study. *Br Med J* 2008; **337**: a439.

Physical exercise in primary prevention

Hamer M, Chida Y. Walking and primary prevention: a meta-analysis of prospective cohort studies. *Br J Sports Med* 2008; **42**: 238–43.

Vanhees L, Sutter J De, Gelada SN, et al. Importance of characteristics and modalities of physical activity and exercise in defining the benefits to cardiovascular health within the general population: recommendations from the EACPR (Part I). *Eur J Prev Cardiol* 2012; **19**: 670–86.

World Health Organization. *Steps to health: a European framework to promote physical activity for health*, 2007. Copenhagen: WHO Regional Office for Europe.

Exercise interventions in cardiovascular diseases

American Association of Cardiovascular and Pulmonary Rehabilitation *Guidelines for cardiac rehabilitation and secondary prevention programs*, 5th edition, 2013. Champaign, IL: Human Kinetics.

American College of Sports Medicine, Chodzko-Zajko WJ, Proctor DN, Fiatarone Singh MA., et al. American College of Sports Medicine position stand. Exercise and physical activity for older adults. *Med Sci Sports Exerc* 2009; **41**: 1510–30.

Butchart EG, Gohlke-Bärwolf C, Antunes MJ, et al. Working Groups on Valvular Heart Disease, Thrombosis, and Cardiac Rehabilitation and Exercise Physiology, European Society of Cardiology. Recommendations for the management of patients after heart valve surgery. *Eur Heart J* 2005; **26**: 2463–71.

Dahabreh IJ, Paulus JK. Association of episodic physical and sexual activity with triggering of acute cardiac events: systematic review and meta-analysis. *J Am Med Assoc* 2011; **305**: 1225–33.

Daniels KM, Arena R, Lavie CJ, et al. Cardiac rehabilitation for women across the lifespan. *Am J Med* 2012; **125**: 937.e1–7.

Joint Task Force on the Management of Valvular Heart Disease of the European Society of Cardiology (ESC), European Association for Cardio-Thoracic Surgery (EACTS), Vahanian A, Alfieri O, Andreotti F, et al. Guidelines on the management of valvular heart disease (version 2012). *Eur Heart J* 2012; **33**: 2451–96.

Piepoli MF, Corrà U, Benzer W, et al/, Cardiac Rehabilitation Section of the European Association of Cardiovascular Prevention and Rehabilitation. Secondary prevention through cardiac rehabilitation: from knowledge to implementation. A position paper from the Cardiac Rehabilitation Section of the European Association of Cardiovascular Prevention and Rehabilitation. *Eur J Cardiovasc Prev Rehabil* 2010; **17**: 1–17.

Piepoli MF, Conraads V, Corrà U, et al. Exercise training in heart failure: from theory to practice. A consensus document of the Heart Failure Association and the European Association for Cardiovascular Prevention and Rehabilitation. *Eur J Heart Fail* 2011; **13**: 347–57.

Piepoli MF, Corrà U, Adamopoulos S, et al. Secondary prevention in the clinical management of patients with cardiovascular diseases. Core components, standards and outcome measures for referral and delivery. *Eur J Prev Cardiol* 2012; **21**: 664–81.

Primary Panel: Moe GW, Ezekowitz JA, O'Meara E, et al., Secondary Panel: Arnold JMO, Ashton T, D'Astous M, et al. The 2013 Canadian Cardiovascular Society heart failure management guidelines update: focus on rehabilitation and exercise and surgical coronary revascularization. *Can J Cardiol* 2014; **30**: 249–63.

Smith SC Jr, Benjamin EJ, Bonow RO, et al. AHA/ACCF secondary prevention and risk reduction therapy for patients with coronary and other atherosclerotic vascular disease: 2011 update: a guideline from the American Heart Association and American College of Cardiology Foundation endorsed by the World Heart Federation and the Preventive Cardiovascular Nurses Association. *J Am Coll Cardiol* 2011; **58**: 2432–46.

Williams MA, Fleg JL, Ades PA, et al. Secondary prevention of coronary heart disease in the elderly (with emphasis on patients > or = 75 years of age): an American Heart Association scientific statement from the Council on Clinical Cardiology Subcommittee on Exercise, Cardiac Rehabilitation, and Prevention. *Circulation* 2002; **105**: 1735–43.

References

1 Wen CP, Wai JPM, Tsai MK, et al. Minimum amount of physical activity for reduced mortality and extended life expectancy: a prospective cohort study. *Lancet* 2011; **378**: 1244–53.

2 Taylor RS, Brown A, Ebrahim S, et al. Exercise-based rehabilitation for patients with coronary heart disease: systematic review and meta-analysis of randomized controlled trials. *Am J Med* 2004; **116**: 682–92.

3 Heran BS, Chen JM, Ebrahim S, et al. Exercise-based cardiac rehabilitation for coronary heart disease. *Cochrane Database Syst Rev* 2011; (7): D001800.

4 Chow CK, Jolly S, Rao-Melacini P, et al. Association of diet, exercise, and smoking modification with risk of early cardiovascular events after acute coronary syndromes. *Circulation* 2010; **121**: 750–8.

5 Piepoli MF, Davos C, Francis DP, et al. Exercise training meta-analysis of trials in patients with chronic heart failure (ExTraMATCH). *Br Med J* 2004; **328**: 189.

6 O'Connor CM, Whellan DJ, Lee KL, et al. Efficacy and safety of exercise training in patients with chronic heart failure: HF-ACTION randomized controlled trial. *J Am Med Assoc* 2009; **301**: 1439–50.

7 Edelmann F, Gelbrich G, Düngen H-D, et al. Exercise training improves exercise capacity and diastolic function in patients with heart failure with preserved ejection fraction: results of the Ex-DHF (Exercise training in Diastolic Heart Failure) pilot study. *J Am Coll Cardiol* 2011; **58**: 1780–91.

8 Mereles D, Ehlken N, Kreuscher S, et al. Exercise and respiratory training improve exercise capacity and quality of life in patients with severe chronic pulmonary hypertension. *Circulation* 2006; **114**: 1482–9.

9 Gielen S, Schuler G, Hambrecht R. Exercise training in coronary artery disease and coronary vasomotion. *Circulation* 2001; **103**: E1–E6.

10 Gielen S, Schuler G, Adams V. Cardiovascular effects of exercise training: molecular mechanisms. *Circulation* 2010; **122**: 1221–38.

11 Neel JV. Diabetes mellitus: a 'thrifty' genotype rendered detrimental by 'progress'? *Am J Hum Genet* 1962; **14**: 353–62.

12 Neel JV, Weder AB, Julius S. Type II diabetes, essential hypertension, and obesity as 'syndromes of impaired genetic homeostasis': the 'thrifty genotype' hypothesis enters the 21st century. *Perspect Biol Med* 1998; **42**: 44–74.

13 Suvorava T, Lauer N, Kojda G. Physical inactivity causes endothelial dysfunction in healthy young mice. *J Am Coll Cardiol* 2004; **44**: 1320–7.

14 Blair SN, Jackson AS. Physical fitness and activity as separate heart disease risk factors: a meta-analysis. *Med Sci Sports Exerc* 2001; **33**: 762–4.

15 Williams PT. Physical fitness and activity as separate heart disease risk factors: a meta-analysis. *Med Sci Sports Exerc* 2001; **33**: 754–61.

16 Morris JN, Everitt MG, Pollard R, et al. Vigorous exercise in leisure-time: protection against coronary heart disease. *Lancet* 1980; **2**: 1207–10.

17 Paffenbarger RJ Jr, Hyde RT, Wing AL, et al. Physical activity, all-cause mortality, and longevity of college alumni. *N Engl J Med* 1986; **314**: 605–13.

18 Sesso HD, Paffenbarger RS, Lee IM. Physical activity and coronary heart disease in men: the Harvard Alumni Health Study. *Circulation* 2000; **102**: 975–80.

19 Slattery ML, Jacobs DR, Nichaman ZM. Leisure time physical activity and coronary heart disease death; the US railroad study. *Circulation* 2001; **79**: 304–11.

20 Blair SN, Kampert JB, Kohl HW, et al. Influences of cardiorespiratory fitness and other precursors on cardiovascular disease and all-cause mortality in men and women. *J Am Med Assoc* 1996; **276**: 205–10.

21 Myers J, Prakash M, Froelicher V, et al. Exercise capacity and mortality among men referred for exercise testing. *N Engl J Med* 2002; **346**: 793–801.

22 Lee I-M, Sesso HD, Oguma Y, et al. Relative intensity of physical activity and risk of coronary heart disease. *Circulation* 2003; **107**: 1110–16.

23 Gibbons RJ, Balady GJ, Bricker JT, et al. ACC/AHA 2002 guideline update for exercise testing: a report of the American College of Cardiology/American Heart Association Task Force on Practice Guidelines (Committee on Exercise Testing). *J Am Coll Cardiol* 2002; **40**: 1531–40.

24 Mieres JH, Shaw LJ, Arai A, et al., Cardiac Imaging Committee, Council on Clinical Cardiology, and the Cardiovascular Imaging and Intervention Committee, Council on Cardiovascular Radiology and Intervention, American Heart Association. Role of noninvasive testing in the clinical evaluation of women with suspected coronary artery disease: consensus statement from the Cardiac Imaging Committee, Council on Clinical Cardiology, and the Cardiovascular Imaging and Intervention Committee, Council on Cardiovascular Radiology and Intervention, American Heart Association. *Circulation* 2005; **111**: 682–96.

25 Wasserman K, Hansen JE, Sue DY, et al. *Principles of exercise testing and interpretation: including pathophysiology and clinical applications*, 5th edn, 2012. Philadelphia, PA: Lippincott, Williams & Wilkins.

26 Myers J, Bellin D. Ramp exercise protocols for clinical and cardiopulmonary exercise testing. *Sports Med* 2000; **30**: 23–9.

27 Mezzani A, Agostoni P, Cohen-Solal A, et al. Standards for the use of cardiopulmonary exercise testing for the functional evaluation of cardiac patients: a report from the Exercise Physiology Section of the European Association for Cardiovascular Prevention and Rehabilitation. *Eur J Cardiovasc Prev Rehabil* 2009; **16**: 249–67.

28 Guazzi M, Adams V, Conraads V, et al., EACPR, AHA. EACPR/AHA Joint Scientific Statement. Clinical recommendations for cardiopulmonary exercise testing data assessment in specific patient populations. *Eur Heart J* 2012; **33**: 2917–27.

29 Kokkinos P, Myers J, Faselis C, et al. Exercise capacity and mortality in older men: a 20-year follow-up study. *Circulation* 2010; **122**: 790–7.

30 Michaelides AP, Tousoulis D, Raftopoulos LG, et al. The impact of novel exercise criteria and indices for the diagnostic and prognostic ability of exercise testing. *Int J Cardiol* 2010; **143**: 119–23.

31 Sharma K, Kohli P, Gulati M. An update on exercise stress testing. *Curr Probl Cardiol* 2012; **37**: 177–202.

32 Kavanagh T, Mertens DJ, Hamm LF, et al. Prediction of long-term prognosis in 12 169 men referred for cardiac rehabilitation. *Circulation* 2002; **106**: 666–71.

33 Mezzani A, Hamm LF, Jones AM, et al. Aerobic exercise intensity assessment and prescription in cardiac rehabilitation: a joint position statement of the European Association for Cardiovascular Prevention and Rehabilitation, the American Association of Cardiovascular and Pulmonary Rehabilitation and the Canadian Association of Cardiac Rehabilitation. *Eur J Prev Cardiol* 2013; **20**: 442–67.

34 Eckart RE, Field ME, Hruczkowski TW, et al. Association of electrocardiographic morphology of exercise-induced ventricular arrhythmia with mortality. *Ann Intern Med* 2008; **149**: 451–60, W82.

35 Sumiyoshi M, Nakata Y, Yasuda M, et al. Clinical and electrophysiologic features of exercise-induced atrioventricular block. *Am Heart J* 1996; **132**: 1277–81.

36 Howley ET, Bassett DR Jr, Welch HG. Criteria for maximal oxygen uptake: review and commentary. *Med Sci Sports Exerc* 1995; **27**: 1292–301.

37 Hamm LF, Crow RS, Stull GA, et al. Safety and characteristics of exercise testing early after acute myocardial infarction. *Am J Cardiol* 1989; **63**: 1193–7.

38 Tristani FE, Hughes CV, Archibald DG, et al. Safety of graded symptom-limited exercise testing in patients with congestive heart failure. *Circulation* 1987; **76**: VI54–V158.

39 Myers J, Arena R, Franklin B, et al., American Heart Association Committee on Exercise, Cardiac Rehabilitation, and Prevention of the Council on Clinical Cardiology, the Council on Nutrition, Physical Activity, and Metabolism, and the Council on Cardiovascular Nursing. Recommendations for clinical exercise laboratories: a scientific statement from the American Heart Association. *Circulation* 2009; **119**: 3144–61.

40 European Stroke Organisation, Tendera M, Aboyans V, Bartelink M-L, et al., ESC Committee for Practice Guidelines. ESC Guidelines on the diagnosis and treatment of peripheral artery diseases: document covering atherosclerotic disease of extracranial carotid and vertebral, mesenteric, renal, upper and lower extremity arteries: the Task Force on the Diagnosis and Treatment of Peripheral Artery Diseases of the European Society of Cardiology (ESC). *Eur Heart J* 2011; **32**: 2851–906.

41 Ehrman JK, American College of Sports Medicine. *ACSM's resource manual for guidelines for exercise testing and prescription*, 2010. Philadelphia, PA: Wolters Kluwer Health/Lippincott Williams & Wilkins.

42 American College of Sports Medicine, Durstine JL, Moore, G, et al. *ACSM's exercise management for persons with chronic diseases and disabilities*, 3rd edn, 2009. Champaign, IL: Human Kinetics.

43 Meyer T, Broocks A. Therapeutic impact of exercise on psychiatric diseases: guidelines for exercise testing and prescription. *Sports Med Auckl NZ* 2000; **30**: 269–79.

44 Ruiz JR, Sui X, Lobelo F, et al. Association between muscular strength and mortality in men: prospective cohort study. *Br Med J* 2008; **337**: a 439.

45 Metter EJ, Talbot LA, Schrager M, Conwit R. Skeletal muscle strength as a predictor of all-cause mortality in healthy men. *J Gerontol A Biol Sci Med Sci* 2002; **57**: B359–B365.

46 Rantanen T, Harris T, Leveille SG, et al. Muscle strength and body mass index as long-term predictors of mortality in initially healthy men. *J Gerontol A Biol Sci Med Sci* 2000; **55**: M168–M173.

47 Rantanen T, Volpato S, Ferrucci L, et al. Handgrip strength and cause-specific and total mortality in older disabled women: exploring the mechanism. *J Am Geriatr Soc* 2003; **51**: 636–41.

48 Gale CR, Martyn CN, Cooper C, et al. Grip strength, body composition, and mortality. *Int J Epidemiol* 2007; **36**: 228–35.

49 Ling CHY, Taekema D, Craen AJM de, et al. Handgrip strength and mortality in the oldest old population: the Leiden 85-plus study. *Can Med Assoc J* 2010; **182**: 429–35.

50 Fried LP, Tangen CM, Walston J, et al., Cardiovascular Health Study Collaborative Research Group. Frailty in older adults: evidence for a phenotype. *J Gerontol A Biol Sci Med Sci* 2001; **56**: M146–M156.

51 Gielen S, Sandri M, Kozarez I, et al. Exercise training attenuates MuRF-1 expression in the skeletal muscle of patients with chronic heart failure independent of age: the randomized Leipzig Exercise Intervention in Chronic Heart Failure and Aging catabolism study. *Circulation* 2012; **125**: 2716–27.

52 Anker SD, Ponikowski P, Varney S, et al. Wasting as independent risk factor for mortality in chronic heart failure. *Lancet* 1997; **349**: 1050–3.

53 Strassburg S, Springer J, Anker SD. Muscle wasting in cardiac cachexia. *Int J Biochem Biol* 2005; **37**: 1938–47.

54 Haehling S von, Lainscak M, Springer J, et al. Cardiac cachexia: a systematic overview. *Pharmacol Ther* 2009; **121**: 227–52.

55 Anker SD, Swan JW, Volterrani M, et al. The influence of muscle mass, strength, fatiguability, and blood flow on exercise capacity in cachectic and non-cachectic patients with chronic heart failure. *Eur Heart J* 1997; **18**: 259–69.

56 Pu CT, Johnson MT, Forman DE, et al. Randomized trial of progressive resistance training to counteract the myopathy of chronic heart failure. *J Appl Physiol* 2001; **90**: 2341–50.

57 Peolsson A, Hedlund R, Oberg B. Intra- and inter-tester reliability and reference values for hand strength. *J Rehabil Med* 2001; **33**: 36–41.

58 Härkönen R, Piirtomaa M, Alaranta H. Grip strength and hand position of the dynamometer in 204 Finnish adults. *J Hand Surg* 1993; **18**: 129–32.

59 Beaton DE, O'Driscoll SW, Richards RR. Grip strength testing using the BTE work simulator and the Jamar dynamometer: a comparative study. Baltimore Therapeutic Equipment. *J Hand Surg* 1995; **20**: 293–8.

60 Crosby CA, Wehbé MA, Mawr B. Hand strength: normative values. *J Hand Surg* 1994; **19**: 665–70.

61 Ploutz-Snyder LL, Giamis EL. Orientation and familiarization to 1RM strength testing in old and young women. *J Strength Cond Res* 2001; **15**: 519–23.

62 Smith SA, Montain SJ, Matott RP, et al. Creatine supplementation and age influence muscle metabolism during exercise. *J Appl Physiol* 1998; **85**: 1349–56.

63 Bjarnason-Wehrens B, Mayer-Berger W, Meister ER, et al. Recommendations for resistance exercise in cardiac rehabilitation. Recommendations of the German Federation for Cardiovascular Prevention and Rehabilitation. *Eur J Cardiovasc Prev Rehabil* 2004; **11**: 352–61.

64 Hammond MD, Bauer KA, Sharp JT, et al. Respiratory muscle strength in congestive heart failure. *Chest* 1990; **98**: 1091–4.

65 Mancini DM, Henson D, LaManca J, et al. Respiratory muscle function and dyspnea in patients with chronic congestive heart failure. *Circulation* 1992; **86**: 909–18.

66 Meyer FJ, Borst MM, Zugck C, et al. Respiratory muscle dysfunction in congestive heart failure: clinical correlation and prognostic significance. *Circulation* 2001; **103**: 2153–8.

67 Mancini DM, Henson D, LaManca J, et al. Benefit of selective respiratory muscle training on exercise capacity in patients with chronic congestive heart failure. *Circulation* 1995; **91**: 320–9.

68 Perk J, Backer G De, Gohlke H, et al., European Association for Cardiovascular Prevention and Rehabilitation (EACPR), ESC Committee for Practice Guidelines (CPG). European guidelines on cardiovascular disease prevention in clinical practice (version 2012). The Fifth Joint Task Force of the European Society of Cardiology and other societies on Cardiovascular Disease Prevention in Clinical Practice (constituted by representatives of nine societies and by invited experts). *Eur Heart J* 2012; **33**: 1635–701.

69 Nocon VM, Hiemann T, Müller-Riemenschneider F, et al. Association of physical activity with all-cause and cardiovascular mortality: a systematic review and meta-analysis. *Eur J Cardiovasc Prev Rehabil* 2008; **15**: 239–46.

70 World Health Organization. *Which are the known causes of and consequences of obesity, and how can it be prevented?*, 2004. Copenhagen: WHO Regional Office for Europe.

71 World Health Organization. *Steps to health: a European framework to promote physical activity for health*, 2007. Copenhagen: WHO Regional Office for Europe.

72 O'Donovan G, Blazevich AJ, Boreham C, et al. The ABC of physical activity for health: a consensus statement from the British Association of Sport and Exercise Sciences. *J Sports Sci* 2010; **28**: 573–91.

73 Vanhees L, Sutter J De, Gelada SN, et al. Importance of characteristics and modalities of physical activity and exercise in defining the benefits to cardiovascular health within the general population: recommendations from the EACPR (Part I). *Eur J Prev Cardiol* 2012; **19**: 670–86.

74 Sluijs EMF van, McMinn AM, Griffin SJ. Effectiveness of interventions to promote physical activity in children and adolescents: systematic review of controlled trials. *Br Med J* 2007; **335**: 703.

75 Daley AJ. Can exergaming contribute to improving physical activity levels and health outcomes in children? *Pediatrics* 2009; **124**: 763–71.

76 National Institute for Health and Care Excellence. *Promoting physical activity in the workplace: full guidance*, 2008. London: NICE. Available from: < http://guidance.nice.org.uk/PH13/Guidance/pdf/English >

77 Goetzel RZ, Ozminkowski RJ, Bruno JA, et al. The long-term impact of Johnson & Johnson's Health & Wellness Program on employee health risks. *J Occup Environ Med* 2002; **44**: 417–24.

78 Burton WN, McCalister KT, Chen C-Y, et al. The association of health status, worksite fitness center participation, and two measures of productivity. *J Occup Environ Med* 2005; **47**: 343–51.

79 Hamer M, Chida Y. Walking and primary prevention: a meta-analysis of prospective cohort studies. *Br J Sports Med* 2008; **42**: 238–43.

80 Hamer M, Chida Y. Active commuting and cardiovascular risk: a meta-analytic review. *Prev Med* 2008; **46**: 9–13.

81 Knuth AG, Hallal PC. Temporal trends in physical activity: a systematic review. *J Phys Act Health* 2009; **6**: 548–59.

82 Jenkins A, Christensen H, Walker JG, et al. The effectiveness of distance interventions for increasing physical activity: a review. *Am J Health Promot* 2009; **24**: 102–17.

83 Kahn E, Ramsey L, Brownson R, et al. The effectiveness of interventions to increase physical activity: a systematic review. *Am J Prev Med* 2002; **22** (4 Suppl.): 73–107.

84 Thompson PD, Franklin BA, Balady GJ, et al., American Heart Association Council on Nutrition, Physical Activity, and Metabolism, American Heart Association Council on Clinical Cardiology, American College of Sports Medicine. Exercise and acute cardiovascular events placing the risks into perspective: a scientific statement from the American Heart Association Council on

Nutrition, Physical Activity, and Metabolism and the Council on Clinical Cardiology. *Circulation* 2007; **115**: 2358–68.

85 Borjesson M, Urhausen A, Kouidi E, et al. Cardiovascular evaluation of middle-aged/senior individuals engaged in leisure-time sport activities: position stand from the sections of exercise physiology and sports cardiology of the European Association of Cardiovascular Prevention and Rehabilitation. *Eur J Cardiovasc Prev Rehabil* 2011; **18**: 446–58.

86 European Association of Cardiovascular Prevention and Rehabilitation Committee for Science Guidelines, Corrà U, Piepoli MF, Carré F, et al. Secondary prevention through cardiac rehabilitation: physical activity counselling and exercise training: key components of the position paper from the Cardiac Rehabilitation Section of the European Association of Cardiovascular Prevention and Rehabilitation. *Eur Heart J* 2010; **31**: 1967–74.

87 American Association of Cardiovascular and Pulmonary Rehabilitation. *Guidelines for cardiac rehabilitation and secondary prevention programs*, 5th edn, 2013. Champaign, IL: Human Kinetics.

88 Scheinowitz M, Harpaz D. Safety of cardiac rehabilitation in a medically supervised, community-based program. *Cardiology* 2005; **103**: 113–17.

89 Mittleman MA. Angina in patients with an active lifestyle. *Eur Heart J* 1996; **17** (Suppl. G): 30–5.

90 Dahabreh IJ, Paulus JK. Association of episodic physical and sexual activity with triggering of acute cardiac events: systematic review and meta-analysis. *J Am Med Assoc* 2011; **305**: 1225–33.

91 Pavy B, Iliou MC, Meurin P, et al., Functional Evaluation and Cardiac Rehabilitation Working Group of the French Society of Cardiology. Safety of exercise training for cardiac patients: results of the French registry of complications during cardiac rehabilitation. *Arch Intern Med* 2006; **166**: 2329–34.

92 Niebauer J, Hambrecht R, Velich T, et al. Attenuated progression of coronary artery disease after 6 years of multifactorial risk intervention: role of physical exercise. *Circulation* 1997; **96**: 2534–41.

93 Schuler G, Hambrecht R, Schlierf G, et al. Regular physical exercise and low-fat diet. Effects on progression of coronary artery disease. *Circulation* 1992; **86**: 1–11.

94 Ornish D, Brown SE, Scherwitz LW, et al. Can lifestyle changes reverse coronary heart disease? The Lifestyle Heart Trial. *Lancet* 1990; **336**: 129–33.

95 Haskell WL, Alderman EL, Fair JM, et al. Effects of intensive multiple risk factor reduction on coronary atherosclerosis and clinical cardiac events in men and women with coronary artery disease. The Stanford Coronary Risk Intervention Project (SCRIP). *Circulation* 1994; **89**: 975–90.

96 Sixt S, Beer S, Blüher M, et al. Long- but not short-term multifactorial intervention with focus on exercise training improves coronary endothelial dysfunction in diabetes mellitus type 2 and coronary artery disease. *Eur Heart J* 2010; **31**: 112–19.

97 Hambrecht R, Niebauer J, Marburger C, et al. Various intensities of leisure time physical activity in patients with coronary artery disease: effects on cardiorespiratory fitness and progression of coronary atherosclerotic lesions. *J Am Coll Cardiol* 1993; **22**: 468–77.

98 Stessman J, Hammerman-Rozenberg R, Cohen A, et al. Physical activity, function, and longevity among the very old. *Arch Intern Med* 2009; **169**: 1476–83.

99 Sandvik L, Erikssen J, Thaulow E, et al. Physical fitness as a predictor of mortality among healthy, middle-aged Norwegian men. *N Engl J Med* 1993; **328**: 533–7.

100 Janssen I, Carson V, Lee I-M, et al. Years of life gained due to leisure-time physical activity in the U.S. *Am J Prev Med* 2013; **44**: 23–9.

101 Boden WE, O'Rourke RA, Teo KK, et al. Optimal medical therapy with or without PCI for stable coronary disease. *N Engl J Med* 2007; **356**: 1503–16.

102 Lee I-M, Shiroma EJ, Lobelo F, et al., Lancet Physical Activity Series Working Group. Effect of physical inactivity on major non-communicable diseases worldwide: an analysis of burden of disease and life expectancy. *Lancet* 2012; **380**: 219–29.

103 Willich S, Lewis M, Lowel H, et al. Physical exertion as a trigger of acute myocardial infarction. *N Engl J Med* 1993; **329**: 1684–90.

104 Mittleman MA, Maclure M, Tofler GH, et al. Triggering of acute myocardial infarction by heavy physical exertion. Protection against triggering by regular exertion. Determinants of Myocardial Infarction Onset Study Investigators. *N Engl J Med* 1993; **329**: 1677–83.

105 Smith SC Jr, Benjamin EJ, Bonow RO, et al. AHA/ACCF secondary prevention and risk reduction therapy for patients with coronary and other atherosclerotic vascular disease: 2011 update: a guideline from the American Heart Association and American College of Cardiology Foundation endorsed by the World Heart Federation and the Preventive Cardiovascular Nurses Association. *J Am Coll Cardiol* 2011; **58**: 2432–46.

106 Nelson ME, Rejeski WJ, Blair SN, et al., American College of Sports Medicine, American Heart Association. Physical activity and public health in older adults: recommendation from the American College of Sports Medicine and the American Heart Association. *Circulation* 2007; **116**: 1094–105.

107 Niebauer J, Mayr K, Tschentscher M, et al. Outpatient cardiac rehabilitation: the Austrian model. *Eur J Prev Cardiol* 2013; **20**: 468–79.

108 Piepoli MF, Corrà U, Benzer W, et al., Cardiac Rehabilitation Section of the European Association of Cardiovascular Prevention and Rehabilitation. Secondary prevention through cardiac rehabilitation: from knowledge to implementation. A position paper from the Cardiac Rehabilitation Section of the European Association of Cardiovascular Prevention and Rehabilitation. *Eur J Cardiovasc Prev Rehabil* 2010; **17**: 1–17.

109 Coats AJ. The muscle hypothesis of chronic heart failure. *J Mol Cell Cardiol* 1996; **28**: 2255–62.

110 Conraads VM, Van Craenenbroeck EM, De Maeyer C, et al. Unraveling new mechanisms of exercise intolerance in chronic heart failure: role of exercise training. *Heart Fail Rev* 2013; **18**: 65–77.

111 Van Craenenbroeck EM, Conraads VM. Mending injured endothelium in chronic heart failure: a new target for exercise training. *Int J Cardiol* 2013; **166**: 310–14.

112 Piepoli MF, Guazzi M, Boriani G, et al., Working Group 'Exercise Physiology, Sport Cardiology and Cardiac Rehabilitation', Italian Society of Cardiology. Exercise intolerance in chronic heart failure: mechanisms and therapies. Part I. *Eur J Cardiovasc Prev Rehabil* 2010; **17**: 637–42.

113 Coats AJ, Adamopoulos S, Radaelli A, et al. Controlled trial of physical training in chronic heart failure. Exercise performance, hemodynamics, ventilation, and autonomic function. *Circulation* 1992; **85**: 2119–31.

114 Belardinelli R, Georgiou D, Cianci G, et al. Randomized, controlled trial of long-term moderate exercise training in chronic heart failure: effects on functional capacity, quality of life, and clinical outcome. *Circulation* 1999; **99**: 1173–82.

115 Hambrecht R, Gielen S, Linke A, et al. Effects of exercise training on left ventricular function and peripheral resistance in patients with chronic heart failure: a randomized trial. *J Am Med Assoc* 2000; **283**: 3095–101.

116 Davies EJ, Moxham T, Rees K, et al. Exercise training for systolic heart failure: Cochrane systematic review and meta-analysis. *Eur J Heart Fail* 2010; **12**: 706–15.

117 Haykowsky MJ, Liang Y, Pechter D, et al. A meta-analysis of the effect of exercise training on left ventricular remodeling in heart failure patients: the benefit depends on the type of training performed. *J Am Coll Cardiol* 2007; **49**: 2329–36.

118 Sandri M, Kozarez I, Adams V, et al. Age-related effects of exercise training on diastolic function in heart failure with reduced ejection fraction: the Leipzig Exercise Intervention in Chronic Heart Failure and Aging (LEICA) Diastolic Dysfunction Study. *Eur Heart J* 2012; **33**: 1758–68.

119 van Tol BAF, Huijsmans RJ, Kroon DW, et al. Effects of exercise training on cardiac performance, exercise capacity and quality of life in patients with heart failure: a meta-analysis. *Eur J Heart Fail* 2006; **8**: 841–50.

120 Keteyian SJ, Leifer ES, Houston-Miller N, et al., HF-ACTION Investigators. Relation between volume of exercise and clinical outcomes in patients with heart failure. *J Am Coll Cardiol* 2012; **60**: 1899–905.

121 Wisloff U, Stoylen A, Loennechen JP, et al. Superior cardiovascular effect of aerobic interval training versus moderate continuous training in heart failure patients: a randomized study. *Circulation* 2007; **115**: 3086–94.

122 Haykowsky MJ, Timmons MP, Kruger C, et al. Meta-analysis of aerobic interval training on exercise capacity and systolic function in patients with heart failure and reduced ejection fractions. *Am J Cardiol* 2013; **111**: 1466–9.

123 Chen Y-M, Zhu M, Zhang Y-X. Combined endurance-resistance training improves submaximal exercise capacity in elderly heart failure patients: a systematic review of randomized controlled trials. *Int J Cardiol* 2013; **166**: 250–2.

124 Mandic S, Myers J, Selig SE. Resistance versus aerobic exercise training in chronic heart failure. *Curr Heart Fail Rep* 2012; **9**: 57–64.

125 Marzolini S, Oh PI, Brooks D. Effect of combined aerobic and resistance training versus aerobic training alone in individuals with coronary artery disease: a meta-analysis. *Eur J Prev Cardiol* 2012; **19**: 81–94.

126 McMurray JJV, Adamopoulos S, Anker SD, et al., ESC Committee for Practice Guidelines. ESC Guidelines for the diagnosis and treatment of acute and chronic heart failure 2012: the Task Force for the Diagnosis and Treatment of Acute and Chronic Heart Failure 2012 of the European Society of Cardiology. Developed in collaboration with the Heart Failure Association (HFA) of the ESC. *Eur Heart J* 2012; **33**: 1787–847.

127 Piepoli MF, Conraads V, Corrà U, et al. Exercise training in heart failure: from theory to practice. A consensus document of the Heart Failure Association and the European Association for Cardiovascular Prevention and Rehabilitation. *Eur J Heart Fail* 2011; **13**: 347–57.

128 Vanhees L, Schepers D, Heidbuchel H, et al. Exercise performance and training in patients with implantable cardioverter-defibrillators and coronary heart disease. *Am J Cardiol* 2001; **87**: 712–15.

129 Vanhees L, Kornaat M, Defoor J, et al. Effect of exercise training in patients with an implantable cardioverter defibrillator. *Eur Heart J* 2004; **25**: 1120–6.

130 Primary Panel: Moe GW, Ezekowitz JA, O'Meara E, et al., Secondary Panel: Arnold JMO, Ashton T, D'Astous M, et al. The 2013 Canadian Cardiovascular Society heart failure management guidelines update: focus on rehabilitation and exercise and surgical coronary revascularization. *Can J Cardiol* 2014; **30**: 249–63.

131 Tjønna AE, Lee SJ, Rognmo Ø, et al. Aerobic interval training versus continuous moderate exercise as a treatment for the metabolic syndrome: a pilot study. *Circulation* 2008; **118**: 346–54.

132 Laoutaris I, Dritsas A, Brown MD, et al. Inspiratory muscle training using an incremental endurance test alleviates dyspnea and improves functional status in patients with chronic heart failure. *Eur J Cardiovasc Prev Rehabil* 2004; **11**: 489–96.

133 Eagle KA, Guyton RA, Davidoff R, et al., American College of Cardiology, American Heart Association Task Force on Practice Guidelines, American Society for Thoracic Surgery and the Society of Thoracic Surgeons. ACC/AHA 2004 guideline update for coronary artery bypass graft surgery: summary article: a report of the American College of Cardiology/American Heart Association Task Force on Practice Guidelines (Committee to Update the 1999 Guidelines for Coronary Artery Bypass Graft Surgery). *Circulation* 2004; **110**: 1168–76.

134 Eagle KA, Guyton RA, Davidoff R, et al. ACC/AHA guidelines for coronary artery bypass graft surgery: executive summary and recommendations: a report of the American College of Cardiology/American Heart Association Task Force on Practice Guidelines (Committee to revise the 1991 guidelines for coronary artery bypass graft surgery). *Circulation* 1999; **100**: 1464–80.

135 Butchart EG, Gohlke-Bärwolf C, Antunes MJ, et al., Working Groups on Valvular Heart Disease, Thrombosis, and Cardiac Rehabilitation and Exercise Physiology, European Society of Cardiology. Recommendations for the management of patients after heart valve surgery. *Eur Heart J* 2005; **26**: 2463–71.

136 Joint Task Force on the Management of Valvular Heart Disease of the European Society of Cardiology (ESC), European Association for Cardio-Thoracic Surgery (EACTS), Vahanian A, Alfieri O, Andreotti F, et al. Guidelines on the management of valvular heart disease (version 2012). *Eur Heart J* 2012; **33**: 2451–96.

137 Piepoli MF, Corrà U, Adamopoulos S, et al. Secondary prevention in the clinical management of patients with cardiovascular diseases. Core components, standards and outcome measures for referral and delivery. *Eur J Prev Cardiol* 2012; **21**: 664–81.

138 Shi Y, Camici GG, Lüscher TF. Cardiovascular determinants of life span. *Pflüg Arch Eur J Physiol* 2010; **459**: 315–24.

139 North BJ, Sinclair DA. The intersection between aging and cardiovascular disease. *Circ Res* 2012; **110**: 1097–108.

140 Hornsby PJ. Senescence and life span. *Pflüg Arch Eur J Physiol* 2010; **459**: 291–9.

141 Forman DE, Rich MW, Alexander KP, et al. Cardiac care for older adults. Time for a new paradigm. *J Am Coll Cardiol* 2011; **57**: 1801–10.

142 Yanowitz FG, LaMonte MJ. Physical activity and health in the elderly. *Curr Sports Med Rep* 2002; **1**: 354–61.

143 Gremeaux V, Gayda M, Lepers R, et al. Exercise and longevity. *Maturitas* 2012; **73**: 312–17.

144 Mora S, Cook N, Buring JE, et al. Physical activity and reduced risk of cardiovascular events: potential mediating mechanisms. *Circulation* 2007; **116**: 2110–18.

145 American College of Sports Medicine, Chodzko-Zajko WJ, Proctor DN, Fiatarone Singh MA, et al. American College of Sports Medicine position stand. Exercise and physical activity for older adults. *Med Sci Sports Exerc* 2009; **41**: 1510–30.

146 Williams MA, Fleg JL, Ades PA, et al., American Heart Association Council on Clinical Cardiology Subcommittee on Exercise, Cardiac Rehabilitation, and Prevention. Secondary prevention of coronary heart disease in the elderly (with emphasis on patients > or = 75 years of age): an American Heart Association scientific statement from the Council on Clinical Cardiology Subcommittee on Exercise, Cardiac Rehabilitation, and Prevention. *Circulation* 2002; **105**: 1735–43.

147 Sattelmair JR, Pertman JH, Forman DE. Effects of physical activity on cardiovascular and noncardiovascular outcomes in older adults. *Clin Geriatr Med* 2009; **25**: 677–702, viii-ix.

148 Hollmann W, Strüder HK, Tagarakis CVM, et al. Physical activity and the elderly. *Eur J Cardiovasc Prev Rehabil* 2007; **14**: 730–9.

149 Keogh JWL, Kilding A, Pidgeon P, et al. Physical benefits of dancing for healthy older adults: a review. *J Aging Phys Act* 2009; **17**: 479–500.
150 Marques EA, Mota J, Machado L, et al. Multicomponent training program with weight-bearing exercises elicits favorable bone density, muscle strength, and balance adaptations in older women. *Calcif Tissue Int* 2011; **88**: 117–29.
151 Orr R. Contribution of muscle weakness to postural instability in the elderly. A systematic review. *Eur J Phys Rehabil Med* 2010; **46**: 183–220.
152 Ryan AS. Insulin resistance with aging: effects of diet and exercise. *Sports Med* 2000; **30**: 327–46.
153 Hills AP, Shultz SP, Soares MJ, et al. Resistance training for obese, type 2 diabetic adults: a review of the evidence. *Obes Rev* 2010; **11**: 740–9.
154 Physical Activity Guidelines Committee. *Physical Activity Guidelines Advisory Committee report, 2008*, 2008. Washington, DC: US Department of Health and Human Services.
155 Pelliccia A, Maron BJ, Culasso F, et al. Athlete's heart in women. Echocardiographic characterization of highly trained elite female athletes. *J Am Med Assoc* 1996; **276**: 211–15.
156 Carvalho EEV, Crescêncio JC, Elias J, et al. Improved endothelial function and reversal of myocardial perfusion defects after aerobic physical training in a patient with microvascular myocardial ischemia. *Am J Phys Med Rehabil* 2011; **90**: 59–64.
157 Daniels KM, Arena R, Lavie CJ, et al. Cardiac rehabilitation for women across the lifespan. *Am J Med* 2012; **125**: 937.e 1–7.
158 Figueroa A, Park SY, Seo DY, et al. Combined resistance and endurance exercise training improves arterial stiffness, blood pressure, and muscle strength in postmenopausal women. *Menopause* 2011; **18**: 980–4.
159 Committee on Obstetric Practice. ACOG Committee opinion. Exercise during pregnancy and the postpartum period. *Int J Gynaecol Obstet* 2002; **77**: 79–81.
160 Kardel KR, Kase T. Training in pregnant women: effects on fetal development and birth. *Am J Obstet Gynecol* 1998; **178**: 280–6.
161 Juhl M, Andersen PK, Olsen J, et al. Physical exercise during pregnancy and the risk of preterm birth: a study within the Danish National Birth Cohort. *Am J Epidemiol* 2008; **167**: 859–66.
162 Juhl M, Kogevinas M, Andersen PK, et al. Is swimming during pregnancy a safe exercise? *Epidemiology* 2010; **21**: 253–8.
163 Zhang C, Solomon CG, Manson JE, et al. A prospective study of pregravid physical activity and sedentary behaviors in relation to the risk for gestational diabetes mellitus. *Arch Intern Med* 2006; **166**: 543–8.
164 Dempsey JC, Sorensen TK, Williams MA, et al. Prospective study of gestational diabetes mellitus risk in relation to maternal recreational physical activity before and during pregnancy. *Am J Epidemiol* 2004; **159**: 663–70.
165 Koltyn KF, Schultes SS. Psychological effects of an aerobic exercise session and a rest session following pregnancy. *J Sports Med Phys Fitness* 1997; **37**: 287–91.
166 Jakicic JM, Clark K, Coleman E, et al., American College of Sports Medicine. American College of Sports Medicine position stand. Appropriate intervention strategies for weight loss and prevention of weight regain for adults. *Med Sci Sports Exerc* 2001; **33**: 2145–56.
167 Donnelly JE, Blair SN, Jakicic JM, et al., American College of Sports Medicine. American College of Sports Medicine Position Stand. Appropriate physical activity intervention strategies for weight loss and prevention of weight regain for adults. *Med Sci Sports Exerc* 2009; **41**: 459–71.
168 Zeni AI, Hoffman MD, Clifford PS. Energy expenditure with indoor exercise machines. *J Am Med Assoc* 1996; **275**: 1424–7.
169 Poirier P, Després JP. Exercise in weight management of obesity. *Cardiol Clin* 2001; **19**: 459–70.
170 Washburn RA, Donnelly JE, Smith BK, et al. Resistance training volume, energy balance and weight management: rationale and design of a 9 month trial. *Contemp Clin Trials* 2012; **33**: 749–58.
171 Colberg SR, Albright AL, Blissmer BJ, et al., American College of Sports Medicine, American Diabetes Association. Exercise and type 2 diabetes: American College of Sports Medicine and the American Diabetes Association: joint position statement. Exercise and type 2 diabetes. *Med Sci Sports Exerc* 2010; **42**: 2282–303.
172 Chakravarthy MV, Booth FW. Eating, exercise, and 'thrifty' genotypes: connecting the dots toward an evolutionary understanding of modern chronic diseases. *J Appl Physiol* 2004; **96**: 3–10.
173 Leon AS, Connett J, Jacobs DR Jr, et al. Leisure-time physical activity levels and risk of coronary heart disease and death. The Multiple Risk Factor Intervention Trial. *J Am Med Assoc* 1987; **258**: 2388–95.
174 Manson JE, Greenland P, LaCroix AZ, et al. Walking compared with vigorous exercise for the prevention of cardiovascular events in women. *N Engl J Med* 2002; **347**: 716–25.
175 Williams MA. Exercise testing in cardiac rehabilitation. Exercise prescription and beyond. *Cardiol Clin* 2001; **19**: 415–31.

CHAPTER 13

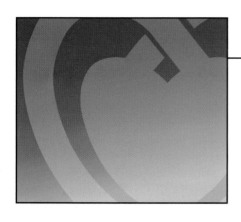

Overweight, obesity, and abdominal adiposity

Gabriele Riccardi and Maria Masulli

Contents

Summary

Obesity is a serious chronic disease of epidemic and global proportions; it is often associated, particularly when body fat is predominantly visceral, with cardiovascular risk factors such as dyslipidaemia (high triglycerides, low high-density lipoprotein cholesterol, and abnormal low-density lipoprotein composition, i.e. the presence of small, dense low-density lipoprotein particles), hypertension and left ventricular hypertrophy and impaired glucose tolerance/diabetes, a cluster making up metabolic syndrome. The incidence of cardiovascular diseases (CVD) is increased in obese people. Since overweight and obesity are associated with decreased lifespan, weight loss might be expected to improve long-term survival and have beneficial effects on CVD risk. The therapeutic approaches to obesity are lifestyle changes, drugs, and bariatric surgery. Lifestyle modifications focused on modest (5–10%) weight loss and moderate-intensity physical activity can significantly reduce the incidence of type 2 diabetes and other cardiometabolic risk factors. A low-fat (low saturated fat) diet, rich in fruit and vegetables as well as legumes and whole grains and poor in sugars, should be advised for its beneficial impact on weight and cardiovascular risk. The three main weight-reducing drugs are orlistat (currently available) and sibutramine and rimonabant, which have been withdrawn from the market as a result of cardiovascular and neuropsychiatric effects, respectively. Bariatric surgery represents an effective treatment for severe obesity and has a beneficial impact on survival, cardiovascular risk factors, prevention/remission of chronic diseases (hypertension, hyperlipidaemia, and diabetes), and cardiovascular events. Prevention of obesity at the population level will probably play a major role in combating the current obesity epidemic. Combining different intervention strategies is probably the best choice for maximizing the effects and minimizing the costs.

Case study

A 60-year-old white man goes to his general practitioner (GP) for a check-up. He works for an insurance company, doesn't smoke, and doesn't drink alcohol regularly. His family history is positive for type 2 diabetes (mother), obesity and hypertension (mother and father), and cardiovascular disease (his father suffered a myocardial infarction at the age of 59). His past medical history is negative for metabolic disorders, cardiovascular, renal, or liver disease. At the physical examination he has a BMI of 28 kg/m^2 and a waist circumference of 107 cm. The patient refers to a weight gain of several kilograms over the past 2 years; he does not follow any specific diet and eats out at restaurants or has fast food several times a week. Moreover, he works long hours and has a sedentary lifestyle. His blood pressure is 144/92 mmHg. The

(continued)

Case study *(continued)*

rest of the physical examination is unremarkable. The GP prescribes laboratory tests which show thyroid, renal, and hepatic function to be within normal limits. Metabolic assessment shows: fasting blood glucose 95 mg/dl; total cholesterol 260 mg/dl; triglycerides 190 mg/dl; low-density lipoprotein 181 mg/dl; high-density lipoprotein 38 mg/dl.

You need to consider the following questions:

- What is the diagnosis?
- What is the calculated 10-year risk for a cardiovascular event in this patient?
- What is the best therapeutic approach?

Introduction

Obesity is a serious chronic disease of epidemic and global proportions: the prevalence of obesity has been increasing at a frightening rate over the past few decades. This multifactorial disease particularly threatens the health of younger generations. Overweight and obesity represent risk factors for the onset of different chronic diseases that are responsible for 60% of deaths worldwide. Globally, about 1.5 billion adults are overweight, and among these 500 million are obese [1]. These numbers have doubled since 1980, and projections estimate that by 2015 about 2.5 billion adults will be overweight and 700 million obese. Globalization may exacerbate the uneven dietary development between rich and poor: while high-income groups in developing countries enjoy the benefits of a more dynamic marketplace, lower-income groups may experience convergence towards poor-quality diets. Many developing countries are in a 'nutrition transition' implicated in the rapid rise of obesity and diet-related chronic diseases worldwide.

Overweight, obesity, and life expectancy

Obesity is associated with many severe comorbidities. Metabolic abnormalities, such as dyslipidaemia, hypertension, and left ventricular hypertrophy, impaired glucose tolerance, and diabetes, form a cluster known as metabolic syndrome, a predictor of atherosclerosis and cardiovascular disease (CVD). Other diseases, such as non-alcoholic fatty liver disease and cholelithiasis, cancer, sleep apnoea/sleep-disordered breathing, and osteoarthritis are also a consequence of obesity, and may induce significant physical disability.

Quality of life is often impaired in obese people due to the presence of comorbidities and social limitations. Life expectancy is also reduced: large epidemiological studies such as the Prospective Studies Collaboration, the Cancer Prevention Study II, and the European Prospective Study, have shown that overweight and obesity are associated with increased all-cause mortality [2].

The relationship between mortality and overweight or obesity is controversial. There is a J-shaped relationship between body mass index (BMI) and the risk of death, with the highest risk in the lowest and the highest BMI categories. A possible confounder in the relationship between underweight and mortality could be represented by smoking, since this is associated with a lower BMI and an increased risk of cardiovascular, respiratory, and neoplastic death. Results from an analysis of pooled data from 19 prospective studies (➲ Fig. 13.1), including 1.46 million white adults aged 19 to 84 years followed up for 10 years, has confirmed the J-shaped relationship between obesity and all-cause mortality. Among healthy people who have never smoked, the hazard ratios (HRs) for all-cause mortality (taking normal weight individuals as the reference group) were 1.47 (95% CI 1.33–1.62) in underweight people, 1.13 (95% CI 1.09–1.17) in overweight subjects, 1.44 (95% CI 1.38–1.50) for those in obesity class I (BMI 30–34.9 kg/m^2), 1.88 (95% CI 1.77–2.00) for those in obesity class II (BMI 35–39.9 kg/m^2), and 2.51 (95% CI 2.30–2.73) for those in obesity class III (BMI 40.0–49.9 kg/m^2). The increased HR in underweight people reduced as the length of follow-up increased. This finding can be explained by the confounding effect of pre-existing (undiagnosed or unreported) diseases and disease-related weight loss that could contribute to the excess mortality in underweight people. The association between underweight and mortality was also attenuated in participants who reported higher levels of physical activity. The HR per five-unit increase in BMI was 1.31 (95% CI 1.29–1.33) for the BMI range of 25 to 50 kg/m^2 [3].

An obese person with a BMI between 30 and 35 kg/m^2 has a life expectancy that is 4–5 years lower than the life expectancy of a person of normal weight. A recent study conducted in the US population has also predicted that if the prevalence of obesity continues to grow at the present rate, by year 2050 average life expectancy will have to be adjusted downward by at least 5 years. In other words, the trend towards higher rates of obesity in United States over time will have a negative impact on the health of the population (longevity and quality of life) which will outweigh any benefits resulting from the continued reductions in the number of smokers [4].

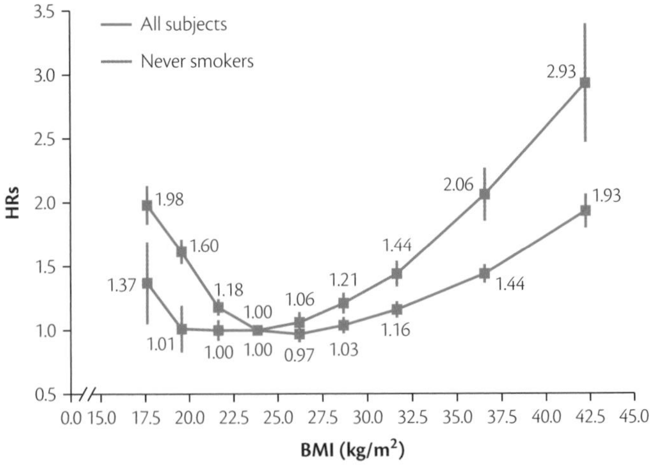

Fig. 13.1 Estimated hazard ratios for death according to increasing BMI categories.

Source: data from Flegal KM, Kit BK, Orpana H, Graubard BI. Association of all-cause mortality with overweight and obesity using standard body mass index categories: a systematic review and meta-analysis. *JAMA* 2013 Jan 2; **309**(1): 71–82.

Obesity, and in particular abdominal adiposity, affects lifespan mostly because it is associated with an increased risk of metabolic, cardiovascular, and cancer events. However, there is a large and continually growing body of evidence indicating that excess body weight is associated with a more favourable prognosis in patients with CVD, including heart failure [5,6]. This phenomenon has been called the 'obesity paradox'. Observational studies consistently show that patients with heart failure who are overweight or obese have a significantly lower mortality risk compared with those of normal weight.

There are several potential explanations for the obesity paradox. First, selection bias may be a contributing factor: excess body weight can cause dyspnoea/peripheral oedema for reasons not related to heart failure, thus leading to an early diagnosis of heart failure at a stage when myocardial impairment is not yet severe. This could also explain why obese patients with heart failure are managed more effectively, and enjoy a better prognosis. Alternatively, only the healthiest of the obese patients may be surviving for long enough to develop heart failure. In addition, potential confounders such as smoking, unrecognized systemic illness, or unintentional weight loss may potentially account for paradoxical results.

On the other hand, it is possible that excess body weight really is protective in relation to cardiovascular mortality. Chronic heart failure is a catabolic state, and the development of wasting, characterized by loss of muscle, bone, and fat, is a marker of more severe disease. Many patients with heart failure are malnourished, whereas moderately obese patients with chronic heart failure may tolerate the metabolic stress better than lean individuals. Moreover, altered cytokine and neuroendocrine profiles of obese patients play a role in modulating the progression of heart failure.

Keypoints

Overweight and obesity are associated with increased all-cause mortality. There is a J-shaped relation between BMI and the risk of death, with the highest risk in the lowest and highest categories of BMI.

Overweight in patients with heart failure is associated with a lower risk of mortality and better prognosis. This phenomenon is called the 'obesity paradox'.

Cardiovascular events in people with overweight, obesity, and abdominal adiposity

Both cross-sectional and prospective studies have shown a close relationship between excessive body fat and premature cardiovascular morbidity and mortality [7,8].

In the 1980s, the Framingham Heart Study, a large 26-year follow-up prospective study, showed that the BMI was an important predictor of cardiovascular disease (myocardial infarction and stroke), particularly among the younger members of the cohort [9]. This finding was confirmed by a more recent study, the MELANY study, suggesting that overweight children and adolescents are at increased risk of diabetes and coronary heart disease, independently of their adult BMI [10]. In particular, this study showed that adolescent BMI is a significant predictor of the incidence of angiography-proven coronary heart disease in adult life across the entire BMI range: the risk of coronary heart disease increases by 12% for each one-unit increment in BMI.

Several studies have clearly shown that the distribution of body fat, especially abdominal fat, is predictive of both prevalent and incident coronary heart disease and cerebrovascular disease, this relation being largely independent of total body fat. Since BMI provides a crude measurement of total adiposity, and is an inadequate index of regional body fat distribution, measures of central obesity, such as waist circumference and waist-to-hip ratio, have to be utilized in order to get a more accurate prediction of the cardiovascular risk associated with excessive accumulation of body fat in the splanchnic region, even in subjects with a normal BMI [8].

Central obesity is recognized as a key driver of metabolic syndrome, a clustering of multiple cardiovascular and metabolic abnormalities, including atherogenic dyslipidaemia, hypertension, elevated fasting insulin/insulin resistance, hyperglycaemia, plus a pro-thrombotic and pro-inflammatory state. Metabolic syndrome has been recognized as a predictor of diabetes and CVD. Multiple definitions have been proposed for the syndrome since it was first postulated. The definitions of the World Health Organization (WHO) [11] and the European Group for the Study of Insulin Resistance (EGIR) [12] emphasize the presence of insulin resistance for the diagnosis. The definition of the International Diabetes Federation (IDF) [13] requires the presence of central obesity for the diagnosis. The definition of the Adult Treatment Panel III (ATP III) [14] is more clinically oriented and is based on the presence of at least three factors among the five listed in ➲ Table 13.1.

Table 13.1 Criteria for the definition of metabolic syndrome according to the Adult Treatment Panel III (ATP III) [14]

Components of metabolic syndrome	ATP III definition*
Waist circumference	M: >102 cm F: >88 cm
Triglycerides	≥150 mg/dl
HDL cholesterol	M: <40 mg/dl F: <50 mg/dl
Systolic/diastolic blood pressure	≥130/≥85 mmHg or antihypertensive drugs
Fasting glycaemia	≥100 mg/dl or antihyperglycaemic drugs

*At least three of the components required.

M, males; F, females.

From Grundy SM, Cleeman JI, Daniels SR, Donato KA, Eckel RH, Franklin BA, Gordon DJ, Krauss RM, Savage PJ, Smith SC Jr, Spertus JA, Costa F; American Heart Association; National Heart, Lung, and Blood Institute. Diagnosis and management of the metabolic syndrome: an American Heart Association/National Heart, Lung, and Blood Institute Scientific Statement. *Circulation*. 2005 Oct 25; **112**(17): 2735–52.

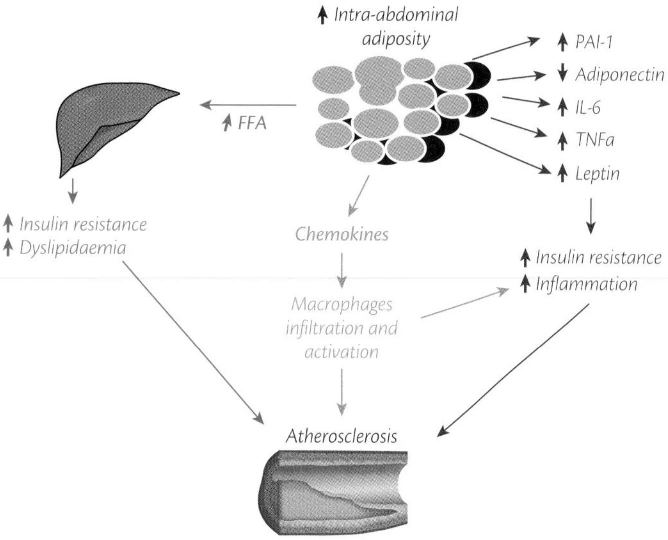

Fig. 13.2 Intra-abdominal adiposity promotes insulin resistance and increases the cardiovascular risk [15].

Increased waist circumference is a marker of the accumulation of visceral fat: impaired insulin sensitivity has been proposed as the link between obesity, and in particular visceral adiposity, and cardiovascular risk factors clustering in the metabolic syndrome; they contribute to the increased rate of events observed in obesity, particularly when fat is predominantly found in the abdominal region.

The mechanisms by which abdominal adiposity leads to atherosclerosis are shown in ➲ Fig. 13.2. Excess body fat leads to an alteration in the profile of hormones secreted by adipose tissue (adipokines) that cause insulin resistance and vascular inflammation; they promote activation of macrophages and their infiltration in the vessel wall, facilitating the atherosclerotic process. Visceral adiposity is often associated with endothelial upregulation of the adhesion molecules and hypercoagulability. The inflammatory background is also probably promoted by a concomitant deficit of nitric oxide, which also appears to decrease the vasodilator properties of perivascular adipose tissue, leading to hypoxia, inflammation, and oxidative stress. Increased visceral adiposity leads to increased mobilization of free fatty acids (FFA) into the portal vein, resulting in hepatic insulin resistance [15].

Keypoints

Obesity, and in particular visceral obesity, is associated with an increased rate of cardiovascular events.

Overweight and obesity in childhood predict the risk of coronary heart disease and diabetes in adulthood independently of the adult BMI.

Visceral adiposity is the key driver of metabolic syndrome, that is a clustering of multiple cardiovascular and metabolic abnormalities (dyslipidaemia, hypertension, elevated fasting insulin/insulin resistance, hyperglycaemia, and pro-thrombotic and pro-inflammatory state).

Metabolic syndrome has been recognized as a predictor of diabetes and CVD.

Cardiovascular risk factors in people with overweight, obesity, and abdominal adiposity

Many epidemiological studies have clearly shown that obesity, particularly of the abdominal type, increases the risk of CVD both directly and by promoting the occurrence of comorbid conditions such as diabetes, hyperlipidaemia, and hypertension.

Overweight, obesity, and diabetes

Obesity is strictly related to type 2 diabetes mellitus. Longitudinal studies have demonstrated that a higher BMI is a strong predictor for developing type 2 diabetes, with a linear increase in diabetes risk across the whole spectrum of BMI but highest in obese subjects with BMI > 30 kg/m^2. Moreover, individuals who were obese as adolescents (versus adult onset) are more likely to have diabetes in young adulthood, independent of current body weight, with the highest risk being among those with persistent obesity from their teens to adult years [10].

In a multivariate model adjusted for age, family history of diabetes, systolic and diastolic blood pressure, physical activity, and glucose and triglyceride levels, adolescent BMI was a predictor of incident diabetes, with a significantly increased risk observed for the three highest BMI deciles (HR in the highest BMI group versus the lowest 2.76, 95% CI 2.11–3.58) (➲ Fig. 13.3). The risk of diabetes increased by 9.8% for each one-unit increment in BMI.

For a given BMI, the distribution of visceral rather than subcutaneous body fat confers greater risk of metabolic abnormalities, and in particular of type 2 diabetes. Prospective studies have shown that waist circumference is a better predictor of the risk of developing diabetes than most other measures of adiposity (BMI, waist-to-hip ratio, iliac circumference) [16].

Overweight, obesity, and hypertension

Obesity is recognized as one of the most important risk factors for the development of hypertension. The relation between adiposity and blood pressure appears to be linear. Obese individuals exhibit higher levels of office as well as ambulatory blood pressure. Obese subjects have higher blood pressure than non-obese individuals even in the normotensive range. Many large epidemiological studies have shown a relationship between body weight and blood pressure. In the Framingham Study, the prevalence of hypertension in obese individuals was twice that in subjects of normal weight. This relationship has been demonstrated in both sexes, in all age groups, and in several ethnic groups [17].

There are several mechanisms linking obesity and hypertension. Clinical and experimental studies have demonstrated the presence of sympathetic hyperactivity, accelerated regional kinetics of catecholamines, excited neuromuscular activity, dysregulation in sodium-modulator hormones, and pre-clinical left ventricular dysfunction in obese subjects. These factors contribute to the development of arterial hypertension. Moreover, the renin–angiotensin–aldosterone system and abnormal renal sodium handling play a critical role in the regulation of cardiovascular homeostasis.

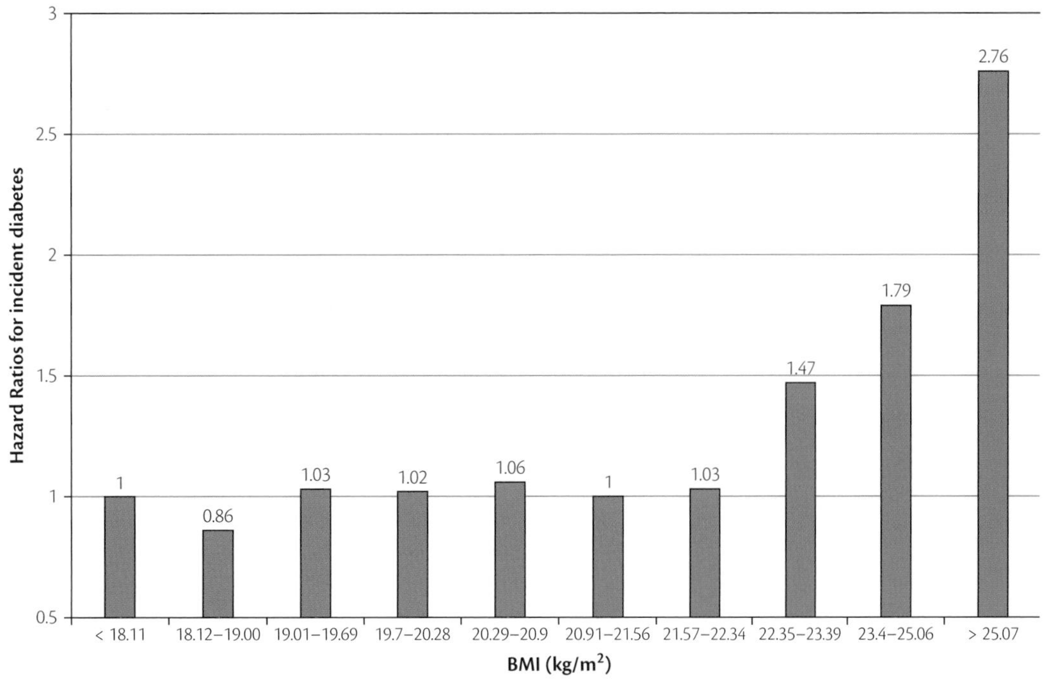

Fig. 13.3 Hazard ratios (HR) for incident diabetes in adulthood according to BMI categories in adolescence. In a multivariate model (adjusted for age, family history of diabetes, systolic and diastolic blood pressure, physical activity, and glucose and triglyceride levels), adolescent BMI was a predictor of incident diabetes, with a significantly increased risk observed for the three highest BMI deciles (HR in the highest BMI group versus the lowest is 2.76, 95% CI 2.11–3.58).

Overweight, obesity, and dyslipidaemia

Obese people often have increased triglycerides, decreased levels of high-density lipoprotein (HDL), and abnormal low-density lipoprotein (LDL) composition (a higher proportion of small, dense LDL particles) [18]. The pathogenesis of dyslipidaemia associated with obesity is closely related to insulin resistance (➲ Fig. 13.4); it plays a major role in the development of atherosclerosis and CVD in obese individuals.

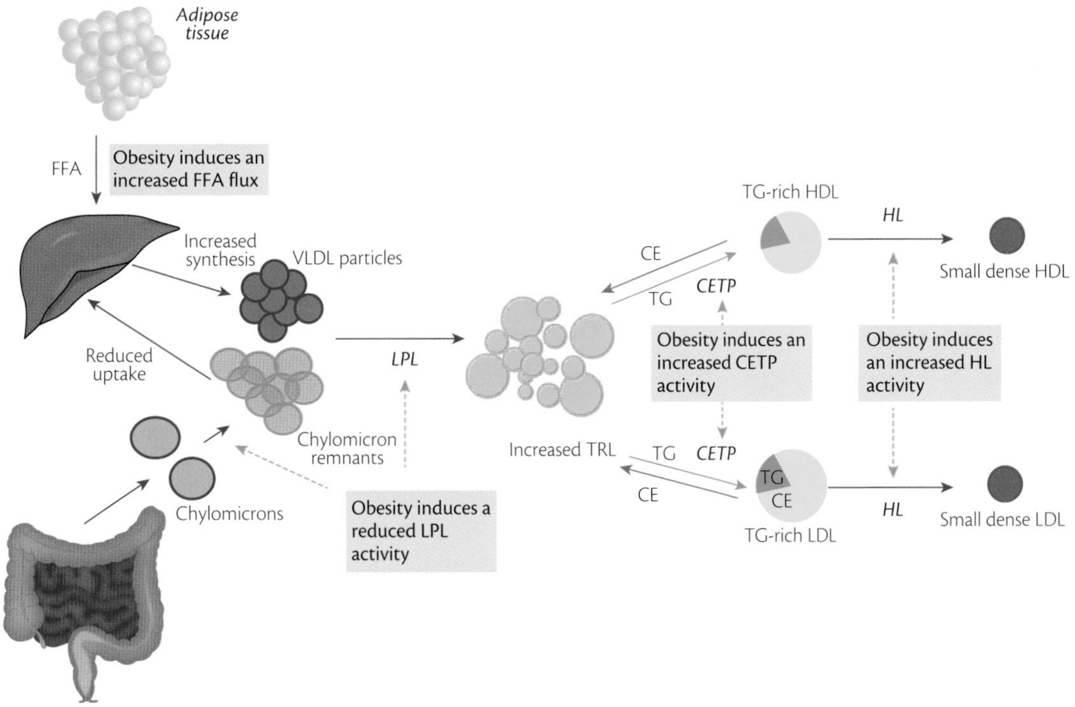

Fig. 13.4 Major abnormalities in lipid metabolism induced by obesity. FFA, free fatty acids; VLDL, very low-density lipoprotein; LPL, lipoprotein lipase; TRL, triglyceride-rich lipoprotein; CETP, cholesterol ester transfer protein; CE, cholesterol ester; TG, triglycerides; LDL, low-density lipoprotein; HL, hepatic lipase; HDL, high-density lipoprotein.

Obesity is always associated with increases in plasma triglycerides. The hepatic overproduction of very low-density lipoprotein (VLDL) appears to be the primary impairment in an insulin-resistant state. Inability to suppress hepatic glucose production, impaired muscle glucose uptake and oxidation, and inability to suppress release of FFA from adipose tissue are the most important consequences of insulin resistance in liver, muscle, and adipose tissue, respectively. These events induce an increased flux of FFA to the liver (FFA being an important regulator of hepatic VLDL production). In addition to increased VLDL synthesis, obesity and insulin resistance are also associated with a decreased clearance of VLDL particles. Since lipoprotein lipase (LPL) activity and mass are decreased in insulin-resistant subjects, the clearance of VLDL is also decreased.

Obesity is also associated with decreased HDL cholesterol. A difference in 10 mg/dl (0.26 mmol/L) in HDL has been found between normal weight and obese subjects. Longitudinal data obtained from the Framingham Offspring Study have confirmed this association, and have shown that the increase of 1 BMI unit is associated with a decrease in HDL cholesterol of 3 mg/dl (0.08 mmol/L) over an 8-year follow-up period.

The effects of obesity on LDL concentrations are less consistent. Several studies have demonstrated that obesity is associated with a change in LDL composition—LDL particles in overweight/obese subjects are smaller and denser, and therefore more atherogenic, than in subjects of normal weight.

Keypoints

The typical dyslipidaemia associated with obesity, and in particular with abdominal adiposity, is characterized by high triglycerides, low HDL cholesterol, and abnormal LDL composition (the presence of small, dense LDL particles).

This pattern of dyslipidaemia associated with obesity is closely related to the impairment of insulin sensitivity and is predictive of atherosclerosis and increased cardiovascular risk.

Benefits of weight reduction on cardiovascular events in overweight or obese people

Since overweight and obesity are associated with a decreased lifespan, increased prevalence of cardiovascular risk factors, and higher rates of cardiovascular events, weight loss might be expected to improve long-term survival and to have many beneficial effects on cardiovascular risk factors.

The relation between weight loss and mortality is debated, with observational studies suggesting no change, reduced, or improved mortality subsequent to weight loss. This discrepancy concerning the effects of weight loss on mortality has been particularly related to the inability of observational studies to discriminate between intentional and unintentional weight loss. Thus, weight loss might be the consequence of conditions that lead to death (e.g. cancer) rather than the cause of increased mortality. However, observational epidemiological studies based on American Cancer Society data have suggested that intentional weight loss is associated with decreased mortality, although the information on intentionality was based on retrospective, self-reported data collected at baseline [19–21].

The therapeutic approaches used for the treatment of obesity are lifestyle changes (diet and physical activity), drugs, and bariatric surgery.

Lifestyle changes

Weight loss obtained by lifestyle intervention has been proven to be effective in reducing the incidence of diabetes and other cardiovascular risk factors. A modest decrease in body weight appears to be able to increase insulin sensitivity, and therefore improve the overall profile of metabolic derangements and cardiovascular risk factors clustering with insulin resistance.

The first report was by Pan et al. from China [22]. They showed a reduction in the incidence of new cases of diabetes of 31% with dietary changes, 46% with exercise, and 42% with both after 6 years of follow-up. The first scientifically robust evidence on the impact of weight reduction on incidence of type 2 diabetes came from Finland in 2001 [23] and the United States in 2002 [24], establishing beyond doubt that type 2 diabetes can be prevented in people at increased risk.

Both studies demonstrated that intensive lifestyle modifications in people with impaired glucose tolerance who were overweight reduced the risk of developing type 2 diabetes by approximately 60%. The interventions differed slightly but included a modest reduction in weight, frequent moderate exercise, and a healthy diet.

In both studies, dietary change involved a reduction in the intakes of fats and refined carbohydrates (e.g. sweets) and increased consumption of fruit, vegetables, and wholegrain cereals; neither adopted a target for reducing calorie intake. By contrast, there were targets for weight loss. In the Finnish study, the target was a reduction of 5% of the baseline weight. After 1 year, mean weight loss was 4.7% (4.2 kg) in the intervention group and 0.9% (0.8 kg) in controls; after 2 years the intervention group regained some weight (mean loss from baseline 3.9%, 3.5 kg) but controls were unchanged. Mean waist circumference also decreased more in the intervention group (by 4.4 cm versus 1.3 cm). The US study set a more ambitious target of a 7% reduction of the baseline weight; among those receiving intensive lifestyle advice, 50% achieved the target at 24 weeks but only 38% sustained this at the last visit (i.e. after up to 4 years). Mean weight loss during the study was 0.1 kg with standard lifestyle advice, 2.1 kg with the addition of metformin, and 5.6 kg with intensive lifestyle advice. Towards the end of the study mean body weights remained substantially different among the three intervention groups, but they were beginning to converge.

The Diabetes Prevention Program Outcomes Study (DPPOS) is a long-term (10 years) follow-up of the US Diabetes Prevention Program (DPP) designed to investigate whether the delay in development of diabetes seen during the DPP could be sustained and to assess the long-term effects of the interventions on health [25]. This study has shown that the cumulative incidence of diabetes remained lower in the lifestyle and metformin groups than in the placebo group. During follow-up, the incidence rate of diabetes in the lifestyle group was reduced by 34% (95% CI 24–42) and in the metformin group by 18% (95% CI 7–28) compared with placebo. The lifestyle effect was greatest in participants aged 60–85 years at randomization (49% rate reduction), in whom metformin had no significant effect. In this study, onset of diabetes was delayed by about 4 years by lifestyle intervention and 2 years by metformin compared with placebo. The lifestyle intervention also resulted in improved blood pressure and plasma lipid concentrations despite a reduction in drug treatment.

The Finnish Diabetes Prevention Study used an approach similar to that in the DPP lifestyle group. During the 4-year active intervention, diabetes incidence was reduced by 58%. Although the intervention was not actively delivered during the 3-year follow-up it remained effective, with a 39% reduction in incidence of diabetes during the observation period.

Together, these studies demonstrate that relatively modest changes in diet, but particularly a reduction in fat intake, an increase in exercise, and a reduction in body weight, are associated with substantial reductions in cardiovascular risk factor profiles in people at high risk of diabetes.

A 20-year follow-up was reported from the Da Qing Prevention Trial [26] in 577 Chinese individuals with impaired glucose tolerance. After 6 years of treatment, cumulative diabetes incidences were similar with all three interventions. Treatment and regular follow-up were discontinued after 6 years, but cumulative incidence over 20 years, gathered largely from clinical and historical data, remained lower in the intervention groups than in the usual care group.

The Japanese Diabetes Prevention Programme and the Indian Diabetes Prevention Programme also reported reduced rates of conversion to diabetes of 57.4% over 4 years and 28.5% over 3 years, respectively [27,28].

It is important to note that a reduction in body weight in overweight individuals also has beneficial effects by reducing the occurrence and/or the severity of the development of diseases related to diabetes, including arterial hypertension and dyslipidaemia.

A recent study conducted in a population of dysmetabolic subjects has demonstrated that a lifestyle intervention inducing a modest reduction in BMI and waist circumference was able to substantially reduce the prevalence of metabolic syndrome (−31%) and of multiple metabolic/inflammatory abnormalities (−41%) [29].

The challenge facing public health professionals is how to implement the lifestyle changes achieved in these intervention trials in markedly varying sociocultural settings, and how to identify and target people with impaired glucose tolerance on a mass scale. Furthermore, although long-term benefits might be anticipated, the impact of these changes on clinical outcomes such as CVD and mortality remains unknown.

Weight loss is also associated with a lowering of blood pressure. Many clinical trials have clearly demonstrated the effect of weight loss on reducing blood pressure. The Hypertension Prevention Trial [30] documented that in individuals with borderline elevations in blood pressure a mean weight loss of 5 kg was associated with a decrease of 5 mmHg in systolic blood pressure. Lifestyle interventions based on a low-calorie diet and associated with weight loss are associated with a reduction in blood pressure. Even modest weight loss (i.e. 10% of body weight) reduces blood pressure [31].

Studies examining the effects of weight loss on lipid patterns indicate that reduction in body weight is associated with a modest, but statistically significant, decrease in total and LDL cholesterol, whereas the effects on triglycerides are usually more pronounced.

A systematic review of 70 studies [32] designed to induce weight reduction and detect changes in plasma lipids indicated that weight loss per se (average 16 kg or 16% from baseline weight) is associated with a mean decrease in plasma total cholesterol of about 30 mg/dl (0.78 mmol/L), with LDL and VLDL cholesterol dropping in equal proportions. Overall, significant correlations are found between the degree of weight reduction and the decrease in plasma total cholesterol, LDL, and VLDL cholesterol, and triglyceride concentrations. For every kilogram decrease in body weight, total and LDL cholesterol are reduced by 2 mg/dl (0.05 mmol/L) and 0.8 mg/dl (0.02 mmol/L), respectively. Furthermore, a 0.3 mg/dl (0.008 mmol/L) reduction in HDL cholesterol occurs for subjects who actively lose weight, whereas a 0.4 mg/dl (0.01 mmol/L) increase occurs for subjects at a stabilized weight reduction.

Improvements in HDL cholesterol and in plasma triglycerides tend to be greater in overweight or obese subjects on a low-carbohydrate diet, whereas change in LDL cholesterol levels were more favourable in subjects on low-fat diets.

The Look AHEAD Trial [33,34], which enrolled over 5000 patients with diabetes, has shown that lifestyle intervention aimed to obtain an average 1-year weight loss of at least 7% is associated with improvement in lipids, blood pressure, and glycaemic control across all BMI categories. Nearly 40% of severely obese patients lost more than 10% of their initial body weight at 1 year. Additionally, 42% achieved the American Diabetes Association goal for LDL cholesterol, 66% for blood pressure, and 71% for glycaemic control, all significantly greater than at baseline and comparable with individuals with a BMI < 40 kg/m^2. These promising findings suggest that severely obese individuals with type 2 diabetes can be successfully treated with behavioural weight loss programmes.

Observational studies indicate that the impact of physical activity on lipid fractions is greatest for HDL cholesterol, which tends to increase, and for triglycerides, which tend to decrease, in active individuals compared with sedentary subjects. The increase in HDL cholesterol associated with physical activity varies from 9 to 50% and triglyceride reduction ranges from 19 to 50%. By contrast, changes in plasma total and LDL cholesterol are less consistent and wane in many studies after adjustment for other lifestyle components (dietary habits, smoking, and alcohol consumption).

Aerobic physical activity with total energy expenditure of 1500–2200 kcal/week (which corresponds to jogging about 24–32 km/week) may increase plasma HDL cholesterol levels by 3.5–6 mg/dl (0.09–0.16 mmol/L) and lower plasma triglyceride levels by 7–20 mg/dl (0.08–0.23 mmol/L). A further 16 km/week would trigger an additional 3 mg/dl (0.08 mmol/L) increase in plasma HDL cholesterol and an additional 3–8 mg/dl (0.03—0.09 mmol/L) decrease in plasma triglycerides [35].

In the context of the lifestyle interventions, dietary factors may directly influence cardiovascular risk factors, such as lipid levels, blood pressure, and glucose levels.

Keypoints

Lifestyle modification focused on a modest (5–10%) weight loss and moderate-intensity physical activity can significantly reduce the incidence of type 2 diabetes and cardiometabolic risk factors in high-risk individuals, with benefits sustained for at least 10 years.
Weight loss, even modest (i.e. 10% of body weight) is associated with a lowering of blood pressure.
In most available studies, weight loss significantly reduces plasma total and LDL cholesterol, and, even more, plasma triglycerides. HDL cholesterol levels tend to rise on sustained weight loss.
Regular aerobic activity induces an increase in plasma HDL cholesterol and a decrease in plasma triglycerides, whereas the effects on total and LDL cholesterol are modest.

Dietary modifications to reduce body weight

Obesity develops when energy intake is greater than energy expenditure: overall it is a consequence of low physical activity and increased consumption of energy-dense foods. To achieve weight loss, energy intake must be less than the energy expenditure: in order to obtain a weight loss of 1 kg/week, a calorie deficit of 1000 kcal/day would be needed, on the basis of predictions based on the laws of thermodynamics. In practice, a much lower weight reduction is observed, since weight reduction influences not only fat mass but also muscles, and therefore the energy expenditure progressively declines. The minimum energy required by an adult of normal weight who stays in bed is approximately 0.8–0.9 kcal/min (1150 kcal/day); this maintains body temperature, function of the heart and other organs, and tissue repair. High levels of physical activity can increase energy expenditure four- to eightfold.

Reduced-calorie diets can vary in energy intake, and can be adopted according to clinical judgement: very low-calorie diets (less than 800 kcal/day) should be used only when more rapid weight loss is needed and require strict medical monitoring; low-calorie (800–1500 kcal/day) or moderate diets (about 300–500 kcal less than the typical daily intake) are also used (➲ Table 13.2).

Exercise is recommended as a weight loss intervention, particularly when combined with dietary changes (➲ Table 13.3). The combination of increased physical activity and caloric restriction result in more relevant and sustained weight reduction and changes in body composition (fat versus lean mass) than diet or physical activity alone. While short-term weight loss depends mainly on caloric restriction, maintenance of weight loss mostly depends on the level of physical activity. For most people long-term success is still difficult to achieve, and current therapies for obesity do not provide sufficient support for patients to adhere to the required lifestyle changes.

The body has multiple mechanisms for modifying energy balance to re-establish the original body weight. Weight loss induces a reduction in energy expenditure, hindering maintenance of weight loss—failure to maintain weight loss in the long term is a common problem.

Table 13.2 Practical examples of how to lose 1 kg of body weight in 1 month by reducing energy intake by about 300 kcal/day

Food items corresponding to approximately 300 kcal
◆ A portion of fried potatoes
◆ An aperitif with nibbles
◆ A slice of cake
◆ A bag of potato crisps
◆ A hot dog
◆ A cheeseburger
◆ Three glasses of wine
◆ A chocolate bar
◆ An ice cream
◆ A pastry
◆ A muffin

Table 13.3 Energy expenditure for different types of physical activity

Activity	Energy (kcal/min)
Sleeping	0.9
Sitting	1.0
Standing	1.1
Using the computer	1.3
Brisk walking (4 km/h)	2.5–3.5
Washing the floor	3.6
Ironing	3.5–4.2
Plastering a wall	4.1–5.5
Shovelling	6.0
Tilling the land	5.5–7.0
Cleaning and beating carpets	7.8
Bicycle riding (22 km/h)	11.1
Running (12 km/h)	15.0

There is currently strong disagreement on the optimal composition of a weight-reducing diet; in particular it is debated whether low-fat diets, recommended by the American Heart Association and the US National Institutes of Health, are still the best choice. As a matter of fact, low-carbohydrate diets have recently become very popular for weight loss, and a number of intervention trials have evaluated their effects in overweight people. Comparisons of low-carbohydrate diets (≤45% of energy from carbohydrates) and low-fat diets (≤30% of energy from fats) have been attempted, with many studies evaluating their impact on body weight and relevant metabolic risk factors; however, since many clinical trials have small sample sizes and insufficient statistical power to detect small changes in metabolic risk factors that may have public health importance, meta-analyses of randomized controlled trials have been undertaken in order to perform an overall comparison between these two approaches.

In a paper published in 2012 by Hu et al. [36], 23 trials from multiple countries with a total of 2788 participants were included in a meta-analysis on the effects of low-carbohydrate versus low-fat diets in overweight people. Both types of dietary interventions lowered weight and improved metabolic risk factors; however, compared with participants on low-fat diets, those on low-carbohydrate diets experienced a slightly (but statistically significant) lower reduction in total and LDL cholesterol but a greater increase in HDL cholesterol and decrease in triglycerides. Reductions in body weight, waist circumference, and other metabolic risk factors were not significantly different between the two diets. These findings suggest that low-carbohydrate diets are as effective as low-fat diets in reducing weight and improving metabolic risk factors. Studies demonstrating long-term effects of low-carbohydrate diets on cardiovascular events are warranted. So far, preliminary data from the follow-up of dietary interventions seem to indicate that in the long term the impact of low-carbohydrate diets on body weight disappears more rapidly than with other dietary approaches, particularly those based on the Mediterranean model with plenty of dietary fibre (vegetables, fruit, and wholegrain cereal foods).

Keypoints

General recommendations for a healthy diet:
- Limit energy intake from total fats
- Replace saturated fats with unsaturated fats
- Increase consumption of fruit and vegetables as well as legumes and whole grains
- Reduce the intake of sugars (particularly in beverages)

Prevention of obesity

At the population level, preventing obesity is probably more effective than treating it. In this respect, the lifestyle trends of people living in the western world and in countries where economic conditions are rapidly improving need to go in the direction of the rediscovery and implementation of a concept of nutrition and lifestyle that is associated with 'quality' rather than 'quantity' (➲ Table 13.4): a reduction of the amount of food

Table 13.4 Food choices for controlling body weight

	To be preferred	To be eaten in moderation	To be eaten occasionally and in small amounts
Cereals	Whole grains (not exceeding portion size)	Refined bread, rice and pasta, biscuits, cornflakes	Pastries, muffins, pies, croissants
Vegetables	Raw and cooked vegetables		Vegetables prepared in butter or cream
Legumes	All (including soy and soy protein)		
Fruit	Fresh or frozen fruit	Dried fruit, jelly, jam, sorbets	Canned fruit, popsicles
Sweet foods and sweeteners	Non-caloric sweeteners		Cakes, ice creams, sucrose, honey, fructose, glucose, chocolate, candies
Meat and fish	Lean and oily fish, poultry without skin, lean cuts of beef, lamb, pork, or veal,	Seafood, shellfish, ham	Sausages, salami, bacon, spare ribs, hot dogs, offal
Dairy food and eggs	Skimmed milk and yoghurt, egg white	Low-fat milk, low-fat cheese, and other milk products	Regular cheese, cream, egg yolk, whole milk and yoghurt, ice cream
Cooking fat and dressings	Vinegar, ketchup, mustard, fat-free dressing	Vegetable oils, soft margarines, salad dressing, mayonnaise (two tablespoons a day)	Butter, solid margarines, trans-fats, palm and coconut oils, lard, bacon fat, dressing made with egg yolks
Nuts/seeds		All	Coconut
Drinks	Water, sparkling water, coffee, tea, soft drinks with artificial sweeteners	Wine or beer (not more than one glass a day)	Spirits, fruit juices, aperitifs, soft drinks
Cooking procedures	Grilling, boiling, steaming	Stir-frying, roasting	Frying

that is consumed has to be balanced by greater attention to taste and gastronomic pleasure, changing the relationship between people and food (with the rediscovery of the social and cultural values linked with the act of eating). Similarly, the quality of living standards (with significant time devoted to physical activity and a less stressful daily routine) might also play a significant role in preventing weight gain. Obviously, this requires a total paradigm shift starting from pre-school children through to adolescence. This phase of life is important for developing healthy eating habits and behaviours that can continue into adulthood. Achieving a healthy diet in children is also a step on the path to a broader education, helping to improve tastes for different foods and facilitating a willingness to accept those that are appropriate for health (e.g. fish and vegetables) but not always favoured by children and adolescents. The gradual introduction of these foods into the daily diet becomes crucial for the development of perceptions and beliefs that can be maintained into adulthood.

A strong communication effort by governments, scientific societies, the medical profession, and private companies is needed to give people a greater awareness of the importance of dietary habits and, more generally, lifestyle in preventing obesity. Governments can help people change their lifestyle by making new healthy options available or by making existing ones more accessible and affordable. Alternatively, they can use persuasion, education, and information to make healthy options more attractive. The latter approach is more expensive and difficult to implement; conversely, regulations and fiscal measures have high political and welfare costs since they involve all consumers indiscriminately. So far, governments in the OECD area have been actively involved in disseminating nutritional guidelines and health promotion messages to school-age children; in particular, 'active transport' (cycling and walking) and active leisure have been emphasized. Other initiatives were aimed at changes in school meals and regulations on vending machines in schools, and at promoting better facilities for physical activity. Since 2010 there has also been an increased partnership between governments and the food and beverage industry (e.g. in the UK and Switzerland) in the design and implementation of actions to fight obesity. This has contributed to the re-formulation of some products in order to avoid unhealthy ingredients and to limit portion sizes; moreover, advertisements to vulnerable groups like children have been reduced [37].

Keypoints

Prevention of obesity is very important at the population level. Lifestyle changes have to be promoted from pre-school age through to adolescence.

The importance of a healthy diet and increased physical activity are important health promotion messages for school-age children.

Drugs for treating obesity

The three main drug options for the long-term treatment of obesity are orlistat, which is currently available, sibutramine, which was withdrawn from the market in 2010 due to cardiovascular side effects, and rimonabant, withdrawn from the market in 2008 due to neuropsychiatric effects. None of these drugs produces weight losses of 5–10% that are recommended to improve the cardiovascular risk profile and reduce the risk of diabetes. However, combined with lifestyle modification, weight-loss thresholds of 5–10% are achievable by most patients.

Orlistat is a gastric and pancreatic lipase inhibitor that reduces absorption of dietary fat by around 30%. Treatment with orlistat has been demonstrated to be associated with an improvement in cardiovascular risk factors, such as glucose control, plasma lipids, and hypertension.

Using data from the clinical trials of orlistat, Heymsfield et al. [38] pooled information on 675 subjects from three studies. During treatment, 6.6% of the patients taking orlistat converted from normal to impaired glucose tolerance (IGT), compared with 10.8% in the placebo treated group. None of the patients in the orlistat arm who originally had normal glucose tolerance developed diabetes, compared with 1.2% in the placebo group. Of those who initially had IGT, 7.6% in the placebo group and 3.0% in the orlistat group developed diabetes. The effect of orlistat in preventing diabetes was assessed in a 4-year study. In this trial weight was reduced by 2.8 kg (95% CI 1.1–4.5) compared with placebo, and the conversion rate to diabetes was reduced from 9% to 6% (HR 0.63, 95% CI 0.46–0.86). The incidence of new cases was also reduced from 10.9% to 5.2% ($p < 0.05$) during a 3-year period in which overweight patients were treated with orlistat and lifestyle changes or lifestyle changes alone.

Orlistat therapy is also associated with a reduction in total cholesterol of –13.1 mg/dl (–0.34 mmol/L) [95% CI –15.8 (–0.41) to –1.04 mg/dl (–0.027 mmol/l)] and LDL cholesterol of –11.2 mg/dl (–0.29 mmol/L) [95% CI –13.1 (–0.34) to –8.6 mg/dl (–0.24 mmol/L)], a reduction in systolic (–2.02 mmHg, 95% CI –2.87 to –1.17 mmHg) and diastolic blood pressure (–1.64 mmHg, 95% CI –2.20 to –1.09), and a small improvement in glycaemic control in diabetic patients [reduction in glycated haemoglobin (HbA1c) of –0.17%, 95% CI –0.24 to –0.10%].

Originally developed as an antidepressant, sibutramine is a centrally acting monoamine re-uptake inhibitor that mainly acts to increase satiety. In long-term studies, sibutramine has had little effect on concentrations of LDL cholesterol and glycaemic control, and has had conflicting effects (no change to mild improvement) on concentrations of triglycerides and HDL cholesterol. Furthermore the SCOUT (Sibutramine Cardiovascular Outcomes Trial) study [39] showed that subjects with pre-existing cardiovascular disease receiving long-term sibutramine treatment had an increased risk of non-fatal myocardial infarction and non-fatal stroke (HR for non-fatal infarction 1.28, 95% CI 1.04–1.57, $p = 0.02$; HR for non-fatal stroke 1.36, 95% CI 1.04–1.77, $p = 0.03$), leading to concerns about potential cardiovascular toxic effects. The drug was therefore withdrawn in 2010.

Rimonabant is a potent CB1 (endocannabinoid receptor 1) receptor blocker that acts at the level of the central nervous system by inhibiting food intake and promoting satiety. Potential peripheral mechanisms include enhanced thermogenesis via increased oxygen consumption in skeletal muscle, diminished hepatic and adipocyte lipogenesis, augmentation of adiponectin concentrations, promotion of vagally mediated cholecystokinin-induced satiety, inhibition of pre-adipocyte proliferation, and increased adipocyte maturation without lipid accumulation. Compared with placebo, rimonabant reduced body weight by 4.6 kg (95% CI 4.3–5.0 kg), reduced waist circumference, and improved triglyceride and HDL cholesterol profiles. LDL cholesterol did not improve and blood pressure was either unchanged or slightly reduced. The presence of metabolic syndrome was reduced in subjects treated with rimonabant. The CRESCENDO Study (Comprehensive Rimonabant Evaluation Study of Cardiovascular Endpoints and Outcomes) [40], which investigated the cardiovascular safety of rimonabant, showed an excess of neuropsychiatric effects in the rimonabant arm and so the trial was prematurely terminated. The drug was withdrawn from the market in 2008.

Keypoints

The three main drug options for the long-term treatment of obesity are orlistat which is currently available and sibutramine and rimonabant, which have been withdrawn from the market for their cardiovascular and neuropsychiatric side effects, respectively. None of these drugs produces weight losses of 5–10%, as recommended to improve the cardiovascular risk profile and the risk of diabetes. However, this target is achievable by most patients when a weight-reducing drug is used in combination with lifestyle modifications.

Orlistat therapy is associated with a decreased incidence of diabetes, a reduction in total and LDL cholesterol, a reduction in systolic and diastolic blood pressure, and a small improvement in glycaemic control in diabetic patients.

Bariatric surgery

Bariatric surgery has a favourable impact on several medical comorbidities and is considered the only intervention to offer substantial and long-term weight loss for obese patients. Bariatric surgery is associated with prevention and remission of type 2 diabetes, reduced cancer incidence, and improved all-cause mortality. Emerging data also suggest a role in the reduction of cardiovascular risk [41–44]. The Swedish Obese Subjects (SOS) Study [45], a trial focused primarily on long-term mortality following bariatric surgery, involved 4047 obese participants, 2010 of whom had bariatric surgery (vertical banded gastroplasty, gastric banding, and gastric bypass) and 2037 matched controls who received conventional weight loss therapy. Over a period of up to 16 years there were 129 deaths in the control group (6.3%) compared with 101 in the bariatric surgery group (5.0%), representing an unadjusted HR of 0.76 (95% CI 0.59–0.99, $p = 0.04$).

After 10 years from randomization in the SOS study, the surgical group had a higher rate of remission of diabetes, hypertriglyceridaemia, and hypertension compared with the control group. There were no statistical differences between groups with regards to remission of hypercholesterolaemia. Incidence rates of new cases of diabetes and hypertriglyceridaemia were lower in the surgical group than in the controls.

Over a 15-year follow-up, bariatric surgery was associated with a reduction in the number of cardiovascular deaths and first cardiovascular events (fatal and non-fatal) after controlling for the cardiometabolic risk profile at baseline. Compared with controls, the adjusted HR of bariatric surgery for total cardiovascular events was 0.67 (95% CI 0.54–0.83, $p < 0.001$) and the adjusted HR for fatal cardiovascular events was 0.47 (95% CI 0.29–0.76, $p = 0.02$). There have been similar findings in obese patients with type 2 diabetes who underwent bariatric surgery.

In a smaller subsample of the SOS study, cardiac and vascular structure and function were examined at baseline and after 1–4 years of follow-up. The systolic and diastolic blood pressure, left ventricular mass, and relative wall thickness were reduced by bariatric surgery, whereas the left ventricular ejection fraction and the diastolic function, estimated from the E/A ratio, were improved. The rate of increase in intima–media thickness was normalized in the surgical group, and a reduction in various cardiovascular symptoms (dyspnoea, chest discomfort) was found. Subjects in the bariatric arm also experienced less sleep apnoea, joint pain and fractures, and biliary disease, and had an improved quality of life.

In total, 89% of all operations in the SOS study were undertaken as open surgery. Over the first 90 days after inclusion in the intervention study, five deaths (0.25%) were observed in the surgery group and two (0.1%) in the control group. Amongst the 2010 patients in the surgery group, four died during the primary hospital stay (three due to anastomotic leaks with general organ failure and one due to myocardial infarction). The fifth surgical patient died 60 days post-surgery from an acute myocardial infarction. Amongst the patients in the surgery group, 292 (14.5%) had at least one non-fatal complication over the first 90 days. Pulmonary complications were the most common (total 5.2%, including thromboembolism in 0.8%) followed by vomiting (3.0%), wound infection (2.1%), haemorrhage (1.3%), and anastomotic leak (1.2%). In 2.9% of the patients these complications were serious enough to require a second operation during the first 90 days.

Keypoints

Retrospective mortality studies and the SOS prospective mortality study have reported higher survival in patients who have undergone bariatric surgery compared with matched severely obese, non-operated controls.

Improvement in cardiovascular risk factors, remission of chronic disease (hypertension, hyperlipidaemia, and diabetes), and reduced incidence of diabetes have been reported after bariatric surgery.

Patients who undergo bariatric surgery have a reduction in the risk of total cardiovascular events of 33% and fatal cardiovascular events of 53%.

Conclusions

In the European guidelines on cardiovascular disease prevention in clinical practice (2012 version) is clearly stated that 'weight reduction in overweight and obese people is recommended as this is associated with favourable effects on blood pressure and dyslipidaemia, which may lead to less CVD'. This recommendation is classified as class 1, level A, grade strong. However, despite this recommendation obesity is becoming of epidemic proportions worldwide in both children and adults. If the projected trends for obesity from 2005 to 2020 continue, obesity will increasingly counterbalance the beneficial effects of declining rates of smoking on CVD.

The role of overweight as a major cardiovascular risk factor is clearly established. The observation in many epidemiological studies that after multivariable adjustment the association between weight and cardiovascular risk tends to become less significant should not be interpreted as evidence that body weight is not important; conversely, since it exerts its effect on risk by influencing multiple risk factors it represents an important link between lifestyle and CVD.

As well as its effects on cardiovascular events, overweight plays a relevant role in the global risk of diseases and disabilities. In 2010 obesity ranked as the sixth most important risk factor for the global burden of disease, as recently reported in a very authoritative study [46], and is a major contributor to years of healthy life lost (DALYs). It is striking that in 2010 high BMI was a more important cause of poor health worldwide than childhood underweight, whereas childhood underweight was a much more prominent risk factor than high BMI in 1990. Evidence that increased cardiovascular risk starts at a young age has accumulated over past decades. Although children are at very low absolute risk of developing CVD, those at relatively high risk have a higher probability of experiencing a cardiovascular event later in life because of 'tracking' of risk factors (i.e. two-thirds of the adolescents who are obese will remain obese in their adult life). The wide availability and easy access to food with a high caloric density and an increasingly sedentary lifestyle represent the two main features of an environment favouring overweight and obesity (the so-called 'obesogenic environment'). Every individual can easily adopt certain behaviours to limit these aspects, but this is not going to be the solution to the global problem at the population level. People should be able to effectively make healthy choices and adopt the correct behaviours; therefore actions are required which depend on a set of public and private actors. Combining different interventions not only for the treatment of obesity but also for its prevention can provide an effective solution to a major health problem at a sustainable cost.

Solution to the case study

What is the diagnosis?

The patient is overweight with abdominal adiposity and has metabolic syndrome. Visceral fat is the key driver of metabolic syndrome, a clustering of multiple cardiovascular and metabolic abnormalities (dyslipidaemia, hypertension, elevated fasting insulin/insulin resistance, hyperglycaemia, pro-thrombotic and pro-inflammatory state). In this patient the diagnosis is based on the presence of abdominal adiposity, high blood pressure, hypertriglyceridaemia, and low HDL cholesterol.

What is the calculated 10 year risk for a cardiovascular event of that patient?

Metabolic syndrome has been recognized as a predictor of diabetes and cardiovascular diseases. Many epidemiological studies have clearly shown that obesity, particularly of the abdominal type, increases the risk of CVD both directly and by promoting the occurrence of comorbid conditions. These abnormalities, even if mild, contribute to a significant increase in the cardiovascular risk. According to the SCORE charts for countries with low CVD rates, this patient has a risk of developing a fatal cardiovascular event in 10 years of about 5%. His risk could be further increased because of the presence of metabolic syndrome and a family history of premature cardiovascular disease.

What is the best therapeutic approach?

The best approach for this patient is advice on a low-calorie diet plus recommendations to increase physical activity. Weight loss obtained with lifestyle intervention, even if modest (i.e. 5–10% of body weight), has been proven to be effective in reducing the incidence of diabetes and other cardiovascular risk factors. A modest decrease in body weight appears to be able to increase insulin sensitivity and, therefore, improves the overall metabolic profile and the cardiovascular risk factors that cluster with insulin resistance. The first approach to an overweight patient should be to improve his or her lifestyle, by promoting greater physical activity and a healthier diet, moderately reduced in its energy content, low in total fat, and in particular trans and saturated fat, low in salt, rich in fibre, and poor in sugar (particularly by limiting sweet beverages). In primary prevention the pharmacological approach to the associated conditions (hypercholesterolaemia and hypertension) can be considered as a second-line therapy.

Follow-up

The patient returns to his GP 3 months later. He has lost 5 kg and his waist circumference is 5 cm smaller. His blood pressure is 136/84 mmHg. Plasma lipids are improved: total cholesterol 229 mg/dl; triglycerides 138 mg/dl; low-density lipoprotein 158 mg/dl; high-density lipoprotein 43 mg/dl. His cardiovascular risk, as assessed by the SCORE charts, has now reduced to 3%.

This case illustrates several issues:

- Abdominal adiposity is often associated with other metabolic abnormalities and cardiovascular risk factors that have to be sought out in each obese/overweight patient.
- The metabolic abnormalities associated with obesity/overweight, even if only mild, increase the global cardiovascular risk.
- Promotion of a healthy lifestyle focused on a modest (5–10%) weight loss and moderate-intensity physical exercise can significantly reduce the risk of type 2 diabetes and the magnitude of the cardiometabolic risk factors in overweight individuals.

Further reading

Perk J, De Backer G, Gohlke H, et al. European guidelines on cardiovascular disease prevention in clinical practice (version 2012). *Eur Heart J* 2012; **33**: 1635–701.

Mancini M, Ordovas JM, Riccardi G, et al. *Nutritional and metabolic bases of cardiovascular disease*. Oxford: Wiley-Blackwell.

References

1 World Health Organization. *Preventing chronic diseases: a vital investment. WHO global report*, 2005. URL: <http://www.who.int/chp/chronic_disease_report>
2 Flegal KM, Kit BK, Orpana H, et al. Association of all-cause mortality with overweight and obesity using standard body mass index categories: a systematic review and meta-analysis. *J Am Med Assoc* 2013; **309**: 71–82.
3 Berrington de Gonzalez A, Hartge P, Cerhan JR, et al. Body-mass index and mortality among 1.46 million white adults. *N Engl J Med* 2010; **363**: 2211–19.
4 Stewart ST, Cutler DM, Rosen AB. Forecasting the effects of obesity and smoking on U.S. life expectancy. *N Engl J Med* 2009; **361**: 2252–60.
5 Oreopoulos A, Padwal R, Kalantar-Zadeh K, et al. Body mass index and mortality in heart failure: a meta-analysis. *Am Heart J* 2008; **156**: 13–22.
6 Arena R, Lavie CJ. The obesity paradox and outcome in heart failure: is excess bodyweight truly protective? *Future Cardiol* 2010; **6**: 1–6.
7 Emerging Risk Factors Collaboration, Wormser D, Kaptoge S, Di Angelantonio E, et al. Separate and combined associations of body-mass index and abdominal adiposity with cardiovascular disease: collaborative analysis of 58 prospective studies. *Lancet* 2011; **377**: 1085–95.
8 Coutinho T, Goel K, Corrêa de Sá D, et al. Central obesity and survival in subjects with coronary artery disease: a systematic review of the literature and collaborative analysis with individual subject data. *J Am Coll Cardiol* 2011; **57**: 1877–86.
9 Hubert HB, Feinleib M, McNamara PM, et al. Obesity as an independent risk factor for cardiovascular disease: a 26-year follow-up of participants in the Framingham Heart Study. *Circulation* 1983; **67**: 968–77.
10 Tirosh A, Shai I, Afek A, et al. Adolescent BMI trajectory and risk of diabetes versus coronary disease. *N Engl J Med* 2011; **364**: 1315–25.
11 World Health Organization. *Definition, diagnosis and classification of diabetes mellitus and its complications. Part 1: diagnosis and classification of diabetes mellitus. Report of a WHO consultation*, WHO/NCD/NCS/99.2, 1999. Geneva: World Health Organization.
12 Balkau B, Charles MA; the European Group for the Study of Insulin Resistance (EGIR): Comment on the provisional report from the WHO consultation. *Diabet Med* 1999; **16**: 442–3.
13 Alberti KG, Zimmet P, Shaw J, IDF Epidemiology Task Force Consensus Group. The metabolic syndrome—a new worldwide definition. *Lancet* 2005; **366**: 1059–62.
14 Grundy SM, Cleeman JI, Daniels SR, et al; American Heart Association; National Heart, Lung, and Blood Institute. Diagnosis and management of the metabolic syndrome: an American Heart Association/National Heart, Lung, and Blood Institute Scientific Statement. *Circulation* 2005; **112**: 2735–52.
15 Hussain A, Hydrie MZI, Claussen B, et al. Type 2 diabetes and obesity: a review. *J Diabetol* 2010; **2**: 1
16 The Diabetes Prevention Program Research Group. Relationship of body size and shape to the development of diabetes in the diabetes prevention program. *Obesity* 2006; **14**: 2107–17.
17 Chang L, Milton H, Eitzman DT, et al. Paradoxical roles of perivascular adipose tissue in atherosclerosis and hypertension. *Circ J* 2012; **77**: 11–18.
18 Howard BV, Ruotolo G, Robbins DC. Obesity and dyslipidemia. *Endocrinol Metab Clin North Am* 2003; **32**: 855–67.
19 French SA, Jeffery RW, Folsom AR, et al. Relation of weight variability and intentionality of weight loss to disease history and health-related variables in a population-based sample of women aged 55–69 years. *Am J Epidemiol* 1995; **142**: 1306–14.
20 Williamson DF, Pamuk E, Thun M, et al. Prospective study of intentional weight loss and mortality in overweight white men aged 40–64 years. *Am J Epidemiol* 1999; **149**: 491–503.
21 Williamson DF, Thompson TJ, Thun M, et al. Intentional weight loss and mortality among overweight individuals with diabetes. *Diabetes Care* 2000; **23**: 1499–504.
22 Pan XR, Li GW, Hu YH, et al. Effects of diet and exercise in preventing NIDDM in people with impaired glucose tolerance. The Da Qing IGT and Diabetes Study. *Diabetes Care* 1997; **20**: 537–44.
23 Tuomilehto J, Lindström J, Eriksson JG, et al; Finnish Diabetes Prevention Study Group. Prevention of type 2 diabetes mellitus by changes in lifestyle among subjects with impaired glucose tolerance. *N Engl J Med* 2001; **344**: 1343–50.
24 Knowler WC, Barrett-Connor E, Fowler SE, et al; Diabetes Prevention Program Research Group. Reduction in the incidence of type 2 diabetes with lifestyle intervention or metformin. *N Engl J Med* 2002; **346**: 393–403.
25 Diabetes Prevention Program Research Group, Knowler WC, Fowler SE, Hamman RF, et al. 10-year follow-up of diabetes incidence and weight loss in the Diabetes Prevention Program Outcomes Study. *Lancet* 2009; **374**: 1677–86.
26 Li G, Zhang P, Wang J, et al. The long-term effect of lifestyle interventions to prevent diabetes in the China Da Qing Diabetes Prevention Study: a 20-year follow-up study. *Lancet* 2008; **371**: 1783–9.
27 Kosaka K, Noda M, Kuzuya T. Prevention of type 2 diabetes by lifestyle intervention: a Japanese trial in IGT males. *Diabetes Res Clin Pract* 2005; **67**: 152–62.
28 Ramachandran A, Snehalatha C, Mary S, et al; Indian Diabetes Prevention Programme (IDPP). The Indian Diabetes Prevention Programme shows that lifestyle modification and metformin prevent type 2 diabetes in Asian Indian subjects with impaired glucose tolerance (IDPP-1). *Diabetologia* 2006; **49**: 289–97.
29 Bo S, Ciccone G, Baldi C, et al. Effectiveness of a lifestyle intervention on metabolic syndrome. A randomized controlled trial. *J Gen Intern Med* 2007; **22**: 1695–703.
30 Hypertension Prevention Trial Research Group. The Hypertension Prevention Trial: three-year effects of dietary changes on blood pressure. *Arch Intern Med* 1990; **150**: 153–62.

31 Siebenhofer A, Jeitler K, Berghold A, et al. Long-term effects of weight-reducing diets in hypertensive patients. *Cochrane Database Syst Rev* 2011; (9): CD008274.

32 Dattilo AM, Kris-Etherton PM. Effects of weight reduction on blood lipids and lipoproteins: a meta-analysis. *Am J Clin Nutr* 1992; **56**: 320–8.

33 Unick JL, Beavers D, Jakicic JM, et al; Look AHEAD Research Group. Effectiveness of lifestyle interventions for individuals with severe obesity and type 2 diabetes: results from the Look AHEAD trial. *Diabetes Care* 2011; **34**: 2152–7.

34 Unick JL, Beavers D, Bond DS, et al; Look AHEAD Research Group. The long-term effectiveness of a lifestyle intervention in severely obese individuals. *Am J Med* 2013; **126**: 236–42.

35 Poli A, Marangoni F, Paoletti R, et al; Nutrition Foundation of Italy. Non-pharmacological control of plasma cholesterol levels. *Nutr Metab Cardiovasc Dis* 2008; **18**: S1–S16.

36 Hu T, Mills KT, Yao L, et al. Effects of low-carbohydrate diets versus low-fat diets on metabolic risk factors: a meta-analysis of randomized controlled clinical trials. *Am J Epidemiol* 2012; **176** (Suppl. 7): S44–S54.

37 Cecchini M., Sassi F, Lauer JA, et al. Tackling of unhealthy diets, physical inactivity, and obesity: health effects and cost-effectiveness. *Lancet* 2010; **376**: 1775–84.

38 Heymsfield SB, Segal KR, Hauptman J, et al. Effects of weight loss with orlistat on glucose tolerance and progression to type 2 diabetes in obese adults. *Arch Intern Med* 2000; **160**: 1321–6.

39 James WP, Caterson ID, Coutinho W, et al; SCOUT Investigators. Effect of sibutramine on cardiovascular outcomes in overweight and obese subjects. *N Engl J Med* 2010; **363**: 905–17.

40 Topol EJ, Bousser MG, Fox KA, et al; CRESCENDO Investigators. Rimonabant for prevention of cardiovascular events (CRESCENDO): a randomised, multicentre, placebo-controlled trial. *Lancet* 2010; **376**: 517–23.

41 Carlsson LM, Peltonen M, Ahlin S, et al. Bariatric surgery and prevention of type 2 diabetes in Swedish obese subjects. *N Engl J Med* 2012; **367**: 695–704.

42 Romeo S, Maglio C, Burza MA, et al. Cardiovascular events after bariatric surgery in obese subjects with type 2 diabetes. *Diabetes Care* 2012; **35**: 2613–17.

43 Moustarah F, Gilbert A, Després JP, et al. Impact of gastrointestinal surgery on cardiometabolic risk. *Curr Atheroscler Rep* 2012; **14**: 588–96.

44 Adams TD, Davidson LE, Litwin SE, et al. Gastrointestinal surgery: cardiovascular risk reduction and improved long-term survival in patients with obesity and diabetes. *Curr Atheroscler Rep* 2012; **14**: 606–15.

45 Sjöström L. Review of the key results from the Swedish Obese Subjects (SOS) trial—a prospective controlled intervention study of bariatric surgery. *J Intern Med* 2013; **273**: 219–34.

46 Lim SS, Vos T, Flaxman AD, et al. A comparative risk assessment of burden of disease and injury attributable to 67 risk factors and risk factor clusters in 21 regions, 1990-2010: a systematic analysis for the Global Burden of Disease Study 2010. *Lancet* 2012; **380**: 2224–60.

CHAPTER 14

Blood pressure

Robert Fagard, Giuseppe Mancia, and
Renata Cifkova

Contents

Summary

Prevention of hypertension can help prevent cardiovascular disease and renal complications. Obesity, a high sodium and low potassium intake, physical inactivity, and high alcohol consumption all contribute to the development of hypertension, and randomized controlled trials have shown that appropriate lifestyle modifications are able to reduce blood pressure and/or prevent the development of hypertension. The major complications of hypertension are stroke, coronary heart disease, heart failure, peripheral artery disease, and chronic kidney disease. Multiple randomized controlled trials and their meta-analyses have shown that treatment with antihypertensive drugs reduces the incidence of fatal and non-fatal cardiovascular events. In addition meta-analyses have shown that there are no clinically relevant differences in the effects of the five major drug classes on outcome, so all of them are considered suitable for the initiation and maintenance of antihypertensive therapy. Nevertheless, the therapeutic approach in the elderly, women, and patients with diabetes, cerebrovascular, cardiac, or renal disease deserves special attention.

Introduction

Hypertension is a major, if not the major, risk factor for cardiovascular (CV) disease (CVD) in Europe and worldwide. Hypertension is found in around 30–45% of the general European population with no systematic trends towards blood pressure (BP) changes in the last decade [1]. BP bears an independent continuous relationship with the incidence of CV events, such as stroke, coronary heart disease (CHD), heart failure, and peripheral artery disease (PAD) as well as end-stage renal disease (ESRD) [2–6]. It is therefore mandatory to prevent the development of hypertension; this is mainly achieved by having a healthy lifestyle and reducing elevated BP by both lifestyle modification and treatment with antihypertensive drugs in order to prevent CV and renal complications.

Classification of blood pressure levels

Office blood pressure

Hypertension is defined as office systolic BP (SBP) ≥ 140 mmHg and/or diastolic BP (DBP) ≥ 90 mmHg [1]. ➲ Table 14.1 summarizes the current definition and classification of BP levels, including isolated systolic hypertension. The diagnosis of hypertension

Table 14.1 Definitions and classification of office blood pressure (BP) levels (mmHg)*

Category	Systolic BP (mmHg)		Diastolic BP (mmHg)
Optimal	<120	and	<80
Normal	120–129	and/or	80–84
High normal	130–139	and/or	85–89
Grade 1 hypertension	140–159	and/or	90–99
Grade 2 hypertension	160–179	and/or	100–109
Grade 3 hypertension	≥180	and/or	≥110
Isolated systolic hypertension	≥140	and	<90

*The BP category is defined by the highest level of BP, whether systolic or diastolic. Isolated systolic hypertension should be graded 1, 2, or 3 according to systolic BP values in the ranges indicated.

should be based on at least two BP measurements on at least two visits. Additional recommendations for proper BP measurement are outlined in the 2013 European Society of Hypertension (ESH)/ European Society of Cardiology (ESC) guidelines for the management of arterial hypertension [1].

Out-of-office blood pressure

Out-of-office BP is commonly assessed by ambulatory or home BP monitoring; its measurement provides information about BP away from the medical environment [7,8]. Definitions of hypertension by office and out-of-office BP levels are summarized in ➲ Table 14.2 [1,7,8]. For ambulatory BP monitoring, average daytime, night-time, and 24-hour BP are the most commonly used variables in clinical practice. Home BP is usually the average of two BP measurements in the morning and two in the evening on at least four to seven consecutive days. White-coat hypertension refers to the condition in which BP is abnormally high in the office and normal out of the office, usually based on daytime ambulatory BP or home BP, and masked hypertension refers to the reverse condition. There is ample evidence that hypertension-induced asymptomatic organ damage and CV and renal morbidity and/or mortality are more closely related to out-of-office BP than to office BP [9–11]. Whereas the prognosis of masked hypertension is similar to that of sustained hypertension, white-coat hypertension has a better prognosis, which appears to be similar to that of true normotension in most of the outcome studies [12–14]. Office BP remains the cornerstone for screening, diagnosis, and management of hypertension. Out-of-office BP is an important adjunct to office BP and is indicated to identify white-coat or masked hypertension, when there is considerable variability in office BP, suspicion of hypotensive episodes, or resistance to antihypertensive treatment [1,7,8].

Table 14.2 Definitions of hypertension by office and out-of-office blood pressure (BP) levels

Category	Systolic BP (mmHg)		Diastolic BP (mmHg)
Office BP	≥140	and/or	≥90
Ambulatory BP			
Daytime (or awake)	≥135	and/or	≥85
Nighttime (or asleep)	≥120	and/or	≥70
24-hour	≥130	and/or	≥80
Home BP	≥135	and/or	≥85

Prevention of hypertension by lifestyle modification

Lifestyle modifications are the cornerstone for the prevention of hypertension. Clinical studies show that the BP-lowering effects of lifestyle modifications can be equivalent to drug monotherapy [15] and should always be advised for patients receiving antihypertensive drugs as they may reduce the dose and number of drugs needed to achieve control of BP. Beside their BP-lowering effect, lifestyle changes contribute to the control of other CV risk factors and clinical conditions [16].

Weight reduction

A substantial and largely consistent body of evidence from observational studies and clinical trials documents that body weight is directly related to BP. In a meta-analysis of randomized controlled trials (RCTs), mean BP reductions associated with an average weight loss of 5.1 kg amounted to 4.4/3.6 mmHg [17]. The relationship between weight loss and reduction in BP appears to be linear (➲ Fig. 14.1). Major guidelines recommend weight loss as an initial intervention in the treatment of hypertension in hypertensive patients who are overweight or obese, but weight maintenance may be a reasonable goal for many of them. Two large meta-analyses of observational studies assessing optimal body mass index (BMI) provided conflicting results. The Prospective Studies Collaboration [18] concluded that mortality was lowest at

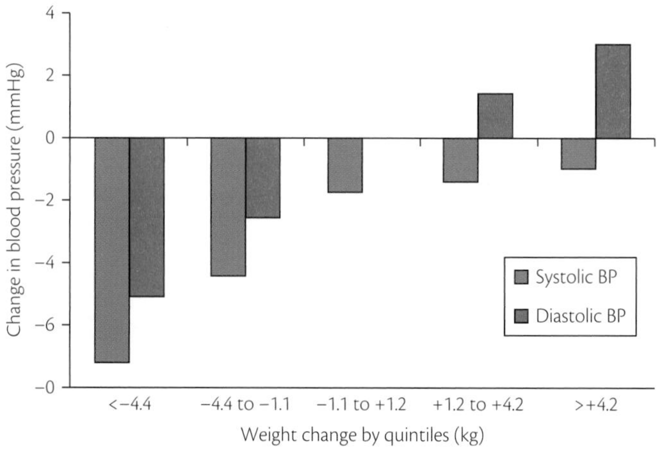

Fig. 14.1 Weight and blood pressure appear to be correlated in a linear relationship.
Source: Frisoli TM et al. *Eur Heart J* 2011; **32**: 3081–3087.

a BMI of about 22.5–25 kg/m^2 whereas a more recent meta-analysis concluded that mortality was lowest in overweight subjects [19]. Weight loss should employ a multidisciplinary approach that optimally includes dietary changes and regular physical exercise. Weight loss programmes are often not successful and their effect on BP may be overestimated. Furthermore, short-term results are often not maintained over the long term.

Dietary minerals

Sodium

The effect of sodium intake on BP is well established. The usual salt intake in many European countries is between 9 and 12 g/day whereas the maximum intake recommended by the World Health Organization for adults is 5 g/day. Processed foods are an important source of dietary sodium. The meta-analysis by He et al. [20], including only randomized controlled trials (RCTs) with a duration of ≥4 weeks or more, predicted a BP-lowering effect of 7/4 mmHg in hypertensive patients and 4/2 mmHg in normotensives with 6 g/day reduction in salt intake (➲ Fig. 14.2). The effect of sodium restriction is greater in black people, the elderly, and in individuals with diabetes, metabolic syndrome, or chronic kidney disease (CKD) [21]. Salt restriction may reduce the number and dose of antihypertensive drugs. There are no data from RCTs on clinical outcome, but observational follow-up of the participants in the Trials of Hypertension Prevention (TOHP) study showed a 25% lower risk of CV events in the sodium restriction group [22]. To reduce sodium intake, consumers should choose foods low in sodium and limit the amount of added salt. Any effective strategy to reduce sodium intake must involve the cooperation of food manufacturers and restaurants, which should progressively reduce the sodium added to their products.

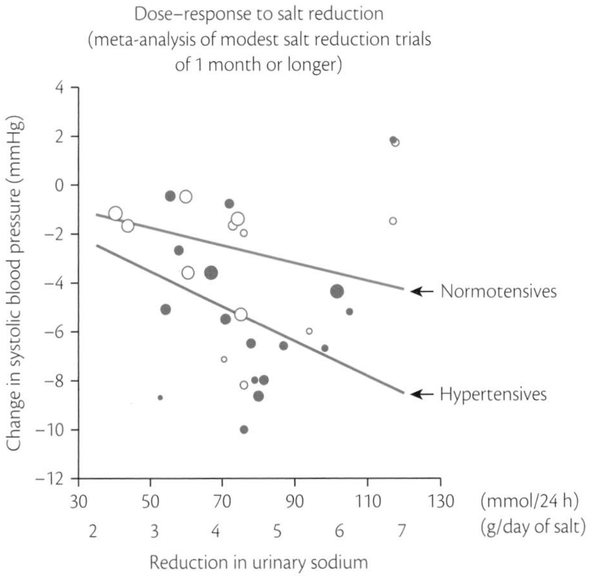

Fig. 14.2 Relationship between the reduction in 24-hour urinary sodium and the change in systolic blood pressure in a meta-analysis of trials of modest salt reduction.
Source: He FJ et al. *Eur Heart J* 2011; **32**: 3073–3080.

Potassium

A high intake of potassium is associated with lower BP. While data from individual trials have been inconsistent, meta-analyses have documented that increased potassium intake lowers BP in normotensive (1.0/0.3 mmHg) and hypertensive individuals (3.5/2.5 mmHg) [23]. In a meta-analysis of 32 trials, potassium supplementation was associated with a fall in BP of 3.1/2.0 mmHg, with a greater effect in patients with a higher salt intake [24]. Potassium appears to reduce BP to a greater extent in blacks than whites. The main sources of potassium are fruits and vegetables; generally, 200 g of fruits (two or three servings a day) and 200 g of vegetables (two or three servings a day) are recommended.

Calcium and magnesium

In a meta-analysis of RCTs, calcium supplementation reduced BP significantly by 1.9/1.0 mmHg, without a significant difference by initial BP level, but with a somewhat larger reduction in BP (2.6/1.3 mmHg) in people with a low calcium intake [25]. Magnesium supplementation did not significantly reduce BP in another meta-analysis, but an apparent dose-dependent effect of magnesium was observed, prompting adequately powered trials with sufficiently high doses of magnesium supplements [26].

Other dietary changes

The landmark study Dietary Approaches to Stop Hypertension (DASH) showed that a diet rich in fruits and vegetables with a fat content typical for the US population lowered BP by 2.8/1.1 mmHg compared with a control diet. When such a diet also incorporated low-fat dairy products and low saturated and total fat, BP decreased by 5.5/3.0 mmHg. The BP decrease was more pronounced in hypertensive patients (11.4/5.5 mmHg) [27]. A number of studies and meta-analyses have reported on the protective CV effect of the Mediterranean diet [28,29]. Fresh fruit is recommended with caution in overweight patients because their sometimes high carbohydrate content may promote weight gain. Patients with hypertension should be advised to eat fish at least twice a week.

Physical exercise

Physical exercise can be divided into two broad categories, namely dynamic aerobic endurance training and resistance training. Meta-analyses of RCTs have concluded that regular dynamic exercise at moderate intensity significantly reduces BP [30,31]. Training induced significant net reductions in resting and daytime ambulatory BP of 3.0/2.4 and 3.3/3.5 mmHg, respectively [31]. The reduction in resting BP was more pronounced in the hypertensive study groups (−6.9/4.9 mmHg) than in the others (−1.9/1.6 mmHg). In addition, body weight decreased by 1.2 kg, waist circumference by 2.8 cm, percentage body fat by 1.4%, and the Homeostasis Model Assessment (HOMA) index of insulin resistance by 0.31 U; high-density lipoprotein cholesterol increased by 0.032 mmol/L [31]. However, the optimal characteristics of such a training programme are still a matter of debate, particularly with regard to the intensity of exercise. In a meta-regression analysis, interstudy differences in the changes in BP were not related to exercise intensity, which ranged from approximately 45% to 85% of maximal exercise capacity [31]. When the effects of training at 33% and 66% of heart rate reserve were compared in one RCT, SBP at rest and during submaximal exercise were reduced with both intensities by about 5 to 6 mmHg, without significant differences in BP reduction between the two intensities [32]. Aerobic interval training has also been shown to significantly reduce BP [33]. A recent meta-analysis of RCTs on resistance training, designed to increase muscular strength, power and/or endurance, found a significant reduction in resting BP by 3.9/3.6 mmHg [34].

Based on current evidence, the following exercise prescription is recommended for hypertensive patients, taking into account their increased CV risk [1,35]:

- frequency—on at least five and preferably every day of the week
- intensity—moderate intensity
- time—at least 30 minutes of physical activity per day
- type—primarily endurance physical activity, supplemented by dynamic resistance exercise.

Finally, all exercising patients should be advised on exercise-related warning symptoms, such as chest pain or discomfort, abnormal dyspnoea, dizziness, or malaise, which would necessitate consulting a qualified physician.

Moderation of alcohol consumption

Longitudinal studies have shown a strong linear relationship between alcohol consumption and BP. Regular alcohol use raises BP in treated hypertensive patients [36]. Heavy drinking is associated with a higher prevalence of hypertension, haemorrhagic stroke, and cardiomyopathy [37], whereas moderate drinking is associated with a lower prevalence of CHD, ischaemic stroke, and sudden cardiac death. In a meta-analysis, decreased consumption of alcohol (–76%, median reduction) was associated with a reduction in BP of 3.3/2.0 mmHg in normotensive and hypertensive individuals [38]. Hypertensive men who drink alcohol should be advised to limit their consumption to no more than 20–30 g ethanol per day, and hypertensive women to no more than 10–20 g ethanol per day.

Smoking cessation

Smoking cessation, although it may not be associated with a decrease in BP, represents the most important preventive measure. In smokers, atherosclerosis develops 10 years earlier than in non-smokers.

Combined modalities

Simultaneous interventions (e.g. to address smoking cessation, reduce dietary salt intake, and increase physical activity) may be more effective than addressing each behaviour sequentially. Attempting to meet one physical activity or dietary goal may actually enhance the chances of attaining the second such goal. In patients who lost weight and reduced their sodium intake, onset of hypertension was more delayed than in those who only lost weight or

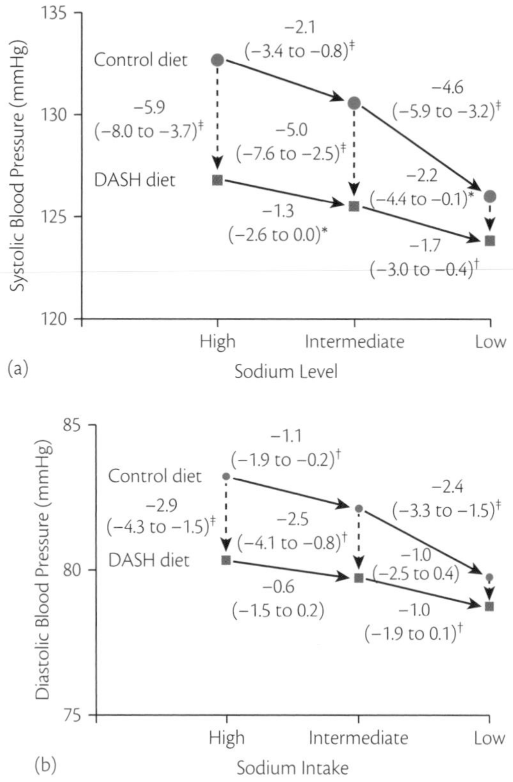

Fig. 14.3 Combining modalities for reducing BP can have additive effects: DASH diet plus salt restriction reduced BP differentially for each level of salt intake. *P < 0.05, †P < 0.01, ‡P < 0.001.
Source: Frisoli TM et al. *Eur Heart J* 2011; **32**: 3081–3087.

only reduced sodium intake. Combining the DASH diet with a low salt intake is associated with a greater decline in BP than each intervention alone (➲ Fig. 14.3) [39]. In patients with elevated BP, combination of the DASH diet with exercise and weight loss resulted in a greater reduction in BP and left ventricular mass than with the DASH diet alone.

Prevention of cardiovascular complications by drug therapy

Evidence of benefit

Trials comparing active treatment versus placebo or no treatment

High BP increases the incidence of fatal and non-fatal CVD, and a substantial number of RCTs comparing antihypertensive treatment with placebo or no treatment have shown that drug therapy is beneficial [40]. In a meta-analysis of RCTs in patients with diastolic hypertension [41], active treatment significantly reduced total mortality by 14% and CV mortality by 21%, mostly due to a reduction in fatal stroke (–45%). The reduction in the odds of any fatal or non-fatal stroke was 42% and in total CHD 14%. In younger and middle-aged patients with diastolic hypertension, treatment was significantly better for all-cause (-17%), CV (-18%), and cerebrovascular mortality (–45%), but not for CHD

(−9%) [42]. As for combined morbidity and mortality, both cerebrovascular events (−33%) and CHD (−16%) were significantly reduced. In elderly patients (aged 60 or older) with diastolic hypertension included in RCTs, active treatment reduced CV, cerebrovascular, and coronary mortality by, respectively, 22, 33, and 26% [43], and in patients with isolated systolic hypertension antihypertensive treatment reduced all-cause mortality by 17% and CV mortality by 25% [44]. The reduction in all fatal and non-fatal CV events, strokes, and coronary events amounted to 32, 37, and 25%, respectively.

Risk for CV events, particularly CHD, differs greatly between men and women. A meta-analysis of individual patient data from RCTs concluded that, in women, odds ratios favouring treatment were significant for fatal strokes (−29%) and combined fatal and non-fatal CV events (−26%) and strokes (−38%), but not for other outcomes. However, the risk ratios between the treated and control groups did not differ between men and women regardless of outcome, and there were no significant interactions between treatment effect and gender [45].

In the very elderly, that is patients aged 80 years and above, a meta-analysis on patients included in RCTs showed that the incidence of major CV events (−22%), fatal and non-fatal stroke (−34%), and heart failure (−39%) was significantly lower in the active treatment group [46]. Later on, the benefit of antihypertensive therapy in the very elderly was confirmed in the properly designed HYVET trial [47]. Active treatment reduced total (−21%) and CV mortality (−23%), any CV event (−34%), stroke (−30%), and heart failure (−64%).

Trials comparing more and less intensive blood pressure lowering

The BP Lowering Treatment Trialists' Collaboration (BPLTTC) reviewed RCTs in which patients were allocated to treatment regimens targeting different BP goals [48]. The difference in BP between more and less intensive treatment was 4/3 mmHg, and was associated with a significantly lower incidence of major CV events (15%) and stroke (23%) but not for other outcomes. Further analysis indicated that for the primary outcome, total major CV events, there was no evidence of a difference in reduction in relative risk in different age groups for BP-lowering regimens compared with less active controls [49].

Trials comparing active treatments

When the beneficial effects of antihypertensive treatment had been shown convincingly, RCTs compared the effects of newer drugs with older drugs or, subsequently, with other newer drugs. In the BPLTTC meta-analysis there were no significant differences in mortality, total major CV events, or CHD between regimens based on angiotensin-converting enzyme (ACE) inhibitors, calcium channel blockers (CCBs), or diuretics or beta-blockers [48]. There was evidence of some differences between active regimens in their effects on stroke and heart failure: regimens based on CCBs appeared to be less effective at preventing heart failure and more effective at preventing stroke. Additional analyses concluded that there was no strong evidence that protection against major CV events by different drug classes varied substantially with age [49] or with gender [50]. Law et al. [51] performed a meta-analysis on RCTs of BP-lowering drugs, in which CHD events or stroke were recorded. They concluded that among the five main drug classes [diuretics, beta-blockers, CCBs, ACE inhibitors and angiotensin II receptor blockers (ARBs)] there was no advantage of any one drug over another in the prevention of CHD. For stroke, however, the preventive effect was greater for CCBs than for other drugs and less for beta-blockers, but CCBs were less effective for the prevention of heart failure. Furthermore, the preventive effect of drugs on CHD and stroke did not differ between people with and without a history of CVD on entry. In a more recent meta-analysis, Fretheim et al. [52] specifically compared the effectiveness of antihypertensive medications for primary prevention of CVD and concluded that there seemed to be little or no difference between commonly used BP-lowering medications for the primary prevention of CVD. In conclusion, a large proportion of the benefits of antihypertensive drugs is accounted for by the BP reduction per se, and comprehensive meta-analyses of RCTs comparing the effects of the five major antihypertensive drug classes on outcome do not show clinically relevant differences. Therefore, they are all considered suitable for initiation and maintenance of antihypertensive treatment.

Therapeutic approach

When to initiate antihypertensive treatment?

Overwhelming evidence from RCTs shows that in patients with a markedly elevated BP, i.e. those with grade 2 or 3 hypertension, antihypertensive drug treatment is associated with a substantial reduction in the incidence of hypertension-related CV complications (stroke, CHD, and heart failure), as well as with a delayed progression of renal damage to ESRD in patients with diabetic or non-diabetic nephropathy [53]. RCTs have also shown, albeit less extensively, that treatment is beneficial in grade 1 hypertension, provided that patients have a high CV risk profile. Less trial-based evidence exists, on the other hand, on whether antihypertensive drug treatment is beneficial in grade 1 hypertension with a low to moderate CV risk or in those aged 65 and above. However, subgroup or post-hoc analyses of several trials have reported that antihypertensive drug treatment may have a beneficial effect in these patients too [54]. It can thus be concluded that prompt antihypertensive drug treatment is mandatory in all patients with grade 2 or 3 hypertension as well as in grade 1 hypertension associated with a high total CV risk. Antihypertensive drug treatment should be also considered, however, in grade 1 hypertension with a mild-to-moderate CV risk, perhaps after a suitable time (weeks or months) of testing whether BP can be effectively reduced by lifestyle changes alone [1].

No data from outcome trials suggest initiation of antihypertensive drug treatment in patients with a high normal BP (i.e. 130–139 mmHg SBP and/or 85–89 mmHg DBP), irrespective of their higher or lower CV risk status, although in these patients antihypertensive drugs may be prescribed for evidence of beneficial effects other than due to BP reduction. Antihypertensive drugs have also been proposed as a means to reduce the risk of developing hypertension, which is greater at high-normal BP [55]. The evidence is still limited, however, and the main strategy against progression to this condition remains the adoption of lifestyle changes that minimize the impact of predictors of hypertension, as already outlined.

Blood pressure goals

The recommendation that most appropriately reflects the currently available evidence is to reduce BP to <140/90 mmHg in patients at both high and low to moderate CV risk, possibly with a lower diastolic target (<85 mmHg) in diabetes [1]. Recommended BP targets in the elderly are discussed in the section 'Therapeutic approach in special conditions'. No information is so far available on the target ambulatory and home BP values to be reached with treatment because this has never been explored by outcome trials with a randomized design.

Choice of antihypertensive drugs

Based on the large number of RCTs of antihypertensive drug therapy and their meta-analyses, it is justifiable to consider several drug classes, i.e. diuretics, beta-blockers, CCBs, ACE inhibitors, and ARBs, as suitable for initiation and maintenance of antihypertensive treatment [48–53,56]. In addition, multiple therapeutic options increase the chance of finding an effective monotherapy in a larger fraction of the hypertensive population [57], taking into account compelling and possible contraindications (➲ Table 14.3) and specific indications (➲ Table 14.4) for the use of antihypertensive drugs [1].

Combination therapy

The administration of a single antihypertensive drug has a limited BP-lowering effect in a noticeable number of patients [58,59]. This low percentage can be substantially increased by the addition of a second or even a third drug, which makes combination treatment a strategy of paramount importance in the management of high BP [60]. Drugs to be combined should have different and complementary mechanisms of action, and evidence should be available that the combination has a greater BP-lowering effect than any of the combination components alone, possibly also with a more favourable tolerability profile and a greater protection against organ damage and CV events [57]. Several combinations fit these requirements partially or totally and can thus be recommended for use: a blocker of the renin–angiotensin system (RAS) (ACE inhibitor or ARB) with a CCB, a RAS blocker with a diuretic, a beta-blocker with a dihydropyridine CCB, and a CCB with a diuretic. A thiazide diuretic, a CCB, and a RAS blocker together appear to be the most rational combination when three drugs are necessary. Whenever failure to reach BP control prompts the use of additional drugs, mineralocorticoid receptor antagonists, alpha-1-blockers, or central agents can be considered. The combination of a beta-blocker and a thiazide diuretic should not be preferred

Table 14.3 Compelling and possible contraindications to the use of antihypertensive drugs

Drug	Compelling	Possible
Diuretics (thiazides)	Gout	Metabolic syndrome Glucose intolerance Pregnancy Hypercalcaemia Hypokalaemia
Beta-blockers	Asthma A–V block (grade 2 or 3)	Metabolic syndrome Glucose intolerance Athletes and physically active patients Chronic obstructive pulmonary disease (except for vasodilator beta-blockers)
Calcium antagonists (dihydropyridines)		Tachyarrhythmia Heart failure
Calcium antagonists (verapamil, diltiazem)	A–V block (grade 2 or 3, trifascicular block) Severe LV dysfunction Heart failure	
ACE inhibitors	Pregnancy Angioneurotic oedema Hyperkalaemia Bilateral renal artery stenosis	Women at risk of pregnancy
Angiotensin receptor blockers	Pregnancy Hyperkalaemia Bilateral renal artery stenosis	Women at risk of pregnancy
Mineralocorticoid receptor antagonists	Acute or severe renal failure (eGFR < 30 ml/min) Hyperkalaemia	

LV, left ventricular; eGFR, estimated glomerular filtration rate.

Table 14.4 Drugs to be preferred in specific conditions

Condition	Drug
Asymptomatic organ damage	
LVH	ACE inhibitor, calcium antagonist, ARB
Asymptomatic atherosclerosis	Calcium antagonist, ACE inhibitor
Microalbuminuria	ACE inhibitor, ARB
Renal dysfunction	ACE inhibitor, ARB
Clinical event	
Previous stroke	Any agent effectively lowering BP
Previous MI	Beta-blocker, ACE inhibitor, ARB
Angina pectoris	Beta-blocker, calcium antagonist
Heart failure	Diuretic, beta-blocker, ACE inhibitor, ARB, mineralocorticoid receptor antagonists
Aortic aneurysm	Beta-blockers
Atrial fibrillation	Consider ARB, ACE inhibitor and beta-blockers or mineralocorticoid receptor antagonist
For ventricular rate control	Beta-blocker, non-dihydropyridine calcium antagonist
ESRD/proteinuria	ACE inhibitor, ARB
Peripheral artery disease	ACE inhibitor, calcium antagonist
Other	
ISH (elderly)	Diuretic, calcium antagonist
Metabolic syndrome	ACE inhibitor, ARB, calcium antagonist
Diabetes mellitus	ACE inhibitor, ARB
Pregnancy	Methyldopa, beta-blocker, calcium antagonist
Blacks	Diuretic, calcium antagonist

LVH, left ventricular hypertrophy; ISH, isolated systolic hypertension.

in patients with a high risk of developing diabetes because the two drugs together may have a noticeable diabetogenic effect [61]. Although particularly effective against a predictor of renal and CV events such as proteinuria and microalbuminuria, the combination of two RAS blockers should also be avoided because the greater antiproteinuric effect that follows their combined administration is associated with a greater risk of hyperkalaemia and renal impairment.

Multiple antihypertensive therapy should usually be adopted after experiencing the inability of monotherapy to control BP. Hypertension guidelines, however, recommend that combination treatment is considered as first step in patients with severe hypertension or at high CV risk. It is believed, although not proven by RCTs, that under these circumstances the risk of an early CV event makes early BP control desirable. Initiating treatment with two drugs has been reported to reduce discontinuation of treatment in a real-life setting, possibly because early BP control favours patient adherence to the prescribed regimen. This may help to increase BP control, which is notoriously low in the hypertensive population worldwide.

Therapeutic approach in special conditions

The elderly

Advice on appropriate lifestyle modifications is also mandatory in elderly patients. As already mentioned, antihypertensive drug treatment is beneficial in elderly and very elderly patients [43,44,46,47]. Based on RCTs there is strong evidence that antihypertensive treatment should be initiated in elderly individuals with SBP ≥ 160 mmHg and that BP should be lowered to <150 mmHg. In elderly individuals younger than 80 years antihypertensive treatment may be considered at SBP > 140 mmHg and aimed at <140 mmHg if individuals are fit and treatment is well tolerated. It is also recommended that hypertensive individuals over 80 should be given antihypertensive treatment if their initial SBP is ≥160 mmHg and that their SBP be reduced to <150 mmHg provided that they are in good physical and mental condition. In frail elderly patients decisions on antihypertensive treatment should be left to the treating physician and based on monitoring the clinical effects of treatment [1].

There is evidence from RCTs in favour of diuretics, beta-blockers, CCBs, ACE inhibitors, and ARBs [49]. The three trials on isolated systolic hypertension in the elderly used a diuretic or a CCB as first-line therapy [44]. In the only RCT in patients aged 80 or above active treatment consisted of the diuretic indapamide, to which the ACE inhibitor perindopril could be added if necessary to achieve the target BP of 150/80 mmHg [47].

Women

There is no evidence that men and women obtain different levels of protection from the lowering of BP or that regimens based on ACE inhibitors, CCBs, ARBs, or diuretics/beta-blockers are more effective in one sex than the other [45,50]. In women of child-bearing potential, particularly without reliable contraception, RAS blockers are contraindicated as angiotensin II is needed for foetal development. While foetal toxicity has been documented for ACE inhibitors and ARBs, there has not been a single case report of exposure to the direct renin inhibitor aliskiren in pregnancy.

Oral contraceptives

Use of oral contraceptives (OCs) is associated with a small but significant increase in BP and with development of hypertension in about 5% of OC users [62,63]. These studies evaluated older-generation OCs with relatively higher oestrogen doses than those currently used. The risk of developing hypertension decreased quickly with cessation of OCs, and past users appeared to have only a slightly increased risk [63]. Similar results were also shown later for second- and third-generation OCs. Earlier prospective studies in OC users consistently showed an increased risk of myocardial infarction (MI) (particularly in smokers) and stroke. There are no CV outcome data available for the newest-generation hormonal contraception formulations developed for non-oral (injectable, topical, and vaginal) routes. Risks and benefits should be weighed in each individual patient before initiating OCs [64]. Women aged 35 years and above should be assessed for CV risk factors including hypertension. It is not recommended to use OCs in women with uncontrolled hypertension. Discontinuation of combined OCs in women with hypertension may improve their BP control. In smokers aged over 35, OCs should be prescribed with caution [65].

Hormone replacement therapy

Hormone replacement therapy (HRT) and selective oestrogen receptor modulators (SERMs) should not be used for the primary or secondary prevention of CVD [66]. If, on occasion, younger, perimenopausal women are being treated for severe menopausal symptoms, the benefits should be weighed against potential risks of HRT. The probability that BP will increase with HRT in menopausal hypertensive women is low.

Pregnancy

Hypertensive disorders in pregnancy have been recently reviewed in ESC guidelines on the management of CVD during pregnancy [67]. While there is consensus that drug treatment of severe hypertension in pregnancy (SBP > 160 mmHg and/or DBP > 110 mmHg) is required and beneficial, the benefits of antihypertensive therapy for mildly to moderately elevated BP in pregnancy (≤160/110 mmHg), either pre-existing or pregnancy-induced, have not been demonstrated in clinical trials, except for a lowered risk of developing severe hypertension [68]. Despite lack of evidence, the 2013 ESH/ESC guidelines [1] continue to suggest initiation of antihypertensive treatment at 140/90 mmHg in women with:

- gestational hypertension (with or without proteinuria)
- pre-existing hypertension with the superimposition of gestational hypertension
- hypertension with subclinical organ damage or symptoms at any time during pregnancy.

In any other circumstances, initiation of drug treatment is recommended in all women with persistent elevation of BP ≥ 150/95 mmHg.

Pre-eclampsia is a pregnancy-specific syndrome occurring after mid-gestation, defined by de novo appearance of hypertension accompanied by new-onset proteinuria; it is the most frequent cause of maternal death worldwide. Based on a recent meta-analysis [69], women at risk of pre-eclampsia are advised to take 75 mg of aspirin daily from 12 weeks' gestation until delivery [70].

Long-term cardiovascular consequences of pregnancy-induced hypertension

A large meta-analysis found that women with a history of pre-eclampsia have approximately double the risk of subsequent CHD, stroke, and venous thromboembolic events over 5–15 years after pregnancy [71]; the risk of developing hypertension is almost fourfold. Therefore, lifestyle modifications and regular checkups of BP and metabolic factors are recommended after delivery to reduce CV risk in the future.

Diabetes mellitus

High BP is common in patients with type 2 diabetes, and in diabetic patients reduction of BP by drug treatment effectively lowers hypertension-related macrovascular complications [58,72]. Renal microvascular complications are also reduced, whereas the effect of antihypertensive treatment on diabetic neuropathy and retinopathy is uncertain. In diabetic patients antihypertensive drug treatment should be considered together with appropriate lifestyle changes whenever SBP is ≥140 mmHg or DBP ≥ 90 mmHg, with the goal of reducing BP to <140/85 mmHg [1]. No evidence exists that further benefit can be obtained by reducing SBP to <130 mmHg [54]. All major antihypertensive drug classes have been shown to reduce CV risk in diabetes and can thus be considered for treatment, their use in combination being often necessary [56,73]. Unless contraindicated, the combination should always include an ACE inhibitor or an ARB because in type 1 and 2 diabetes these drugs have a BP-independent ability to delay the appearance of proteinuria, exert a greater antiproteinuric effect, and reduce the rate of renal deterioration when nephropathy is present [57,74]. Double blockade of RAS should, on the other hand, be avoided, particularly in patients with impaired renal function because of the increased risk of hyperkalaemia and ESRD [75,76].

Cerebrovascular disease

Acute stroke

There is currently no evidence that lowering of BP has a beneficial effect in acute stroke. However, clinical judgement should be used to manage very high SBP.

Previous stroke or transient ischaemic attack

Prevention of stroke is the most consistent benefit of antihypertensive therapy observed in RCTs, and all drug regimens are acceptable for stroke prevention provided BP is effectively reduced. Meta-analyses [48,51] suggest that CCBs may have a slightly greater effectiveness in stroke prevention, but two successful trials in secondary stroke prevention used a diuretic or a diuretic in combination with an ACE inhibitor. Initiation of antihypertensive drug treatment in patients with a history of stroke or transient ischaemic attack is recommended for SBP ≥ 140 mmHg. A SBP of <140 mmHg should be considered as the goal in these patients.

Cognitive dysfunction and white matter lesions

White matter lesions are known to be associated with increased risk of stroke, cognitive decline, and dementia. A small substudy of the HYVET trial [77] and a recent prospective observational study [78] suggest that a decrease in white matter hyperintensity is possible by lowering BP, but this suggestion requires verification in large RCTs.

Coronary heart disease and heart failure

Antihypertensive treatment is beneficial in patients with CHD in whom it lowers the recurrence of a coronary event as well as of other CV complications. Drug treatment should be implemented whenever BP is ≥140/90 mmHg with the aim of lowering BP below these values; lowering BP to <130/80 mmHg should not be pursued because of an increased risk [79]. Beta-blockers should be preferred in patients with a recent MI, although a few months after the event all drugs can be used. For symptomatic reasons beta-blockers and CCBs should be the preferred drugs in angina pectoris [57].

Prevention of heart failure has been obtained with all major drug classes, although in comparison trials CCBs have apparently been less effective than other drugs, particularly diuretics. Because the difference can be accounted for, at least in part, by the ability of diuretics to mask early symptoms of heart failure (and of CCBs to favour an erroneous diagnosis because of peripheral oedema) the prevailing opinion is that the risk of new-onset heart failure can be substantially reduced, irrespective of the type of treatment employed, provided that BP is effectively lowered. No RCTs have been performed in heart failure patients with current or previous hypertension with the aim of testing whether a reduction in BP is beneficial or harmful. Use of beta-blockers, RAS blockers, and mineralocorticoid receptor antagonists can be recommended, however, because of the ability of these agents to prevent death and hospitalization when left ventricular systolic function is impaired. Although previous and current hypertension is rather common in patients with preserved ejection fraction, no evidence is available on whether a reduction in BP may be protective—the only available trial reported no reduction of CV outcomes by an ARB versus placebo [80].

Renal disease

Antihypertensive treatment exerts a nephroprotective effect, and it should thus be implemented at all stages of CKD. As in other clinical conditions, drug treatment should start at SBP ≥ 140 mmHg. A desirable SBP is <140 mmHg, but SBP < 130 mmHg may be pursued in the presence of persistent proteinuria. Antihypertensive treatment should also be implemented in patients with ESRD and dialysis, although the optimal BP target in such cases is unknown. In diabetic and non-diabetic nephropathy, treatment usually consists of a combination of two or more drugs because renal disease is one of the clinical conditions in which BP control is particularly difficult. The preferred combinations include a RAS blocker (mandatory in the presence of proteinuria) with a CCB and/or a diuretic, thiazides being replaced by loop diuretics in the presence of a marked deterioration (<30 ml/min) in glomerular filtration rate. Double blockade of the RAS and use of mineralocorticoid receptor antagonists should be avoided because of the risk of hyperkalaemia and excessive reduction in renal function [1].

Further reading

Appel LJ, Moore TJ, Obarzanek E, et al. A clinical trial of the effects of dietary patterns on blood pressure. DASH Collaborative Research Group. *N Engl J Med* 1997; **336**: 1117–24.

Beckett NS, Peters R, Fletcher A, et al. Treatment of hypertension in patients 80 years of age or older. *N Engl J Med* 2008; **358**: 1887–98.

Blood Pressure Lowering Treatment Trialists' Collaboration. Effects of different blood pressure-lowering regimens on major cardiovascular events in individuals with and without diabetes mellitus. Results of prospectively designed overviews of randomized trials. *Arch Intern Med* 2005; **165**: 1410–19.

Blood Pressure Lowering Treatment Trialists' Collaboration. Effects of different blood pressure lowering regimens on major cardiovascular events: results of prospectively-designed overviews of randomized trials. *Lancet* 2003: **362**: 1527–35.

Blood Pressure Lowering Treatment Trialists' Collaboration. Effects of different regimens to lower blood pressure on major cardiovascular events in older and younger adults: meta-analysis of randomised trials. *Br Med J* 2008; **336**: 1121–3.

Cornelissen VA, Fagard RH. Effects of endurance training on blood pressure, blood pressure regulating mechanisms and cardiovascular risk factors. *Hypertension* 2005; **46**: 667–75.

Elliott WJ, Meyer PM. Incident diabetes in clinical trials of antihypertensive drugs: a network meta-analysis. *Lancet* 2007; **369**: 201–7.

Elmer PJ, Obarzanek E, Vollmer WM, et al. Effects of comprehensive lifestyle modification on diet, weight, physical fitness, and blood pressure control: 18-month results of a randomized trial. *Ann Intern Med* 2006; **144**: 485–95.

Estruch R, Ros E, Salas-Salvadó J, et al. The PREDIMED Study Investigators. Primary prevention of cardiovascular disease with a Mediterranean diet. *N Engl J Med* 2013; **368**: 1279–90.

Fagard RH. Exercise therapy in hypertensive cardiovascular disease. *Prog Cardiovasc Dis* 2011; **53**: 404–11.

Graudal NA, Hubeck-Graudal T, Jurgens G. Effects of low-sodium diet vs. high-sodium diet on blood pressure, renin, aldosterone, catecholamines, cholesterol, and triglyceride (Cochrane review). *Am J Hypertens* 2012; **25**: 1–15.

Geleijnse JM, Kok FJ, Grobbee DE. Blood pressure response to changes in sodium and potassium intake: a metaregression analysis of randomised trials. *J Hum Hypertens* 2003; **17**: 471–80.

Law MR, Morris JK, Wald NJ. Use of blood pressure lowering drugs in the prevention of cardiovascular disease: meta-analysis of 147 randomised trials in the context of expectations from prospective epidemiological studies. *Br Med J* 2009; **338**: b 1665.

Lewington S, Clarke R, Qizilbash N, et al. Age-specific relevance of usual blood pressure to vascular mortality: a meta-analysis of individual data for one million adults in 61 prospective studies. *Lancet* 2002; **360**: 1903–13.

Mancia G, Fagard R, Narkiewicz K, et al. The Task Force for the management of arterial hypertension of the European Society of Hypertension (ESH) and of the European Society of Cardiology (ESC). 2013 ESH/ESC guidelines for the management of arterial hypertension. *Eur Heart J* 2013; **31**: 1281–357.

Mancia G, Laurent S, Agabiti-Rosei E, et al. Reappraisal of European guidelines on hypertension management: a European Society of Hypertension Task Force document. *J Hypertens* 2009; **27**: 2121–58.

Neter JE, Stam BE, Kok FJ, et al. Influence of weight reduction on blood pressure: a meta-analysis of randomized controlled trials. *Hypertension* 2003; **42**: 878–84.

Perk J, De Backer G, Gohlke H, et al. European Guidelines on cardiovascular disease prevention in clinical practice (version 2012): The Fifth Joint Task Force of the European Society of Cardiology and Other Societies on Cardiovascular Disease Prevention in Clinical Practice (constituted by representatives of nine societies and by invited experts). * Developed with the special contribution of the European Association for Cardiovascular Prevention and Rehabilitation (EACPR). *Eur Heart J* 2012; **33**: 1635–701.

Regitz-Zagrosek V, Blomstrom Lundqvist C, Borghi C, et al. European Society of Gynecology; Association for European Paediatric

Cardiology; German Society for Gender Medicine. ESC Guidelines on the management of cardiovascular diseases during pregnancy: the Task Force on the Management of Cardiovascular Diseases during Pregnancy of the European Society of Cardiology (ESC). *Eur Heart J* 2011; **32**: 3147–97.

Shufelt CL, Merz NB. Contraceptive hormone use and cardiovascular disease. *J Am Coll Cardiol* 2009; **53**: 221–31.

Turnbull F, Woodward M, Neal B, et al. The Blood Pressure Lowering Treatment Trialists' Collaboration. Do men and women respond differently to blood pressure-lowering treatment? Results of prospectively designed overviews of randomized trials. *Eur Heart J* 2008; **29**: 2669–80.

Wald DS, Law M, Morris JK, et al. Combination therapy versus monotherapy in reducing blood pressure: meta-analysis on 11,000 participants from 42 trials. *Am J Med* 2009; **122**: 290–300.

Xin X, He J, Frontini MG, et al. Effects of alcohol reduction on blood pressure: a meta-analysis of randomized controlled trials. *Hypertension* 2001; **38**: 1112–17.

Zanchetti A, Grassi G, Mancia G. When should antihypertensive treatment be initiated and to what levels should systolic blood pressure be lowered? A critical reappraisal. *J Hypertens* 2009; **27**: 923–34.

References

1 Mancia G, Fagard R, Narkiewicz K, et al. The Task Force for the management of arterial hypertension of the European Society of Hypertension (ESH) and of the European Society of Cardiology (ESC). 2013 ESH/ESC Guidelines for the management of arterial hypertension. *Eur Heart J* 2013; **31**: 1281–357.

2 Lewington S, Clarke R, Qizilbash N, et al. Age-specific relevance of usual blood pressure to vascular mortality: a meta-analysis of individual data for one million adults in 61 prospective studies. *Lancet* 2002; **360**: 1903–13.

3 Britton KA, Gaziano JM, Djousse L. Normal systolic blood pressure and risk of heart failure in US male physicians. *Eur J Heart Fail* 2009; **11**: 1129–34.

4 Kalaitzidis RG, Bakris GL. Prehypertension: is it relevant for nephrologists? *Kidney Int* 2010; **77**: 194–200.

5 Lawes CM, Rodgers A, Bennett DA, et al. Blood pressure and cardiovascular disease in the Asia Pacific region. *J Hypertens* 2003; **21**: 707–16.

6 Brown DW, Giles WH, Greenlund KJ. Blood pressure parameters and risk of fatal stroke, NHANES II mortality study. *Am J Hypertens* 2007; **20**: 338–41.

7 O'Brien E, Parati G, Stergiou G, et al. on behalf of the European Society of Hypertension Working Group on Blood Pressure Monitoring. European Society of Hypertension position paper on ambulatory blood pressure monitoring. *J Hypertens* 2013; **31**: 1731–68.

8 Parati G, Stergiou GS, Asmar R, et al. European Society of Hypertension practice guidelines for home blood pressure monitoring. *J Hum Hypertens* 2010; **24**: 779–85.

9 Boggia J, Li Y, Thijs L, et al. Prognostic accuracy of day versus night ambulatory blood pressure: a cohort study. *Lancet* 2007; **370**: 1219–29.

10 Fagard RH, Celis H, Thijs L, et al. Daytime and nighttime blood pressure as predictors of death and cause-specific cardiovascular events in hypertension. *Hypertension* 2008; **51**: 55–61.

11 Ward AM, Takahashi O, Stevens R. Home measurement of blood pressure and cardiovascular disease: systematic review and meta-analysis of prospective studies. *J Hypertens* 2012; **30**: 449–56.

12 Fagard RH, Cornelissen VA. Incidence of cardiovascular events in white-coat, masked and sustained hypertension versus true normotension: a meta-analysis. *J Hypertens* 2007; **25**: 2193–8.

13 Pierdomenico SD, Cuccurullo F. Prognostic value of white-coat and masked hypertension diagnosed by ambulatory monitoring in initially untreated subjects: an updated meta-analysis. *Am J Hypertens* 2011; **24**: 52–8.

14 Franklin SS, Thijs L, Hansen TW, et al. Significance of white-coat hypertension in older persons with isolated systolic hypertension: a meta-analysis using the International Database on Ambulatory Blood Pressure Monitoring in Relation to Cardiovascular Outcomes population. *Hypertension* 2012; **59**: 564–71.

15 Elmer PJ, Obarzanek E, Vollmer WM, et al. Effects of comprehensive lifestyle modification on diet, weight, physical fitness, and blood pressure control: 18-month results of a randomized trial. *Ann Intern Med* 2006; **144**: 485–95.

16 Perk J, De Backer G, Gohlke H, et al. European Guidelines on cardiovascular disease prevention in clinical practice (version 2012): The Fifth Joint Task Force of the European Society of Cardiology and Other Societies on Cardiovascular Disease Prevention in Clinical Practice (constituted by representatives of nine societies and by invited experts). * Developed with the special contribution of the European Association for Cardiovascular Prevention and Rehabilitation (EACPR). *Eur Heart J* 2012; **33**: 1635–701.

17 Neter JE, Stam BE, Kok FJ, et al. Influence of weight reduction on blood pressure: a meta-analysis of randomized controlled trials. *Hypertension* 2003; **42**: 878–84.

18 Prospective Studies Collaboration. Body-mass index and cause-specific mortality in 900 000 adults: collaborative analyses of 57 prospective studies. *Lancet* 2009; **373**: 1083–96.

19 Flegal KM, Kit BK, Orpana H, et al. Association of all-cause mortality with overweight and obesity using standard body mass index categories. A systematic review and meta-analysis. *J Am Med Assoc* 2013; **309**: 71–82.

20 He FJ, MacGregor GA. Effect of modest salt reduction on blood pressure: a meta-analysis of randomized trials. Implications for public health. *J Hum Hypertens* 2002; **16**: 761–70.

21 Graudal NA, Hubeck-Graudal T, Jurgens G. Effects of low-sodium diet vs. high-sodium diet on blood pressure, renin, aldosterone, catecholamines, cholesterol, and triglyceride (Cochrane review). *Am J Hypertens* 2012; **25**: 1–15.

22 Cook NR, Cutler JA, Obarzanek E, et al. Long term effects of dietary sodium reduction on cardiovascular disease outcomes: observational follow-up of the trials of hypertension prevention (TOHP). *Br Med J* 2007; **334**: 885–8.

23 Geleijnse JM, Kok FJ, Grobbee DE. Blood pressure response to changes in sodium and potassium intake: a metaregression analysis of randomised trials. *J Hum Hypertens* 2003; **17**: 471–80.

24 Whelton PK, He J, Cutler JA, et al. Effects of oral potassium on blood pressure. Meta-analysis of randomized controlled clinical trials. *J Am Med Assoc* 1997; **277**: 1624–32.

25 van Mierlo LA, Arends LR, Streppel MT, et al. Blood pressure response to calcium supplementation: a meta-analysis of randomized controlled trials. *J Hum Hypertens* 2006; **20**: 571–80.

26 Jee SH, Miller ER, Guallar E, et al. The effect of magnesium supplementation on blood pressure: a meta-analysis of randomized clinical trials. *Am J Hypertens* 2002; **15**: 891–6.

27 Appel LJ, Moore TJ, Obarzanek E, et al. A clinical trial of the effects of dietary patterns on blood pressure. DASH Collaborative Research Group. *N Engl J Med* 1997; **336**: 1117–24.

28 Sofi F, Abbate R, Gensini GF, et al. Accruing evidence on benefits of adherence to the Mediterranean diet on health: an updated systematic review and meta-analysis. *Am J Clin Nutr* 2010; **92**: 1189–96.

29 Estruch R, Ros E, Salas-Salvadó J, et al. The PREDIMED Study Investigators. Primary prevention of cardiovascular disease with a Mediterranean diet. *N Engl J Med* 2013; **368**: 1279–90.

30 Whelton SP, Chin A, Xin X, et al. Effects of aerobic exercise on blood pressure: a meta-analysis of randomised, controlled trials. *Ann Intern Med* 2002; **136**: 493–503.

31 Cornelissen VA, Fagard RH. Effects of endurance training on blood pressure, blood pressure regulating mechanisms and cardiovascular risk factors. *Hypertension* 2005; **46**: 667–75.

32 Cornelissen VA, Arnout J, Holvoet P, et al. Influence of exercise at lower and higher intensity on blood pressure and cardiovascular risk factors at older age. *J Hypertens* 2009; **27**: 753–62.

33 Molmen-Hansen HE, Stolen T, Tjonna AE, et al. Aerobic interval training reduces blood pressure and improves myocardial function in hypertensive patients. *Eur J Prev Cardiol* 2012; **19**: 151–60.

34 Cornelissen VA, Fagard RH, Coeckelberghs E, et al. Impact of resistance training on blood pressure and other cardiovascular risk factors: a meta-analysis of randomized, controlled trials. *Hypertension* 2011; **58**: 950–8.

35 Fagard RH. Exercise therapy in hypertensive cardiovascular disease. *Prog Cardiovasc Dis* 2011; **53**: 404–11.

36 Puddey IB, Beilin LJ, Vandongen R. Regular alcohol use raises blood pressure in treated hypertensive subjects. A randomised controlled trial. *Lancet* 1987; **1**: 647–51.

37 Klatsky AL.Alcohol and stroke: an epidemiological labyrinth. *Stroke* 2005; **36**: 1835–6.

38 Xin X, He J, Frontini MG, et al. Effects of alcohol reduction on blood pressure: a meta-analysis of randomized controlled trials. *Hypertension* 2001; **38**: 1112–17.

39 Sacks FM, Svetkey LP, Vollmer WM, et al. Effects on blood pressure of reduced dietary sodium and the dietary approaches to stop hypertension (DASH) diet. DASH-Sodium Collaborative Research Group. *N Engl J Med* 2001; **344**: 3–10.

40 Fagard RH, Staessen JA, Thijs L. Results of intervention trials of antihypertensive treatment vs placebo, no or less intensive treatment. In: Mancia G, Chalmers J Julius SC et al. (eds) *Manual of hypertension*, 2002, pp. 21–33. London: Churchill Livingstone.

41 Collins R, Peto R, MacMahon S, et al. Blood pressure, stroke and coronary heart disease. Part 2. *Lancet* 1990; **335**: 827–38.

42 Mulrow CD, Cornell JA, Herrera CR, et al. Hypertension in the elderly. Implications and generalizability of randomized trials. *J Am Med Assoc* 1994; **272**: 1932–8.

43 Thijs L, Fagard R, Lijnen P, et al. A meta-analysis of outcome trials in elderly hypertensives. *J Hypertens* 1992; **10**: 1103–10.

44 Staessen JA, Wang JG, Thijs L, et al. Overview of the outcome trials in older patients with isolated systolic hypertension. *J Hum Hypertens* 1999; **13**: 859–63.

45 Gueyffier F, Boutitie F, Bouissel JP, et al. The effect of antihypertensive drug treatment on cardiovascular outcomes in women and men. Results from a meta-analysis of individual patient data in randomized controlled trials. *Ann Intern Med* 1997; **126**: 761–7.

46 Gueyffier F, Bulpitt C, Boissel JP, et al. Antihypertensive drugs in very old people: a subgroup analysis of randomized controlled trials. *Lancet* 1999; **353**: 793–6.

47 Beckett NS, Peters R, Fletcher A, et al. Treatment of hypertension in patients 80 years of age or older. *N Engl J Med* 2008; **358**: 1887–98.

48 Blood Pressure Lowering Treatment Trialists' Collaboration. Effects of different blood pressure lowering regimens on major cardiovascular events: results of prospectively-designed overviews of randomized trials. *Lancet* 2003; **362**: 1527–35.

49 Blood Pressure Lowering Treatment Trialists' Collaboration. Effects of different regimens to lower blood pressure on major cardiovascular events in older and younger adults: meta-analysis of randomised trials. *Br Med J* 2008; **336**: 1121–3.

50 Turnbull F, Woodward M, Neal B, et al. The Blood Pressure Lowering Treatment Trialists' Collaboration. Do men and women respond differently to blood pressure-lowering treatment? Results of prospectively designed overviews of randomized trials. *Eur Heart J* 2008; **29**: 2669–80.

51 Law MR, Morris JK, Wald NJ. Use of blood pressure lowering drugs in the prevention of cardiovascular disease: meta-analysis of 147 randomised trials in the context of expectations from prospective epidemiological studies. *Br Med J* 2009; **338**: b 1665.

52 Fretheim A, Odgaard-Jensen J, Brors O, et al. Comparative effectiveness of antihypertensive medication for primary prevention of cardiovascular disease: systematic review and multiple treatments meta-analysis. *BMC Med* 2012; **10**: 33.

53 Mancia G, De Backer G, Dominiczak A, et al. 2007 Guidelines for the Management of Arterial Hypertension: the Task Force for the Management of Arterial Hypertension of the European Society of Hypertension (ESH) and the European Society of Cardiology (ESC). *Eur Heart J* 2007; **28**: 1462–536.

54 Zanchetti A, Grassi G, Mancia G. When should antihypertensive treatment be initiated and to what levels should systolic blood pressure be lowered? A critical reappraisal. *J Hypertens* 2009; **27**: 923–34.

55 Julius S, Nesbitt SD, Egan BM, et al. Feasibility of treating prehypertension with an angiotensin-receptor blocker. *N Engl J Med* 2006; **354**: 1685–97.

56 Blood Pressure Lowering Treatment Trialists' Collaboration. Effects of different blood pressure-lowering regimens on major cardiovascular events in individuals with and without diabetes mellitus. Results of prospectively designed overviews of randomized trials. *Arch Intern Med* 2005; **165**: 1410–19.

57 Mancia G, Laurent S, Agabiti-Rosei E, et al. Reappraisal of European guidelines on hypertension management: a European Society of Hypertension Task Force document. *J Hypertens* 2009; **27**: 2121–58.

58 Tarnow L, Rossing P, Gall MA, et al. Prevalence of arterial hypertension in diabetic patients before and after the JNC-V. *Diabetes Care* 1994; **17**: 1247–51.

59 Morgan TO, Anderson AIE, MacInnis RJ. ACE inhibitors, betablockers, calcium blockers, and diuretics for the control of systolic hypertension. *Am J Hypertens* 2001; **14**: 241–7.

60 Wald DS, Law M, Morris JK, et al. Combination therapy versus monotherapy in reducing blood pressure: meta-analysis on 11,000 participants from 42 trials. *Am J Med* 2009; **122**: 290–300.

61 Elliott WJ, Meyer PM. Incident diabetes in clinical trials of antihypertensive drugs: a network meta-analysis. *Lancet* 2007; **369**: 201–7.

62 Dong W, Colhoun HM, Poulter NR. Blood pressure in women using oral contraceptives results from the Health Survey for England1994. *J Hypertens* 1997; **15**: 1063–8.

63 Chasan-Taber L, Willett WC, Manson JE, et al. Prospective study of oral contraceptives and hypertension among women in the United States. *Circulation* 1996; **94**: 483–9.

64 Shufelt CL, Merz NB. Contraceptive hormone use and cardiovascular disease. *J Am Coll Cardiol* 2009; **53**: 221–31.

65 ACOG Committee on Practice Bulletins—Gynecology. ACOG practice bulletin no. 73: use of hormonal contraception in women with coexisting medical conditions. *Obstet Gynecol* 2006; **107**: 1453–72.

66 Mosca L, Benjamin EJ, Berra K, et al. Effectiveness-based guidelines for the prevention of cardiovascular disease in women—2011 update: a guideline from the American Heart Association. *J Am Coll Cardiol* 2011; **57**: 1404–23.

67 Regitz-Zagrosek V, Blomstrom Lundqvist C, Borghi C, et al. European Society of Gynecology; Association for European Paediatric Cardiology; German Society for Gender Medicine. ESC Guidelines on the management of cardiovascular diseases during pregnancy: the Task Force on the Management of Cardiovascular Diseases during Pregnancy of the European Society of Cardiology (ESC). *Eur Heart J* 2011; **32**: 3147–97.

68 Abalos E, Duley L, Steyn DW, et al. Antihypertensive drug therapy for mild to moderate hypertension during pregnancy. *Cochrane Database Syst Rev* 2001; (2): CD002252.

69 Bujold E, Roberge S, Lacasse Y, et al. Prevention of preeclampsia and intrauterine growth restriction with aspirin started in early pregnancy: a meta-analysis. *Obstet Gynecol* 2010; **116** : 402–14.

70 National Institute for Health and Care Excellence. *Hypertension in pregnancy: the management of hypertensive disorders during pregnancy*. NICE Clinical Guidelines no. 107 London: NICE, 2010 (last modified January 2011).

71 Bellamy L, Casas JP, Hingorani AD, et al. Pre-eclampsia and risk of cardiovascular disease and cancer in later life: systematic review and meta-analysis. *Br Med J* 2007; **335**: 974.

72 UK Prospective Diabetes Study Group. Tight blood pressure control and risk of macrovascular and microvascular complications in type 2 diabetes: UKPDS 38. *Br Med J*. 1998; **317**: 703–13.

73 Mancia G, Schumacher H, Redon J, et al. Blood pressure targets recommendations by guidelines and incidence of cardiovascular and renal events in the Ongoing Telmisartan Alone and in combination with Ramipril Global Endpoint Trial (ONTARGET). *Circulation* 2011; **124**: 1727–36.

74 Kunz R, Friedrich C, Wolbers M, et al. Meta-analysis: effect of monotherapy and combination therapy with inhibitors of the renin-angiotensin system on proteinuria in renal disease. *Ann Intern Med* 2008; **138**: 30–48.

75 Mann JFE, Schmieder RE, McQueen M, et al. on behalf of the ONTARGET investigators. Renal outcomes with telmisartan, ramipril, or both, in people at high risk (the ONTARGET study): a multicentre, randomized, double-blind, controlled trial. *Lancet* 2008; **372**: 547–53.

76 Parving HH, Brenner BM, McMurray JJV, et al. Cardiorenal end points in a trial of aliskiren for type 2 diabetes. *N Engl J Med* 2012; **367**: 2204–13.

77 Peters R, Beckett N, Forette F, et al. Incident dementia and blood pressure lowering in the HYpertension in the Very Elderly Trial cognitive function assessment (HYVET-COG): a double-blind, placebo controlled trial. *Lancet Neurol* 2008; **7**: 683–9.

78 Dufouil C, Godin O, Chalmers J, et al. Severe cerebral white matter hyperintensities predict severe cognitive decline in patients with cerebrovascular disease history. *Stroke* 2009; **40**: 2219–21.

79 Messerli FH, Mancia G, Conti CR, et al. Dogma disputed: can aggressive lowering blood pressure in hypertensive patients with coronary artery disease be dangerous? *Ann Intern Med* 2006; **144**: 884–93.

80 Massie BM, Carson PE, McMurray JJ, et al. Irbesartan in patients with heart failure and preserved ejection fraction. *N Eng J Med* 2008; **359**: 2456–67.

CHAPTER 15

Lipids

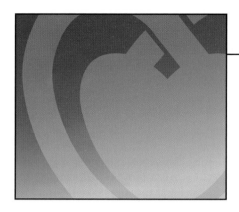

Željko Reiner, Olov Wiklund, and
John Betteridge

Contents

Summary

Increased total plasma cholesterol (TC) and low-density lipoprotein (LDL) cholesterol (LDL-C) is one of the main risk factors for cardiovascular (CV) disease (CVD). It is recommended that TC is used for the estimation of total CV risk when using the SCORE (Systematic COronary Risk Evaluation) algorithm but not as a target for treatment. It should only be considered as a treatment target if LDL-C is not available. High triglycerides (TG), and particularly low high-density lipoprotein (HDL) cholesterol (HDL-C), are also independent CVD risk factors. HDL-C is also used for risk estimation. In general, TC should be below 5 mmol/L (~190 mg/dl) and LDL-C should be below 3 mmol/L (~115 mg/dl). In patients with a very high risk of CVD [i.e. established CVD, diabetes (type 1 or type 2) with one or more other CVD risk factor(s) and/or target organ damage, moderate to severe chronic kidney disease (CKD) or a SCORE level ≥ 10%] the target for LDL-C is <1.8 mmol/L (< ~70 mg/dl) and/or a ≥50% reduction in LDL-C when the target level cannot be reached. In patients at high risk of CVD (i.e. diabetes but no other CV risk factor nor target organ damage, markedly elevated single risk factors, a SCORE level ≥5% to <10%) a target for LDL-C of <2.5 mmol/L (< ~100 mg/dl) should be considered. In subjects at moderate risk (SCORE level >1% to ≤5%) a LDL-C target of <3.0 mmol/L (< ~115 mg/dl) should be considered. All patients with familial hypercholesterolaemia (FH) should be recognized as being at high risk and should be treated by lipid-lowering therapy. There are no specific targets for TG or HDL-C as evidence from outcome studies is lacking, but on the basis of epidemiological data TG levels should be <1.7 mmol/L (150 mg/dl) and HDL-C should be >1.0 (~40 mg/dl) in men and >1.2 (~46 mg/dl) in women. Appropriate modification of lifestyle and particularly diet has a significant impact on improving lipoproteins and an enormous potential for CVD prevention. If lifestyle intervention is not enough, statins are the drugs of choice for hypercholesterolaemia, and statin therapy has a proven beneficial effect on CVD outcomes. Fibrates are the drugs of choice for decreasing high TG and increasing low HDL-C. If monotherapy with a statin at the highest tolerable dose is not sufficient to achieve the target values for LDL-C or an adequate decrease in TG, and an increase in HDL-C cannot be achieved with a fibrate, combination therapy is recommended either with a statin and another LDL-lowering drug in the first case or a statin plus a fibrate in the latter.

Clinical case

A 48-year-old man who works as a lorry driver was advised to have a cholesterol check following the death of his older brother following an acute myocardial infarction (MI) at the age of 56. His father had had his first MI at 46 years and underwent a coronary artery bypass graft (CABG) at the age of 54. He died at the age of 62 after an acute coronary event. The father had continued to smoke, was hypertensive, and was not concordant with medical therapy which included antihypertensives and aspirin from the time of the CABG and, more latterly, a statin.

The patient is not a current smoker, having stopped 10 years previously (giving him a 25 pack-year history). He drinks about 35 units of alcohol each week, mainly in the form of beer, and does not undertake any physical activity. There is no relevant past history and no cardiovascular symptoms. His BMI is 28 kg/m^2 and waist circumference 103 cm. Examination shows no stigmata of hyperlipidaemia and his blood pressure is 152/94 mmHg. The rest of the cardiovascular system is normal.

At his initial check his fasting lipid profile showed a plasma TC of 8.4 mmol/L, TG of 6.7 mmol/L, and HDL-C 0.8 mmol/L. LDL-C could not be calculated because of the high TG which precludes the use of the Friedewald formula to calculate LDL-C. Fasting blood glucose was in the impaired fasting glucose range at 6.1 mmol/L. Thyroid and renal function were normal but alanine aminotransferase was slightly raised. He was started on simvastatin 40 mg/day by his family physician and referred to the lipid clinic for further assessment and management.

At the lipid clinic his fasting lipid profile shows that since taking the simvastatin his TC has fallen to 6 mmol/L and TG to 4.7 mmol/l, and HDL-C is 0.9 mmol/L. Fasting blood glucose is 6.0 mmol/L and alanine aminotransferase 1.5 times the upper limit of normal. Apolipoprotein B is high at 1.28 g/L but lipoprotein(a) (Lp(a)) is <0.03 g/L. His ApoE phenotype is E3E3. A provisional diagnosis of familial combined hyperlipidaemia is made, which is exacerbated by his diet and lifestyle habits. Glucose intolerance and insulin resistance are commonly associated with this condition. Plans for further management are discussed with the patient and his wife and the screening of his two children aged 24 and 22 is arranged. What should be done?

Lipids and CVD risk

A plethora of epidemiological, genetic, and pathological as well as observational and interventional studies have undoubtedly established the crucial role of changed serum lipoprotein concentrations or dyslipidaemias, especially increased serum cholesterol or hypercholesterolaemia, as the most important risk factor in the development of CVD. Therefore it is quite understandable that serum levels of lipids, lipoproteins, apolipoproteins, and various derived ratios are most important in predicting CVD risk. This is particularly true for plasma TC and LDL-C, but also for HDL-C. However, perception, awareness, and knowledge of the importance of dyslipidaemia as an important CVD risk factor is not always adequate and it should be significantly increased in order to improve CVD prevention [1–4].

Which lipid parameters should be measured?

Atherogenic lipoproteins which participate significantly in the aetiopathology of CVD are the apolipoprotein B (ApoB)-containing LDL (particularly small dense LDL), very low-density lipoprotein (VLDL), and intermediate density lipoprotein (IDL). High levels of these lipoproteins are therefore associated with an increased risk of CVD. HDL, on the other hand, is associated with reduced risk, and the main apolipoprotein of HDL is ApoA-I (➲ Table 15.1).

Several lipid parameters are measured to evaluate CVD risk, as described in the following subsections.

Plasma total cholesterol

TC is the main lipid parameter included in the SCORE algorithm [5–8]. It should therefore always be measured to evaluate total CV risk. TC measures all cholesterol-containing lipoproteins, both the atherogenic LDL and VLDL as well as the protective HDL. About 80% of plasma cholesterol is transported in LDL. TC therefore gives a good estimate of the atherogenic lipoproteins. However, in patients with very high HDL-C, TC may overestimate the CVD risk. This is especially true in women, who often have high HDL-C.

Plasma LDL cholesterol

This should always be measured. It is the main atherogenic lipoprotein cholesterol and should be the main lipid parameter for

Table 15.1 Physical and chemical characteristics of the major lipoprotein classes

Lipoproteins	Density (g/ml)	Diameter (nm)	TG (%)	Cholesterol esters (%)	PL (%)	Cholesterol (%)	Major apolipoproteins
Chylomicrons	<0.95	80–100	90-95	2–4	2–6	1	ApoB-48
VLDL	0.95–1.006	30–80	50-65	8–14	12–16	4–7	ApoB-100
IDL	1.006–1.019	25–30	25-40	20–35	16–24	7–11	ApoB-100
LDL	1.019–1.063	20–25	4-6	34–35	22–26	6–15	ApoB-100
HDL	1.063–1.210	8–13	7	10–20	25	5	ApoA-I

VLDL, very low density lipoprotein; IDL, intermediate-density lipoprotein; LDL, low-density lipoprotein; HDL, high-density lipoprotein.

evaluating CVD risk. LDL-C can be calculated using the Friedewald formula* from total TC, TG, and HDL-C, unless TG are significantly elevated (>4.5 mmol/L or 400 mg/dl), but there are also methods that measure LDL-C directly in plasma.

Plasma triglycerides

Plasma TG are associated with CVD risk [9,10]. TG should always be measured. However, since TG are often correlated with other risk factors, such as HDL-C, body weight, hypertension, and diabetes, they might not be a strong risk factor after correction for other risk factors.

Plasma HDL-cholesterol

Plasma HDL-C is associated with reduced risk and in the most recent version of the SCORE algorithm HDL-C is included for evaluation of total CVD risk [5]. Low HDL-C is often associated with metabolic syndrome, type 2 diabetes, obesity, and/or insulin resistance. HDL-C should always be analysed when CVD risk is estimated [6,9,11].

Non-HDL-cholesterol

Non-HDL-C, which measures all ApoB-containing lipoprotein cholesterol, including VLDL-C, IDL-C, and LDL-C, could be recommended as an alternative analysis, especially in patients with high TG, such as in metabolic syndrome and type 2 diabetes [8,9,12].

Apolipoprotein B

ApoB is a direct measure of ApoB-containing lipoproteins. The information obtained from measurement of plasma ApoB is similar to that obtained from non-HDL-C, and could be recommended as an alternative analysis to non-HDL-C in the same group of patients (i.e. with high TG) [9,13–15].

Apolipoprotein A-I

ApoA-I, the main protein component of HDL, and measurement of ApoA-I is an alternative to HDL-C, giving similar information.

Lipoprotein(a)

Lp(a), is a fraction of LDL, characterized by an additional protein, apolipoprotein(a). High Lp(a) is associated with increased CVD risk [16]. The level of Lp(a) is highly genetically determined, and the analysis of Lp(a) is recommended in patients with a strong familial history of CVD. High Lp(a) may indicate the need for more active prevention measures.

Ratios between lipoproteins

Ratios between lipoproteins such as LDL-C/HDL-C, TC/HDL-C or ApoB/ApoA-I have been shown in several studies to be good markers for CVD risk given in one simple figure [8,15]. The ratios do not add information beyond that given by their components, but they may be practical to use, especially in screening situations.

*In mmol/L: LDL-C = TC − HDL-C − TG/2.2. In mg/dl: LDL-C = TC − HDL-C − TG/5.

Other emerging measures

A number of new parameters have been suggested as additional risk markers. So far these have not been shown to add any information to that provided by the parameters already discussed, particularly not in everyday practice. Such analyses are the level of small dense LDL [17,18], lipoprotein-associated phospholipase A2 [8,19], oxidized LDL, and antibodies against oxidized LDL [20].

Genetics of dyslipidaemia

Plasma lipoprotein levels are determined both by genetic and environmental factors, which often interact [21]. A number of genetic variations have been found to be correlated with plasma lipid levels. In most subjects plasma lipids are influenced by interaction of several genes. However, some dyslipidaemias are monogenic disorders associated with specific mutations.

Familial hypercholesterolaemia

Familial hypercholesterolaemia (FH) is a monogenic dominant genetic disease characterized by high levels of LDL-C and a greatly increased risk for premature CVD [22,23]. The prevalence of heterozygous FH is very high at about 1 in 250–500, while for homozygous FH the prevalence is about one in a million. In most cases the disease is caused by a mutation in the LDL receptor gene. However, a similar clinical syndrome can be caused by a mutation in *APOB*, in the gene for PCSK9 and probably also by other rare mutations in other genes. In heterozygous FH plasma TC is in the range of 8–12 mmol/L and in homozygous FH plasma TC is often over 20 mmol/L. Heterozygous FH is associated with about a ten-fold higher risk for premature CVD. In homozygous patients, CVD starts to develop in childhood and untreated patients often die from CVD before the age of 20. The criteria for a clinical diagnosis of heterozygous FH are shown in ➲ Table 15.2. DNA testing gives a good diagnosis even in patients with borderline cholesterol levels, in children, and in screening for new cases in families. The diagnosis of FH should always be considered in young MI patients and in subjects with a family history of premature CVD. From index cases a cascade screening in the family is recommended. Treatment of homozygous FH should be started as early as possible with dietary modifications and statins, while treatment of heterozygous FH should be started at the latest in adolescence or best in childhood. If adequately treated, patients with heterozygous FH will have a normal life expectancy [24]. Homozygous FH should be diagnosed in early childhood and referred to special clinics and treated with apheresis and statins.

Familial combined hyperlipidaemia

Familial combined hyperlipidaemia (FCH) is a common disorder affecting 0.5–1% of the population [25]. The genetic background is complex and involves several susceptibility genes and interaction with the environment. FCH is a major cause of premature CVD. The lipid pattern is variable, and comprises both high TG and LDL-C in varying constellations, often varying within the

Table 15.2 Diagnostic criteria for the clinical diagnosis of heterozygous familial hypercholesterolaemia (FH)

	Criteria	Score
Family history	First-degree relative known with premature CAD* and/or first-degree relative with LDL-C > 95th percentile	1
	First-degree relative with tendon xanthomata and/or children aged under 18 with LDL-C > 95th percentile	2
Clinical history	Patient has premature CAD*	2
	Patient has premature cerebral/peripheral vascular disease	1
Physical examination	Tendon xanthomata	6
	Arcus cornealis below the age of 45	4
LDL-cholesterol	>8.5 mmol/L (>330 mg/dl)	8
	6.5–8.4 mmol/L (250–329 mg/dl)	5
	5.0–6.4 mmol/L (190–249 mg/dl)	3
	4.0–4.9 mmol/L (155–189 mg/dl)	1
Definite FH		Score > 8
Probable FH		Score 6–8
Possible FH		Score 3–5
No diagnosis		Score < 3

*Premature coronary artery disease (CAD) or cardiovascular disease (CVD) (i.e. men before 55 and women before 60 years of age).

From: Reiner Ž, Catapano AL, De Backer G, et al. ESC/EAS guidelines for the management of dyslipidaemias: the Task Force for the management of dyslipidaemias of the European Society of Cardiology (ESC) and the European Atherosclerosis Society (EAS). *Eur Heart J* 2011; **32**: 1769–1818 and *Atherosclerosis* 2011; **217S**: 1769–1818.

individual and within the same family. Typically FCH patients have high levels of small dense LDL and high levels of ApoB. FCH has an overlapping background with type 2 diabetes and metabolic syndrome.

Dysbetalipoproteinaemia (type III dyslipidaemia)

Dysbetalipoproteinaemia (type III dyslipidaemia) is an uncommon disease characterized by severe combined hyperlipidaemia with both TC and TG in the range of 8–12 mmol/L [26]. Cutaneous xanthoma are often seen, and lipid depositions in the palmar creases are most characteristic. The disease is caused by a homozygosity for the ApoE-2 isoform of apolipoprotein E. The penetrance is variable, and the disease can be manifested by factors such as obesity or diabetes. The disease is associated with an increased risk for CVD. Hyperlipidaemia often responds well to diet, weight reduction, and also to fibrate treatment.

Severe hypertriglyceridaemia

Severe hypertriglyceridaemia may be caused by a number of genetic disorders. One is defective lipoprotein lipase or its activator ApoC-II. This leads to severe hypertriglyceridaemia with the accumulation of chylomicrons. TG levels in plasma are often above 20 mmol/l and there is a high risk of acute pancreatitis [27].

Lifestyle and dyslipidaemia

Lifestyle characteristics significantly affect plasma lipid levels. Diet has a major influence on lipids but they are also affected by other factors.

Diet and cholesterol

TC and LDL-C are affected by several dietary components. A major determinant is the intake of saturated fatty acids (SFAs) [28]. It is estimated that a 1% increase in dietary SFAs increases LDL-C levels by 0.02–0.04 mmol/L (~0.8–1.5 mg/dl) [29]. The recommended fat intake is 25–35% of caloric intake, of which SFAs should constitute less than 10%. Trans fatty acids increase LDL-C but also decrease HDL-C and TG [30]. The major source of trans fatty acids are partially hydrogenated fatty acids of industrial origin. A 2% increase in energy intake from trans fatty acids is associated with a 23% increase in coronary events.

Diet and triglycerides

A high intake of simple carbohydrates leads to an increase in TG. In particular a high intake of fructose may increase TG by 30%. Fructose is often used as sweetener in soft drinks.

Body weight, alcohol, and exercise

Overweight and obesity are associated with high TG and low HDL-C.

A high alcohol intake increases plasma TG. For subjects with normal TG a moderate intake of alcohol is seldom a problem. Indeed, a moderate alcohol intake may even increase HDL-C [31].

Physical activity increases insulin sensitivity and contributes to weight reduction, it reduces TG and may also increase HDL-C [32].

Other causes of dyslipidaemia

Dyslipidaemia in diabetes and the metabolic syndrome

Metabolic syndrome is a cluster of symptoms associated with insulin resistance and closely linked to type 2 diabetes. Metabolic syndrome includes dyslipidaemia, hypertension, overweight, abdominal obesity, and insulin resistance. Both metabolic syndrome and type 2 diabetes are associated with an increased risk for CVD, which to a large extent may be explained by the dyslipidaemia. Dyslipidaemia associated with these states is characterized by: hypertriglyceridaemia, low HDL-C, and large number of small dense LDL particles [33,34]. This is a lipoprotein pattern which is regarded as highly atherogenic.

Dyslipidaemia in chronic kidney disease

Dyslipidaemia is common in CKD, and lipid abnormalities worsen with declining glomerular filtration rate (GFR) [5,35]. The early stages of CKD are associated with increased TG and reduced HDL-C. With advancing renal disease TC and LDL-C also increase. Severe combined hyperlipidaemia becomes common and represents a highly atherogenic lipid profile.

Other causes of dyslipidaemia

Dyslipidaemia occurs commonly secondary to other diseases or can be caused by drugs. Examples of some common causes of secondary hyperlipidaemia are given in ➲ Table 15.3.

Table 15.3 Common causes of secondary hyperlipidaemia

Causes of secondary hypercholesterolaemia or hyperlipidaemia	Causes of secondary hypertriglyceridaemia
Hypothyroidism	Hypothyroidism
Nephrotic syndrome	Type 2 diabetes
Pregnancy	Pregnancy
Cushing's syndrome	Diet high in simple carbohydrates
Anorexia nervosa	Renal disease
Immunosuppressive agents	Obesity
Corticosteroids	High alcohol consumption
	Autoimmune disorders
	Multiple medications, including: corticosteroids, oestrogens, tamoxifen, antihypertensives, isotretinoin, ciclosporin, protease inhibitors

Table 15.5 Recommendations for treatment targets in CVD prevention

Recommendations	Class	Level
In patients at ***very high*** CV risk (established CVD, diabetes (type 1 or type 2) with one or more CV risk factors and/or target organ damage, moderate to severe CKD or a SCORE level ≥10%) the LDL-C goal is <1.8 mmol/L (<~70 mg/dl) and/or ≥50% reduction in LDL-C when the target level cannot be reached	I	A
In patients at ***high*** CV risk (markedly elevated single risk factors, diabetes (type 1 or type 2) but without CV risk factors or target organ damage, a SCORE level ≥5 to <10%) a LDL-C goal of <2.5 mmol/L (<~100 mg/dl) should be considered	IIa	A
In subjects at ***moderate*** risk (SCORE level > 1 to <5%) a LDL-C goal of <3.0 mmol/L (<~115 mg/dl) should be considered	IIa	C

From: Reiner Ž, Catapano AL, De Backer G, et al. ESC/EAS guidelines for the management of dyslipidaemias: the Task Force for the management of dyslipidaemias of the European Society of Cardiology (ESC) and the European Atherosclerosis Society (EAS). *Eur Heart J* 2011; **32**: 1769–1818 and *Atherosclerosis* 2011; **217S**: 1769–1818.

When to initiate treatment for dyslipidaemia

The decision to initiate treatment for dyslipidaemia in CVD prevention should be based on total CVD risk as well as on the lipoproteins level [5,6] (➲ Table 15.4). Although SCORE is a good basis for risk determination, several other risk factors outside the SCORE algorithm should be taken into consideration when treatment options are considered. These factors are body weight, abdominal obesity, diabetes, CKD, Lp(a) level, physical activity, and family history. Familial dyslipidaemias such as FH, FCH, and dysbetalipoproteinaemia should always be treated, irrespective of the SCORE value.

Goals of treatment

Reduction of LDL-C reduces the risk for CVD in all subjects, irrespective of risk level. However, the absolute risk reduction is greater in higher-risk subjects. The treatment goals are therefore adapted to the risk level. Based upon meta-analyses of statin trials it has been demonstrated that a reduction of 1 mmol/L in LDL-C results in a 22% reduction in risk [36,37]. Recommended treatment targets are given in ➲ Table 15.5. Alternative treatment goals may be ApoB and non-HDL-C, especially in hypertriglyceridaemia, metabolic syndrome, and type 2 diabetes. The target level for non-HDL should be 0.8 mmol/L above the target for LDL-C. The target for ApoB is 0.8 mg/ml in very high-risk subjects and 1.0 in high-risk patients. Ratios

Table 15.4 Treatment guidelines for dyslipidaemia

Total CV risk (SCORE level, %)	LDL-C level				
	<70 mg/dL <1.8 mmol/L	**70 to <100 mg/dL 1.8 to <2.5 mmol/L**	**100 to <155 mg/dL 2.5 to <4.0 mmol/L**	**155 to <190 mg/dL 4.0 to <4.9 mmol/L**	**>190 mg/dL >4.9 mmol/L**
<1	No lipid intervention	No lipid intervention	Lifestyle intervention	Lifestyle intervention	Lifestyle intervention, consider drug if uncontrolled
Class/level	I/C	I/C	I/C	I/C	IIa/A
≥1 to <5	Lifestyle intervention	Lifestyle intervention	Lifestyle intervention, consider drug if uncontrolled	Lifestyle intervention, consider drug if uncontrolled	Lifestyle intervention, consider drug if uncontrolled
Class/level	I/C	I/C	IIa/A	IIa/A	I/A
>5 to <10, or high risk	Lifestyle intervention, consider drug	Lifestyle intervention, consider drug	Lifestyle intervention and immediate drug intervention	Lifestyle intervention and immediate drug intervention	Lifestyle intervention and immediate drug intervention
Class/level	IIa/A	IIa/A	IIa/A	I/A	I/A
≥10 or very high risk	Lifestyle intervention, consider drug	Lifestyle intervention and immediate drug intervention	Lifestyle intervention and immediate drug intervention	Lifestyle intervention and immediate drug intervention	Lifestyle intervention and immediate drug intervention
Class/level	IIa/A	IIa/A	I/A	I/A	I/A

From: Reiner Ž, Catapano AL, De Backer G, et al. ESC/EAS guidelines for the management of dyslipidaemias: the Task Force for the management of dyslipidaemias of the European Society of Cardiology (ESC) and the European Atherosclerosis Society (EAS). *Eur Heart J* 2011; **32**: 1769–1818 and *Atherosclerosis* 2011; **217S**: 1769–1818.

such as LDL/HDL or ApoB/ApoA-I are not recommended as treatment targets.

There are no specific targets for TG or HDL-C because evidence from outcomes studies is lacking. However, on the basis of epidemiological data, TG levels should be <1.7 mmol/L (150 mg/dl) and HDL-C should be >1.0 mmol/L (~40 mg/dl) in men and >1.2 mmol/L (~46 mg/dl) in women. Lp(a) above 50 mg/dl is associated with increased CVD risk.

Therapeutic approaches

Lifestyle modification

Diet

Appropriate modification of diet and lifestyle has enormous potential for the prevention of CVD on a population basis but also for the individual patient with dyslipidaemia. Individualized diet and lifestyle programmes on top of drug therapy have the potential for enhanced control of the lipid profile which should translate into further CVD risk reduction (this is in addition to the benefits on CVD risk beyond those related to plasma lipids).

Dietary fats

Saturated fatty acids

The proportion of saturated fats in the diet is the most important influence on the level of TC, LDL-C, and HDL-C, and to a lesser degree VLDL and TG. Saturated fat is sometimes referred to as animal fat, but this can be misleading because some important plant products such as palm and coconut oils are rich in SFAs.

The commonest SFAs are lauric (C12:0), myristic (C14:0), palmitic (C16:0), and stearic (C18:0) acids. Myristic acid appears to have the strongest effect in increasing LDL-C and HDL-C, whereas stearic acid appears neutral. Dairy produce, beef, pork, lamb, coconut, and palm oil products are rich in SFAs. Food-based recommendations are clearly more practical than nutrient-based advice, but although epidemiological studies point to a high intake of processed meat products (rich in SFAs) as being a CVD risk factor, the evidence linking a higher intake of dairy produce to CVD is not consistent. The effects of specific foods cannot be determined by their fatty acid content alone [38].

For every 1% of calorie intake contributed by saturated fat, TC increases by 0.07 mmol/L. Similarly, it has been calculated from an amalgamation of various sources of evidence, including epidemiological, clinical, and mechanistic studies, that the replacement of 1% of energy derived from saturated fats with polyunsaturated fatty acids (PUFAs) will reduce CHD by 2–3%. On this basis, consumption of SFAs should be reduced to a maximum of 10% of energy intake.

Dietary cholesterol

Unlike dietary fat, which is almost completely digested and absorbed, only about 50% (30–60%) of dietary cholesterol is absorbed. This is partly influenced by genetic factors such as apolipoprotein E phenotype, being highest in those with apolipoprotein E4 alleles and lowest in those with E2 alleles. Incomplete cholesterol absorption may explain why the impact of increasing dietary cholesterol on TC concentrations is small. Moving from a dietary intake of 200–300 to 300–400 mg/1000 calories would increase plasma cholesterol by 0.12 and 0.11 mmol/L, respectively [39]. Reducing SFAs will also reduce cholesterol intake. US guidelines recommend a cholesterol intake of <300 mg/day [6].

Trans fatty acids

Trans fatty acids are isomers of *cis* PUFAs, the hydrogen atoms attached at the double bonds being on opposite sides, which straightens the chain. This structure is more similar to that of saturated fats. Partial hydrogenation of PUFAs has been used in the food industry to raise the melting point (hardening) of vegetable fats for use in spreads and bakery products. Some trans-fat in the diet comes from ruminant fat in dairy and meat products. Elaidic acid, the *trans* isomer of oleic acid, is the most common dietary trans-fat.

The replacement of 1% of energy derived from trans-fats with either saturated, monounsaturated, or PUFAs would reduce the TC/HDL-C ratio by 0.31, 0.54, and 0.67, respectively [40]. Reducing trans-fats will decrease TC and LDL-C and increase HDL-C. Many manufacturers now produce products that are virtually free of trans-fats. However, as food labelling varies in different countries, patients should be counselled to check food labels for the amount of hydrogenated fat if trans-fats are not mentioned. No more than 1% of total energy should be derived from trans fatty acids, and the less the better.

Unsaturated fatty acids

PUFAs consist of two main subgroups. n-6 fatty acids are characterized by the presence of a double bond six carbon atoms from the methyl end of the chain. The major sources of PUFAs are plants such as sunflower, soy bean, and maize and include the essential fatty acid linoleic acid (C18:2n-6). n-3 fatty acids (the first double bond is at the third carbon atom from the methyl end of the chain) include the essential fatty acid alpha-linolenic acid (C18:3n-3) together with very long chain n-3 fatty acids. Alpha-linolenic acid is found in rapeseed, flaxseed, and soy bean oils and lower plants such as algae, and is the precursor of the n-3 group. Fish that feed on algae in plankton are able to make n-3 fatty acids with more double bonds, including eicosapentaenoic acid (C20:5) and docosahexaenoic acid (C20:6). Oleic acid (C18:1) is the main dietary monounsaturated fatty acid as it is a major component of vegetable oils but is also found in dairy produce and meat. It is the principal fatty acid in olive oil and rapeseed oil.

PUFAs are an excellent replacement for saturates as part of a cholesterol-lowering strategy [41]. Replacing 1% of dietary energy from saturates by PUFAs decreases plasma LDL-C by 0.051 mmol/L while HDL-C also decreases slightly [40]. Replacing saturates with monounsaturates on a similar basis decreases LDL-C by 0.041 mmol/L with a more or less neutral effect on HDL-C. A high intake of monounsaturates is associated with a reduction in TG.

Intake of PUFAs in the form of linoleic and alpha-linolenic acid should account for approximately 6–11% of energy based on a total fat content of 30% of food energy. A minimum intake of fish should be two portions per week as a source of long-chain n-3 fatty acids. This modest increase would reduce CHD mortality by 36% and all-cause mortality by 17%. Use of oleic acid (a non-essential fatty acid) is recommended as simply providing the difference between total fat intake and the sum of polyunsaturates and saturates which approximates to 8–13% of energy.

Carbohydrates and fibre

Carbohydrate is a major component of the diet but there is no clear-cut evidence that replacing saturated fat with carbohydrate will reduce CHD. This is likely to be explained by the failure in most studies to differentiate the type of carbohydrate. A 5% lower energy intake from saturated fat with a concomitant higher energy intake from carbohydrates is associated with a small but significant increase in coronary risk [42]. A positive association between substitution of saturated fat for carbohydrate with a high glycaemic index (GI) and coronary risk [hazard ratio (HR) 1.33, 95% confidence interval (CI) 1.08–1.64] was shown. In contrast there was a non-significant trend to a reduced coronary risk with substitution of carbohydrates with a low GI (HR 0.88, 95% CI 0.72–1.07) [43]. The GI ranks carbohydrates in terms of their ability to increase blood glucose measured as the area under the curve compared with a standard 50-g load of a reference carbohydrate such as glucose.

High-GI foods such as white bread, white rice, pizza, and sugars are rapidly digested and absorbed. This leads to high blood glucose and high insulin to glucagon ratio followed by hypoglycaemia, the secretion of counter-regulatory hormones, and increased concentrations of free fatty acids. These effects will promote hypertriglyceridaemia and lower HDL-C. Individuals with metabolic syndrome and dyslipidaemia will respond more adversely to these processes. These effects are not observed with low-GI, high-fibre carbohydrate. Excess dietary fructose (e.g. high-fructose corn syrup and sucrose) should be avoided as this is associated with a greater drop in HDL-C. An increased intake of dietary fibre (non-starch polysaccharides and other components which are not absorbed) reduces TC and LDL-C and the risk of coronary events.

The carbohydrate content of a prudent diet for patients with dyslipidaemia should be composed of low-GI foods and a high fibre content such as wholegrain cereals, fruit, vegetables, and legumes with a daily intake of 5–15 g of soluble fibre.

Alcohol and smoking

There is a wealth of evidence from population studies showing an effect of alcohol on coronary events and ischaemic stroke. The relationship is J-shaped, with heavy drinkers and non-drinkers at highest risk of CHD mortality and light to moderate drinkers at lowest risk. It is likely that it is the alcohol content that is related to risk and there is no epidemiological evidence of benefit of one form of alcohol, for example red wine, over another. Alcohol can exacerbate hypertriglyceridaemia, and a reduction in alcohol ingestion is an important part of the management of this condition. Moderate alcohol intake is associated with higher concentrations of HDL-C. Therefore, in general, alcohol should be limited to two drinks per day (20 g) for men and one drink per day (10 g) for women, except for patients with high TG who should abstain.

Strong advice to quit smoking with appropriate counselling and pharmacological assistance is a crucial part of the management of all smokers [44]. In terms of dyslipidaemia, smoking cessation improves insulin sensitivity and increases HDL-C.

Weight reduction and physical exercise

Weight reduction is an important component in the management of dyslipidaemia. The main impact of weight reduction is on reducing TG and increasing HDL-C, and even modest reductions in the region of 5–10% of body weight will improve the lipid profile. Weight reduction reduces TG by 20–30% and may also increase HDL-C by 0.01 mmol/L per kilogram lost.

Achieving weight reduction in clinical practice is not easy and requires structured, intensive lifestyle education. The intake of energy-rich foods such as saturated fats and refined carbohydrates should be reduced to achieve a mild calorie deficit and appropriate regular physical activity of moderate intensity should be encouraged. In practice, patients often comment that despite increasing their activity their weight has not changed. In this situation measurement of waist circumference gives a better estimate of benefit reflecting changes in body composition.

Low-fat diets (20%) and high-carbohydrate diets (20% fat, 15% protein, and 65% carbohydrate) reduce LDL-C more than high-fat diets or low-carbohydrate diets (5% versus 1%, $p = 0.001$); highest carbohydrate versus the lowest (96% versus 15%, $p = 0.01$) [45]. The lowest-carbohydrate diet (40% fat, 15% protein, 35% carbohydrate) increases HDL-C more than the highest-carbohydrate diet (20% fat, 15% protein, 65% carbohydrate) (9% versus 6%, $p = 0.02$). All these diets decrease plasma triglycerides to a similar degree, namely 12–17% [45].

Patients with dyslipidaemia should perform regular physical activity and aerobic exercise as an important part of their overall management. This is important for assisting with weight reduction and in addition increases HDL-C and reduces TG [46]. In patients without CVD it is recommended that physical activity or aerobic exercise training of moderate intensity lasting 2.5–5 hours every week should be undertaken. In those with established coronary disease or stable chronic heart failure it is recommended that they undergo moderate to vigorous intensity exercise at least three times a week.

Functional foods

Products containing plant stanols or sterols are useful in addition to, but not as a substitute for, appropriate dietary and lifestyle advice [47,48]. These products decrease the intestinal absorption of cholesterol. With amounts of 2 g/day, LDL-C falls on average by 10%. However, there is a marked variation in effect amongst different individuals, presumably related to the degree to which they absorb cholesterol. Their effects are additive to other dietary and drug interventions.

Adoption and maintenance of dietary and lifestyle measures

It is clear that individualized dietary and lifestyle interventions can have a potentially favourable impact on plasma lipid and lipoprotein concentrations on top of pharmacotherapy. However, in clinical practice it is often difficult to achieve optimal implementation of lifestyle changes, and even more difficult to achieve behavioural change in the long term [49] (➲ Table 15.6).

Table 15.6 Recommendations for counselling individuals to promote dietary changes and physical activity (PA) to reduce CVD risk

Cognitive-behavioural strategies for promoting behaviour change

Class I:

- Design interventions to target dietary and PA behaviours with specific, proximal goals (goal setting). Level of evidence: A
- Provide feedback on progress toward goals. Level of evidence: A
- Provide strategies for self-monitoring. Level of evidence: A
- Establish a plan for frequency and duration of follow-up contacts (e.g. in person, oral, written, electronic) in accordance with individual needs to assess and reinforce progress toward goal attainment. Level of evidence: A
- Utilize motivational interviewing strategies, particularly when an individual is resistant or ambivalent about dietary and PA behaviour change. Level of evidence: A
- Provide for direct or peer-based long-term support and follow-up, such as referral to ongoing community-based programmes, to offset the common occurrence of declining adherence that typically begins at 4–6 months in most behaviour change programmes. Level of evidence: B
- Incorporate strategies to build self-efficacy into the intervention. Level of evidence: A
- Use a combination of two or more of the above strategies (e.g. goal setting, feedback, self-monitoring, follow-up, motivational interviewing, self-efficacy) in an intervention. Level of evidence: A

Class II:

- Use incentives, modelling, and problem solving strategies. Level of evidence: B

Intervention processes and/or delivery strategies

Class I:

- Use individual- or group-based strategies. Level of evidence: A
- Use individual-oriented sessions to assess where the individual is in relation to behaviour change, to jointly identify the goals for risk reduction or improved cardiovascular health, and to develop a personalized plan to achieve it. Level of evidence: A
- Use group sessions with cognitive–behavioural strategies to teach skills to modify the diet and develop a PA programme, to provide role modelling and positive observational learning, and to maximize the benefits of peer support and group problem solving. Level of evidence: A
- For appropriate target populations, use Internet- and computer-based programmes to target dietary and PA change; evidence is less good for targeting PA alone; adding a form of e-counselling improves outcomes. Level of evidence: B

Class IIa:

- Use individualized rather than non-individualized print- or media-only delivery strategies. Level of evidence: A
- Address cultural and social context variables that influence behavioural change. Level of evidence: A

Class IIb:

- Utilize church, community, work, or clinic settings for delivery of interventions. Level of evidence: B
- Use a multiple-component delivery strategy that includes a group component rather than individual-only or group-only approaches. Level of evidence: A
- Use culturally adapted strategies, including the use of peer or lay health advisors to increase trust; tailor health messages and counselling strategies to be sensitive to the cultural beliefs, values, language, literacy, and customs of the target population. Level of evidence: A
- Use problem solving to address barriers to PA and dietary change, such as lack of access to affordable healthier foods, lack of resources for PA, transportation barriers, and poor local safety. Level of evidence: B

Reproduced from: Scientific Statement from AHA: Interventions to Promote Physical Activity and Dietary Lifestyle Changes for Cardiovascular Risk Factor Reduction in Adults: A Scientific Statement From the American Heart Association. *Circulation* 2010; **122**: 406–441, with permission of Wolters Kluwer Health.

Pharmacotherapy of dyslipidaemias

Pharmacotherapy for high LDL-C

Statins should be used as the drugs of first choice in patients with high LDL-C. Their mechanism of action is based upon reducing synthesis of cholesterol in the liver by competitively inhibiting HMG-CoA reductase activity. The reduction in intracellular cholesterol concentration induces expression of low-density lipoprotein receptor (LDLR) on the hepatocyte cell surface, resulting in a decrease of up to 65% in circulating LDL-C concentration and an increased extraction of LDL-C from the blood, but also a decrease in TG and increased HDL-C.

A number of large-scale clinical trials have undoubtedly demonstrated that statins substantially reduce CV morbidity and mortality as well as the need for coronary artery interventions [36, 50,51]. In high doses statins have also been shown to slow the progression or even promote regression of coronary atherosclerosis [52].

In general, the safety profile of statins is very acceptable. Higher activity of liver enzymes in plasma is occasional and in most cases reversible. The incidence of myopathy is low and rhabdomyolysis is extremely rare. An elevation of creatine kinase (CK) is the best indicator of statin-induced myopathy. The risk of myopathy can be minimized by identifying vulnerable patients and/or by avoiding interactions of statins with specific drugs (➲ Table 15.7). Because statins are prescribed on a long-term basis, possible interactions with other drugs deserve particular attention, as many patients will receive pharmacological therapy for concomitant conditions [53]. The benefits of statin treatment for primary CVD

Table 15.7 Selected drugs that may increase risk of myopathy and rhabdomyolysis when used concomitantly with a statin (CYP3A4 inhibitors/substrates or other mechanisms)

Ciclosporin, tacrolimus
Macrolides (azithromycin, clarithromycin, erythromycin)
Azole antifungals (itraconazole, ketoconazole, fluconazole)
Calcium antagonists (mibefradil, diltiazem, verapamil)
Nefazodone
HIV protease inhibitors (amprenavir, indinavir, nelfinavir, ritonavir, saquinavir)
Sildenafil
Others: digoxin, niacin, fibrates (particularly gemfibrozil)

prevention far outweigh the mildly increased risk of developing diabetes which has been described as a possible adverse effect of long-term high-dose treatment, even among those at risk for diabetes [54]. Although there have been some reports suggesting otherwise, statins do not confer an increased risk of cancer or cognitive decline [55,56].

Bile acid sequestrants (cholestyramine, colestipol, colesevelam) prevent the entry of bile acid into the blood by binding bile acids and thereby remove a large portion of the bile acids from the enterohepatic circulation. This leads to an increase in cholesterol catabolism to bile acids, resulting in a compensatory increase in hepatic LDLR activity, clearing LDL-C from the circulation and thus reducing LDL-C levels. At the top doses these drugs reduce LDL-C by 18–25%. They have no major effect on HDL-C, while TG may increase in some patients. However, data from studies with hard end-points are sparse. Bile acid sequestrants have adverse gastrointestinal effects which seriously decrease compliance. They also have important interactions with many commonly prescribed drugs and should therefore be administered either 4 h before or 1 h after other drugs [57].

Cholesterol absorption inhibitors (ezetimibe) inhibit the intestinal uptake of dietary and biliary cholesterol. In response to reducing the amount of lipoprotein cholesterol circulated to the liver, the liver reacts by upregulating LDLR, which in turn leads to increased clearance of LDL-C from the blood. The recommended dose of ezetimibe is 10 mg/day. It reduces LDL-C by 15–22% but it is rarely used as monotherapy. Most recently it has been shown that adding ezetimibe to a statin causes a modest additional benefit in reducing cardiovascular events in high-risk patients.

Pharmacotherapy of high triglycerides

Fibrates should be used as the drugs of first choice. They are agonists of peroxisome proliferator-activated receptor-alpha acting via transcription factors regulating various steps in lipid and lipoprotein metabolism. The reduction in TG is variable, ranging from 10 to 50%. Fibrates also increase low HDL-C and moderately decrease LDL-C, particularly decreasing the very atherogenic small dense LDL. The data from major trials with fibrates have shown consistent decreases in the rates of non-fatal MI (although in some cases from post hoc analyses), the effect being most robust in subjects with elevated TG/low HDL-C [58]. They are generally well tolerated. Myopathy, liver enzyme elevations, and cholelithiasis represent the most well-known safety issues. Whether the increase in serum creatinine which has also been reported reflects kidney dysfunction or not is a matter of ongoing debate. The increase of homocysteine by fibrates has been considered to be relatively innocent with respect to CVD risk.

Nicotinic acid (niacin) is no longer approved in Europe. It reduces TG but also moderately reduces LDL-C and increases HDL-C [59]. Flushing, associated with itching and tingling, is the main adverse effect of niacin and significantly affects compliance.

Prescription n-3 PUFAs, particularly ethyl esters, in doses of 3–4 g/day safely reduces serum TG by modulating VLDL and chylomicron metabolism [60]. Each 1-g increase in daily n-3 PUFA intake per day decreases TG by approximately 8 mg/dl. The response is curvilinear, with individuals with lower baseline TG showing less of a TG-lowering effect (20% versus 30% for higher TG levels). TC is not significantly affected by n-3 PUFAs, although LDL-C concentrations tend to rise by 5–10% and HDL–C by 1-3%. However, an ethyl eicosapentaenoic acid preparation seems to also decrease LDL-C [61]. Data from studies with hard end-points are not conclusive.

Pharmacotherapy of combined hyperlipidaemia

Combined hyperlipidaemia, i.e. an increase in both LDL-C and TG, can be treated with statins since they decrease not only TC and LDL-C but also, to a lesser extent, TG. The most potent TG reduction is obtained with the more potent statins in high dose. In severe hypertriglyceridaemia (>10 mmol/L) statins have no effect. If both LDL-C and TG are very high, lipid-lowering drug combinations of a statin and TG-lowering agent will be the best option for reaching the treatment goals.

Drug combinations for treatment of dyslipidaemias

Many patients with dyslipidaemia, particularly those with familial dyslipidaemia, combined hyperlipidaemia, established CVD, diabetes, or metabolic syndrome, but also asymptomatic high-risk individuals, may not always reach treatment targets with only one drug. Therefore combination treatment may be needed [62].

Combination of a statin and a bile acid sequestrant or a combination of a statin and ezetimibe can be used for greater reduction of LDL-C than can be achieved with either drug alone. Another advantage of combination therapy is that lower doses of statins can be used, thus diminishing the risk of adverse effects associated with high doses. However, statins should be used in the highest tolerable doses to reach the LDL-C target level before combination therapy is considered. A recently published study with simvastatin in combination with ezetimibe supports the view that the combination can offer additional risk reduction to the single drug treatment.

Fibrates, particularly fenofibrate, are useful in combination with statin when TG remains elevated even during statin treatment. Furthermore fibrates may also increase low HDL-C, and further lower LDL-C, particularly small dense LDL, when applied together with a statin [58,63,64]. Other drugs metabolized through cytochrome P450 should be avoided when this combination is prescribed to decrease the risk of adverse effects. Fibrates should preferably be taken in the morning and statins in the evening to minimize peak dose concentrations and decrease the risk of myopathy, although this adverse effect is very rare. It is advisable to avoid the addition of gemfibrozil to a statin regimen [65].

Combination therapy with statins and prescription n-3 PUFAs is more effective than monotherapy with each drug alone, causing a greater reduction of TG and an increase in HDL-C compared with statins alone. Combination therapy with fenofibrate and prescription n-3 PUFAs reduces TG concentration by 60%. Prescription n-3 PUFAs may be used safely in combination with both statins and fibrates.

The possible beneficial effects of new lipid-lowering drugs such as mipomersen, lomitapide, and monoclonal antibodies to PSCK9 on preventing cardiovascular events remain yet to be evaluated.

Follow-up and safety control

Response to therapy can be assessed at 6–8 weeks from initiation or dose increases for statins, but response to fibrates and lifestyle may take longer. Lipids should, of course, be tested before starting lipid-lowering drug treatment by performing at least two measurements, taken with a 1–12 week interval, with the exception of conditions where immediate drug treatment is suggested, such as in acute coronary syndrome. Lipids should be checked 8 (±4) weeks after starting drug treatment. Once a patient has reached his or her target lipid level, lipids should be checked annually unless there are problems with adherence or another specific reason for more frequent reviews.

When statin treatment is used, safety blood tests are advised including alanine aminotransferase (ALT) and CK at baseline to identify the limited number of patients in whom treatment is contraindicated.

Liver enzymes (ALT) should therefore be measured in all patients taking lipid-lowering drugs before starting drug treatment. They should also be measured 8 weeks after starting drug treatment or after any dose increase and should be less than three times the upper limit of normal (ULN). If values rise to three or more times ULN, the lipid-lowering drug should be stopped or the dose reduced and liver enzymes rechecked within 4–6 weeks. After ALT has returned to normal, cautious reintroduction of therapy may be considered. It is not necessary to routinely monitor liver enzymes in all patients taking lipid-lowering therapy since it has been shown that such monitoring is not effective for detecting or preventing serious liver injury.

CK should be measured before starting lipid-lowering treatment in all patients, but if this is not possible at least in those patients with an increased risk for myopathy such as the very elderly with comorbidities, patients with earlier muscle symptoms, or patients on interacting drugs. If the baseline CK level is more than five times ULN, drug therapy should not be started but the CK value should be rechecked. It is not necessary to routinely monitor CK in patients taking lipid-lowering therapy. CK should only be checked if a patient develops myalgia. If CK becomes raised to more than five times ULN in a person taking lipid-lowering drugs, lipid-lowering treatment should be stopped, renal function checked, and CK monitored fortnightly. The possibility of transient CK elevation for other reasons such as muscle exertion should be considered, as well as secondary causes of myopathy if CK remains elevated. If CK returns to five or more times ULN and there are no muscle symptoms, statin treatment can be continued but patients should be alerted to report muscle symptoms and further checks of CK should be considered. If muscle symptoms are still present although CK is less than or equal to fives times ULN, they should be monitored and CK should be regularly checked. If the muscle pains cease on withdrawal of the statin and recur when it is reintroduced, especially if this is tried several times, a causal relationship is more or less proven. In this case, the use of a very low dose of a statin two or three times a week with a very gradual increase in dosage can be effective [66].

Solution to the clinical case

The patient should be referred to a dietician for lifestyle advice to reinforce the physician's explanation of its central importance in management. The focus should be primarily on reduction in alcohol intake, saturated fat, salt, and refined carbohydrate together with the adoption of some regular physical activity. Simvastatin could be changed to atorvastatin or rosuvastatin 40 mg/day as more intensive statin therapy is needed, given the residual mixed lipaemia and the high ApoB. An ultrasound of the abdomen should be performed to confirm fatty liver, which is expected. Statin therapy is not contraindicated in fatty liver. Arrangements should be made for follow-up in the clinic for 4 months with a further visit to the dietician. A target weight reduction of 5 kg should be discussed.

At review the patient's fasting lipid profile showed a TC of 5.1 mmol/L, TG 2.4 mmol/L, HDL-C 1.1 mmol/L and calculated LDL-C 2.9 mmol/L. He had been successful in reducing his alcohol intake to about 16 units each week and BMI was 26.7 kg/m^2. On average he was walking briskly for 35 minutes three times a week. His fasting glucose was 5.8 mmol/L and the ALT had improved to just two units above normal. Given his high risk, more intensive therapy was instigated to further reduce his LDL-C and non-HDL-C. Rather than increase the atorvastatin to 80 mg/day, which would result in a reduction of only about 5%, ezetimibe 10 mg/day was added. His blood pressure had fallen to 136/84 mmHg with the reduction in salt, alcohol, and weight.

He responded well to the addition of ezetimibe and his LDL-C had fallen to 2.3 mmol/L when he was next seen. He admitted to feeling better, having lost a little more weight and felt that he would be able to maintain his improved diet and lifestyle supported by his wife and family.

Further reading

Artinian NT, Fletcher GF, Mozaffarian D, et al. Interventions to promote physical activity and dietary lifestyle changes for cardiovascular risk factor reduction in adults. A scientific statement from the American Heart Association. *Circulation* 2010; **122**: 406–41.

Chapman MJ, Ginsberg HN, Amarenco P, et al. Triglyceride-rich lipoproteins and high-density lipoprotein cholesterol in patients at high risk of cardiovascular disease: evidence and guidance for management. *Eur Heart J* 2011; **32**: 1345–61.

Emerging Risk Factors Collaboration. Major lipids, apolipoproteins, and risk of vascular disease. *J Am Med Assoc* 2009; **302**: 1993–2000.

European Heart Network. *Diet, physical activity and cardiovascular prevention in Europe*. Summary report, November 2011. Brussels: European Heart Network. URL: <http://www.ehnheart.org/publications/publications/publication/521-diet-physical-activity-and-cardiovascular-disease-prevention.html>

Fruchart JC, Sacks F, Hermans MP, et al. The Residual Risk Reduction Initiative: a call to action to reduce residual vascular risk in dyslipidemic patients. A position paper by the Residual Risk Reduction Initiative (R[3]I). *Diabetes Vasc Dis Res* 2008; **4**: 319–35.

Goldberg AC, Hopkins PN, Toth PP, et al. National Lipid Association Expert Panel on Familial Hypercholesterolemia. Familial hypercholesterolemia: screening, diagnosis and management of pediatric and adult patients: clinical guidance from the National Lipid Association Expert Panel on Familial Hypercholesterolemia. *J Clin Lipidol* 2011; **5** (3 Suppl.): S1–S8.

Hooper L, Summerbell CD, Thompson R, et al. Reduced or modified dietary fat for preventing cardiovascular disease. *Cochrane Database Syst Rev* 2011; (7): CD002137.

Lichtenstein AH, Appel LJ, Brands M, et al. A Scientific Statement from the American Heart Association Nutrition Committee. Diet and Lifestyle recommendations revision 2006. *Circulation* 2006; **114**: 82–96.

Marcus BH, Williams DM, Dubbert PM, et al. Scientific Statement from the American Heart Association Council on Nutrition, Physical Activity and Metabolism (Subcommittee on Physical Activity); Council on Cardiovascular Disease in the Young; and the Interdisciplinary Working Group on Quality of Care and Outcomes Research. *Circulation* 2006; **114**: 2739–52.

Mead A, Atkinson G, Albin D, et al. Dietetic guidelines on food and nutrition in the secondary prevention of cardiovascular disease—evidence from systematic reviews of randomized controlled trials (second update, January 2006). *J Hum Nutr Diet* 2006; **19**: 401–19.

Nordestgaard BG, Chapman MJ, Ray K, et al. Lipoprotein(a) as a cardiovascular risk factor: current status. *Eur Heart J* 2010; **31**: 2844–53.

Perk J, De Backer G, Gohlke H, et al. European guidelines on cardiovascular disease prevention in clinical practice (version 2012): the Fifth Joint Task Force of the European Society of Cardiology and Other Societies on Cardiovascular Disease Prevention in Clinical Practice (constituted by representatives of nine societies and by invited experts). *Eur Heart J* 2012; **33**: 1635–701.

Reiner Ž, Catapano AL, De Backer G, et al. ESC/EAS guidelines for the management of dyslipidaemias: the task force for the management of dyslipidaemias of the European Society of Cardiology (ESC) and the European Atherosclerosis Society (EAS). *Eur Heart J* 2011; **32**: 1769–818.

Reiner Ž. Combined therapy in the treatment of dyslipidemia. *Fundam Clin Pharmacol* 2010; **24**: 19–28.

Reiner Ž. Statins in the primary prevention of cardiovascular disease. *Nat Rev Cardiol* 2013; **10**: 453–64.

Vanhees L, Geladas N, Hansen D, et al; on behalf of the writing group. Importance of characteristics and modalities of physical activity and exercise in the management of cardiovascular health in individuals with cardiovascular risk factors: recommendations from the EACPR (Part II). *Eur J Prev Cardiol* 2012; **19**: 1005–33.

Zannad F, Dallongeville J, Macfadyen RJ, et al. Prevention of cardiovascular disease guided by total risk estimations—challenges and opportunities for practical implementation: highlights of a CardioVascular Clinical Trialists (CVCT) workshop of the ESC Working Group on CardioVascular Pharmacology and Drug Therapy. *Eur J Prev Cardiol* 2012; **19**: 1454–64.

References

1 Reiner Ž. How to improve cardiovascular diseases prevention in Europe? *Nutr Metab Cardiovasc Dis* 2009; **19**: 451–4.

2 Reiner Ž, Sonicki Z, Tedeschi-Reiner E. Physicians' perception, knowledge and awareness of cardiovascular risk factors and adherence to prevention guidelines: the PERCRO-DOC survey. *Atherosclerosis* 2010; **213**: 598–603.

3 Reiner Ž, Sonicki Z, Tedeschi-Reiner E. Public perceptions of cardiovascular risk factors in Croatia: the PERCRO survey. *Prev Med* 2010; **51**: 494–6.

4 Reiner Ž, Sonicki Z, Tedeschi-Reiner E. The perception and knowledge of cardiovascular risk factors among medical students. *Croat Med J* 2012; **53**: 278–84.

5 Catapano AL, Reiner Z, De Backer G, et al. ESC/EAS guidelines for the management of dyslipidaemias. The Task Force for the management of dyslipidaemias of the European Society of Cardiology (ESC) and the European Atherosclerosis Society (EAS). *Atherosclerosis* 2011; **217**: 3–46.

6 Perk J, De Backer G, Gohlke H, et al. European guidelines on cardiovascular disease prevention in clinical practice (version 2012): the Fifth Joint Task Force of the European Society of Cardiology and Other Societies on Cardiovascular Disease Prevention in Clinical Practice (constituted by representatives of nine societies and by invited experts). *Atherosclerosis* 2012; **223**: 1–68.

7 Prospective Studies Collaboration, Lewington S, Whitlock G, Clarke R, et al. Blood cholesterol and vascular mortality by age, sex, and blood pressure: a meta-analysis of individual data from 61 prospective studies with 55,000 vascular deaths. *Lancet* 2007; **370**: 1829–39.

8 Emerging Risk Factors Collaboration, Di Angelantonio E, Gao P, Pennells L, et al. Lipid-related markers and cardiovascular disease prediction. *J Am Med Assoc* 2012; **307**: 2499–2506.

9 Chapman MJ, Ginsberg HN, Amarenco P, et al. Triglyceride-rich lipoproteins and high-density lipoprotein cholesterol in patients at high risk of cardiovascular disease: evidence and guidance for management. *Eur Heart J* 2011; **32**: 1345–61.

10 Triglyceride Coronary Disease Genetics Consortium and Emerging Risk Factors Collaboration, Sarwar N, Sandhu MS, Ricketts SL, et al. Triglyceride-mediated pathways and coronary disease: collaborative analysis of 101 studies. *Lancet* 2010; **375**: 1634–9.

11 Cooney MT, Dudina A, De Bacquer D, et al. How much does HDL cholesterol add to risk estimation? A report from the SCORE Investigators. *Eur J Cardiovasc Prev Rehabil* 2009; **16**: 304–14.

12 Robinson JG, Wang S, Smith BJ, et al. Meta-analysis of the relationship between non-high-density lipoprotein cholesterol reduction and coronary heart disease risk. *J Am Coll Cardiol* 2009; **53**: 316–22.

13 Charlton-Menys V, Betteridge DJ, Colhoun H, et al. Targets of statin therapy: LDL cholesterol, non-HDL cholesterol, and apolipoprotein B in type 2 diabetes in the Collaborative Atorvastatin Diabetes Study (CARDS). *Clin Chem* 2009; **55**: 473–80.

14 Taskinen MR, Barter PJ, Ehnholm C, et al. Ability of traditional lipid ratios and apolipoprotein ratios to predict cardiovascular risk in people with type 2 diabetes. *Diabetologia* 2010; **53**: 1846–55.

15 Emerging Risk Factors Collaboration, Di Angelantonio E, Sarwar N, et al. Major lipids, apolipoproteins, and risk of vascular disease. *J Am Med Assoc* 2009; **302**: 1993–2000.

16 Nordestgaard BG, Chapman MJ, Ray K, et al. Lipoprotein(a) as a cardiovascular risk factor: current status. *Eur Heart J* 2010; **31**: 2844–53.

17 Packard CJ. Small dense low-density lipoprotein and its role as an independent predictor of cardiovascular disease. *Curr Opin Lipidol* 2006; **17**: 412–17.

18 Mora S, Szklo M, Otvos JD, et al. LDL particle subclasses, LDL particle size, and carotid atherosclerosis in the Multi-Ethnic Study of Atherosclerosis (MESA). *Atherosclerosis* 2007; **192**: 211–17.

19 Davidson MH, Corson MA, Alberts MJ, et al. Consensus panel recommendation for incorporating lipoprotein-associated phospholipase A2 testing into cardiovascular disease risk assessment guidelines. *Am J Cardiol* 2008; **101**: 51F–57F.

20 Taleb A, Tsimikas S. Lipoprotein oxidation biomarkers for cardiovascular risk: what does the future hold? *Expert Rev Cardiovasc Ther* 2012; **10**: 399–402.

21 Nordestgaard BG, Tybjærg-Hansen A. Genetic determinants of LDL, lipoprotein(a), triglyceride-rich lipoproteins and HDL: concordance and discordance with cardiovascular disease risk. *Curr Opin Lipidol* 2011; **22**: 113–22.

22 Liyanage KE, Burnett JR, Hooper AJ, et al. Familial hypercholesterolemia: epidemiology, Neolithic origins and modern geographic distribution. *Crit Rev Clin Lab Sci* 2011; **48**: 1–18.

23 Goldberg AC, Hopkins PN, Toth PP, et al. National Lipid Association Expert Panel on Familial Hypercholesterolemia. Familial hypercholesterolemia: screening, diagnosis and management of pediatric and adult patients: clinical guidance from the National Lipid Association Expert Panel on Familial Hypercholesterolemia. *J Clin Lipidol* 2011; **5**(3 Suppl.): S1–S8.

24 Versmissen J, Oosterveer DM, Yazdanpanah M, et al. Efficacy of statins in familial hypercholesterolaemia: a long term cohort study. *Br Med J* 2008; **337**: a2423.

25 Veerkamp MJ, de Graaf J, Bredie SJ, et al. Diagnosis of familial combined hyperlipidemia based on lipid phenotype expression in 32 families: results of a 5-year follow-up study. *Arterioscler Thromb Vasc Biol* 2002; **22**: 274–82.

26 Eichner JE, Dunn ST, Perveen G, et al. Apolipoprotein E polymorphism and cardiovascular disease: a HuGE review. *Am J Epidemiol* 2002; **155**: 487–95.

27 Ewald N, Hardt PD, Kloer HU. Severe hypertriglyceridemia and pancreatitis: presentation and management. *Curr Opin Lipidol* 2009; **20**: 497–504.

28 Mozaffarian D, Micha R, Wallace S. Effects on coronary heart disease of increasing polyunsaturated fat in place of saturated fat: a systematic review and meta-analysis of randomized controlled trials. *PLoS Med* 2010; 7 (3): e1000252.

29 Mensink RP, Zock PL, Kester AD, et al. Effects of dietary fatty acids and carbohydrates on the ratio of serum total to HDL cholesterol and on serum lipids and apolipoproteins: a meta-analysis of 60 controlled trials. *Am J Clin Nutr* 2003; **77**: 1146–55.

30 Mozaffarian D, Aro A, Willett WC. Health effects of trans-fatty acids: experimental and observational evidence. *Eur J Clin Nutr* 2009; **63**: S5–S21.

31 Rimm EB, Williams P, Fosher K, et al. Moderate alcohol intake and lower risk of coronary heart disease: meta-analysis of effects on lipids and haemostatic factors. *Br Med J* 1999; **319**: 1523–28.

32 Shaw K, Gennat H, O'Rourke P, et al. Exercise for overweight or obesity. *Cochrane Database Syst Rev* 2006; (4): CD003817.

33 Adiels M, Olofsson SO, Taskinen MR, et al. Overproduction of very low-density lipoproteins is the hallmark of the dyslipidemia in the metabolic syndrome. *Arterioscler Thromb Vasc Biol* 2008; **28**: 1225–36.

34 Scott R, O'Brien R, Fulcher G, et al; Fenofibrate Intervention and Event Lowering in Diabetes (FIELD) Study Investigators. Effects of fenofibrate treatment on cardiovascular disease risk in 9,795 individuals with type 2 diabetes and various components of the metabolic syndrome: the Fenofibrate Intervention and Event Lowering in Diabetes (FIELD) study. *Diabetes Care* 2009; **32**: 493–8.

35 Jenkins M, Goldsmith D. Statins and kidney disease: is the study of heart and renal protection at the cutting edge of evidence? *Curr Opin Cardiol* 2012; **27**: 429–40.

36 Cholesterol Treatment Trialists' (CTT) Collaboration, Baigent C, Blackwell L, Emberson J, et al. Efficacy and safety of more intensive lowering of LDL cholesterol: a meta-analysis of data from 170,000 participants in 26 randomised trials. *Lancet* 2010; **376**: 1670–81.

37 Cholesterol Treatment Trialists' (CTT) Collaborators. The effects of lowering LDL cholesterol with statin therapy in people at low risk of vascular disease: meta-analysis of individual data from 27 randomised trials. *Lancet* 2012; **380**: 581–90.

38 Astrup A, Dyerberg J, Elwood P, et al. The role of reducing intakes of saturated fat in the prevention of cardiovascular disease: where does the evidence stand in 2010? *Am J Clin Nutr* 2011; **93**: 684–8.

39 Keys A. Serum cholesterol response to dietary cholesterol. *Am J Clin Nutr* 1984; **40**: 351–9.

40 Mensink RP, Zock PL, Kester ADM, et al. Effects of dietary fatty acids and carbohydrates on the ratio of serum total to HDL cholesterol and on serum lipids and apolipoproteins: a meta-analysis of 60 controlled trials. *Am J Clin Nutr* 2003; **77**: 1146–55.

41 He K, Song Y, Daviglus ML, et al. Accumulated evidence on fish consumption and coronary heart disease mortality: a meta-analysis of cohort studies. *Circulation* 2004; **109**: 2705–11.

42 Jakobsen MU, O'Reilly EJ, Heitman BL, et al. Major types of dietary fat and risk of coronary heart disease: a pooled analysis of 11 cohort studies. *Am J Clin Nutr* 2009; **89**: 1425–32.

43 Jakobsen MU, Dethlefsen C, Joenson AM, et al. Intake of carbohydrates compared with intake of saturated fatty acids and risk of myocardial infarction: importance of the glycaemic index. *Am J Nutr* 2010; **91**: 1764–8.

44 US Centers for Disease Control and Prevention. *Targeting tobacco use at a glance 2008*, 2008 Atlanta, GA: US Centers for Disease Control and Prevention.

45 Sacks FM, Bray G, Carey VJ, et al. Comparison of weight-loss diets with different compositions of fat, protein and carbohydrates. *N Engl J Med* 2009; **360**: 859–73.

46 Vanhees L, Geladas N, Hansen D, et al; on behalf of the writing group. Importance of characteristics and modalities of physical activity and exercise in the management of cardiovascular health in individuals with cardiovascular risk factors: recommendations from the EACPR (Part II). *Eur J Prev Cardiol* 2012; **19**: 1005–33.

47 Law M. Plant sterol and stanol margarines and health. *Br Med J* 2000; **320**: 861–4.

48 Schonfeld G. Plant sterols in atherosclerosis prevention. *Am J Nutr* 2010; **92**: 3–4.

49 Artinian NT, Fletcher GF, Mozaffarian D, et al; American Heart Association Prevention Committee of the Council on Cardiovascular Nursing. Interventions to promote physical activity and dietary lifestyle changes for cardiovascular risk factor reduction in adults: a scientific statement from the American Heart Association. *Circulation* 2010; **122**: 406–41.

50 Brugts JJ, Yetgin T, Hoeks SE, et al. The benefits of statins in people without established cardiovascular disease but with cardiovascular risk factors: meta-analysis of randomised controlled trials. *Br Med J* 2009; **338**: b2376.

51 Mills EJ, Rachlis B, Wu P, et al. Primary prevention of cardiovascular mortality and events with statin treatments. A network meta-analysis involving more than 65,000 patients. *J Am Coll Cardiol* 2008; **52**: 1769–81.

52 Fellström BC, Jardine AG, Schmieder RE, et al; AURORA Study Group. Rosuvastatin and cardiovascular events in patients undergoing hemodialysis. *N Engl J Med* 2009; **360**: 1395–407.

53 Reiner Ž, Galic M, Hanzevacki M, et al. Concomitant use of statins and cytochrome P 450 inhibitors in Croatia. *Lijec Vjesn* 2005; **127**: 65–8.

54 Ridker PM, Pradhan A, MacFadyen JG, et al. Cardiovascular benefits and diabetes risks of statin therapy in primary prevention: an analysis from the JUPITER trial. *Lancet* 2012; **380**: 565–71.

55 Jakovljević M, Reiner Ž, Miličić D. Mental disorders, treatment response, mortality and serum cholesterol: a new holistic look at old data. *Psychiatr Danub* 2007; **19**: 279–90.
56 Jukema JW, Cannon CP, de Craen AJM, et al. The controversies of statin therapy: weighing the evidence. *J Am Coll Cardiol* 2012; **60**: 875–81.
57 Levy P. Review of studies on the effect of bile acid sequestrants in patients with type 2 diabetes mellitus. *Metab Syndr Relat Disord* 2010; 8 (Suppl. 1): S9–S13.
58 Jun M, Foote C, Lu J, et al. Effects of fibrates on cardiovascular outcomes: a systematic review and meta-analysis. *Lancet* 2010; **375**: 1875–84.
59 Kamann VS, Kashyap ML. Mechanism of action of niacin. *Am J Cardiol* 2008; **101**: 20B–26B.
60 Mozaffarian D, Wu JH. Omega-3 fatty acids and cardiovascular disease: effects on risk factors, molecular pathways, and clinical events. *J Am Coll Cardiol* 2011; **58**: 2047–67.
61 Ballantyne CM, Bays HE, Kastelein JJ, et al. Efficacy and safety of eicosapentaenoic acid ethyl ester (AMR101) therapy in statin-treated patients with persistent high triglycerides (from the ANCHOR Study). *Am J Cardiol* 2012; **110**: 984–92.
62 Reiner Ž. Combined therapy in the treatment of dyslipidemia. *Fundam Clin Pharmacol* 2010; **24**: 19–28.
63 Vakkilainen J, Steiner G, Ansquer JC, et al; DAIS Group. Relationships between low-density lipoprotein particle size, plasma lipoproteins, and progression of coronary artery disease: the Diabetes Atherosclerosis Study (DAIS). *Circulation* 2003; **107**: 1733–7.
64 ACCORD Study Group, Ginsberg HN, Elam MB, Lovato LC, et al. Effects of combination lipid therapy in type 2 diabetes mellitus. *N Engl J Med* 2010; **362**: 1563–74.
65 Jones PJ, Davidson MH. Reporting rate of rhabdomyolysis with fenofibrate + statin versus gemfibrozil + any statin. *Am J Cardiol* 2005; **95**: 120–2.
66 Reiner Ž. Resistance and intolerance to statins. *Nutr Metab Cardiovasc Dis* 2014; **24**: 1057–66.

CHAPTER 16

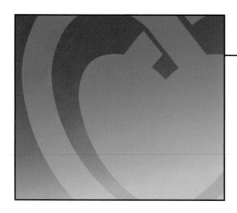

Glucose intolerance and diabetes

Christina Jarnert, Linda Mellbin, Lars Rydén, and Jaakko Tuomilehto

Contents

Summary

Diabetes dramatically increases the risk of cardiovascular disease (CVD). Diabetes is defined by elevated glucose in the circulating blood. The level of glycaemia has a graded relation with CVD risk, and diabetes is very frequent in people with CVD. When CVD patients without previously diagnosed diabetes are tested for glycaemia, the proportion of those found to have disturbed glucose metabolism is 60–70%. In the general population, half of people with type 2 diabetes are undiagnosed due to the lack of specific symptoms and a lack of systematic early detection efforts. Yet efficient methods exist for population screening. Despite considerable improvements in the management of CVD, patients with disturbed glucose metabolism have not benefited to the same extent as those without diabetes. Possible explanations for this are higher blood pressure, dyslipidaemia, advanced atherosclerosis, insufficient use of evidence-based CVD management, or inadequate glycaemic control. In patients with CVD and cardiometabolic disorder it is not sufficient to focus on the CVD manifestations alone—simultaneous actions directed towards the underlying complex metabolic disorder are required together with attention to other existing concomitant risk factors. Primary and secondary prevention in people with diabetes and other disturbances in glucose metabolism must be multifactorial and treatment targets stricter than for patients without glucose aberrations. Increased collaboration between different therapeutic disciplines, including diabetologists, cardiologists, general practitioners, and dieticians, is key to improved management for this large and high-risk population. Some important aspects of these issues are presented in this chapter.

Introduction

Diabetes mellitus (DM) is a condition defined and diagnosed by an elevated level of glucose in the blood. Recently, high glycated haemoglobin (HbA1c) has also been accepted for a diagnosis of DM. Despite considerable progress in care for patients with cardiovascular disease (CVD) there is an increasing challenge concerning the prevention and treatment of CVD in people with DM or disturbed glucose metabolism, who are at high risk of CVD.

The International Diabetes Federation (IDF) estimated that in Europe in 2011 53 million people aged 20–79 years had DM; that number is expected to exceed 64 million

Table 16.1 Burden of diabetes mellitus (DM) in Europe in 2011 and predictions for 2030

Variable	2011	2030
Total population (millions)	899	931
Adults (20–79 years; millions)	653	673
DM (20–79 years)		
European prevalence (%)	8.1	9.5
Number with DM (millions)	52.8	64.2
Impaired glucose tolerance (20–79 years)		
Regional prevalence (%)	9.6	10.6
Number with IGT (millions)	63.0	71.5
Type 1 DM in children (0–14 years)		
Number with type 1 DM (thousands)	116.1	–
Number newly diagnosed/year (thousands)	17.9	–
DM mortality (20–79 years)		
Number of deaths; men (thousands)	282.4	–
Number of deaths; women (thousands)	317.6	–
Healthcare expenditure due to DM (people aged 20–79 years, Europe)		
Total expenditure (billions of €)	994.7	1195.9

Source: data from IDF *Diabetes Atlas*, version 5, edition 2012.

by 2030. In addition 63 million Europeans had impaired glucose tolerance (IGT) in 2011 (➲ Table 16.1). The continuous increase in the prevalence of DM is not only due to an ageing population, but also to changing lifestyles leading to an unhealthy diet, increased prevalence of overweight, and physical inactivity [1]. The World Health Organization (WHO) multinational study of vascular disease in DM (➲ Fig. 16.1) revealed that the majority of deaths in people with DM are caused by CVD, and this is a global pattern [2]. DM is a major burden on society; approximately 15%

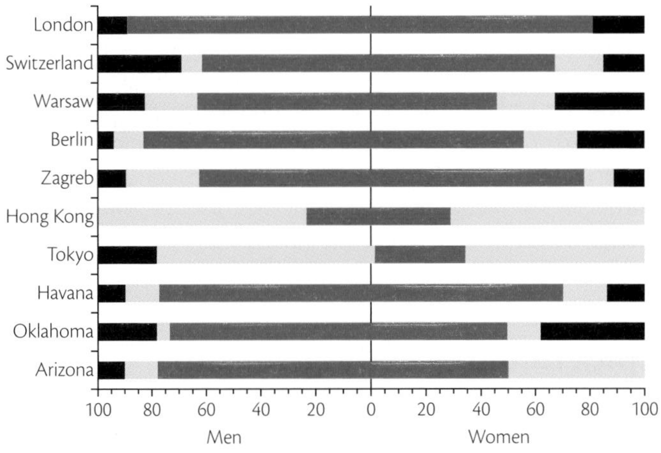

Fig. 16.1 WHO data on reasons for mortality in diabetes: red, ischaemic heart disease; pink, cerebrovascular disease; black, other.
Springer and *Diabetologia*, **44**, 2001, S19, An analysis of serial Minnesota ECG code changes in the London cohort of the WHO multinational study of vascular disease in diabetes, H. Keen, Fig. 3B, With kind permission from Springer Science and Business Media.

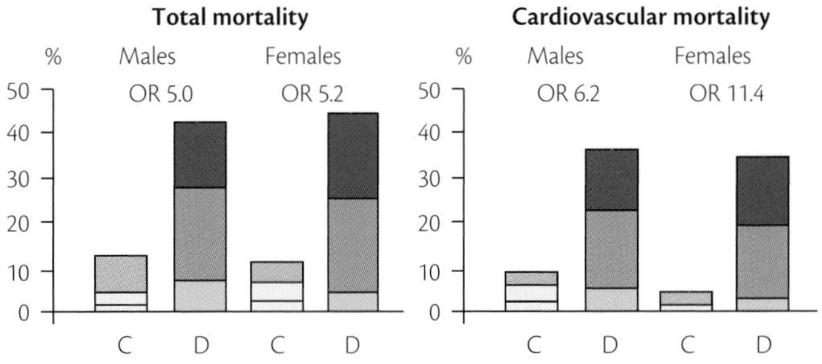

Fig. 16.2 Mortality and morbidity in males and females over 15 years in patients with newly detected type 2 diabetes (D) and non-diabetic controls (C). In each bar the different gradations of shading (from the bottom) represent follow-up during 5, 10, and 15 years, respectively. OR, odds ratio.
Source: data from Niskanen L, Turpeinen A, Penttilä I, Uusitupa MI. Hyperglycemia and compositional lipoprotein abnormalities as predictors of cardiovascular mortality in type 2 diabetes: a 5-year follow-up from the time of diagnosis. *Diabetes Care* 1998; **21**: 1861–1869.

of all healthcare expenses in Europe are due to DM, mostly a result of CVD complications.

In the recent years DM and its precursor states have become important aspects in the prevention and care of CVD. The 2012 Joint European Society guideline on CVD prevention recommended classifying people with DM and at least one other CVD risk factor or target organ damage as being at very high risk for developing a CVD event, and all other people with DM as being at high risk [3]. More detailed risk estimates may be performed by means of so-called risk engines, i.e. statistical models that are used to predict a disease event. One was developed on the basis of the United Kingdom Prospective Diabetes Study (UKPDS) [4], and the most recent is based on information from 24 000 patients in the Swedish National Diabetes Registry followed from 2002 to 2007 [5]. It takes into account treatment targets and modalities and is available at the Swedish National Diabetes Registry website (<http://www.ndr.nu/risk/>). The increased CVD risk is particularly apparent in women, as illustrated by a Finnish study in which patients aged 45–64 years with newly detected type 2 diabetes (T2DM) were followed for 15 years [6]. Total mortality was considerably higher among men and women with T2DM than in those without (men 44% versus 13%; women 44% versus 11%); the risk of CVD death in men with DM was increased six-fold and in women eleven-fold (➲ Fig. 16.2).

Classification and diagnosis of DM and other disorders of glucose metabolism

The uniform classification and diagnostic criteria for DM are based on recommendations outlined by the WHO Expert Committee in 1980 and further refined by WHO consultation groups and the expert groups of the American Diabetes Association (ADA) over the years [7–11]. HbA1c has recently been recommended as a diagnostic test for DM [11,12]. The currently recommended thresholds for fasting plasma glucose (FPG), 2-hour post-challenge plasma glucose (2-hPG) after a standard 75-g

Table 16.2 Diagnostic criteria for glucose perturbations as defined by World Health Organization (WHO) and American Diabetes Association (ADA)

Diagnosis/ measurement	WHO 2006/WHO 2011	ADA 2013
Diabetes		
HbA1c	Can be used. If measured ≥6.5% (48 mmol/mol)	Recommended ≥6.5% (48 mmol/mol)
FPG	Recommended ≥7.0 mmol/L (≥126 mg/dl) OR use 2-hPG	≥7.0 mmol/L (≥126 mg/dl) OR use 2-hPG
2-hPG	≥11.1 mmol/L (≥200 mg/dl)	≥11.1 mmol/L (≥200 mg/dl)
IGT		
FPG	<7.0 mmol/L (<126 mg/dl)	<7.0 mmol/L (<126 mg/dl)
2-hPG	≥7.8 to <11.1 mmol/L (≥140 to <200 mg/dl)	Not required. If measured 7.8–11.0 mmol/L (140–198 mg/dl)
IFG		
FPG	If measured 6.1–6.9 mmol/L (110–125 mg/dl)	5.6–6.9 mmol/L (100–125 mg/dl)
2-hPG	<7.8 mmol/L (<140 mg/dl)	

FPG, fasting plasma glucose; 2-hPG, 2-hour post-load plasma glucose; IGT, impaired glucose tolerance; IFG, impaired fasting glucose.

Source: data from World Health Organization (WHO) Consultation. Definition and diagnosis of diabetes and intermediate hyperglycaemia, 2006. <http://www.who.int/diabetes/publications/Definition%20and%20diagnosis%20of%20diabetes_new.pdf>

World Health Organization (WHO), Abbreviated report of a WHO consultation. Use of glycated hemoglobin (HbA1c) in the diagnosis of diabetes mellitus, 2011 <http://www.who.int/diabetes/publications/diagnosis_diabetes2011/en/index.html>

Inzucchi SE, Bergenstal RM, Buse JB, et al. Management of hyperglycaemia in type 2 diabetes: a patient-centered approach. Position statement of the American Diabetes Association (ADA) and the European Association for the Study of Diabetes (EASD). *Diabetologia* 2012; **55**: 1577–1596.

oral glucose tolerance test (OGTT), and HbA1c are shown in ➲ Table 16.2. It must be kept in mind that FPG and HbA1c have a lower sensitivity to identify people with DM and people at risk of DM compared with 2-hPG [13,14]. Therefore the WHO guideline emphasizes the use of a 2-hour OGTT and stresses that a HbA1c value of <6.5% does not exclude the presence of DM that may be detected by blood glucose measurement, and has no interpretation regarding classification and diagnosis of hyperglycaemic states [12].

There are two main aetiological categories of DM: type 1 diabetes (T1DM) and T2DM. Both of them have a strong genetic susceptibility, but the genes associated with them are largely different [7–11]. Other categories also exist: 'other specific types' (mainly due to monogenic mutations) and 'gestational DM' [7,9]. Insulin is a peptide hormone that is essential for maintaining whole body glucose homeostasis and promoting efficient glucose utilization.

T1DM is characterized by insulin deficiency due to destructive lesions of pancreatic beta-cells, progressing towards absolute insulin deficiency. It typically occurs in young people of normal weight presenting with polyuria, thirst, and weight loss with a propensity to ketosis. However, T1DM may occur at any age [15], sometimes with slow progression (often also called 'latent autoimmune diabetes in adults' or LADA) [16]. European people with T1DM often have autoantibodies to pancreatic beta-cell proteins that may be detected before the clinical manifestation of the disease [17,18]. Compared with other ethnicities and geographical regions, T1DM is more common in Europid (Caucasian) populations [19]. Finland has by far the highest incidence of childhood-onset T1DM in the world, and other populations in northern Europe and Canada also have a high incidence. The incidence of T1DM is increasing globally at a rate of approximately 3% a year [19].

T2DM is a progressive disease which most often develops after middle age, but there is a trend towards a decreasing age of onset in many populations. Over 90% of adults with DM have T2DM. It is characterized by a combination of insulin resistance and beta-cell dysfunction/failure, often but not always in association with obesity (typically with an abdominal distribution of adiposity) and sedentary lifestyle, the two major and most well-known risk factors for T2DM. Many other lifestyle factors also contribute to the risk of T2DM [20]. Interestingly, the vast majority of genes that have been confirmed to be associated with T2DM have an action related to pancreatic beta-cell function or insulin secretion [21]. There is a hyperbolic relationship between insulin sensitivity (resistance) in peripheral tissues and insulin secretion from the pancreas [22]. When insulin secretion becomes inadequate in relation to insulin resistance, glucose intolerance and T2DM occur [23,24]. An impaired first phase of insulin secretion, causing post-prandial hyperglycaemia, typically characterizes the early stage of T2DM. This is followed by a deteriorating second-phase insulin response and persistent hyperglycaemia, which is apparent even in the fasting state [23–26]. The level of HbA1c is only increased following increased long-lasting elevated blood glucose concentrations, and therefore high HbA1c is secondary to sustained elevation of blood glucose. Although it may look as if HbA1c is easier to measure, it has problems with standardization and its use will inevitably delay the diagnosis of asymptomatic T2DM [27].

Impaired glucose metabolism (also called pre-diabetes), i.e. impaired fasting glucose (IFG) and impaired glucose tolerance (IGT), refers to an intermediate state in the progression from normal glucose homeostasis to DM. Studies suggest that IGT is associated with insulin resistance in muscle and defective insulin secretion, resulting in less efficient disposal of the glucose load during an OGTT, while IFG is associated with impaired insulin secretion and impaired suppression of hepatic glucose output [26].

Epidemiology of dysglycaemia in CVD

Prevalence

T2DM remains undetected in approximately half of the people who suffer from it [28] because hyperglycaemia does not cause specific symptoms until it has been present for a long time and glucose levels are very high. That is why the condition remains unrecognized for years if no proper screening takes place. The progression from asymptomatic hyperglycaemia to frank T2DM may take 10–15 years [29]. There are indeed more people with undiagnosed T2DM and other disorders of glucose metabolism than with diagnosed T2DM [28]. Since systematic assessments over time have only been carried out in very few countries (and with variable methods), the prevalence of T2DM reported by bodies such as the IDF is certainly underestimated. Moreover the prevalence is rapidly increasing making 'old' data inaccurate. A Turkish study carried out in 2010 is so far the only nationwide prevalence study of DM and other disorders of glucose metabolism carried out in Europe with the standard methodology recommended by the WHO at the time [30]. The overall prevalence of DM was 16.5%, with 7.5% screen detected DM; the prevalence was higher in women than in men. The prevalence of isolated IFG, isolated IGT, and combined pre-diabetes was 14.7, 7.9, and 8.2%, respectively. Compared with a previous national prevalence study carried out in 1997–98 the increase in the prevalence of DM was 90% and in IGT 106%. In 2010, only about 20% of Turkish people above the age of 65 were free from disorders of glucose metabolism. Another very large study from China published in 2013 reported that the estimated prevalence of DM among a representative sample of Chinese adults was 12% and that of pre-diabetes 50% [31], while in 2001 prevalence of DM was 5.5% [32]; thus there was an increase of over 100% in 10 years. The vast majority of Chinese with DM in the more recent study had not been diagnosed previously. In a recent Finnish population-based study among people aged 45–74, also using the WHO criteria, the prevalence of DM and other disorders of glucose metabolism was almost 40%, and higher in men (42%) than in women (33%) [33]. In most populations DM seems to be more common in men than in women until the age of 65.

Cardiovascular risk

People with previously undetected T2DM and IGT have an increased risk of CVD. Convincing evidence for such a relation was provided by the DECODE study which analysed several European cohort studies with baseline OGTT data [34–36]; these findings were subsequently confirmed by other investigators [37–39]. Increased mortality and CVD risk were observed in people with DM and IGT identified by 2-hPG, but not in people with IFG identified by FPG. People with IGT have an approximately 30% increased risk of CVD, while those with previously undiagnosed T2DM have a risk of CVD almost as high as those with previously diagnosed T2DM [35]. The increase in risk with 2-hPG is graded, the higher the glucose the higher the CVD mortality. All manifestations of CVD are increased in people with T2DM [40]: CHD, stroke, peripheral artery disease, heart failure, and cardiomyopathy due to diabetes. At the population level post-challenge or post-prandial glucose is a better predictor of CVD than fasting glucose [41], even within the 'normoglycaemic' range [42]. The glucose concentration in blood varies markedly during a normal day, mostly reflecting the intake of food, carbohydrates in particular, and physical activity. Actually, fasting glucose is a reflection of the lowest glucose level during the day, but people are spending most of the day in the post-prandial or post-absorptive state with higher blood glucose than after an overnight fast [44].

The cut-points defining DM have been determined mainly on the basis of DM-induced retinopathy [7–10], a condition that is very specific for hyperglycaemia. The cut-points defining other disorders of glucose metabolism are mainly based on the rate of progression to DM. Macrovascular complications associated with hyperglycaemia do, however, start to develop before the currently defined thresholds of DM [39]. The DECODE data also showed that a J-shaped relation exists between mortality and glucose concentrations for both FPG and 2-hPG, except for the relation between 2-hPG and CVD mortality, where the relation is graded and increasing (➲ Fig. 16.3). That high fasting and 2-hPG concentrations are associated with increased risk of mortality is now unequivocally confirmed. A high 2-hPG predicted all-cause and CVD mortality after adjustment for other major cardiovascular risk factors while a high FPG alone was not predictive once 2-hPG was taken into account, in both European and Asian populations [35,44]. At the population level the highest number of excess CVD deaths occurred in people with IGT

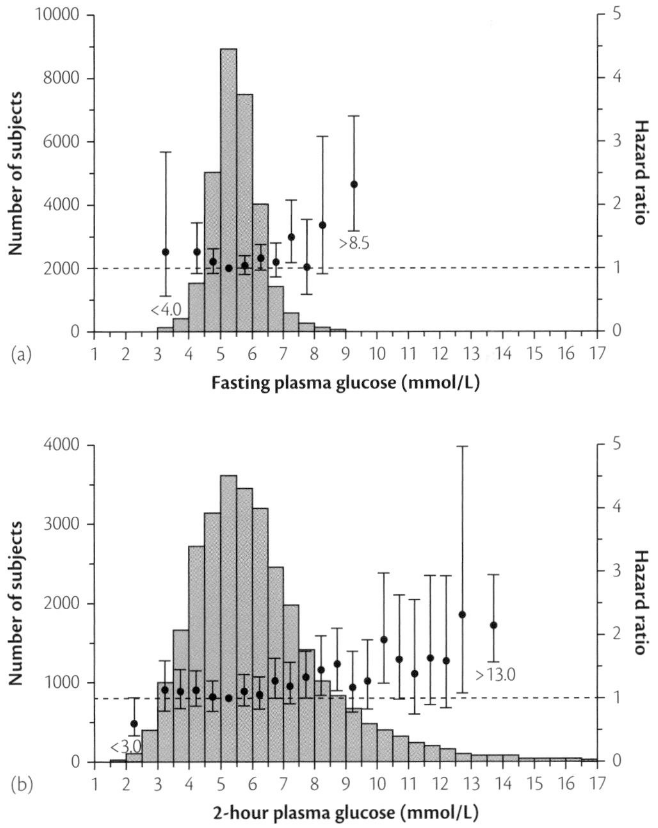

Fig. 16.3 Distributions of fasting plasma glucose (a), 2-hour post-load plasma glucose (b), and hazard ratios for CVD mortality with 95% confidence intervals (bars) according to glucose intervals of 0.5 mmol/L in people without a previous history of diabetes, adjusted for age, sex, cohort, serum cholesterol, systolic blood pressure, body mass index, and smoking.

Source: data from DECODE Study Group. Glucose tolerance and cardiovascular mortality. *Arch Intern Med* 2001; **161**: 397–404.

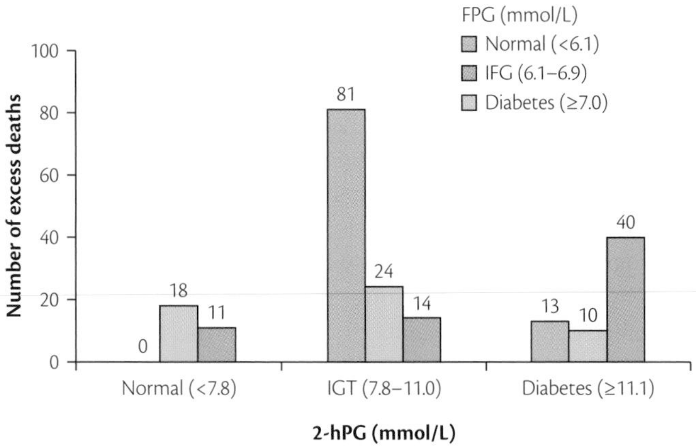

Fig. 16.4 Number of excess deaths by fasting plasma glucose (FPG) and 2-hour post-load plasma glucose (2-hPG) category. The comparison group is the one with both normal FPG and 2-hPG where the number of excess deaths was set to zero.

Source: data from DECODE Study Group. Glucose tolerance and mortality: comparison of WHO and American Diabetes Association diagnostic criteria. *Lancet* 1999; **354**: 617–621.

[34], since the number of such people is highest in the hyperglycaemic population (➲ Fig. 16.4).

Screening for DM and other disturbances in glucose metabolism

Random testing of blood glucose among people without known DM to determine CVD risk has not been recommended due to a lack of affirmative evidence that the prognosis of CVD related to T2DM can be improved by early detection and treatment [45,46]. Screening for hyperglycaemia should therefore be selectively targeted to high-risk individuals. Screening may, however, facilitate CVD risk reduction by multifactorial management, and early detection may allow interventions that retard the progression of microvascular disease, which may make screening for T2DM beneficial [47]. In addition, there is an interest in identifying people with IGT since most will progress to T2DM, and this progression can be retarded by lifestyle interventions [48–52].

A stepwise approach for early detection of T2DM and other disorders of glucose metabolism in the general population is currently recommended [53]. The first step is to use questionnaire-based information, i.e. a non-laboratory risk score that provides summary information on the presence of certain aetiological risk factors for T2DM. In the second step people with a high risk score will be referred for further testing of dysglycaemia and other CVD risk factors. Such a first step is not needed in people with pre-existing CVD and pregnant women, who all should be tested for dysglycaemia following the current guidelines [40,54]. Several DM risk scores have been developed. Most of them perform well, and it does not matter which one is used, as underlined by recent systematic reviews [55]. An example is the FINnish Diabetes RIsk SCore (FINDRISC; <http://www.diabetes.fi/english>) [56] which is commonly used to screen for DM risk in Europe (➲ Fig. 16.5).

Pathophysiological relation between dysglycaemia and CVD

There are several factors contributing to the development of CVD among people with DM. These are the same as in people without DM, but hyperglycaemia adds further to the risk, either directly or through other mechanisms due to the elevated blood glucose [40]. Hyperglycaemia is associated with an atherogenic lipid profile, high blood pressure, low-grade inflammation, renal disorder, etc., all of which increase CVD risk.

In the United Kingdom Prospective Diabetes Study (UKPDS) an increase of 1% in HbA1c resulted in a 14% higher risk of developing myocardial infarction and a 21% higher risk of death [57]. A recent meta-analysis summarized findings from 112 studies comprising almost 700 000 people followed for a mean period of 11 years [58]. The increased risk was more apparent in women than in men and in younger age groups, non-smokers, and those in the lower range of elevated blood pressure. Thus, it seems that people who otherwise have a relatively low CVD risk profile are proportionally more exposed to CVD when they have disorders of glucose metabolism. This is partly due to the fact that among them the risk in the comparison group without DM is very low, leading to a high increase in relative risk among people with DM, even though the absolute risk may not be very high.

It has been discussed whether hyperglycaemia is harmful in itself or if it should be seen as a marker of other pathophysiological mechanisms of importance for the development of CVD. In favour of a direct influence is that hyperglycaemia causes oxidative stress, which is considered as a central trigger for many processes that are harmful to vascular walls, for example endothelial dysfunction, chronic inflammation, neovascularization, and arteriolar and capillary narrowing disturbing collateral circulation [59]. In addition, T2DM and its preceding stages are characterized by other factors that may promote injury to vascular walls and atherothrombotic disease. Among them are decreased insulin sensitivity together with increased thrombogenesis and reduced fibrinolytic capacity. Another example of the influence of dysmetabolism is that less myocardial energy is produced by glucose oxidation and more by the energy-demanding beta-oxidation of free fatty acids. This may, particularly during myocardial ischaemia and adrenergic stress, contribute to myocardial dysfunction [59].

Screening for dysglycaemia in patients with CVD

The Glucose And Myocardial Infarction (GAMI) study, which recruited 181 patients, showed the high prevalence of glucose perturbations in people with acute coronary syndrome (ACS) without a history of DM [60]. They were all subjected to an OGTT about 5 days after onset of symptoms. Only 33% had normal glucose tolerance, while 34% had IGT and 33% previously undetected T2DM. The Euro and China Heart Surveys [61,62] recruited patients with stable and unstable coronary artery disease (CAD), and confirmed the results of the GAMI study in larger

Type 2 diabetes risk assessment form

Circle the right alternative and add up your points.

1. Age
0 p. Under 45 years
2 p. 45-54 years
3 p. 55-64 years
4 p. Over 64 years

2. Body mass Index
0 p. Lower than 25 kg/m^2
1 p. 25-30 kg/m^2
3 p. Higher than 30 kg/m^2

3. Waist circumference measured below the ribs (usually at the level of the navel)

	MEN	WOMEN
0 p.	Less than 94 cm	Less than 80 cm
3 p.	94-102 cm	80-88 cm
4 p.	More than 102 cm	More than 88 cm

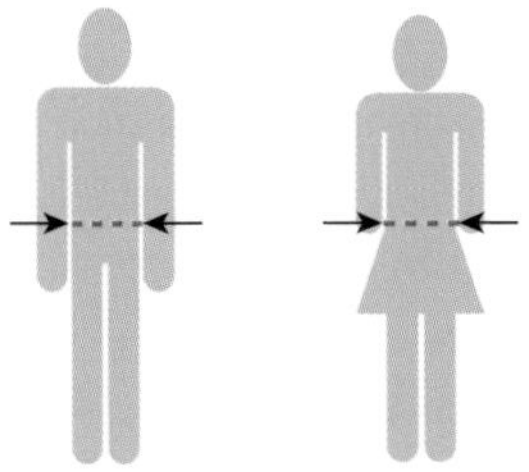

4. Do you usually have daily at least 30 min of physical activity at work and/or during leisure time (including normal daily activity)?
0 p. Yes
2 p. No

5. How often do you eat vegetables, fruit, or berries?
0 p. Every day
1 p. Not every day

6. Have you ever taken anti-hypertensive medication regularly?
0 p. No
2 p. Yes

7. Have you ever been found to have high blood glucose (e.g. in a health examination, during an illness, during pregnancy)?
0 p. No
5 p. Yes

8. Have any of the members of your immediate family or other relatives been diagnosed with diabetes (type 1 or type 2)?
0 p. No
3 p. Yes: grandparent, aunt, uncle, or first cousin (but not own parent, brother, sister or child)
5 p. Yes: parent, brother, sister, or own child

Total risk score

☐ **The risk of developing type 2 diabetes within 10 years is**

Lower than 7	**Low:** estimated 1 in 100 will develop disease
7-11	**Slightly elevated:** estimated 1 in 25 will develop disease
12-14	**Moderate:** estimated 1 in 6 will develop disease
15-20	**High:** estimated 1 in 3 will develop disease
Higher than 20	**Very High:** estimated 1 in 2 will develop disease

Test designed by Professor Jaakko Tuomilehto. Department of Public Health, University of Helsinki, and Dr Jaana Lindstrom, MFS, National Public Health Institute.

Fig. 16.5 The FINnish Diabetes Risk Score (FINFRISC) for the assesement of the 10-year risk of developing type 2 diabetes in adults.
With permission from the Finnish Diabetes Association, accessed from <http://www.diabetes.fi/english>

populations from several countries, including people with acute and stable CAD. In the Euro Heart Survey on Diabetes and the Heart (n = 4961, 25 countries) the prevalence of known DM was 31%, while 12% had newly detected DM, 25% IGT, and 3% IFG, leaving only 32% with normal glucose regulation (➲ Fig. 16.6). In a study in India among people with ACS and without a history of DM, 84% had glucose perturbations: IFG or IGT in 46% and undiagnosed DM in 38% [63]. These studies all demonstrated that a substantial proportion of people with glucose disturbances would have remained undetected without an OGTT [64]. A similar pattern has subsequently been shown in patients with cerebrovascular and peripheral vascular disease [65]. In an Austrian study, 238 consecutively admitted acute stroke patients were screened for glucose perturbations using an OGTT in the first and second weeks after the stroke event: 20% had normal glucose levels, 20% had previously known DM, 16% were classified as having newly diagnosed DM, 23% IGT, and 1% IFG. The remaining 20% had transient hyperglycaemia or missing data in the second OGTT. Subsequently it was shown that newly detected glucose disturbances in these studies had a negative prognostic implication in ACS and stroke [65,66].

HbA1c has been recommended as a diagnostic tool for DM in the general population [11,12]. HbA1c, like other parameters of glycaemia, shows a graded association with CVD risk [67–69]. Studies that compared all three main glycaemic parameters—FPG, 2-hPG, and HbA1c—simultaneously for mortality and CVD risk have revealed that the association is strongest for 2-hPG, and that the risk observed with FPG and HbA1c is no longer significant after controlling for the effect of 2-hPG [70,71].

The use of HbA1c in people with CVD and without a history of DM to detect previously unrecognized T2DM or other disorders of glucose metabolism has not been well studied in the past. An Indian study reported that 27% of newly diagnosed ACS patients with DM had HbA1c < 6.0% [65]. Recently, Hage et al. [72]

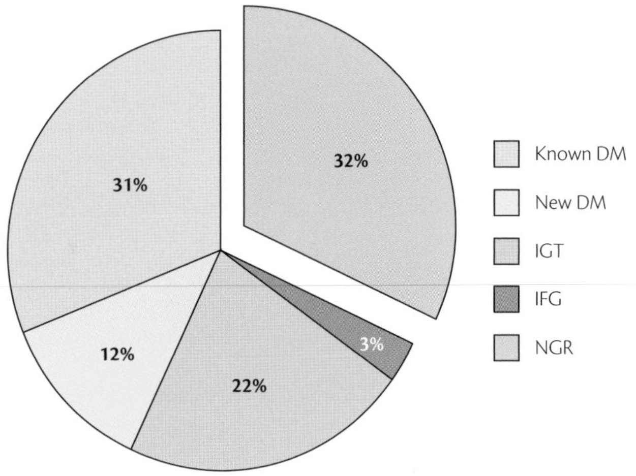

Fig. 16.6 The prevalence of abnormal glucose regulation in patients with established coronary artery disease investigated in the Euro Heart Survey on Diabetes and the Heart: DM, diabetes mellitus; IGT, impaired glucose tolerance; IFG, impaired fasting glucose; NGR, normal glucose regulation.
Source: data from Genuth S, Alberti KG, Bennett P, et al. Follow-up report on the diagnosis of diabetes mellitus. *Diabetes Care* 2003; **26**(11): 3160–3167.

screened 174 patients with ACS, of whom 27 had T2DM according to the OGTT. FPG failed to detect 63% and HbA1c 93% of these patients (➲ Fig. 16.7). Similar findings have been reported in patients with ACS selected for further investigation due to elevated admission glucose [73] and in patients referred for coronary angiography [74]. There are many pros and cons to be considered when deciding which test for glycaemia will be used. HbA1c is clearly the least sensitive test for identifying glycaemic perturbations, and there are many additional issues besides blood glucose concentration that may lead to an artificial increase or decrease in HbA1c, especially factors or disorders influencing red blood cell turnover [75].

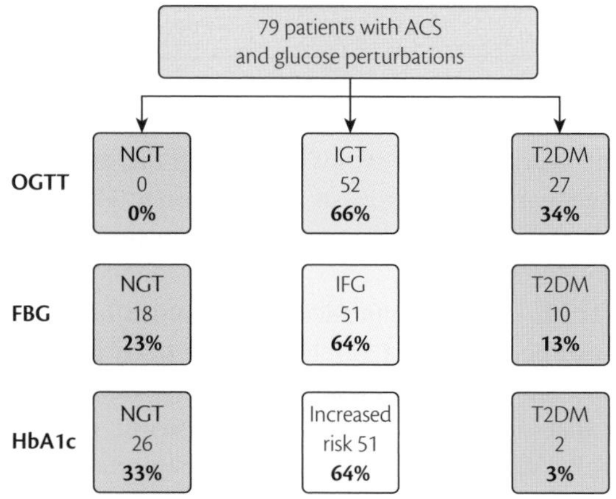

Fig. 16.7 The pattern of glucose perturbation in 79 patients with acute coronary syndrome (ACS) if screened by oral glucose tolerance test (OGTT), fasting blood glucose (FBG), or glycated haemoglobin A1c (HbA1c). NGT, normal glucose tolerance; IGT, impaired glucose tolerance; IFG, impaired fasting glucose; T2DM, type 2 diabetes mellitus. See text for further explanation.
Reproduced from Hage C, Lundman P, Rydén L, Mellbin L. Fasting glucose, HbA1c or oral glucose tolerance testing for the detection of glucose abnormalities in patients with acute coronary syndromes. *Eur J Prev Cardiol* 2013; **20**: 549–554 by permission of SAGE.

In summary, DM and IGT are common conditions in patients with CVD and influence their prognosis negatively; a 2-h OGTT is needed when screening patients with CVD for glucose perturbations since both FPG and HbA1c are very insensitive. However, screening may be initiated with HbA1c and/or FPG assays, but needs to be followed by an OGTT if these laboratory investigations do not provide a clear diagnosis as recommended in the 2013 ESC and EASD guidelines on diabetes, pre-diabetes, and CVD [40].

Delaying or preventing the onset of DM

A modest weight loss in combination with increased physical activity prevents or retards the progression towards DM in people with IGT, underlining the importance of structured lifestyle counselling. DM prevention trials, especially the European trials, have shown a preventive effect in a range of 50–60% with 3–5 years of intervention (➲ Table 16.3) [48–50,52,53]. It has been estimated that the provision of such lifestyle counselling among six high-risk individuals over 3 years will prevent one case of DM [52]. A long-term follow-up of participants in a Chinese DM prevention study showed a persistent reduction in the incidence of T2DM, a 17% trend towards a reduction in cardiovascular mortality, and a 47% reduction of severe retinopathy in the intervention group after 20 years [51]. A favourable impact of a DM prevention programme was also reported from a 12-year follow-up of a Swedish study [76]. Men with IGT subjected to lifestyle counselling had lower all-cause mortality than those in the routine care group (6.5 versus 14.0 per 1000 person-years; $p = 0.009$).

Management of DM

Multifactorial management

The great importance of multifactorial management of people with T2DM was demonstrated by the landmark STENO 2 trial randomizing the participants to intensive, target-driven multifactorial therapy at a specialized clinic or to conventional care. Targets included lifestyle counselling, HbA1c, blood lipids, and blood pressure. Moreover, all patients in the intensive group were prescribed a renin–angiotensin system (RAS) inhibitor and aspirin. Even if all treatment targets were not fully met, intensively treated patients were considerably better managed than those offered standard care. After 7.8 years of follow-up there was a 50% reduction in micro- and macrovascular events in the intensively treated group. Thereafter target-driven management was recommended for all participants, who were followed for a total of 13 years. By that time patients originally allocated to the intensively managed group had an absolute mortality reduction of 20%, an absolute reduction of cardiovascular events of 29%, and diabetes-induced nephropathy and progression of retinopathy was substantially less prevalent

Table 16.3 Efficacy of the prevention of type 2 diabetes in high-risk people with impaired glucose tolerance in randomized controlled trials

Study	Intervention	Patients (*n*)	Dropouts (%)	Follow-up (years)	RRR (%)
Da-Qing Study, China [51]	Diet	130	8	6	31
	Exercise	141			46
	Diet + exercise	126			42
	Control	133			
Diabetes Prevention Study, Finland [48]	Diet + PA	265	8	3.2	58
	Control	257			
US Diabetes Prevention Program, USA [49]	Diet + PA	1079	8	2.8	58
	Metformin	1073			31
	Placebo	1082			
SLIM study, the Netherlands [50]	Diet + PA	74	8	3	58
	Control	73			
EDIPS-Newcastle, UK [52]	Diet + PA	51	19	3.1	55
	Control	51			

RRR, relative risk reduction; PA, physical activity.

[77,78]. The intensive management turned out to be more cost-effective than conventional care [79]. Further support for a multifactorial treatment approach came from the Euro Heart Survey on Diabetes and the Heart. Among 1425 patients with DM and coronary artery disease, 44% had been subjected to comprehensive evidence-based therapy (a combination of aspirin, beta-blockade, RAS inhibitors, and statins), and these patients had significantly lower all-cause mortality (3.5% versus 7.7%, $p = 0.001$) and fewer combined cardiovascular events (11.6% versus 14.7%, $p = 0.05$) after 1 year of follow-up [80].

Target-driven treatment

Lifestyle

Lifestyle advice is the cornerstone of management for people with glucose perturbations. Advice should focus on a diet rich in fruits, vegetables, wholegrain cereals, and low-fat protein sources and a reasonable restriction of total energy intake [81]. Total fat intake should be <35%, saturated fat <10%, and monounsaturated fatty acids >10% of total energy, and dietary fibre intake should be >40 g/day. Weight stabilization is recommended before weight reduction, at least in non-obese people. Sodium restriction is also strongly recommended, without any specified target. Moderate to vigorous physical activity for at least 150 minutes a week is recommended, preferably as a combination of aerobic and resistance training [82]. Smoking cessation is obligatory, and structured advice, including pharmacological support, should be offered those who are smokers. Details on effective support can be found in the 2013 European guidelines for diabetes, pre-diabetes, and CVD [40].

Glucose control

Microvascular complications increase almost linearly with an increasing HbA1c and with no clear threshold in both T1DM and T2DM [83,84]. Glycaemic control, targeting a HbA1c of 6.0–7.0% (42–53 mmol/mol) decreases this progression in both T1DM and T2DM (but less obviously in T2DM) [85]. Macrovascular complications are also decreased, but less convincingly so and only after long periods of observation. A meta-analysis of cardiovascular outcomes from major clinical trials suggests that a 1% lowering of HbA1c reduces the relative risk for non-fatal myocardial infarction by 15%. However, it had no impact on stroke or all-cause mortality [86]. This analysis also revealed that, seen from the perspective of preventing macrovascular complications, a short duration of DM, freedom from cardiovascular disease, and a low HbA1c at the start of treatment seemed to make strict glycaemic control more rewarding.

The ADA and the European Association for the Study of Diabetes (EASD) recently recommended that glycaemic control should be applied in an individualized manner taking age, duration of DM, and history of cardiovascular disease into account [85]. Tight glycaemic control targeting a near normal HbA1c of ≤7% (≤53 mmol/mol) is recommended for the prevention of microvascular complications and can also be considered for the prevention of cardiovascular disease. In elderly people with long-standing and/or a complicated disease a less strict target of <7.5–8.0% (<58–64 mmol/mol) may be acceptable following consideration of age, capacity for self-care, and availability of support. There are now a variety of possible pharmacological treatments, and many more are in the pipeline. The general recommendation is to start with metformin and add other therapeutic options when needed in an individualized manner, as outlined in detail in the ADA/EASD recommendations [85].

Blood pressure

Hypertension is more common in people with DM than in the general population: about 50% in T1DM [87,88] and 60–80% in T2DM [89]. Obesity, and renal involvement may explain some of this increase in hypertension in DM. Although pathophysiological mechanisms for the relation between DM and hypertension are not fully understood, they may include: (1) hyperinsulinaemia linked to increased renal reabsorption of sodium, (2) increased sympathetic tone, and (3) increased RAS system activity [90].

Only limited population-based data exist regarding blood pressure trends in people with DM. The proportion of hypertensive people in the United States with DM and poorly controlled blood pressure decreased from the 1970s to the 1990s [91]. Data from the National Health and Nutrition Examination Surveys (NHANES) did not reveal any changes in blood pressure control in patients with DM from 1988–94 to the early 2000s [92] or from 1999 to 2006 [93]. Nevertheless, the NHANES data showed a decrease in mean blood pressure levels among adults with diagnosed DM from 135/72 mmHg in 1988–94 to 131/69 mmHg in 2001–08 [94], while the prevalence of patients with DM and a blood pressure >140/90 mmHg or under antihypertensive drug treatment increased from 64 to 69%.

Recent data from the Swedish National Diabetes register using three cross-sectional samples in 2005, 2007, and 2009 (not all the same patients) showed a decrease of mean blood pressure from 141/77 to 136/76 mmHg and a decrease of inadequately controlled hypertension (≥140/90 mmHg) from 58 to 46% [95]. From 1997 to 2002 the Finnish national chronic disease risk factor surveys showed a decrease in mean blood pressure in middle-aged men with DM on blood pressure-lowering drug treatment from 154/87 to 150/84 mmHg and a decrease from 149/82 to 148/78 mmHg in women [96]. During the same period there was a statistically significant increase from 23 to 34% in the prevalence of controlled blood pressure (<140/90 mmHg), both among patients with DM and antihypertensive drug treatment and people without DM.

The risk of CVD with DM and hypertension combined is additive; hypertension results in a four-fold increase in CVD risk in people with DM [97]. However, CVD risk may not be completely linear with increasing blood pressure level. In a cohort of 34 000 Swedish patients with T2DM aged 35 years or older and free of CVD at baseline followed at primary care centres, 6344 (19%) had a first CVD event and 6235 died (18%) between 1999 and 2008 [98]. The associations between annually updated systolic and diastolic blood pressure and risk of major events were U-shaped. The lowest risk of CVD events was observed at a systolic pressure of 135–139 mmHg and a diastolic pressure of 74–76 mmHg, and the lowest mortality risk at 142–150 mmHg and 78–79 mmHg, respectively.

The lowering of blood pressure in hypertensive people with DM is important for preventing CVD events. In DM the recommended level of blood pressure has been debated. In general, measures to lower raised blood pressure should be applied in all patients due to the substantially enhanced cardiovascular risk associated with increasing blood pressure levels. The recent meta-analysis by Bangalore et al. [99] summarized data from available randomized controlled clinical trials examining the effects of intensive lowering of blood pressure in patients with DM, IFG, or IGT. The findings do not support lowering systolic pressure below 135 mmHg, because there were no significant benefits of further lowering of systolic pressure compared with standard blood pressure control strategy on macro- and microvascular (cardiac, renal, and retinal) events. Results for diastolic blood pressure were less clear, since several controlled trials, even placebo-controlled ones, have unequivocally shown benefits from intensive lowering of diastolic pressure below 80 mmHg, in particular in people with isolated systolic hypertension. Microalbuminuria is an important consequence of hypertension in DM. It can be delayed or reduced by efficient antihypertensive drug treatment—but trials in populations with diabetes, including normotensive and hypertensive people, have been unable to demonstrate that reduction in proteinuria is also accompanied by a reduction in CV outcomes [100–102].

The present recommendation in European guidelines for the management of arterial hypertension is to lower blood pressure to 140/85 [40,103] as summarized below:

1. While initiation of blood pressure-lowering treatment in patients with DM whose systolic blood pressure is ≥160 mmHg is mandatory, it is strongly recommended to start drug treatment when it is >140 mmHg.
2. A systolic blood pressure target of <140 mmHg is recommended in patients with DM.
3. The diastolic blood pressure target in patients with DM is recommended to be <85 mmHg.
4. All classes of blood pressure-lowering drugs can be used in patients with DM; RAS blockers should be preferred, especially in the presence of proteinuria or microalbuminuria.
5. It is recommended that choices of drugs for individuals take comorbidities into account.
6. Simultaneous administration of two blockers of the RAS should be avoided in patients with DM.

Blood lipids

T2DM is frequently associated with dyslipidaemia, which is not always recognized if total serum cholesterol alone is measured since low-density lipoprotein cholesterol (LDL-C) may remain within the normal range. Dyslipidaemia in T2DM may often be better characterized by determining high-density lipoprotein cholesterol (HDL-C). Many people with T2DM have the so-called 'atherogenic lipid triad' of high serum triglycerides (TG), low HDL-C, and a preponderance of small, dense LDL-C particles [40]. There is an inverse relationship between serum levels of HDL-C and TG in T2DM patients, with low serum HDL-C levels possibly representing an independent risk factor for CVD [104]. Small, dense LDL-C particles are highly atherogenic as they are more likely to form oxidized LDL and are less readily cleared, and small, dense LDL-C predicts intima–media thickness in people with T2DM and pre-diabetes [105]. Insulin resistance, which is a common phenotype in T2DM, leads to high levels of very low-density lipoprotein (VLDL), which contains a high concentration of TG, resulting in high serum TG and low serum HDL-C. Nevertheless, a recent meta-analysis that estimated the prospective association of LDL-C on CVD risk among people with T2DM found that LDL-C is an independent risk factor for incident CVD and CVD mortality in T2DM [106, 107]. A total of 30 378 participants (aged 35–64 years) were followed for 15 years in the Chinese Multi-provincial Cohort Study; 65.5% of CHD and 70.2% of ischaemic stroke events occurred in participants with low LDL-C [108].

High triglycerides predicted CHD (hazard ratio 1.74, $p = 0.001$), and low HDL-C predicted ischaemic stroke (hazard ratio 1.54, $p = 0.002$) in participants with low LDL-C. DM predicted CHD in participants with high LDL-C (hazard ratio 2.38, $p = 0.005$), but not in those with low LDL-C.

In people with T1DM and good glycaemic control, the lipid profile is different, with normal serum TG and HDL-C within the upper normal range. In a US multicentre study of young people with DM onset at age <20 years, 1973 participants had HbA1c, fasting total cholesterol, LDL-cholesterol, HDL-cholesterol, and TG measured during the follow-up [109]. There were significant trends of higher levels of total cholesterol (TC), LDL-C, TG, and non-HDL-C (but not HDL-C) with higher HbA1c concentrations for both T1DM and T2DM patients. The slopes of increase in TC were 0.20 mmol/L per unit increase in HbA1c for T1DM and 0.21 mmol/L for T2DM. Levels of TC, LDL-C, TG, and non-HDL-C were all significantly higher in patients with T2DM than T1DM, and HDL-C was lower in T2DM. Among T1DM patients with a poor glycaemic control, 35, 27, and 12% had high concentrations of TC (> 5.2 mmol/L), LDL-C (>3.4 mmol/L), and TG (>2.3 mmol/L), respectively. In T2DM patients with a poor glycaemic control, the corresponding percentages for high levels of TC, LDL-C, and TG were 65, 43, and 40%. Thus, glycaemic control and lipid levels are independently associated with both T1DM and T2DM in young people.

Excess weight gain in T1DM patients is associated with sustained increases in central obesity, insulin resistance, dyslipidaemia, and blood pressure, as well as more extensive atherosclerosis during long-term follow-up [110].

Apolipoprotein A and B (ApoA and ApoB) and the ApoB/ApoA ratio have been proposed as CVD risk markers in T2DM, since the LDL particle size does not affect ApoB levels. In the Emerging Risk Factor Collaboration Study [107], based on 68 studies ($n = 302\,430$ participants without a history of CVD), non-HDL-C and ApoB had a similar association with CHD risk both in people with and without DM. An increase of one standard deviation in HDL-C (0.38 mmol/L) was associated with a 22% lower risk of CHD. Estimated risks for non-HDL and ApoB were similar, and so were the risks estimated for HDL-C and ApoA. Thus, non-HDL-C seems to be the most convenient tool for risk assessment in clinical practice.

Substantial evidence exists for the efficacy of statin therapy in the prevention of CVD in T2DM [106,111]. In a meta-analysis of 14 randomized controlled trials (RCTs) including 18 686 people with DM with 3247 major vascular events, a lowering of LDL-C by 1 mmol/L resulted in a 9% reduction in all-cause mortality and a 21% reduction in the incidence of major vascular outcomes. The benefit was similar to that seen in people without DM, and started at a LDL-C level as low as 2.6 mmol/L [106]. In subgroup analysis among 1466 adult patients in these trials with T1DM, the risk reduction was of the order of 20%, i.e. similar to that in patients with T2DM. RCTs indicate that statin therapy has a cardiovascular benefit among patients with T2DM. Recently, statins were reported to increase the risk of DM by 9% [112]. A recent meta-analysis assessed whether statins deteriorate glycaemic control in T2DM using findings from 26 eligible studies with 3232 participants. Statin therapy had no remarkable influence on HbA1c, FPG, body mass index, fasting insulin, or homeostatic model assessed insulin resistance [113].

Trials aimed at increasing HDL-C and decreasing TG have provided controversial results. The largest recent placebo-controlled trials, FIELD (using fenofibrate) [114] and HPS2-THRIVE (using niacin) [115], did not reveal any reduction in CVD events. Thus, drugs that increase HDL-C (other than statins) are not recommended in T2DM patients for the prevention of CVD.

The present European guidelines for the management of diabetes, pre-diabetes, and CVD [40] provides the following recommendations:

1. Statin therapy should be prescribed to patients with T1DM and T2DM at very high risk (documented CVD or one or more additional CVD risk factors and/or target organ damage) with a LDL-C target of <1.8 mmol/L (<70 mg/dl).
2. Statin treatment is recommended in patients with T2DM without further CVD risk factors with a LDL-C target of <2.5 mmol/L (<100 mg/dl).
3. The use of drugs that increase HDL-C to prevent CVD is discouraged.

Further reading

Anselmino M, Malmberg K, Öhrvik J, et al. Evidence-based medication and revascularization: powerful tools in the management of patients with diabetes and coronary artery disease: a report from the Euro Heart Survey on diabetes and the heart. *Eur J Cardiovasc Prev Rehabil* 2008; **15**: 216–23.

Bangalore S, Kumar S, Lobach I. Blood pressure targets in subjects with type 2 diabetes mellitus/impaired fasting glucose: observations from traditional and Bayesian random-effects meta-analyses of randomized trials. *Circulation* 2011; **123**: 2799–810.

Bartnik M, Rydén L, Malmberg K, et al. Oral glucose tolerance test is needed for appropriate classification of glucose regulation in patients with coronary artery disease. A report from the Euro Heart Survey on diabetes and the heart. *Heart* 2007; **93**: 72–7.

Gaede P, Lund-Andersen H, Parving HH, et al. Effect of a multifactorial intervention on mortality in type 2 diabetes. *N Engl J Med* 2008; **358**: 580–91.

Gaede P, Vedel P, Larsen N, et al. Multifactorial intervention and cardiovascular disease in patients with type 2 diabetes. *N Engl J Med* 2003; **348**: 383–93.

International Diabetes Federation. *IDF diabetes atlas*, 5th edn, 2012 update. Brussels: International Diabetes Federation. URL: <http://www.idf.org/diabetesatlas>

Inzucchi SE, Bergenstal RM, Buse JB, et al. Management of hyperglycaemia in type 2 diabetes: a patient-centered approach. Position statement of the American Diabetes Association (ADA) and the European Association for the Study of Diabetes (EASD). *Diabetologia* 2012; **55**: 1577–96.

Kearney PM, Blackwell L, Collins R, et al. Efficacy of cholesterol-lowering therapy in 18,686 people with diabetes in 14 randomised trials of statins: a meta-analysis. *Lancet* 2008; **371**: 117–25.

Knowler WC, Barrett-Connor E, Fowler SE, et al. Reduction in the incidence of type 2 diabetes with lifestyle intervention or metformin. *N Engl J Med* 2002; **346**: 393–403.

Mancia G, Fagard R, Narkiewicz K, et al. 2013 ESH/ESC Guidelines for the management of arterial hypertension: the Task Force for the management of arterial hypertension of the European Society of Hypertension (ESH) and of the European Society of Cardiology (ESC). *J Hypertens* 2013; **31**: 1281–357.

Mann JI, De Leeuw I, Hermansen K, et al. Diabetes and Nutrition Study Group of the European Association: evidence-based nutritional approaches to the treatment and prevention of diabetes mellitus. *Nutr Metab Cardiovasc Dis* 2004; **14**: 373–94.

Perk J, De Backer G, Golke H, et al. European guidelines on cardiovascular disease prevention in clinical practice (version 2012). *Eur Heart J* 2012; **33**: 1635–701.

Rydén L, Grant PJ, Anker SD, et al. European guidelines on diabetes, pre-diabetes, and cardiovascular disease (developed in collaboration with EASD). *Eur Heart J* 2013; **34**: 3035–87.

Tuomilehto J, Lindstrom J, Eriksson JG, et al. Prevention of type 2 diabetes mellitus by changes in lifestyle among subjects with impaired glucose tolerance. *N Engl J Med* 2001; **344**: 1343–50.

Turnbull FM, Abraira C, Anderson RJ, et al. Intensive glucose control and macrovascular outcomes in type 2 diabetes. *Diabetologia* 2009; **52**: 2288–98.

World Health Organization. *Abbreviated report of a WHO consultation. Use of glycated hemoglobin (HbA1c) in the diagnosis of diabetes mellitus*, 2011. URL: <http://www.who.int/diabetes/publications/diagnosis_diabetes2011/en/index.html>

References

1 International Diabetes Federation. *IDF diabetes atlas*, 5th edn, 2012 update. Brussels: International Diabetes Federation. URL: <http://www.idf.org/diabetesatlas>

2 Morrish NJ, Wang SL, Stevens LK, et al. Mortality and causes of death in the WHO multinational study of vascular disease in diabetes. *Diabetologia* 2001; **44**: S14–S21.

3 Perk J, De Backer G, Golke H, et al. European guidelines on cardiovascular disease prevention in clinical practice (version 2012). *Eur Heart J* 2012; **33**: 1635–701.

4 Stevens RJ, Kothari V, Adler AI, et al. The UKPDS risk engine: a model for the risk of coronary heart disease in type II diabetes (UKPDS 56). *Clin Sci* 2001; **101**: 671–9.

5 Cederholm J, Eeg-Olofsson K, Eliasson B, et al. Risk prediction of cardiovascular disease in type 2 diabetes: a risk equation from the Swedish national diabetes register. *Diabetes Care* 2008; **31**: 2038–43.

6 Niskanen L, Turpeinen A, Penttilä I, et al. Hyperglycemia and compositional lipoprotein abnormalities as predictors of cardiovascular mortality in type 2 diabetes: a 5-year follow-up from the time of diagnosis. *Diabetes Care* 1998; **21**: 1861–9.

7 World Health Organization Consultation. *Definition, diagnosis and classification of diabetes mellitus and its complications. Part 1: diagnosis and classification of diabetes mellitus*, 1999. Geneva: World Health Organization. URL: <http://whqlibdoc.who.int/hq/1999/who_ncd_ncs_99.2.pdf>

8 World Health Organization Consultation. *Definition and diagnosis of diabetes and intermediate hyperglycaemia*, 2006. URL: <http://www.who.int/diabetes/publications/Definition%20and%20diagnosis%20of%20diabetes_new.pdf>

9 Report of the Expert Committee on the Diagnosis and Classification of Diabetes Mellitus. *Diabetes Care* 1997; **20**: 1183–97.

10 Genuth S, Alberti KG, Bennett P, et al. Follow-up report on the diagnosis of diabetes mellitus. *Diabetes Care* 2003; **26**: 3160–7.

11 American Diabetes Association. Diagnosis and classification of diabetes mellitus. *Diabetes Care* 2012; **35** (Suppl. 1): S64–S71.

12 World Health Organization. *Abbreviated report of a WHO consultation. Use of glycated hemoglobin (HbA1c) in the diagnosis of diabetes mellitus*, 2011. URL: <http://www.who.int/diabetes/publications/diagnosis_diabetes2011/en/index.html>

13 Costa B, Barrio F, Cabre JJ, et al. Shifting from glucose diagnostic criteria to the new HbA criteria would have a profound impact on prevalence of diabetes among a high-risk Spanish population. *Diabet Med* 2011; **28**: 1234–7.

14 Pajunen P, Peltonen M, Eriksson JG, et al. HbA in diagnosing and predicting type 2 diabetes in impaired glucose tolerance: the Finnish Diabetes Prevention Study. *Diabet Med* 2011; **28**: 36–42.

15 Laakso M, Pyorala K. Age of onset and type of diabetes. *Diabetes Care* 1985; **8**: 114–7.

16 Pozzilli P, Di Mario U. Autoimmune diabetes not requiring insulin at diagnosis (latent autoimmune diabetes of the adult): definition, characterization and potential prevention. *Diabetes Care* 2001; **24**: 1460–7.

17 Gottsater A, Landin-Olsson M, Fernlund P, et al. Beta-cell function in relation to islet cell antibodies during the first 3 yr after clinical diagnosis of diabetes in type II diabetic patients. *Diabetes Care* 1993; **16**: 902–10.

18 Tuomilehto J, Zimmet P, Mackay IR, et al. Antibodies to glutamic acid decarboxylase as predictors of insulin-dependent diabetes mellitus before clinical onset of disease. *Lancet* 1994; **343**: 1383–5.

19 WHO DIAMOND Project. Incidence and trends of childhood Type 1 diabetes worldwide 1990-99. *Diabet Med* 2006; **23**: 857–66.

20 Ma RC, Chan JC. Type 2 diabetes in East Asians: similarities and differences with populations in Europe and the United States. *Ann N Y Acad Sci* 2013; **1281**: 64–91.

21 Morris AP, Voight BF, Teslovich TM, et al. Large-scale association analysis provides insights into the genetic architecture and pathophysiology of type 2 diabetes. *Nat Genet* 2012; **44**: 981–90.

22 Kahn SE. The importance of beta-cell failure in the development and progression of type 2 diabetes. *J Clin Endocrinol Metabol* 2001; **86**: 4047–58.

23 Ahren B, Pacini G. Age-related reduction in glucose elimination is accompanied by reduced glucose effectiveness and increased hepatic insulin extraction in man. *J Clin Endocrinol Metabol* 1998; **83**: 3350–6.

24 Mari A, Tura A, Natali A, et al. Impaired beta cell glucose sensitivity rather than inadequate compensation for insulin resistance is the dominant defect in glucose intolerance. *Diabetologia* 2010; **53**: 749–56.

25 Weyer C, Bogardus C, Pratley RE. Metabolic characteristics of individuals with impaired fasting glucose and/or impaired glucose tolerance. *Diabetes* 1999; **48**: 2197–203.

26 Abdul-Ghani MA, Jenkinson CP, Richardson DK, et al. Insulin secretion and action in subjects with impaired fasting glucose and impaired glucose tolerance—results from the Veterans Administration genetic epidemiology study. *Diabetes* 2006; **55**: 1430–5.

27 Hare MJ, Shaw JE, Zimmet PZ. Current controversies in the use of haemoglobin A1c. *J Intern Med* 2012; **271**: 227–36.

28 DECODE Study Group. Age- and sex-specific prevalences of diabetes and impaired glucose regulation in 13 European cohorts. *Diabetes Care* 2003; **26**: 61–9.

29 Harris MI, Klein R, Welborn TA, et al. Onset of NIDDM occurs at least 4-7yr before clinical diagnosis. *Diabetes Care* 1992; **15**: 815–19.

30 Satman I, Omer B, Tutuncu Y, et al. Twelve-year trends in the prevalence and risk factors of diabetes and prediabetes in Turkish adults. *Eur J Epidemiol* 2013; **28**: 169–80.

31 Xu Y, Wang L, He J, et al. Prevalence and control of diabetes in Chinese adults. *J Am Med Assoc* 2013; **310**: 948–58.

32 Gu D, Reynolds K, Duan X, et al. Prevalence of diabetes and impaired fasting glucose in the Chinese adult population. *Diabetologia* 2003; **46**: 1190–8.

33 Saaristo TE, Barengo NC, Korpi-Hyovalti E, et al. High prevalence of obesity, central obesity and abnormal glucose tolerance in the middle-aged Finnish population. *BMC Publ Health* 2008; **8**: 423.

34 DECODE Study Group. Glucose tolerance and mortality: comparison of WHO and American Diabetes Association diagnostic criteria. *Lancet* 1999; **354**: 617–21.

35 DECODE Study Group. Glucose tolerance and cardiovascular mortality. *Arch Intern Med* 2001; **161**: 397–404.

36 DECODE Study Group. Is the current definition for diabetes relevant to mortality risk from all causes and cardiovascular and noncardiovascular diseases? *Diabetes Care* 2003; **26**: 688–96.

37 Levitan EB, Song Y, Ford ES, et al. Is nondiabetic hyperglycemia a risk factor for cardiovascular disease? A meta-analysis of prospective studies. *Arch Intern Med* 2004; **164**: 2147–55.

38 Esposito K, Giugliano D, Nappo F, et al. Regression of carotid atherosclerosis by control of postprandial hyperglycemia in type 2 diabetes mellitus. *Circulation* 2004; **110**: 214–19.

39 Cavalot F, Petrelli A, Traversa M, et al. Postprandial blood glucose is a stronger predictor of cardiovascular events than fasting blood glucose in type 2 diabetes mellitus, particularly in women: lessons from the San Luigi Gonzaga Diabetes Study. *J Clin Endocrinol Metab* 2006; **91**: 813–19.

40 Rydén L, Grant PJ, Anker SD, et al. European guidelines on diabetes, pre-diabetes, and cardiovascular disease (developed in collaboration with EASD). *Eur Heart J* 2013; **34**: 3035–87.

41 Al Arouj M, Cockram C, Davidson J, et al. *Guideline for management of postmeal glucose*, 2007. Brussels: International Diabetes Federation.

42 Ning F, Tuomilehto J, Pyorala K, et al. Cardiovascular disease mortality in Europeans in relation to fasting and 2-h plasma glucose levels within a normoglycemic range. *Diabetes Care* 2010; **33**: 2211–16.

43 Monnier L. Is postprandial glucose a neglected cardiovascular risk factor in type 2 diabetes? *Eur J Clin Invest* 2000; **30** (Suppl. 2): 3–11.

44 Nakagami T, Qiao Q, Tuomilehto J, et al. Screen-detected diabetes, hypertension and hypercholesterolemia as predictors of cardiovascular mortality in five populations of Asian origin: the DECODA study. *Eur J Cardiovasc Prev Rehabil* 2006; **13**: 555–61.

45 Engelgau MM, Colagiuri S, Ramachandran A, et al. Prevention of type 2 diabetes: issues and strategies for identifying persons for interventions. *Diabetes Technol Ther* 2004; **6**: 874–82.

46 Simmons RK, Echouffo-Tcheugui JB, Sharp SJ, et al. Screening for type 2 diabetes and population mortality over 10 years (ADDITION-Cambridge): a cluster-randomised controlled trial. *Lancet* 2012; **380**: 1741–8.

47 Waugh N, Scotland G, McNamee P, et al. Screening for type 2 diabetes: literature review and economic modeling. *Health Technol Assess* 2007; **11**: 1–125.

48 Tuomilehto J, Lindstrom J, Eriksson JG, et al. Prevention of type 2 diabetes mellitus by changes in lifestyle among subjects with impaired glucose tolerance. *N Engl J Med* 2001; **344**: 1343–50.

49 Knowler WC, Barrett-Connor E, Fowler SE, et al. Reduction in the incidence of type 2 diabetes with lifestyle intervention or metformin. *N Engl J Med* 2002; **346**: 393–403.

50 Roumen C, Corpeleijn E, Feskens EJ, et al. Impact of 3-year lifestyle intervention on postprandial glucose metabolism: the SLIM study. *Diabet Med* 2008; **25**: 597–605.

51 Li G, Zhang P, Wang J, et al. The long-term effect of lifestyle interventions to prevent diabetes in the China Da Qing Diabetes Prevention Study: a 20-year follow-up study. *Lancet* 2008; **371**: 1783–9.

52 Penn L, White M, Oldroyd J, et al. Prevention of type 2 diabetes in adults with impaired glucose tolerance: the European Diabetes Prevention RCT in Newcastle upon Tyne, UK. *BMC Publ Health* 2009; **9**: 342.

53 Paulweber B, Valensi P, Lindstrom J, et al. A European evidence-based guideline for the prevention of type 2 diabetes. *Horm Metab Res* 2010; **42** (Suppl. 1): S3–36.

54 Metzger BE, Gabbe SG, Persson B, et al. International association of diabetes and pregnancy study groups recommendations on the diagnosis and classification of hyperglycemia in pregnancy. *Diabetes Care* 2010; **33**: 676–82.

55 Abbasi A, Peelen LM, Corpeleijn E, et al. Prediction models for risk of developing type 2 diabetes: systematic literature search and independent external validation study. *Br Med J* 2012; **345**: e5900.

56 Schwarz PEH, Lindström J, Kissimova-Skarbek K, et al. The European Perspective of Type2 Diabetes Prevention: Diabetes in Europe-Prevention Using Lifestyle, Physical Activity and Nutritional Intervention (DE-PLAN) Project. *Exp Clin Endocrinol Diabetes* 2008; **116**: 167–72.

57 UK Prospective Diabetes Study (UKPDS) Group. Intensive blood-glucose control with sulphonylureas or insulin compared with conventional treatment and risk of complications in patients with type 2 diabetes. (UKPDS 33). *Lancet* 1998; **352**: 837–53.

58 Sarwar N, Gao P, Seshasai SR, et al. Diabetes mellitus, fasting blood glucose concentration, and risk of vascular disease: a collaborative meta-analysis of 102 prospective studies. *Lancet* 2010; **375**: 2215–22.

59 Brownlee M. The pathophysiology of diabetic complications: a unifying mechanism. *Diabetes* 2005; **54**: 1615–25.

60 Norhammar A, Tenerz Å, Nilsson G, et al. Glucose metabolism in patients with acute myocardial infarction and no previous diagnosis of diabetes mellitus. A prospective study. *Lancet* 2002; **359**: 2140–4.

61 Bartnik M, Rydén L, Ferrari R, et al. The prevalence of abnormal glucose regulation in patients with coronary artery disease across Europe. *Eur Heart J* 2004; **25**: 1880–90.

62 Hu DY, Pan CY, Yu JM; China Heart Survey Group. The relationship between coronary artery disease and abnormal glucose regulation in China: the China Heart Survey. *Eur Heart J* 2006; **27**: 2573–9.

63 Bartnik M, Rydén L, Malmberg K, et al. Oral glucose tolerance test is needed for appropriate classification of glucose regulation in patients with coronary artery disease. A report from the Euro Heart Survey on diabetes and the heart. *Heart* 2007; **93**: 72–7.

64 Ramachandran A, Chamukuttan S, Immaneni S, et al. High incidence of glucose intolerance in Asian-Indian subjects with acute coronary syndrome. *Diabetes Care* 2005; **28**: 2492–6.
65 Matz K, Keresztes K, Tatschl C, et al. Disorders of glucose metabolism in acute stroke patients: an underrecognized problem. *Diabetes Care* 2006; **29**: 792–7.
66 Lenzén M, Rydén L, Öhrvik J, et al. Diabetes known or newly detected, but not impaired glucose regulation has a negative influence on 1-years outcome in patients with coronary artery disease: a report from the Euro Heart Survey on diabetes and the heart. *Eur Heart J* 2006; **27**: 2969–74.
67 Khaw KT, Wareham N, Bingham S, et al. Association of hemoglobin A1c with cardiovascular disease and mortality in adults: the European prospective investigation into cancer in Norfolk. *Ann Intern Med* 2004; **141**: 413–20.
68 Selvin E, Steffes MW, Zhu H, et al. Glycated hemoglobin, diabetes, and cardiovascular risk in nondiabetic adults. *N Engl J Med* 2010; **362**: 800–11.
69 Santos-Oliveira R, Purdy C, da Silva MP, et al. Haemoglobin A1c levels and subsequent cardiovascular disease in persons without diabetes: a meta-analysis of prospective cohorts. *Diabetologia* 2011; **54**: 1327–34.
70 Qiao Q, Dekker JM, de Vegt F, et al. Two prospective studies found that elevated 2-hr glucose predicted male mortality independent of fasting glucose and HbA1c. *J Clin Epidemiol* 2004; **57**: 590–6.
71 Meigs JB, Nathan DM, D'Agostino RB, Sr, et al. Fasting and postchallenge glycemia and cardiovascular disease risk: the Framingham Offspring Study. *Diabetes Care* 2002; **25**: 1845–50.
72 Hage C, Lundman P, Rydén L, et al. Fasting glucose, HbA1c or oral glucose tolerance testing for the detection of glucose abnormalities in patients with acute coronary syndromes. *Eur J Prev Cardiol* 2013; **20**: 549–54.
73 de Mulder M, Oemrawsingh RM, Stam F, et al. Comparison of diagnostic criteria to detect undiagnosed diabetes in hyperglycaemic patients with acute coronary syndrome. *Heart* 2012; **98**: 37–41.
74 Doerr R, Hoffmann U, Otter W, et al. Oral glucose tolerance test and HbA1c for diagnosis of diabetes in patients undergoing coronary angiography the Silent Diabetes Study. *Diabetologia* 2011; **54**: 2923–30.
75 Bonora E, Tuomilehto J. The pros and cons of diagnosing diabetes with A1C. *Diabetes Care* 2011; **34** (Suppl. 2): S184–S190.
76 Eriksson KF, Lindgärde F. No excess 12-year mortality in men with impaired glucose tolerance who participated in the Malmö Preventive Trial with diet and exercise. *Diabetologia* 1998; **41**: 1010–16.
77 Gaede P, Vedel P, Larsen N, et al. Multifactorial intervention and cardiovascular disease in patients with type 2 diabetes. *N Engl J Med* 2003; **348**: 383–93.
78 Gaede P, Lund-Andersen H, Parving HH, et al. Effect of a multifactorial intervention on mortality in type 2 diabetes. *N Engl J Med* 2008; **358**: 580–91.
79 Gaede P, Valentine WJ, Palmer AJ, et al. Cost-effectiveness of intensified versus conventional multifactorial intervention in type 2 diabetes: results and projections from the Steno-2 study. *Diabetes Care* 2008; **31**: 1510–15.
80 Anselmino M, Malmberg K, Öhrvik J, et al. Evidence-based medication and revascularization: powerful tools in the management of patients with diabetes and coronary artery disease: a report from the Euro Heart Survey on diabetes and the heart. *Eur J Cardiovasc Prev Rehabil* 2008; **15**: 216–23.
81 Mann JI, De Leeuw I, Hermansen K, et al. Diabetes and Nutrition Study Group of the European Association: evidence-based nutritional approaches to the treatment and prevention of diabetes mellitus. *Nutr Metab Cardiovasc Dis* 2004; **14**: 373–94.
82 Sigal RJ, Kenny GP, Boule NG, et al. Effects of aerobic training, resistance training, or both on glycemic control in type 2 diabetes: a randomized trial. *Ann Intern Med* 2007; **147**: 357–69.
83 Diabetes Control and Complications Trial Group. The absence of a glycemic threshold for the development of long-term complications: the perspective of the Diabetes Control and Complications Trial. *Diabetes* 1996; **45**: 1289–98.
84 Stratton IM, Adler AI, Neil HA, et al. Association of glycaemia with macrovascular and microvascular complications of type 2 diabetes (UKPDS 35): prospective observational study. *Br Med J* 2000; **321**: 405–12.
85 Inzucchi SE, Bergenstal RM, Buse JB, et al. Management of hyperglycaemia in type 2 diabetes: a patient-centered approach. Position statement of the American Diabetes Association (ADA) and the European Association for the Study of Diabetes (EASD). *Diabetologia* 2012; **55**: 1577–96.
86 Turnbull FM, Abraira C, Anderson RJ, et al. Intensive glucose control and macrovascular outcomes in type 2 diabetes. *Diabetologia* 2009; **52**: 2288–98.
87 Cleary PA, Orchard TJ, Genuth S, et al. The effect of intensive glycemic treatment on coronary artery calcification in type 1 diabetic participants of the Diabetes Control and Complications Trial/Epidemiology of Diabetes Interventions and Complications (DCCT/EDIC) Study. *Diabetes* 2006; **55**: 3556–65.
88 Soedamah-Muthu SS, Colhoun HM, Abrahamian H, et al. Trends in hypertension management in Type I diabetes across Europe, 1989/1990-1997/1999. *Diabetologia* 2002; **45**: 1362–71.
89 Colosia AD, Palencia R, Khan S. Prevalence of hypertension and obesity in patients with type 2 diabetes mellitus in observational studies: a systematic literature review. *Diabetes Metab Syndr Obes* 2013; **6**: 327–38.
90 Redon J, Cifkova R, Laurent S, et al. Mechanisms of hypertension in the cardiometabolic syndrome. *J Hypertens* 2009; **27**: 441–51.
91 Imperatore G, Cadwell BL, Geiss L, et al. Thirty-year trends in cardiovascular risk factor levels among US adults with diabetes: National Health and Nutrition Examination Surveys, 1971–2000. *Am J Epidemiol* 2004; **160**: 531–9.
92 Saydah SH, Fradkin J, Cowie CC. Poor control of risk factors for vascular disease among adults with previously diagnosed diabetes. *J Am Med Assoc* 2004; **291**: 335–42.
93 Cheung BMY, Ong KL, Cherny SS, et al. Diabetes prevalence and therapeutic target achievement in the United States, 1999 to 2006. *Am J Med* 2009; **122**: 443–53.
94 Wang J, Geiss LS, Cheng YJ, et al. Long-term and recent progress in blood pressure levels among U.S. adults with diagnosed diabetes, 1988–2008. *Diabetes Care* 2011; **34**: 1579–81.
95 Nilsson PM, Cederholm J, Zethelius B, et al. Trends in blood pressure control in patients with type 2 diabetes—data from the Swedish National Diabetes Register (NDR). *Blood Press* 2011; **20**: 348–54.
96 Barengo NC, Tuomilehto JO. Blood pressure treatment target in patients with diabetes mellitus—current evidence. *Ann Med* 2012; **44** (Suppl. 1): S36–S42.
97 Mogensen CE. New treatment guidelines for a patient with diabetes and hypertension. *J Hypertens* 2003; **21** (Suppl.): S25–S30.
98 Sundström J, Sheikhi R, Östgren CJ, et al. Blood pressure levels and risk of cardiovascular events and mortality in type-2 diabetes: cohort study of 34 009 primary care patients. *J Hypertens* 2013; **31**: 1603–10.
99 Bangalore S, Kumar S, Lobach I. Blood pressure targets in subjects with type 2 diabetes mellitus/impaired fasting glucose: observations from traditional and Bayesian random-effects meta-analyses of randomized trials. *Circulation* 2011; **123**: 2799–810.
100 Schrier RW, Estacio RO, Esler A. Effects of aggressive blood pressure control in normotensive type 2 diabetic patients on albuminuria, retinopathy and strokes. *Kidney Int* 2002; **61**: 1086–97.

101 ADVANCE Collaborative Group. Effects of a fixed combination of perindopril and indapamide on macrovascular and microvascular outcomes in patients with type 2 diabetes mellitus (the ADVANCE trial): a randomised controlled trial. *Lancet* 2007; **370**: 829–40.

102 Haller H, Ito S, Izzo JL Jr, et al.: ROADMAP Trial Investigators. Olmesartan for the delay or prevention of microalbuminuria in type 2 diabetes. *N Engl J Med* 2011; **364**: 907–17.

103 Mancia G, Fagard R, Narkiewicz K, et al. 2013 ESH/ESC guidelines for the management of arterial hypertension: the Task Force for the management of arterial hypertension of the European Society of Hypertension (ESH) and of the European Society of Cardiology (ESC). *J Hypertens* 2013; **31**: 1281–357.

104 Barter P, Gotto AM, LaRosa JC, et al. HDL cholesterol, very low levels of LDL cholesterol, and cardiovascular events. *N Engl J Med* 2007; **357**: 1301–10.

105 Gerber PA, Thalhammer C, Schmied C, et al. Small, dense LDL particles predict changes in intima media thickness and insulin resistance in men with type 2 diabetes and prediabetes—a prospective cohort study. *PLoS One* 2013; **8**: e72763.

106 Kearney PM, Blackwell L, Collins R, et al. Efficacy of cholesterol-lowering therapy in 18,686 people with diabetes in 14 randomised trials of statins: a meta-analysis. *Lancet* 2008; **371**: 117–25.

107 Emerging Risk Factors Collaboration. Major lipids, apolipoproteins, and risk of vascular disease. *J Am Med Assoc* 2009; **302**: 1993–2000.

108 Liu J, Wang W, Wang M, et al. Impact of diabetes, high triglycerides and low HDL cholesterol on risk for ischemic cardiovascular disease varies by LDL cholesterol level: a 15-year follow-up of the Chinese Multi-provincial Cohort Study. *Diabetes Res Clin Pract* 2012; **96**: 217–24.

109 Guy J, Ogden L, Wadwa RP, et al. Lipid and lipoprotein profiles in youth with and without type 1 diabetes: the SEARCH for Diabetes in Youth case-control study. *Diabetes Care* 2009; **32**: 416–20.

110 Purnell JQ, Zinman B, Brunzell JD; DCCT/EDIC Research Group. The effect of excess weight gain with intensive diabetes mellitus treatment on cardiovascular disease risk factors and atherosclerosis in type 1 diabetes mellitus: results from the Diabetes Control and Complications Trial/Epidemiology of Diabetes Interventions and Complications Study (DCCT/EDIC) study. *Circulation* 2013; **127**: 180–7.

111 Chen YH, Feng B, Chen ZW. Statins for primary prevention of cardiovascular and cerebrovascular events in diabetic patients without established cardiovascular diseases: a meta-analysis. *Exp Clin Endocrinol Diabetes* 2012; **120**: 116–20.

112 Sattar N, Preiss D, Murray HM, et al. Statins and risk of incident diabetes: a collaborative meta-analysis of randomised statin trials. *Lancet* 2010; **375**: 735–42.

113 Zhou Y, Yuan Y, Cai RR, et al. Statin therapy on glycaemic control in type 2 diabetes: a meta-analysis. *Expert Opin Pharmacother* 2013; **14**: 1575–84.

114 Keech A, Simes RJ, Barter P, et al. Effects of long-term fenofibrate therapy on cardiovascular events in 9795 people with type 2 diabetes mellitus (the FIELD study): randomised controlled trial. *Lancet* 2005; **366**: 1849–61.

115 HPS2-THRIVE Collaborative Group. Landray MJ, Haynes R, Hopewell JC, Parish S, Aung T, Tomson J, Wallendszus K, Craig M, Jiang L, Collins R, Armitage J. Effects of extended-release niacin with laropiprant in high-risk patients. *N Engl J Med* 2014; **371**: 203–12.

CHAPTER 17

Coagulation and thrombosis

Kurt Huber and Joao Morais

Contents

Summary

Antithrombotic therapy consisting of antiplatelet agents and/or anticoagulants is an important means of avoiding atherothrombotic complications after acute cardiovascular events such as myocardial infarction, stroke, and peripheral artery obstructions, but also after mechanical interventions (balloon dilatation and/or stent implantation) and bypass surgery in elective patients. This is known as secondary prevention. Primary prevention by antithrombotics usually refers to the prevention of stroke in patients with atrial fibrillation and those with an increased risk for stroke or peripheral thromboembolic events by the use of anticoagulants. In certain situations a combination of anticoagulants and antiplatelet agents is mandatory. The flipside of the coin, however, is bleeding hazards. This chapter explains the pathophysiological background for coagulation and thrombosis, reports on the epidemiology of antithrombotic treatment, and describes the efficacy and safety of preventive antithrombotic measures in different cardiovascular indications including coronary artery disease (stable disease and acute coronary syndrome), patients after coronary bypass grafting, as well as in special situations, i.e. chronic heart failure, artificial valves, and atrial fibrillation (with the simultaneous need for dual antiplatelet therapy). A short paragraph summarizes the current discussion about skipping aspirin in order to reduce the rate and severity of bleeding events.

Clinical case

A76-year-old male patient develops paroxysmal atrial fibrillation 3 months after implantation of a drug-eluting stent in the proximal left anterior descending coronary artery. Stent implantation was performed in a stable clinical situation due to the patient's exercise-inducible ischaemia. Accordingly, the patient is under dual antiplatelet therapy with aspirin (100 mg/day) and clopidogrel (75 mg/day). In addition, he receives a statin (atorvastatin 40 mg/day; with this treatment he had a recent low-density lipoprotein cholesterol measurement of 65 mg/dl), as well as an angiotensin-converting enzyme inhibitor (enalapril 10 mg twice a day). His blood pressure is well controlled and mostly (with a few exceptions) in the normal range. Besides recurrent palpitations related to atrial fibrillation he has no complaints, particularly no chest pain or dyspnoea. His CHADS-VASc score is 4. What is your antithrombotic strategy at this point?

Introduction

Arterial thrombosis is initiated by two main mechanisms, endothelial erosion or plaque rupture; endothelial erosion accounts for about 25% of all cases of fatal coronary thrombosis while plaque rupture causes approximately 75% of cases of major coronary thrombosis. Both mechanisms result in the exposure of thrombogenic material, for example collagen and tissue factor (TF), to the circulation, leading to initial thrombin formation and consecutive activation and aggregation of platelets accompanied by the simultaneous release of vasoactive substances. As a consequence thrombus formation and vasoconstriction occur with myocardial ischaemia and acute coronary syndrome (ACS) as sequelae [1].

Coagulation and thrombus formation are regulated in three overlapping phases, namely initiation, amplification, and propagation [2,3] whereby the process starts on cells exposing TF and continues on the surfaces of activated platelets (➲ Fig. 17.1). Accordingly, both anticoagulants and antiplatelet agents play an important role in the prevention of atherothrombotic cardiovascular events.

Epidemiology of antithrombotic treatment in coronary artery disease

Population-based surveys conducted around the year 2000 in Europe showed that the majority of patients presenting with ACS receive aspirin during hospital admission, and in addition either unfractionated heparin (UFH) or a low-molecular-weight heparin (LMWH) (in similar proportions) [4,5]. The frequency of use of heparin varies little according to the presence of ST elevation on admission or by final diagnosis (Q-wave myocardial infarction, non-Q-wave myocardial infarction, or unstable angina), but there is considerable variation in usage between different European countries. At hospital discharge, most patients are treated with an antithrombotic agent; the majority with aspirin, but warfarin and LMWH have also occasionally been used [5].

In the most recent study, the EUROASPIRE-II study published in 2001, treatment of patients who had undergone a coronary procedure (coronary bypass surgery or percutaneous coronary intervention, PCI) or who had been hospitalized with acute myocardial infarction (MI) or coronary ischaemia, was investigated [6]. On admission, around half the patients were already taking an antiplatelet agent and only a few per cent an oral anticoagulant. On discharge, the majority of patients were prescribed an antiplatelet treatment strategy and about 12% an anticoagulant regimen. Again, there was evidence of dissimilarities in the frequency and type of anticoagulant prescribed in different European countries.

Based on recent guidelines it is expected that in-hospital treatment strategies might change with implementation of recommended anticoagulants such as fondaparinux [recommended in non-ST-segment elevation MI (NSTEMI) ACS patients] and bivalirudin (for all ACS patients, NSTEMI ACS and STEMI alike), although the recommendation for the latter has been reduced for the STEMI cohort in the recent myocardial revascularization guidelines [7]. In addition, oral anticoagulants as an 'add-on' to dual antiplatelet therapy (DAPT) might gain more acceptance in secondary prevention on the basis of the results of the ATLAS-2 trial [8] (see 'Triple therapy in secondary prevention after ACS').

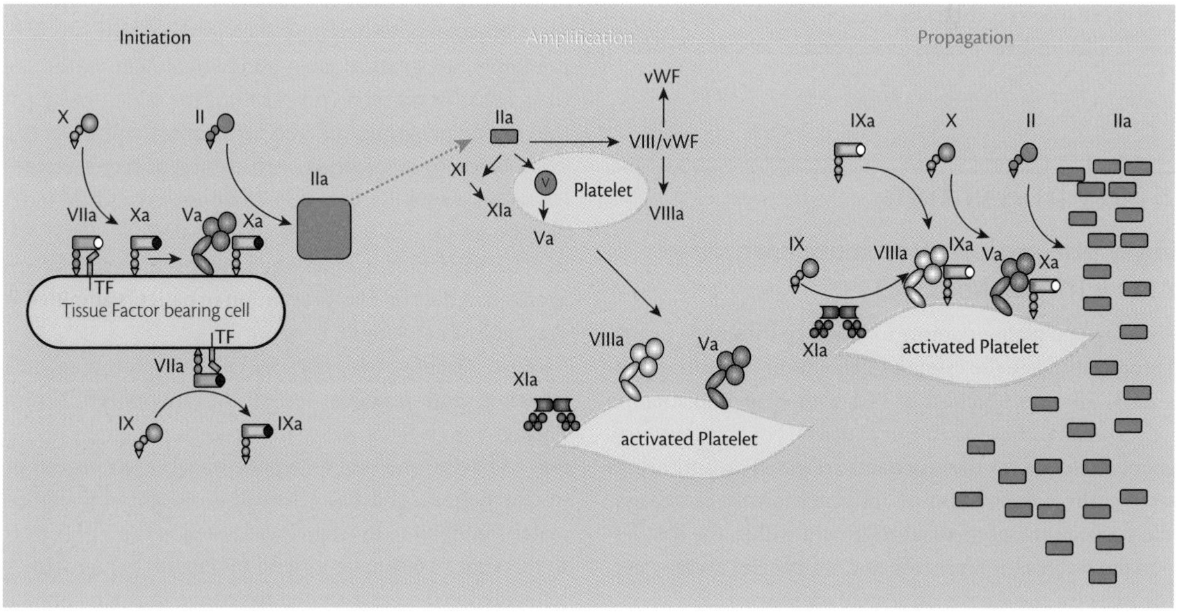

Fig. 17.1 Cell-based model of coagulation.
Adapted from Monroe et al. *Arterioscler Thromb Vasc Biol*, 2002; **22**: 1381–1389.

Primary prevention

Primary prevention of coronary heart disease with warfarin, which during testing had a mean low international normalized ratio (INR) of 1.5 and led to reduced risk of fatal myocardial infarction with an acceptable bleeding risk, has never been part of routine management.

Earlier investigations reported a benefit of acetylsalicylic acid (ASA, aspirin) in primary prevention, but more recent publications have questioned these results [9]. The JPAD (Japanese Primary Prevention of Atherosclerosis with Aspirin for Diabetes) trial showed that low-dose aspirin in primary prevention did not significantly reduce the risk of cardiovascular events while the risk of haemorrhagic stroke and severe gastrointestinal bleeds was similar between the aspirin and non-aspirin treated groups [10]. Furthermore, a huge randomized trial including a general population of roughly 29 000 patients with a low ankle–brachial index showed that primary prevention with aspirin did not significantly reduce vascular events [11]. Finally, the POPADAD (Prevention Of Progression of Arterial Disease And Diabetes) trial did not show a benefit of the use of aspirin or antioxidants in primary prevention of cardiovascular events and mortality in people with diabetes [12]. In the meta-analysis of the Antiplatelet Trialists' Collaboration (ATC), aspirin treatment gave a 12% proportional reduction in serious vascular events per year (0.51% aspirin versus 0.57% control, $p = 0.0001$), which was mainly due to the reduction in non-fatal MIs. However, vascular mortality was not significantly reduced by aspirin treatment, while major gastrointestinal and extracranial bleeds increased significantly (0.10% versus 0.07% per year, $p < 0.0001$) leading to no net clinical benefit for aspirin in primary prevention when major bleeding events were also considered in the risk/benefit assessment [13]. Moreover, when used as primary prevention aspirin failed to reduce the risk of MI or death from cardiovascular causes in healthy women [14].

Based on these more recent trials, the role of aspirin in primary prevention is diminished by its unacceptable efficacy-to-harm ratio.

Secondary prevention

Secondary prevention after acute coronary syndrome with/without PCI

Plaque fissuring and plaque rupture followed by thrombus formation and propagation are the essential elements in the pathophysiology of ACS. The introduction of PCI with stent implantation inside the vessel amplifies the role of platelets. For this reason all management strategies for these patients are based on antithrombotic therapy. The combination of antiplatelets with anticoagulants is the cornerstone of medical treatment within the first few hours up to the stabilization process, and antiplatelet therapy persists as adequate for the long-term secondary process.

Aspirin was the first single oral agent used for the purpose of secondary prevention in this setting in the mid 1980s. Cairns et al. [15] showed the efficacy of aspirin (325 mg four times a day) in a small group of 555 patients classified as having unstable angina. Managed for a mean follow-up of 18 months, 8.6% of the group of patients treated with aspirin suffered cardiac death or acute MI against 17% in the comparator group, representing a risk reduction of 51% ($p = 0.008$). Since then aspirin has become part of all therapeutic regimens and has a major role in all scenarios involving platelets [16].

Antiplatelet therapy was reinvigorated in 2001 with the introduction of the concept of DAPT. The membrane receptor P2Y12, which takes part in the mechanism of platelet activation mediated by ADP, was recognized as a special target for antiplatelets. The combination of drugs acting through both mechanisms (i.e. cyclooxygenase inhibition by aspirin plus ADP receptor inhibition) allowed higher levels of platelet inhibition to be achieved. Ticlopidine was the first ADP receptor inhibitor to be used in combination with aspirin in patients treated with percutaneous coronary angioplasty [17]. Clopidogrel was the second P2Y12 receptor antagonist; it is closely related to ticlopidine but has the great advantage of having been tested in large randomized clinical trials [18].

The concept of DAPT was expanded to the medical management of patients with ACS in the CURE (Clopidogrel in Unstable angina to prevent Recurrent Events) trial [19]: in this trial 12 562 patients who had presented within 24 hours after the onset of symptoms were randomly assigned to receive clopidogrel (300 mg immediately, followed by 75 mg once a day) (6259 patients) or placebo (6303 patients) in addition to aspirin for 3–12 months. The first primary outcome—a composite of death from cardiovascular causes, non-fatal MI, or stroke—occurred in 9.3% of patients in the clopidogrel group and in 11.4% in the placebo group [relative risk (RR) with clopidogrel compared with placebo 0.80, 95% CI 0.72–0.90, $p < 0.001$].

A subgroup analysis named PCI-CURE assessed the efficacy of clopidogrel in patients managed with PCI [20]. A subgroup of 2658 patients undergoing PCI in the CURE study had been randomly assigned double-blind treatment with clopidogrel ($n = 1313$) or placebo ($n = 1345$). Fifty-nine (4.5%) patients in the clopidogrel group suffered the primary end-point (a composite of cardiovascular death, MI, or urgent target-vessel revascularization within 30 days of PCI) compared with 86 (6.4%) in the placebo group (RR 0.70, 95% CI 0.50–0.97, $p = 0.03$). CURE and PCI-CURE definitely established the role of DAPT for acute management and secondary prevention in patients admitted with ACS managed or not with PCI.

More recently two new P2Y12 receptor antagonists were launched and properly tested in randomized clinical trials. Prasugrel is an agent quite similar to clopidogrel with the advantage of having one step of hepatic metabolism instead of two (as in clopidogrel), and has achieved a recognizably higher level of platelet inhibition. Prasugrel was tested in the TRITON trial [21]. In this trial 13 608 patients with moderate- to high-risk ACS with scheduled PCI were assigned to receive prasugrel (a 60 mg loading dose and a 10 mg daily maintenance dose) or clopidogrel (a 300 mg loading dose and a 75 mg daily maintenance dose) for

6–15 months. The primary efficacy end-point occurred in 12.1% of patients receiving clopidogrel and 9.9% of patients receiving prasugrel [hazard ratio (HR) for prasugrel versus clopidogrel 0.81, 95% CI 0.73–0.90, $p < 0.001$], showing the superiority of the new compound.

The second new agent is ticagrelor. Although this also acts through the P2Y12 receptor it is not a thienopyridine like clopidogrel and prasugrel but by definition a pyrimidine. The main pharmacological differences from clopidogrel and prasugrel are the lack of hepatic metabolism and reversibility—ticagrelor is the first reversible oral antiplatelet agent. This drug was tested in the PLATO trial [22]: in this multicentre, double-blind, randomized trial, ticagrelor (180 mg loading dose, 90 mg twice daily thereafter) and clopidogrel (300–600 mg loading dose, 75 mg daily thereafter) were compared for the prevention of cardiovascular events in 18 624 patients admitted to the hospital with ACS, with or without ST-segment elevation. At 12 months, the primary end-point—a composite of death from vascular causes, MI, or stroke—had occurred in 9.8% of patients receiving ticagrelor compared with 11.7% of those receiving clopidogrel (HR 0.84, 95% CI 0.77–0.92, $p < 0.001$).

The introduction of these new agents is assumed by the European guidelines on STEMI [23] and NSTEMI [24] as well as in the recently published ESC guidelines on myocardial revascularization [7] and will contribute to a rapid change in antiplatelet strategies for secondary prevention in cardiovascular diseases [9].

How long DAPT should be used for following an episode of ACS and after stent implantation is a matter of intense debate. Since the CURE trial, 9–12 months has been the magic period of intervention, which has not changed with the recent guidelines on myocardial revascularization [7]. In the chronic phase of cardiovascular disease (more than 12 months after an acute episode) monotherapy with aspirin is recommended [25].

The drawback of DAPT is the risk of bleeding. Despite the variations in incidence and definition of bleeding across studies, older age, female sex, lower body weight, use of invasive procedures, and renal insufficiency have consistently been found to be powerful predictors of bleeding complications in ACS and PCI [26]. Bleeding is a major predictor of an adverse prognosis, including the risk of death. Strategies to reduce the risk of bleeding should be implemented, and adequate use of antithrombotics is the key to success. The right dose for the right time is the main message here.

Triple therapy in secondary prevention after ACS

This type of combination antithrombotic therapy consists at present of two already investigated antithrombotic strategies: (1) a combination of aspirin + clopidogrel + a direct Factor Xa inhibitor (apixaban or rivaroxaban) [27] and (2) a combination of three different antiplatelet agents including aspirin + clopidogrel + the thrombin receptor antagonist vorapaxar [9,28]. In general these antithrombotic combination strategies have not yet been sufficiently tested to be in routine clinical use, and the ideal patient profile for maximum benefit with the lowest bleeding hazard still has to be evaluated.

In the APPRAISE-2 (Apixaban for Prevention of Acute Ischaemic and Safety Events) trial the direct Factor Xa inhibitor apixaban was tested versus placebo in addition to DAPT (aspirin + clopidogrel) in patients after ACS [29]. The dosage of apixaban was 5 mg twice a day (2.5 mg twice a day in patients with reduced kidney function), comparable to the dosage that has been used in patients with non-valvular atrial fibrillation. While the combined primary end-point (cardiovascular mortality, MI, or stroke) was similar in triple antithrombotic therapy compared with DAPT, bleeding hazard was statistically lower in DAPT-treated patients, leading to premature stoppage of the trial.

In contrast, the direct Factor Xa inhibitor rivaroxaban, given in a lower daily dosage (5 mg twice a day or 2.5 mg twice a day) than when used in non-valvular atrial fibrillation, was superior to DAPT with respect to the primary combined end-point (8.9% versus 10.7%, $p = 0.008$) (ATLAS ACS-2-TIMI-51 trial [8]). The lower dosage was also superior to DAPT with respect to the secondary end-points all-cause and cardiovascular death ($p = 0.002$ for both). The rate of spontaneous (non-coronary artery bypass graft-related) severe bleeding complications increased from 0.6% in patients under DAPT to 2.1% in patients under triple therapy ($p < 0.001$), intracranial bleeds increased from 0.2% to 0.6% ($p = 0{,}009$), but fatal bleeds were not statistically elevated (DAPT 0.2%, triple therapy 0.3%; $p = 0.66$). As more than 10% of patients were lost to follow-up, this indication is still under discussion and has so far only been approved by the European Medicines Agency (EMA). Nevertheless, with the availability of stronger P2Y12 receptor inhibitors than clopidogrel (prasugrel, ticagrelor) it might be difficult to define those patient cohorts that would especially benefit from this treatment option.

Triple antithrombotic therapy in secondary prevention after ACS, consisting of three antiplatelet agents (aspirin + clopidogrel + vorapaxar), adds a thrombin receptor antagonist to the usual DAPT, which also inhibits the thrombin-mediated activation of platelets (TRACER trial [30]). Like the APPRAISE-2 trial, the TRACER trial was stopped prematurely due to more frequent severe bleeding hazards, including intracerebral bleeds (1.1% versus 0.2%, $p < 0.001$). On the other hand, the primary combined end-point (cardiovascular mortality, MI, stroke, ischaemia-driven hospitalization, or acute coronary revascularization) was similar for both treatment groups (DAPT 19.9%, triple therapy 18.5%; $p = 0.07$). However, for some secondary end-points like the combination of cardiovascular death, MI, or stroke, triple antiplatelet therapy was superior to DAPT ($p = 0.02$).

Finally, the TRA-2P secondary prevention trial in roughly 25 000 patients with clinically stable coronary artery disease included patients 2 weeks to 12 months after the index event and treated over a medium follow-up period of 30 months [31]. The rate of the combined primary end-point (cardiovascular death, MI, stroke) was significantly lower in vorapaxar-treated patients compared with DAPT only (9.3% versus 10.5%; $p < 0.0001$). Triple therapy was also superior to DAPT with respect to several secondary endpoints. As soon as the results from the TRACER trial were made public, patients with a history of stroke or transitory ischaemic attack were no longer recruited into the TRA-2P trial. Nevertheless the rate of intracerebral bleeding increased significantly in patients receiving triple therapy.

In summary, the present data do not support the wide use of vorapaxar as a third antiplatelet agent in secondary prevention after ACS. However, post hoc analyses of the TRA-2P and TRACER trials might help to differentiate subgroups of patients who might benefit from a triple antiplatelet approach in secondary prevention of ACS.

Secondary prevention after elective PCI

The long-term benefit of DAPT following elective PCI was proven for the first time in the CREDO (Clopidogrel for the Reduction of Events During Observation) trial [32]. Patients were randomly assigned to receive a 300 mg clopidogrel loading dose ($n = 1053$) or placebo ($n = 1063$) 3–24 hours before PCI. Thereafter, all patients received clopidogrel (75 mg/day) through to day 28. From day 29 through to 12 months patients in the loading-dose group received clopidogrel (75 mg/day) and those in the control group received placebo. Both groups received aspirin throughout the study. At 1 year, long-term clopidogrel therapy was associated with a 26.9% relative reduction in the combined risk of death, MI, or stroke (95% CI 3.9–44.4%, $p = 0.02$).

Late stent thrombosis has been emphasized as a major complication after stent implantation, having dramatic implications for survival [33]. A large amount of evidence has been published linking the premature interruption of clopidogrel and the occurrence of stent thrombosis at 30 days or 6 months following intervention [34].

The role of the new antiplatelet agents in non-acute patients is unknown, but current guidelines state a strict minimum of 1 month for patients with a bare metal stent and 6 months for patients with a drug-eluting stent in stable disease and elective PCI [7].

Secondary prevention after coronary artery bypass graft

The long-term role of aspirin is an important component of secondary prevention after surgery in the broad range of patients with stable vascular disease. Beyond this clinical benefit, aspirin started less than 6 hours after surgery has a proven efficacy in reducing graft occlusion without an increase in bleeding [35].

The role of DAPT after coronary artery bypass grafting is unclear and somewhat controversial. A meta-analysis (six randomized clinical trials and six observational registries) including almost 25 000 patients compared aspirin versus aspirin + clopidogrel [36]. In-hospital or 30-day mortality was lower with aspirin + clopidogrel (0.8% versus 1.9%, $p < 0.0001$). Early saphenous graft closure was lower with DAPT (RR = 0.59, 95% CI 0.43–0.82, $p = 0.02$). The observed benefit was blunted by a trend for an increased risk of major bleeding.

In summary, current evidence does not support the use of DAPT after coronary artery bypass grafting and more evidence from randomized controlled trials assessing clinical outcomes is necessary to make definitive recommendations.

Special clinical situations

Chronic heart failure

Heart failure is a special condition in which the risk of embolism is always present, but an effective strategy for prevention is not clear. The Virchow triad, characterized by the presence of abnormal blood flow, abnormalities in the vessel wall, and abnormalities in the blood constituents, is the main pathophysiological explanation for the occurrence of episodes of thromboembolism in this setting [37]. There are many epidemiological data showing a clear link between heart failure and stroke. This link is particularly strong within the first 6 months of an acute episode of heart failure, but it returns later to close to normal [38].

The major criterion to be considered in patients with heart failure regarding antithrombotic prophylaxis is whether or not atrial fibrillation is present. Heart failure is a well-known risk factor for stroke in patients with atrial fibrillation and it is one of the components of the CHADS2 and CHA2DS2-VASc scores [39]. Heart failure in patients with atrial fibrillation is a strong indication (class IA) for the use of oral anticoagulants to prevent stroke and peripheral embolism [40].

The absence of atrial fibrillation defines a totally different scenario. There are a limited number of randomized clinical trials that have tested the efficacy of antithrombotic therapy in patients with heart failure in sinus rhythm. The ESC Heart Failure Association and the ESC Working Group on Thrombosis have published a joint consensus document on this subject [41].

Anticoagulation with vitamin K antagonists (VKAs) was tested in three randomized clinical trials without any convincing result. The WATCH (Warfarin and Antiplatelet Therapy in Chronic Heart failure) [42], HELAS (Heart failure Long-term Antithrombotic Study) [43], and WARCEF (Warfarin versus Aspirin in patients with Reduced Cardiac Ejection Fraction) [44] trials were designed to enrol patients with a clinical history of heart failure and ECG on sinus rhythm. None of the clinical trials showed any overall benefit of warfarin on rates of death or stroke with an increase of major bleeding, and there is no compelling reason to use warfarin routinely for all heart failure patients in sinus rhythm.

A second consideration is the use of antiplatelets, and aspirin in particular. The role of aspirin is well established in special conditions such as heart failure in patients with ischaemic heart disease or post-acute MI. In the subset of patients with heart failure without vascular disease the benefit of aspirin is less clear, and there is no available prospective evidence from long-term studies to recommend routine use of aspirin in heart failure patients living in sinus rhythm.

Another controversial issue is the higher risk of hospital admissions in patients managed with aspirin observed in the WATCH and HELAS trials, pointing towards a suspected negative interaction between ACE inhibitors and aspirin. However, a systematic review published in 2002 showed that the evidence of any reduction in the benefit of ACE inhibitor therapy when added to aspirin was too weak to justify any concern [45].

In summary the joint document [41] states that: '. . . In the absence of a specific indication, such as documented coronary artery disease, aspirin should not be initiated . . .' and '. . . there is currently no compelling reason to use warfarin routinely for all HF patients in sinus rhythm . . .'.

Atrial fibrillation and coronary artery disease

In patients who need DAPT but have atrial fibrillation with an increased stroke risk (CHA2DS2-VASc score ≥ 2) [46] triple therapy consisting of DAPT and an anticoagulant, usually a VKA, is mandatory [40]. Unfortunately this strategy is associated with increased bleeding rates [26,47]. Accordingly, the use of three antithrombotic agents has to be weighed against the individual risk for thromboembolic and bleeding complications.

Until the ESC annual meeting in 2014 there existed two position papers concerning triple therapy in patients with atrial fibrillation and coronary artery disease: one written by European experts [48] and the other by North American experts [49]. Both papers agreed that sufficient data are only available for the combination of aspirin + clopidogrel + VKA and that bare metal stents should be preferred over drug-eluting stents in patients with increased bleeding risk. In most instances warfarin was the anticoagulant tested, and an INR goal of 2.0–2.5 was mandatory to reduce severe bleeding hazards in combination with one or two antiplatelet agents. It was further recommended that the duration of triple therapy should be as short as possible. In this respect, however, the North American and European recommendations were different: while in Europe the safety aspect has highest priority and the longest recommended time for triple therapy was just 6 months, depending on the stent type, the bleeding tendency, and the acuteness and thrombotic risk of coronary disease, experts from North America preferred an approach that was more linked to efficacy [50]. The US experts recommended in certain cases triple therapy for up to 12 months (➲ Figs 17.2 and 17.3). The North American position paper [49] also recommended for the first time the optional use of the new oral anticoagulant (NOAC) dabigatran instead of warfarin in a dosage of 110 mg twice a day.

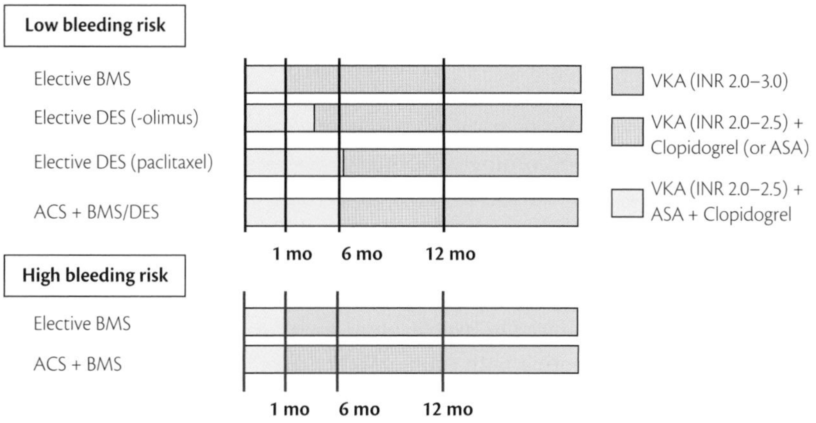

Fig. 17.2 ESC guidelines in patients with atrial fibrillation at moderate to high thromboembolic risk in whom oral anticoagulation is required. BMS, bare metal stent; DES, drug-eluting stent; ACS, acute coronary syndrome; VKA, vitamin K antagonist; INR, international normalized ratio; ASA, acetylsalicylic acid; mo, months.
Source: data from Camm J, et al. *Eur Heart J* 2010; **31**: 2369–2429.

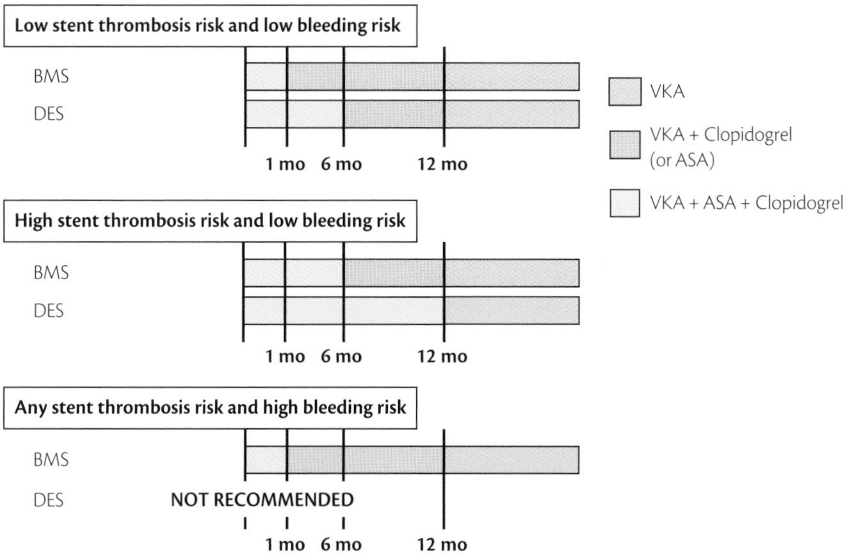

Fig. 17.3 A North American consensus document on antithrombotic therapy in patients with atrial fibrillation and a coronary stent with moderate to high stroke risk (CHADS2 ≥ 2). BMS, bare metal stent; DES, drug-eluting stent; VKA, vitamin K antagonist; ASA, acetylsalicylic acid.; mo, months.
Source: data from Faxon DP, *Circ Cardiovasc Interv* 2011; **4**: 522–534.

The recently published European position paper [51], which updates the former one, and as well as the well-known combination of aspirin + clopidogrel + VKA, allows the use of NOACs expanding to all available agents, dabigatran, rivaroxaban, and apixaban. Importantly, NOACs should be used in the lower tested dosages (dabigatran 110 mg twice a day, apixaban 2 × 2.5 mg twice a day, rivaroxaban 15 mg once a day). In addition, an algorithm has been developed, based on expert opinion, which recommends the duration and composition of dual or triple antithrombotic therapy based on the stroke risk, the bleeding risk, and the acuteness of intervention. There is still no recommendation for using the new P2Y12-inhibitors prasugrel or ticagrelor in combination with any anticoagulant as data are still missing. Ongoing trials might help to bring more knowledge to this problem.

Artificial valves and coronary artery disease

Artificial mechanical heart valves represent one of the major indications for oral anticoagulation. According to the 2012 ESC guidelines on the management of valvular heart disease [52] the target INR should be established based on thrombogenicity of the prosthesis and patient-related risk factors (mitral or tricuspid valve replacement; previous thromboembolism; atrial fibrillation; mitral stenosis; left ventricular ejection fraction < 35%). The INR varies from 2.5 in low-risk patients with a low-thrombogenic valve up to 4.0 in patients with at least one risk factor and a valve with a high thrombogenic profile. The new oral anticoagulants should not be used in this field, and in patients with bioprosthesis warfarin may be avoided.

Aspirin should be considered in patients with concomitant vascular disease, in particular coronary heart disease, and aspirin plus a P2Y12 receptor inhibitor is necessary following coronary stent implantation. The risk of bleeding is too high in patients on triple therapy. For this reason drug-eluting stents to shorten the use of triple therapy should be avoided in patients with an artificial mechanical heart valve [53].

Another situation for the use of aspirin is in the first 3 months after implantation of a bioprosthesis. There is actually no evidence to support the use of antiplatelet agents beyond 3 months in patients with a bioprosthesis who do not have a compelling indication other than the artificial valve itself [54].

DAPT with clopidogrel and aspirin is a widely accepted strategy in patients undergoing transcatheter aortic valve implantation (TAVI); however, this is not a proven strategy and further studies are needed.

Skipping aspirin?

The combination of multiple antithrombotic agents has been more effective than unidirectional therapy but is associated with more bleeding events [26,47], and the stronger P2Y12 receptor inhibitors have not yet been sufficiently tested. It is therefore an open question whether aspirin can be avoided to reduce bleeding risk while maintaining at least similar efficacy to the classical triple therapy. However, ethics committees have so far frequently refused permission to perform studies without aspirin in acute coronary artery disease and/or secondary prevention because it is seen as essential for prevention of atherothrombotic events.

In the WOEST trial [55], a small prospective, randomized controlled study published in 2013 involving just over 500 patients who were on anticoagulants and needed DAPT, aspirin was not given and clopidogrel + VKA was tested in one of two study arms while in the other the classical triple therapy was used. Over a 12-month follow-up, bleeding complications were more than doubled in the triple therapy arm compared with dual antithrombotic treatment with clopidogrel + VKA (44.9 versus 19.5%, $p < 0.001$). Moreover, there was a significant reduction in the combined secondary efficacy end-point (death, MI, target vessel revascularization, stroke, or stent thrombosis) in patients on dual versus on triple antithrombotic therapy (17.7 versus 11.3%, $p = 0.025$). Due to the relatively small number of patients and the fact that the efficacy outcome was not statistically powered, these results are hypothesis generating and should be proven by future studies with sufficient patient numbers. Moreover, this trial has other limitations, for example the long (12 months) duration of combination therapies, which is not recommended in the recent position statements [49,50]. In addition, severe bleeding complications, for example intracerebral bleeds, as defined by the Thrombolysis In Myocardial Infarction (TIMI) classification, were not statistically increased in the triple therapy group.

Accordingly, further studies are needed to find out if aspirin can be avoided in certain indications and combination strategies. As an example, the GLOBAL LEADERS trial will investigate the usual DAPT for 12 months (in elective patients aspirin + clopidogrel, in ACS patients aspirin + ticagrelor) followed by aspirin alone for another 12 months after coronary stenting with the BioMatrix Flex™ stent versus DAPT for only 1 month with aspirin + ticagrelor followed by 23 months of ticagrelor as monotherapy, respectively.

Potential objections against this strategy of avoiding aspirin include the anti-inflammatory action of aspirin in the 100 mg daily dosage, which might be an important preventive mechanism. Moreover, aspirin is an important inhibitor of explosive thromboxane synthesis after plaque rupture in ACS, which leads to thromboxane-induced thrombin formation, a mechanism that cannot be influenced by P2Y12 receptor blockers.

Conclusion

While primary prevention with antithrombotic agents is still a matter of debate and frequently not performed, secondary prevention is necessary in patients with stable and proven coronary artery disease (lifelong aspirin or clopidogrel if there are side effects), in patients after stable, elective stent implantation (DAPT, aspirin + clopidogrel, for different durations based on the chosen stent type), as well as in patients after ACS (aspirin + prasugrel or ticagrelor for 9–12 months). Special indications include patients after aortocoronary bypass surgery (aspirin or clopidogrel or a combination of both), chronic heart failure (VKAs), and patients with an increased CHADS-VASc score (≥1) who develop atrial fibrillation while under DAPT (triple therapy consisting of aspirin + clopidogrel + VKA). Combination antithrombotic therapy in patients with atrial fibrillation after stent implantation (aspirin + clopidogrel + VKA or one of the available NOACs in reduced dosage), but also as secondary prevention strategy (e.g. rivaroxaban + DAPT), is the subject of several investigations, as is skipping of aspirin in favour of a dual antithrombotic strategy in order to reduce bleeding complications.

Solution to the clinical case

Beyond the risk of stent thrombosis related to previous coronary intervention the occurrence of atrial fibrillation is adding a new kind of risk. With a CHA2DS2Vasc2 score of 4 the risk of embolic stroke is too high, requiring an efficient antithrombotic regime based on anticoagulants.

According to the current recommendations triple therapy should be considered, adding warfarin (INR 2.0–2.5) on top of dual antiplatelet therapy for at least three months followed by dual antiplatelets alone. Intervention was performed in a stable condition and a drug-eluted stent was implanted. Then six months of triple therapy is enough.

Further reading

Camm AJ, Lip GY, De Caterina R, et al. 2012 focused update of the ESC guidelines for the management of atrial fibrillation: an update of the 2010 ESC guidelines for the management of atrial fibrillation—developed with the special contribution of the European Heart Rhythm Association. *Eur Heart J* 2012; **33**: 2719–47.

De Caterina R, Husted S, Wallentin L, et al. General mechanisms of coagulation and targets of anticoagulants (Section I). Position Paper of the ESC Working Group on Thrombosis – Task Force on Anticoagulants in Heart Disease. *Thromb Haemost* 2013; **109**: 569–79.

Hamm CW, Bassand J-P, Agewall S, et al. ESC guidelines for the management of acute coronary syndromes in patients presenting without persistent ST-segment elevation. *Eur Heart J* 2011; **32**: 2999–3054.

Lip GY, Windecker S, Huber K, et al. Management of antithrombotic therapy in atrial fibrillation patients presenting with acute coronary syndrome and/or undergoing percutaneous coronary or valve interventions: a joint consensus document of the European Society of Cardiology Working Group on Thrombosis, European Heart Rhythm Association (EHRA), European Association of Percutaneous Cardiovascular Interventions (EAPCI) and European Association of Acute Cardiac Care (ACCA) endorsed by the Heart Rhythm Society (HRS) and Asia-Pacific Heart Rhythm Society (APHRS). *Eur Heart J* 2014; **35**: 3155–79.

Pamukcu B, Huber K, Lip GY. Antiplatelet therapy in atherothrombotic cardiovascular diseases for primary and secondary prevention: a focus on old and new antiplatelet agents. *Curr Pharm Des* 2012; **18**: 850–60.

Patrono C, Andreotti F, Arnesen H, et al. Antiplatelet agents for the treatment and prevention of atherothrombosis. *Eur Heart J* 2011; **32**: 2922–32.

Steg PG, Huber K, Andreotti F, et al. Bleeding in acute coronary syndromes and percutaneous coronary interventions: position paper by the Working Group on Thrombosis of the European Society of Cardiology. *Eur Heart J* 2011; **32**: 1854–64.

Steg PG, James SK, Atar D, et al. ESC guidelines for the management of acute myocardial infarction in patients presenting with ST-segment elevation. *Eur Heart J* 2012; **33**: 2569–619.

Wallentin L, Becker R, Budaj A, et al. for the PLATO Investigators. Ticagrelor versus clopidogrel in patients with acute coronary syndromes. *N Engl J Med* 2009; **361**: 1045–57.

Windecker S, Kolh P, Alfonso F, et al; authors/Task Force members. 2014 ESC/EACTS Guidelines on myocardial revascularization: the Task Force on Myocardial Revascularization of the European Society of Cardiology (ESC) and the European Association for Cardio-Thoracic Surgery (EACTS) developed with the special contribution of the European Association of Percutaneous Cardiovascular Interventions (EAPCI). *Eur Heart J* 2014; **35**: 2541–619.

Wiviott SD, Braunwald E, McCabe CH, et al. Prasugrel versus clopidogrel in patients with acute coronary syndromes. *N Engl J Med* 2007; **357**: 2001–15.

References

1 De Caterina R, Husted S, Wallentin L, et al. Anticoagulants in heart disease—current status and perspectives: Section I—general background on coagulation and targets of anticoagulants. *Thromb Haemostas* 2013; **109**: 569–79.

2 Monroe DM, Hoffman M. What does it take to make the perfect clot? *Arterioscler Thromb Vasc Biol* 2006; **26**: 41–8.

3 Roberts HR, Hoffman M, Monroe DM. A cell-based model of thrombin generation. *Thromb Hemostas* 2006; **32**(Suppl. 1): 32–8.

4 Fox KA, Cokkinos DV, Deckers JW, et al. The ENACT study: a pan-European survey of acute coronary syndromes. European Network for Acute Coronary Treatment. *Eur Heart J* 2000; **21**: 1440–9.

5 Hasdai D, Behar S, Wallentin L, et al. A prospective survey of the characteristics, treatments and outcomes of patients with acute coronary syndromes in Europe and the Mediterranean basin. The Euro Heart Survey of Acute Coronary Syndromes (Euro Heart Survey ACS). *Eur Heart J* 2002; **23**: 1190–201.

6 Wood DA for the EUROASPIRE II Study Group. Lifestyle and risk factor management and use of drug therapies in coronary patients from 15 countries; principal results from EUROASPIRE II. Euro Heart Survey Programme. *Eur Heart J* 2001; **22**: 554–72.

7 Windecker S, Kolh P, Alfonso F, et al.; authors/Task Force members. 2014 ESC/EACTS guidelines on myocardial revascularization: the Task Force on Myocardial Revascularization of the European Society of Cardiology (ESC) and the European Association for Cardiothoracic Surgery (EACTS) developed with the special contribution of the European Association of Percutaneous Cardiovascular Interventions (EAPCI). *Eur Heart J* 2014; **35**: 2541–619.

8 Mega JL, Braunwald E, Wiviott SD, et al. ATLAS ACS 2-TIMI 51 Investigators. Rivaroxaban in patients with a recent acute coronary syndrome. *N Engl J Med* 2012; **366**: 9–19.

9 Pamukcu B, Huber K, Lip GY. Antiplatelet therapy in atherothrombotic cardiovascular diseases for primary and secondary prevention: a focus on old and new antiplatelet agents. *Curr Pharm Des* 2012; **18**: 850–60.

10 Ogawa H, Nakayama M, Morimoto T, et al. The Japanese Primary Prevention of Atherosclerosis With Aspirin for Diabetes (JPAD) Trial Investigators. Low-dose aspirin for primary prevention of atherosclerotic events in patients with type 2 diabetes: a randomized controlled trial. *J Am Med Assoc* 2008; **300**: 2134–41.

11 Fowkes FG, Price JF, Stewart MC, et al. for the Aspirin for Asymptomatic Atherosclerosis Trialists. Aspirin for prevention of cardiovascular events in a general population screened for a low ankle brachial index: a randomized controlled trial. *J Am Med Assoc* 2010; **303**: 841–8.

12 Belch J, MacCuish A, Campbell I, et al. Prevention of Progression of Arterial Disease and Diabetes Study Group; Diabetes Registry Group; Royal College of Physicians Edinburgh. The prevention of progression of arterial disease and diabetes (POPADAD) trial: factorial randomised placebo controlled trial of aspirin and antioxidants in patients with diabetes and asymptomatic peripheral arterial disease. *Br Med J* 2008; **337**: a1840.

13 Antithrombotic Trialists (ATT) Collaboration. Aspirin in the primary and secondary prevention of vascular disease: collaborative meta-analysis of individual participant data from randomised trials. *Lancet* 2009; **373**: 1849–60.

14 Ridker PM, Cook NR, Lee IM. A randomized trial of low-dose aspirin in the primary prevention of cardiovascular disease in women. *N Engl J Med* 2005; **352**: 1293–304.

15 Cairns JA, Gent M, Singer J, et al. Aspirin, sulfinpyrazone, or both in unstable angina. Results of a Canadian multicenter trial. *N Engl J Med* 1985; **313**: 1369–75.

16 Patrono C, Andreotti F, Arnesen H, et al. Antiplatelet agents for the treatment and prevention of atherothrombosis. *Eur Heart J* 2011; **32**: 2922–32.

17 Morice MC, Zemour G, Benveniste E, et al. Intracoronary stenting without coumadin: one month results of a French multicenter study. *Cathet Cardiovasc Diagn* 1995; **35**: 1–7.

18 CAPRIE Steering Committee. A randomised, blinded, trial of clopidogrel versus aspirin in patients at risk of ischaemic events (CAPRIE). *Lancet* 1996; **348**: 1329–39.

19 The Clopidogrel in Unstable Angina to Prevent Recurrent Events Trial Investigators. Effects of clopidogrel in addition to aspirin in patients with acute coronary syndromes without ST-segment elevation. *N Engl J Med* 2001; **345**: 494–502.

20 Mehta SR, Yusuf S, Peters RJ, et al. Effects of pre-treatment with clopidogrel and aspirin followed by long-term therapy in patients undergoing percutaneous coronary intervention: the PCI-CURE study. *Lancet* 2001; **358**: 527–33.

21 Wiviott SD, Braunwald E, McCabe CH, et al. Prasugrel versus clopidogrel in patients with acute coronary syndromes. *N Engl J Med* 2007; **357**: 2001–15.

22 Wallentin L, Becker R, Budaj A, et al. for the PLATO Investigators. Ticagrelor versus clopidogrel in patients with acute coronary syndromes. *N Engl J Med* 2009; **361**: 1045–57.

23 Steg PG, James SK, Atar D, et al. ESC Guidelines for the management of acute myocardial infarction in patients presenting with ST-segment elevation. *Eur Heart J* 2012; **33**: 2569–619.

24 Hamm CW, Bassand J-P, Agewall S, et al. ESC guidelines for the management of acute coronary syndromes in patients presenting without persistent ST-segment elevation. *Eur Heart J* 2011; **32**: 2999–3054.

25 Perk J, De Backer G, Gohlke H, et al. European guidelines on cardiovascular disease prevention in clinical practice (version 2012). The Fifth Joint Task Force of the European Society of Cardiology and Other Societies on Cardiovascular Disease Prevention in Clinical Practice (constituted by representatives of nine societies and by invited experts). Developed with the special contribution of the European Association for Cardiovascular Prevention and Rehabilitation (EACPR). *Eur Heart J* 2012; **33**: 1635–701.

26 Steg PG, Huber K, Andreotti F, et al. Bleeding in acute coronary syndromes and percutaneous coronary interventions: position paper by the Working Group on Thrombosis of the European Society of Cardiology. *Eur Heart J* 2011; **32**: 1854–64.

27 Sinnaeve PR, Adriaenssens T, Höchtl T, et al. New oral anticoagulant agents after ACS. *Eur Heart J Acute Cardiovasc Care* 2012; **1**: 79–86.

28 Hoechtl T, Sinnaeve PR, Adriaenssens T, et al. Oral antiplatelet therapy in acute coronary syndromes: update 2012. *Eur Heart J Acute Cardiovasc Care* 2012; **1**: 87–93.

29 Alexander JH, Lopes RD, James S, et al. for the APPRAISE-2 Investigators. Apixaban with antiplatelet therapy after acute coronary syndromes. *N Engl J Med* 2011; **365**: 699–708.

30 Tricoci P, Huang Z, Held C, et al. Thrombin-receptor antagonist vorapaxar in acute coronary syndromes. *N Engl J Med* 2012; **366**: 20–33.

31 Morrow DA, Braunwald E, Bonaca MP, et al. TRA 2P-TIMI 50 Steering Committee and Investigators. Vorapaxar in the secondary prevention of atherothrombotic events. *N Engl J Med* 2012; **366**: 1404–13.

32 Steinhubl SR, Berger PB, Mann JT, III, et al. for the CREDO Investigators. Early and sustained dual oral antiplatelet therapy following percutaneous coronary intervention. A randomized controlled trial. *J Am Med Assoc* 2002; **288**: 2411–20.

33 Almalla M, Schröder J, Hennings V, et al. Long-term outcome after angiographically proven coronary stent thrombosis. *Am J Cardiol* 2013; **111**: 1289–94.

34 Roy P, Bonello L, Torguson R, et al. Temporal relation between clopidogrel cessation and stent thrombosis after drug-eluting stent implantation. *Am J Cardiol* 2009; **103**: 801–5.

35 Musleh G, Dunning J. Does aspirin 6 h after coronary artery bypass grafting optimise graft patency? *Interact Cardiovasc Thorac Surg* 2003; **2**: 413–15.

36 Deo SV, Dunlay SM, Shah IK, et al. Dual anti-platelet therapy after coronary artery bypass grafting: is there any benefit? A systematic review and meta-analysis. *J Card Surg* 2013; **28**: 109–16.

37 Virchow R. *Virchow's triad*, 1856. Frankfurt: Meidlinger Sohn & Co.

38 Alberts VP, Bos MJ, Koudstaal PJ, et al. Heart failure and the risk of stroke: the Rotterdam Study. *Eur J Epidemiol* 2010; **25**: 807–12.

39 Olesen JB, Torp-Pedersen C, Hansen ML, et al. The value of the CHA2DS2-Vasc score for refining stroke risk stratification in patients with atrial fibrillation with a CHADS2 score 0-1: a nationwide cohort study. *Thromb Haemostas* 2012; **107**: 1172–9.

40 Camm AJ, Lip GY, De Caterina R, et al. 2012 focused update of the ESC guidelines for the management of atrial fibrillation: an update of the 2010 ESC guidelines for the management of atrial fibrillation—developed with the special contribution of the European Heart Rhythm Association. *Eur Heart J* 2012; **33**: 2719–47.

41 Lip GY, Piotrponikowski P, Andreotti F, et al. Thromboembolism and antithrombotic therapy for heart failure in sinus rhythm: an executive summary of a joint consensus document from the ESC Heart Failure Association and the ESC working group on thrombosis. *Thromb Haemostas* 2012; **108**: 1009–22.

42 Massie BM, Collins JF, Ammon SE, et al. WATCH Trial Investigators. Randomized trial of warfarin, aspirin, and clopidogrel in patients with chronic heart failure: the Warfarin and Antiplatelet Therapy in Chronic Heart Failure (WATCH) trial. *Circulation* 2009; **119**: 1616–24.

43 Cokkinos DV, Haralabopoulos GC, Kostis JB, et al. for the HELAS Investigators. Efficacy of antithrombotic therapy in chronic heart failure: the HELAS study. *Eur J Heart Fail* 2006; **8**: 428–32.
44 Homma S, Thompson JL, Pullicino PM, et al. for the WARCEF Investigators. Warfarin and aspirin in patients with heart failure and sinus rhythm. *N Engl J Med* 2012; **366**: 1859–69.
45 Teo KK, Yusuf S, Pfeffer M, et al. for the ACE Inhibitors Collaborative Group. Effects of long-term treatment with angiotensin-converting enzyme inhibitors in the presence or absence of aspirin: a systematic review. *Lancet* 2002; **360**: 1037–43.
46 Lip GY, Nieuwlaat R, Pisters R, et al. Refining clinical risk stratification for predicting stroke and thromboembolism in atrial fibrillation using a novel risk factor-based approach: the Euro Heart Survey on atrial fibrillation. *Chest* 2010; **137**: 263–72.
47 Hansen ML, Sørensen R, Clausen MT, et al. Risk of bleeding with single, dual, or triple therapy with warfarin, aspirin, and clopidogrel in patients with atrial fibrillation. *Arch Intern Med* 2010; **170**: 1433–41.
48 Lip G, Huber K, Andreotti F, et al. Consensus Document of European Society of Cardiology Working Group on Thrombosis. Antithrombotic management of atrial fibrillation patients presenting with acute coronary syndrome and/or undergoing coronary stenting: executive summary—a Consensus Document of the European Society of Cardiology Working Group on Thrombosis, endorsed by the European Heart Rhythm Association (EHRA) and the European Association of Percutaneous Cardiovascular Interventions (EAPCI). *Eur Heart J* 2010; **31**: 1311–18.
49 Faxon DP, Eikelboom JW, Berger PB, et al. Consensus document: antithrombotic therapy in patients with atrial fibrillation undergoing coronary stenting. A North-American perspective. *Thrombos Haemostas* 2011; **106**: 572–84.
50 Huber K, Airaksinen KJ, Cuisset T, et al. Antithrombotic therapy in patients with atrial fibrillation undergoing coronary stenting: similarities and dissimilarities between North America and Europe. *Thromb Haemostas* 2011; **106**: 569–71.
51 Lip GY, Windecker S, Huber K, et al. Management of antithrombotic therapy in atrial fibrillation patients presenting with acute coronary syndrome and/or undergoing percutaneous coronary or valve interventions: a joint consensus document of the European Society of Cardiology Working Group on Thrombosis, European Heart Rhythm Association (EHRA), European Association of Percutaneous Cardiovascular Interventions (EAPCI) and European Association of Acute Cardiac Care (ACCA) endorsed by the Heart Rhythm Society (HRS) and Asia-Pacific Heart Rhythm Society (APHRS). *Eur Heart J* 2014; **35**: 3155–79.
52 Vahanian A, Alfieri O, Andreotti F, et al. Guidelines on the management of valvular heart disease (version 2012). Joint Task Force on the Management of Valvular Heart Disease of the European Society of Cardiology (ESC); European Association for Cardio-Thoracic Surgery (EACTS). *Eur Heart J* 2012; **33**: 2451–96.
53 Camm AJ, Kirchhof P, Lip GY, et al. European Heart Rhythm Association; European Association for Cardio-Thoracic Surgery. Guidelines for the management of atrial fibrillation: the Task Force for the Management of Atrial Fibrillation of the European Society of Cardiology (ESC). *Eur Heart J* 2010; **31**: 2501–55.
54 Gherli T, Colli A, Fragnito C, et al. Comparing warfarin with aspirin after biological aortic valve replacement: a prospective study. *Circulation* 2004; **110**: 496–500.
55 Dewilde W, Oirbasn T, Verheugt FW, et al. The WOEST Trial: first randomised trial comparing two regimens with and without aspirin in patients on oral anticoagulation therapy undergoing coronary stenting. *Lancet* 2013; **381**: 1107–15.

CHAPTER 18

Psychosocial factors in the prevention of cardiovascular disease

Töres Theorell, Chantal Brisson, Michel Vézina, Alain Milot, and Mahée Gilbert-Ouimet

Contents

Summary

This chapter begins by outlining the theoretical sociological, psychological, and physiological framework for the relationships between psychosocial factors and coronary heart disease (CHD). This is followed by a review of the scientific evidence for such an association. Individual behaviours and coping mechanisms as well as environmental conditions of relevance for CHD are described. In particular type A and D behaviour, depressive states, covert coping, social support and social networks, socioeconomic conditions, and theoretical models of the work environment of relevance for CHD (job strain, effort–reward imbalance, organizational justice, and leadership) are discussed. The results from controlled studies of the effects of psychosocial interventions are surveyed. Such interventions can be divided into those that target the individual behaviour and those that target the environment. There are also interventions that target both. Most studies looking at interventions that target the individual have been secondary intervention trials (efforts to reduce the risk of recurrence after a first major CHD event). Although the evidence is mixed, those studies which have used a thorough and long-lasting approach with a long follow-up period have shown significant effects on recurrence rate. There are important gender differences in the patterning of effects. In the second group (environmental interventions) most studies have been work-based and have aimed at improving work organization. There is accumulating evidence from such controlled studies that risk factors for CHD (blood pressure, plasma cortisol and the anabolic/regenerative hormone dehydroepiandrosterone sulphate) can be favourably influenced.

Clinical case

The patient, a 42-year-old woman, is an accountant for a small shop. By the age of 36 she had already suffered a minor stroke with partial paresis of the right hand and expressive aphasia. This episode had occurred during a period when she had decided to break away from a difficult marriage. She had then gone through the divorce, met a new man, and was now pregnant (she had one child from her first marriage). She received conflicting advice from different physicians with regard to legal abortion. One argument against

(*continued*)

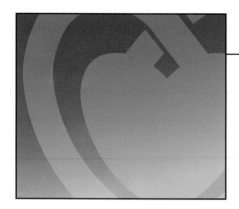

Clinical case *(continued)*

abortion was: 'You owe this new man a child'. The patient had pronounced variations in blood pressure (sometimes hypotension and sometimes blood pressure in the range 200–230 mmHg systolic and 100–130 mmHg diastolic) and it was very difficult to prescribe adequate blood pressure medication. She was prescribed self-monitoring of blood pressure. On doing this she discovered patterns: her circadian blood pressure variation and her blood pressure levels (systolic as well as diastolic) tended to normalize after a vacation but after some weeks of working she saw a pronounced afternoon elevation. This information made it possible for her to lower her medication to optimal levels, with fewer potential adverse effects on her foetus. She gave birth to a normal child. In general she learned some self-regulation of blood pressure from the patterns she discovered for herself, in line with the reported beneficial effects of self-monitoring.

Two years later her blood pressure variations had become more pronounced, and she now also had transitory attacks of neurological symptoms when her blood pressure levels were high—clumsiness in her right hand and difficulties in word finding lasting for some minutes. This mostly occurred during the afternoons, and she related this to her deteriorated work environment. Sometimes she even dropped items on the floor and made strange mistakes in her typing because of her attacks of clumsiness. External financial requirements had become tougher and her boss (the shop owner) had decided to withdraw lunch breaks because of increased workload and reduced income. The shop owner had started to talk about the patient moving to some other job because of her difficulties. This increased her tension. The patient described herself as 'overcommitted' in an overburdened situation at work.

Psychosocial concepts

In this chapter we refer to psychosocial factors as a number of social conditions and psychological processes which are potentially of significance for the development of cardiovascular disease (CVD). The importance of psychosocial factors for the aetiology and clinical course of CVD has been a subject of debate for decades (see for instance [1,2]).

The individual and the environment

➲ Figure 18.1 is a schematic depiction of the interplay between structural and individual factors in psychosocial stress reactions. There are three levels in the diagram—stressors and regenerative factors, coping, and stress/regeneration reactions. Each level theoretically represents a level at which interventions could be made. ➲ Figure 18.1 shows that there are both positive (anabolism or regeneration) and energy mobilization (stress) aspects to the interplay (the black parts represent energy mobilization and the white parts regeneration). The floating border between black and white illustrates that stressors can become anti-stressors and vice versa; that destructive patterns of coping can become constructive and that catabolic reactions could change to anabolic reactions.

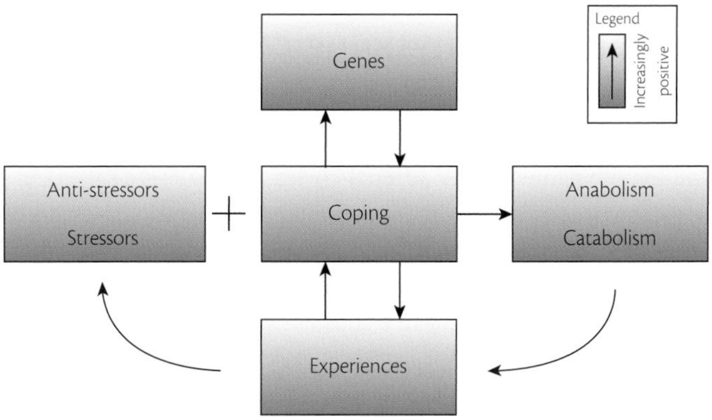

Fig. 18.1 Stressors and anti-stressors, the environmental level—positive and negative aspects. Schematic presentation of the interplay between environment, individual coping, and reactions to the environment. The blue parts represent energy mobilization and the white parts regeneration. The floating border between blue and white illustrates that stressors could become anti-stressors, and vice versa, that destructive patterns of coping could become constructive and that catabolic reactions could change to anabolic.
Theorell, T: Stress Reduction Programs for the work place. In: Gatchel, RJ and Schultz, IZ. Handbook of Occupational Health and Wellness. Springer Science, New York 2012.

Stressors and anti-stressors

Factors in the environment that cause, trigger, or sustain stress reactions or their positive counterparts are labelled *stressors* and *anti-stressors* (or *regenerative factors*), respectively. These are positioned to the left of the diagram in ➲ Fig. 18.1. Social conditions are very important prerequisites for an individual's stressors, but also for his or her positive reactions to the social situation.

Principles for intervention

Psychosocial interventions in the prevention of CVD could address either the external environment (anti-stressors or stressors) or the individual (coping), or both. In line with this, environmental interventions could be directed against the individual's general life situation, and will be exemplified by work intended to improve social networks and social support. It could also be directed to specific areas of life, here exemplified by organizational factors at work. In both cases, reduction of negative stressors or stimulation of positive conditions—or both—could be targets.

Work and other areas of life

An interesting aspect of someone's work situation is that its organization is something that can be changed, hence stimulating conditions for reduced negative stress reactions and improved protection against such reactions. Most of the literature on work organization interventions is devoted to the reduction of negative stressors. An important observation, however, is that the worksite also has a responsibility for creating a positive atmosphere that stimulates creativity and social support. These factors could be labelled as *anti-stressors*. Anti-stressors are likely to stimulate regenerative 'healing' and health promotion processes in employees.

Basic psychophysiological mechanisms

One of the central components of the stress reaction is the hypothalamo–pituitary–adrenocortical (HPA) axis, extending from the hypothalamus to the adrenal cortex (see ➲ Fig. 18.2). If the organism interprets its situation as energy demanding, a chain of reactions starts resulting in raised blood concentration of corticosteroids. These corticosteroids help the organism in a number of ways to sustain its fight in a stressful situation. However, if the stressor is long lasting (for instance weeks or months) those same effects may be damaging to health. There are other components in the immediate stress reaction, some of which occur more immediately (within seconds or less) than the reactions of the HPA system (which take place within minutes), such as those occurring in the sympatho-adrenergic system (noradrenalin) and the sympathomedullary system (adrenalin).

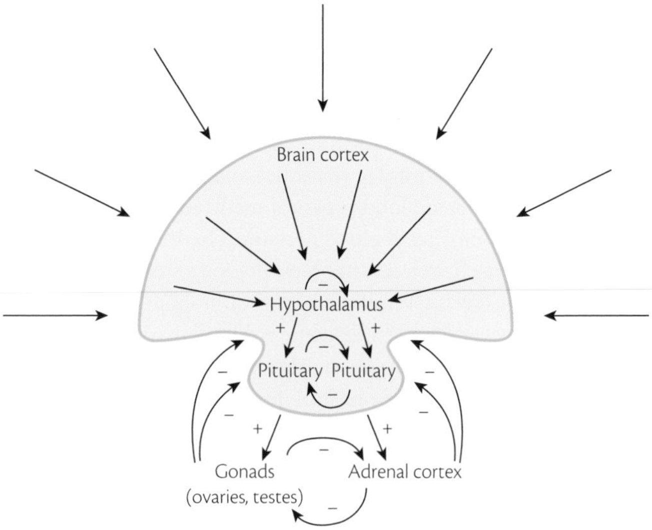

Fig. 18.2 Schematic presentation of the interplay between energy mobilization (right hand side) and regeneration (left hand side) from the hypothalamus through the pituitary to the endocrine end organs. The two sides influence one another.

Theorell, T: Stress Reduction Programs for the work place. In: Gatchel, RJ and Schultz, IZ. Handbook of Occupational Health and Wellness. Springer Science, New York 2012.

Stress reactions of relevance to coronary heart disease

Energy mobilization is associated with a number of other bodily reactions which are important in the mechanisms of CVD (see ➲ Fig. 18.3):

1. Activation of the renin–angiotensin system. The sympathetic nervous system, a primary mediator of the acute stress response, is one of the major pathways activating the renin–angiotensin system. Therefore stress can stimulate the secretion of renin and increase plasma levels of angiotensin II which has significant actions on vessel walls. Angiotensin II causes vasoconstriction, endothelial dysfunction, cellular proliferation, and inflammation, all of which promote atherosclerosis. In conjunction with sympathetic activation and stimulation of the HPA axis, activation of the renin–angiotensin system can lead to hypertension, arterial stiffness, and cardiovascular events [3–5].
2. Inflammatory reactions are stimulated. Such reactions are mirrored for instance in increased plasma concentration of interleukin 6 (IL-6).
3. Coagulation is stimulated, which is mirrored for instance in an increased plasma concentration of fibrinogen.

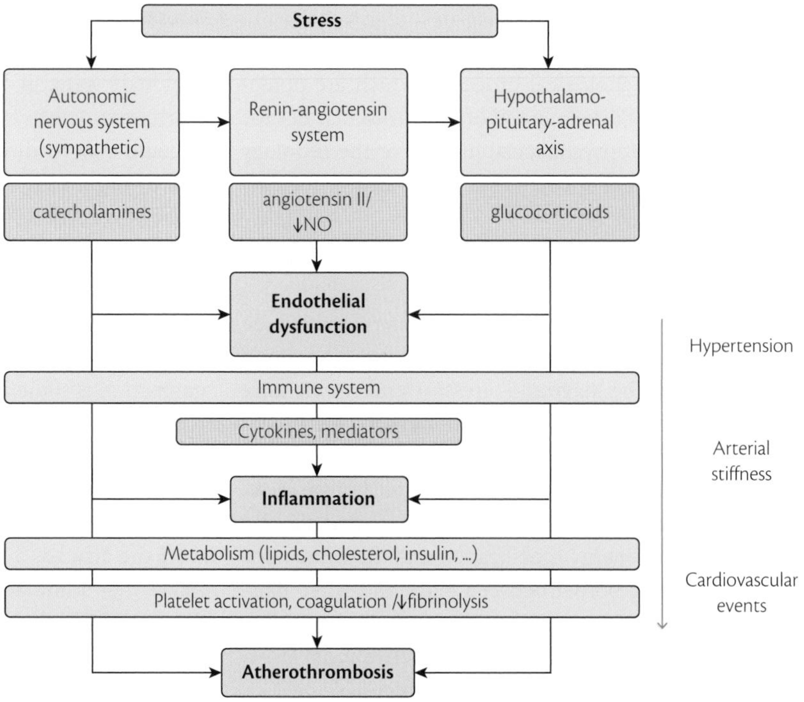

Fig. 18.3 Endocrine and cardiovascular responses to stress. NO, nitric oxide.

Effects on coagulation, blood pressure (BP), and inflammation may give rise to accelerated coronary atherosclerosis and hence influence the buildup of an increased risk of developing CVD. There are also stress-related mechanisms that may increase acute risks. One of those is rupture of atherosclerotic plaques—an acute exacerbation of the atherosclerotic process itself. Another mechanism relates to cardiac arrhythmia:

4. Changes in electrical thresholds in the heart's conductance system may arise due to exposure to catecholamine. This increases the risk of developing arrhythmias.

Counterbalancing stress—the HPG axis

There is also a counterbalancing system (an anti-stress system) which protects against adverse effects of long-lasting stress. This HPG (hypothalamo–pituitary–gonadal) axis is at the same levels as the HPA axis, ranging from the hypothalamus to the gonadal glands. The balance between the HPA and HPG axes is illustrated in ➲ Fig. 18.2. The HPG axis represents the 'regenerative' or 'anabolic' part of metabolism. Testosterone and oestrogen, as well as their precursor dehydroepiandrosterone sulphate (DHEA-S), are examples of corticosteroids with a mainly anabolic/regenerative function. The direct relationship between plasma concentration of DHEA-S and the incidence of myocardial infarction (MI) has not been studied extensively, although one work has shown that there is an increased mortality among women with MI who have a low concentration of DHEA-S [6]. This is in line with the general observation that DHEA-S facilitates regeneration. Other hormones also participate in this, such as the pituitary growth hormone. There is a balance between the HPA axis and the HPG axis. This means that the HPG axis tends to lower its activity when the HPA axis has maximal activity (in stressful situations). It also means that damaging effects of long-lasting stress can be dampened by high activity in the HPG axis. Thus, the balance between HPA and HPG activity is an important principle in health promotion.

The parasympathetic system

It has been know for a long time that the parasympathetic system is central to the counterbalancing mechanism since it stimulates anabolic processes. This is important for the heart muscle itself. In addition, high parasympathetic activity may dampen the atherosclerotic process due to inhibition of the activity of pro-inflammatory cytokines such as IL-6 [7].

Lifestyle and psychosocial factors

Lifestyle factors interact with psychosocial factors: for example, some psychosocial factors (such as low social class) are associated with poor lifestyle habits such as cigarette smoking, lack of physical activity outside work, and poor eating habits. In addition, mental illnesses associated with elevated risk of CVD, such as depression, are associated with psychosocial conditions such as low social class, poor social support, and adverse working conditions.

Controversies in the field of psychosocial factors and cardiovascular disease have arisen concerning the role of lifestyle factors. It has been argued [1] that if the effect of adverse psychosocial conditions on heart disease risk is mediated via effects on lifestyle factors (such as cigarette smoking, eating habits, and physical exercise during leisure) there is no 'real' effect of psychosocial factors at all. However, a large prospective study published in 2012 [8] showed that the effect of 'job strain' (high demands and low control) on risk of MI cannot be totally explained by lifestyle factors. This means that direct physiological stress mechanisms are important. Regardless of this, psychosocial factors are important in primary prevention of CVD since a poor psychosocial situation may decrease an individual's willingness to follow advice on smoking, diet, and physical activity.

Individual psychosocial factors and efforts to improve coping with adverse psychosocial conditions

Coping is the intermediate level in ➲ Fig. 18.1. This corresponds to the individual's interpretation and handling of stressors/anti-stressors. In preventive work it makes good sense to try to improve a patient's coping pattern. Several intervention trials have been performed in which this has been the aim. However, before these are reviewed it should be pointed out that it is preferable in such prevention to work with both environmental factors and coping patterns in parallel processes. For instance, employees may not be motivated to improve their own coping pattern if they feel that the work environment is dysfunctional. And it may turn out to be impossible to obtain sustainable effects on individual coping patterns if the environmental aspects are neglected. Conversely, efforts to improve work organization benefit from discussions with employees regarding individual coping patterns [9].

Specific coping patterns

The following coping patterns have been identified as potential cardiovascular risk factors and are thus possible targets in cardiovascular prevention (in chronological order as they appeared in scientific discussion):

- type A behaviour
- depression/type D personality
- poor stress management.

Principles for intervention in individual counselling on psychosocial factors

A common method used for interventions in individuals is cognitive–behavioural therapy (CBT) or methods related to CBT.

Type A behaviour and its most important component, hostility, have been documented as possible cardiovascular risk factors since the first prospective study was published by Rosenman et al. in 1976 [10]. Since then, some studies have verified type A behaviour as a risk factor, whereas other studies have failed to do so. There is evidence from a meta-analytical study [11] that hostility is an independent risk factor for coronary heart disease (CHD), and it has therefore been suggested that it would be useful to decrease hostile and angry coping patterns by means of CBT in primary prevention of CHD.

That depression is an independent predictor of CHD risk has been shown in a meta-analytic study by Rugulies [12], which showed that the onset of clinical depression was a stronger predictor of CHD risk than depressive symptoms. People with type D personality have a propensity to react with depressive symptoms. This has been mentioned as an important coping pattern that should be taken into account in the treatment of patients with manifest CHD [13].

Poor individual stress management is the general concept underlying most of the intervention programmes that have been proposed in relation to primary prevention of CHD. One aspect of this could, for instance, be covert coping, which has been shown in a recent prospective study to be an independent predictor of MI risk [14]. Covert coping—a tendency to cope passively with unfair treatment at work and not to discuss the problem with colleagues and superiors—is a result of both individual experiences and the working conditions [15]. Covert coping is therefore a potential target to be addressed from the point of view of both the individual and the environment. Outside work, an intervention trial (ENRICHD; Enhancing Recovery in Coronary Heart Disease) has been performed in which efforts to improve social support and the social network were combined with an approach aimed at decreased depressive tendencies [16].

Individual psychosocial interventions in CHD

Evaluations of CHD-related health effects of individual programmes relevant to psychosocial prevention of CHD have been done as secondary preventive trials. The evidence for the feasibility of such programmes in primary prevention is accordingly indirect.

One of the established CHD risk factors, high BP, has been used as an outcome variable in intervention trials. Hypertension and high BP will therefore be included in this review because of the established relationship between high BP and CHD risk—with the underlying hypothesis that interventions that lead to a lowered BP will also decrease CHD risk.

The social network and social support outside work

Lack of a social network and social support are established independent risk factors for CHD in both men and women [17,18]. Accordingly efforts to improve social network/support would be a logical component in primary CHD prevention. The only large-scale random trial that has tested the feasibility and effects of such efforts has been the ENRICHD study [16] mentioned earlier. Since in that study the focus was not just on social networks/support, there is no published large-scale strict evaluation that has tested possible effects of a 'pure' network/support strategy. There have been discussions about whether the mechanism underlying the association between social network/support and CHD risk is direct (i.e. a lack of social support acts as a stressor) or indirect (i.e. good support helps one to cope with stressors).

Family conditions important in the development of CHD

A poor marital relationship has been shown to be of particular significance for the development of CHD in women [19]: a longitudinal study of women who were followed after a first acute coronary event showed that the degree of coronary atherosclerosis according to angiography progressed more rapidly among women who had both job strain and poor marital relationships compared with other working cohabiting women. Interaction between job conditions and family situation was observed. As a consequence, supportive discussions regarding marital conditions were an integral part of a secondary CHD prevention programme [20].

Results of intervention trials based upon strategies outside work

A review by Spence et al. [21] of individualized stress management interventions based upon a systematic literature search came to the conclusion that such interventions (key words in the literature search were 'psychological', 'behavioural', 'cognitive', 'relaxation', 'meditation', 'biofeedback', and 'stress management') are of value in the treatment of high BP. In particular, the authors point out the value of individualized cognitive–behavioural interventions. There are a wide range of non-pharmacological behavioural programmes for stress management, and since Spence et al.'s original work computer-based programmes have been introduced. In 2005 a randomized control trial evaluation [22] of a computer-based stress management programme at work sites showed beneficial effects after 6 months on physiological stress parameters of relevance to CHD as well as regeneration (a significantly better development of DHEA-S plasma concentration in stress management). Self-reported indices of stress-related symptoms also improved significantly during the first 6 months in the intervention group but not in the control group. However, after 12 months none of the significant differences between the groups were sustained. It should therefore be cautioned that many of the evaluation studies in the literature have had relatively short follow-up periods and questions related to the long-lasting sustainability of effects are therefore important. In general these studies do point at the possibility of using individualized stress management programmes in CHD prevention.

The follow-up effects of psychosocial interventions in secondary CHD prevention (i.e. preventing a second heart attack) were summarized by Schneiderman and Orth-Gomer in 2012 [23]. So far there have been six large published prospective studies, three with positive [20,24,25] results and three with null results [16,26,27].

A number of interesting points have been raised in comparisons between the three studies with positive results and those with null results:

1. There is an important interaction between psychosocial interventions and 'conventional' clinical work with patients. When a patient's social and psychological conditions are taken into account it is possible to increase the patient's willingness to follow clinical advice regarding, for example, medication, adopting good eating habits, and doing physical exercise—the dialogue between patient and caregiver becomes more personal and this in itself gives rise to clinical benefits. A 'psychosocial motivation' effect is potentially a very important addendum in preventive work.
2. Some effects of psychosocial interventions may arise after a long time, whereas other effects may disappear rapidly. Therefore a long follow-up is important for judging the usefulness of psychosocial interventions. In the study by Orth-Gomér et al. [20],

the differences in mortality between the intervention group and the control group did not really begin to diverge until after 2 years of follow-up. In the three studies with positive results longer follow-up periods were used than in the other studies.

3. The intensity of the intervention programmes has been an important factor. Two of the successful interventions [24,25] were focused on reduction of type A behaviour (hostility), whereas the third study [20] was directed at improving stress management in general. All these studies had extensively engaging intervention programmes, whereas the programmes in the other three studies were much less extensive. In the study by Berkman et al. [16], the intention was to improve social support. However, that part of the study would have required much more extensive input.
4. There is a clear indication that the programmes need to be gender specific. In the studies published by Frasure-Smith et al. [27] and Berkman et al. [16] there are indications that the women may have been harmed by the intervention. In the Berkman et al. study [16], white men benefitted significantly from the programme with regard to both mortality and incidence of reinfarction whereas women tended to have a worsened risk of recurrence.

To sum this up, there is evidence from some studies that psychosocial interventions aiming at improved coping and stress management may have an important role in CHD prevention programmes. Our patient in the clinical case would probably have benefited from individual stress management counselling. However, the likelihood that such counselling will have sustained effects would have increased had such an intervention taken place concomitantly with an improved work situation.

Psychosocial working conditions in relation to CVD risk

A majority of adults in industrialized countries spend over half of their waking hours at work [28,29]. Work is therefore a major life component. This section will present (1) the most widely used definitions of psychosocial factors at work and the importance of these exposures and (2) the prospective evidence regarding the effect of these psychosocial factors on CVD risk.

Definition and importance of exposure to adverse psychosocial factors at work

Two major theoretical models have been developed to assess the influence on CVD of psychosocial factors at work: the job strain model, developed by Karasek and Theorell [30], and the effort–reward imbalance (ERI) model, elaborated by Siegrist [31]. The two-dimensional job strain model suggests that workers who simultaneously experience high psychological demands and low job control (decision latitude) are more likely to develop stress-related health problems [30]. Psychological demands refer to an excessive work load, having to work very hard or very fast, doing unexpected tasks, and receiving conflicting demands. Job control is a combination of skill discretion (learning new activities, opportunities to develop skills, creativity, variety of activities, nonrepetitive work) and decision authority (taking part in decisions affecting oneself, making one's own decisions, having a say in the job, and freedom as to how the work is accomplished).

Johnson et al. [32] introduced social support at work from supervisors and colleagues as a third component of the job strain model. The combination of the three factors, high psychological demand, low job control, and low social support at work, called iso-strain, is hypothesized to carry an increased risk of illness.

The second model, ERI, proposes that extrinsic efforts should be rewarded in various ways [31,33]. Workers sense a detrimental imbalance when high extrinsic effort is accompanied by low reward. Extrinsic effort refers to intense time pressure, frequent interruptions, numerous responsibilities, increased workload, and mandatory overtime. In order to counteract such efforts, three types of reward were proposed by Siegrist: income, esteem, and occupational status control (job security, promotion prospects, and unforced job change). A third component, over-commitment, a personal coping style expressed through an inability to withdraw from work obligations, impatience, irritability, and a high need for approval, is also included in this model [31].

The high proportion of individuals exposed to such adverse psychosocial factors at work underlies their public health and clinical relevance. Indeed, in studies of large samples in various workplaces in the United States, Europe, and Japan, approximately 20% of workers are exposed to high job strain (see ➲ Fig. 18.4).

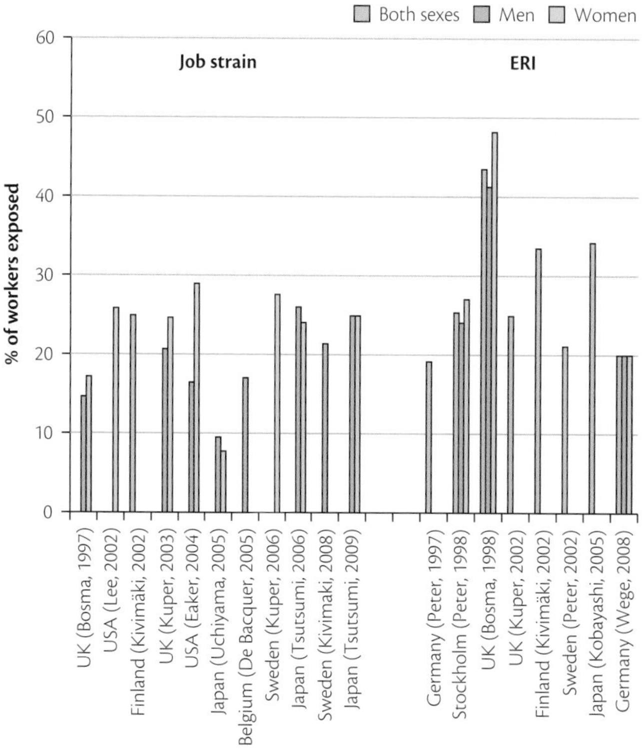

Fig. 18.4 Proportion of workers exposed to job strain or effort–reward imbalance in various countries and workplaces.

Similarly, approximately 20–25% of workers are exposed to ERI. Exposure to these stressors is therefore as prevalent as cigarette smoking (21%), a known CVD risk factor [34].

Psychosocial factors at work and cardiovascular risk

Job strain and CVD risk

The contribution of job strain to the development of CVD has been investigated in prospective studies conducted in the United States, Europe, and Japan (➲ Table 18.1). These studies included general population samples as well as a variety of workplaces. Studies conducted in workplaces were composed of white-collar and industrial employees of various ages. Length of follow-up was typically 5 years or more. Outcomes that have been investigated include all CVD events, fatal CVD, non-fatal MI, stroke, and angina pectoris. Methodological issues and reviews of this literature are provided in references [8,35–37].

Prospective studies using self-reported exposure assessments and conducted in working age populations are presented in ➲ Table 18.1. These studies have avoided the well-documented bias of job title exposure scores [36–38] and older populations.

Table 18.1 Prospective studies of job strain and CVD risk

Author, year	No. of participants and gender	Age at baseline (years), population type, country	Follow-up (years)	Exposure assessment	Event	Results for	RR and 95% CI
Prospective studies using a self-reported measure of exposure to job strain and conducted in a working-age population							
Tsutsumi, 2009 [77]	3191 M, 3363 F	18–65, general working population, Japan	11	Self-reported	Stroke morbidity and mortality	Job strain (M and F)	M: 2.53 (1.08–5.94) F: 1.46 (0.63–3.38)
Kivimaki, 2008 [78]	3160 M	19–65, general working population, Sweden	10	Self-reported	Ischaemic disease	Job strain	1.22 (0.75–1.96)
Tsutsumi, 2006 [79]	3659 M, 3995 F	18–65, general working population, Japan	9.4	Self-reported	CVD mortality	Job strain	1.98 (0.59–6.7)
Kornitzer, 2006 [80]	21 111 M	35–59, general working population, Belgium, Spain, France, Sweden	3.3	Self-reported	Non-fatal and fatal MI, sudden cardiac death, revascularization for acute coronary event	Job strain	1.46 (0.96–2.25)
Kuper, 2006 [81]	48 066 F	30–50, general working population, Sweden	11	Self-reported	Non-fatal MI and fatal CVD	Full-time workers: job strain	1.0 (0.5–1.9)
Netterstrom, 2006 [82]	659 M	30–60, general working population, Denmark	13–14	Self-reported	Incident IHD	Job strain	2.4 (1.0–5.7)
Uchiyama, 2005 [83]	908 M, 707 F	40–65, treated hypertensive workers free of diagnosed CVD, Japan	5.6	Self-reported	Incident CVD	Job strain (M and F)	M: 1.86 (0.51–6.75) F: 9.05 (1.17–69.86)
De Bacquer, 2005 [84]	14 337 M	35–59, men employed in a variety of occupations, Belgium	3.2	Self-reported	Incident CVD	Job strain and iso-strain	Job strain: 1.26 (0.66–2.41) Iso-strain: 1.92 (1.05–3.54)
Kuper, 2002 [48]	6895 M, 3413 F	35–55, white-collar workers, UK	11.2	Self-reported	Non-fatal MI, angina, CVD death	Job strain (M and F combined)	1.38 (1.10–1.75)
Kivimaki, 2002 [49]	545 M, 267 F	18-65, industrial employees, Finland	25.6	Self-reported	CVD mortality	Job strain	2.22 (1.04–4.73)
Bosma, 1998 [50]	6895 M, 3413 F	35–55, white-collar workers, UK (Whitehall Study)	5.3	Self-reported and external assessment	Any CVD event: self-reported angina and diagnosed IHD	Job strain at baseline* (self-report; M and F)	M: 1.45 (1.03–2.06) F: 1.14 (0.76–1.72)
Johnson, 1989 [32]	7219 M	25–65, general working population, Sweden	9	Self-reported	CVD mortality	Iso-strain	1.92 (1.15–3.21)
Alfredsson, 1985 [85]	958 096 M and F	20–64, general working population, Sweden	1	Imputed by job title	Non-fatal MI (hospitalization)	M: aged 20–54; hectic work and few possibilities to learn things. F: aged 20–64; hectic and monotonous work	M: 1.6 (1.3–1.9)† F: 1.6 (1.1–2.3)†

CVD, cardiovascular disease; M, male; F, female; RR, relative risk; CI, confidence interval; IHD, ischaemic heart disease; MI, myocardial infarction.

*RRs for cumulative exposure of job strain are not mentioned in the study. The risk of any incident CVD for cumulative self-reported low job control is 2.

†These measures correspond to relative hospitalization ratio.

Those studies conducted in men and those conducted in both genders have more consistently reported a higher risk in workers with high strain compared with unexposed workers (see ➲ Table 18.1). Among studies reporting a significant effect, the observed relative risks ranged from 1.38 to 2.4. A recent analysis based upon data from 13 European cohorts presented a risk of 1.23 [8]. In this analysis of a large merged cohort the corresponding population attributable risk for high strain was 3.4%, which was markedly less than the population attributable risk for standard risk factors such as smoking (36%), abdominal obesity (20%), and physical inactivity (12%) [39]. However, it should be pointed out that in some countries, for instance in Sweden, antismoking propaganda has been effective, and therefore the prevalence of smoking is markedly lower than it used to be. On a population basis, the results of further reduction of cardiovascular risk based upon reduced smoking will be more limited than in countries with a high prevalence of smoking. However, it is also important to consider that psychosocial factors at work are notoriously difficult to measure and that such measurement limitations generally lead to an underestimation of their true effects [40]. Also, the analysis of these European cohorts is limited by the use of a single baseline measurement of job strain, which has also been shown to underestimate the true effects on CVD risk [37]. Finally, there are other important psychosocial factors at work, such as ERI and other emerging models, which the available evidence suggests are causally related to CVD risk [37,41]. Therefore, comparison with standard risk factors needs to take these relevant issues into account, especially when examining the potential public health benefit for primary prevention by targeting psychosocial factors at work. It is likely that this benefit is more pronounced than what can be measured at present with available empirical studies.

Gender issues

Previous studies found the deleterious effect of job strain on CVD risk less consistently in women than in men (see ➲ Table 18.1) [35,42,43]. However, in 2012 a prospective analysis of a merged European cohort including 197 473 men and women observed similar effects in men and women [8]. Potential explanations for gender differences include the fact that CVD arises on average 10 years later in women leading to low statistical power to detect an effect in some studies, and different occupational trajectories (often characterized by episodes of not working or reduced working hours episodes due to pregnancy or more family responsibilities than men [36,44,45] resulting in less continuous exposure to psychosocial factors at work). It is important to mention that the proportion of women exposed to high strain was consistently higher than that of men in large studies conducted in the United States and Europe (see ➲ Fig. 18.4). High job strain is therefore a frequent psychosocial exposure in women. Its related cardiovascular risk needs to be further investigated.

Socioeconomic status

The deleterious effect of lower socioeconomic status on CVD risk has been well documented [46,47]. Most prospective studies that reported a deleterious effect of high strain on CVD risk controlled for socioeconomic status, therefore showing an independent effect of job strain. In several studies the effect of high strain on CVD risk has been higher in groups with lower socioeconomic status such as blue-collar workers compared with white-collar workers, although diverging results have also been observed [8.]

Effort–reward imbalance and CVD risk

Several prospective studies conducted in Germany, England, and Finland have evaluated the effect of ERI on CVD risk (see ➲ Table 18.2) [48–51, 52]. Outcomes investigated include fatal CVD, fatal and non-fatal MI, and exertional angina. All of these studies used self-reported exposure assessments and were conducted in working age populations. Four out of five of the studies described in ➲ Table 18.2 included both men and women.

All five studies consistently reported an increased CVD risk, which remained significant after controlling for socioeconomic status and standard risk factors, therefore showing an independent effect on CVD risk. Relative risks observed ranged between 1.26 and 4.53. A meta-analysis including four of these studies showed a summary relative risk of 2.05 (95% CI 0.97–4.32) in men and 2.51 (95% CI 1.58–3.98) in women [37]. Moreover, Bosma et al. [50] showed that ERI remained an independent predictor of CHD after controlling for job control. This finding provides support for mutually independent effects of ERI and job strain.

Table 18.2 Prospective studies of effort–reward imbalance (ERI) and risk of CVD

Author, year	No. of participants, gender	Age at baseline (years), population type, country	F-U (years)	Exposure assessment	Event	RR and 95% CIs
Wege 2008, [51]	1069 M, 730 F	45–65, general working population, Germany	5	Self-reported	Angina on exertion	2.04 (1.43–2.92)
Kivimäki, 2002 [49]	545 M, 267 F	≥18, industrial workers, Finland	25.6	Self-reported	CVD death	2.42 (1.2–5.73)
Kuper, 2002 [48]	6895 M, 3413 F	35–55, white-collar, UK	11	Self-reported	Incident CVD	1.26 (1.03–1.55)
Bosma, 1998 [50]	6895 M, 3413 F	35–55, white-collar, UK	5.3	Self-reported	Incident CVD	M: 2.98 (1.48–5.99); F: 3.59 (1.10–11.7)
Siegrist,1990 [52]	416 M	25–55, blue-collar, Germany	6.5	Self-reported	Incident IHD	4.53 (1.43–14.3)*

RR, relative risk; M, male; F, female; CI: confidence interval; CVD: cardiovascular disease; F-U: follow-up; IHD: ischaemic heart disease.
*The RR and 95% CI are taken from [37]. RR is for either high efforts or low rewards.

Job strain, effort–reward imbalance and other cardiovascular outcomes

Blood pressure

Two recent literature reviews evaluated the effects of job strain and ERI on BP [53,54]. The first review is a narrative report of key studies. It presents evidence pointing toward a deleterious relationship between psychosocial factors at work and BP. The second literature review, which is systematic, observed a deleterious effect of psychosocial factors at work in about half of the published studies. However, more consistent effects were observed in studies of higher methodological quality (prospective design and/or ambulatory BP measures)—which strengthens the evidence for a causal relationship. More consistent effects were also observed for men than for women and for ERI compared with job strain. Among studies showing a significant effect, higher mean systolic and diastolic BP (ranging, respectively, from +1.8 to +11 mmHg and from +0.8 to +17.9 mmHg) and higher odds ratios of hypertension (ranging from 1.18 to 5.77) were observed in workers exposed to psychosocial factors at work compared with non-exposed workers.

There is also some evidence showing a stronger effect on BP when workers are exposed to job strain for longer time [2,55–57] and evidence for a lowering of BP when exposure ceases [55,56]. This temporal dimension of the relationship provides further support for a causal relationship.

Metabolic syndrome and obesity

A deleterious effect of job strain has also been observed in prospective studies on metabolic syndrome and obesity. Indeed, Chandola et al. [58] observed that employees with chronic work stress (i.e. three or more exposures to high strain combined with low social support at work over a 14-year follow-up) were more than twice as likely to have metabolic syndrome than those without work stress (odds ratio of 2.25). In addition, five prospective studies have evaluated the effect of job strain or its components on body mass index (BMI) [59–63] or on change in abdominal circumference [59,64]. Four of these studies observed an adverse effect of either high psychological demands [62], low job control [60–62], or both [59–61,64]. Kivimaki et al. [61] pointed out some of the potential causal mechanisms involved by showing that high job strain was prospectively associated with weight gain among men who were overweight (BMI > 27 kg/m^2) at baseline, while it was associated with weight loss among those who had a low weight [61].

Other psychosocial models and CVD risk

Two emerging theoretical models have identified other psychosocial factors at work that may influence employees' health: the organizational injustice model [65] and the leadership model [66].

The organizational injustice model focuses on three dimensions. The first is injustice in the distribution of resources, which is partly included in the ERI model. The other two components are procedural injustice (decision-making procedures) and relational injustice (fair treatment of employees by supervisors) [65]. In a meta-analysis, Kivimaki et al. [37] presented a summary relative risk of CVD of 1.47 when reporting organizational injustice, adjusted for age, gender, and other standard risk factors for CVD, including job strain and ERI (based on two prospective studies including a total of 7246 men and women). A recent systematic review of prospective studies on mental health also pointed out evidence that organizational injustice can be considered a complementary model to the job strain and ERI models [67].

The model of managerial leadership is defined by managers' behaviours such as consideration for individual employees, provision of clarity in goals and role expectations, and supplying information and feedback [68]. In a 9.7-year prospective study on 3122 Swedish male employees a higher leadership score was associated with a lower risk of ischaemic heart disease [68]. This effect was stronger when the duration of exposure was longer. Although improvement of leadership has not been evaluated specifically in primary CHD prevention, two Swedish controlled evaluation studies have shown that it may be possible to reduce HPA activity—lowered morning plasma cortisol paralleled by improved decision authority—in employees after a year-long psychosocial education programme for managers [69] and that it is also possible to stimulate HPG activity—favourable development of DHEA-S paralleled by improved coping and mental condition in employees after another year-long manager intervention programme [70] designed to improve managers' degree of empathy (a programme with artistic components).

Primary psychosocial interventions in the workplace and cardiovascular outcomes

Based on the empirical evidence previously presented in the section 'Psychosocial working conditions in relation to CVD risk', it is reasonable to assume that primary prevention to reduce exposure to these psychosocial factors at work may contribute to lowering CVD risk. Although there have been no psychosocial workplace intervention studies to evaluate the effect of reducing these exposures on CVD risk per se, some studies have evaluated the effects on other cardiovascular outcomes, namely BP [71,72], catecholamine, and lipids [72,73].

A first study conducted among bus drivers in Stockholm [71] observed a significantly lower systolic BP at work in those who benefited from improved working conditions. A second study conducted among Swedish assembly-line workers [72] showed beneficial effects of a flexible form of work organization on systolic BP during work shifts. One of these studies [72], along with another study conducted among Swedish civil servants [73], also showed significantly lower catecholamine and lipids in workers exposed to the psychosocial workplace intervention.

Both studies on BP were limited by the use of casual BP measurements and small samples ($n = 20$ [71] and $n = 65$ [72]) and did not evaluate the effects of reducing exposure to job strain nor ERI.

Interventions targeting exposure to job strain and effort-reward imbalance to improve work organization and blood pressure

The Quebec psychosocial workplace intervention was conducted in partnership with three public organizations. Briefly, these organizations include over 2200 employees aged 18–65. Their main activity is delivering insurance services to the general population. Their jobs encompass the full range of white-collar occupations, including senior and middle managers, professionals, technicians, and office workers.

A quasi-experimental design with a control group and before–after measures was used. The intervention group comprised a total of 1165 workers (718 women and 447 men, representing 80.7% of all workers). The control group mainly comprised workers employed in two comparable organizations (673 women and 508 men, representing 80.2% of all workers). A baseline measurement of psychosocial factors at work and health indicators was performed in each group before the intervention.

The intervention group was assisted by researchers to identify intervention priorities and agreed to engage in intervention activities, while the control group was not assisted by researchers and was not asked to engage in intervention activities. The intervention was defined as all organizational interventions introduced in the workplace with the explicit goal (or the plausible consequence) of improving employees' situation with regard to one of the four adverse psychosocial factors at work that were considered to be part of the intervention. These four psychosocial factors were based on the job strain and ERI models (high psychological demands, low job control, low social support, and low reward). Decisions regarding these changes were made by the managers. However, managers benefited from a systematic a priori risk evaluation and from qualitative focus groups with workers, both conducted by the researchers, to help them identify intervention targets and priorities.

Management implemented various organizational interventions designed to improve the psychosocial work environment. Examples of major interventions were: implementing regular individual employee/manager meetings on day-to-day matters, organizational restructuring aimed at reducing workload, and slowing down the implementation of important changes in work processes and computer software to allow a period of adaptation. The majority of changes implemented corresponded to the initially identified targets for intervention [74]. In addition, the intervention group implemented interventions to reduce the workload, while this psychosocial factor was not acted upon in the control group. A detailed description of the intervention content is provided elsewhere [74].

A second measurement was taken 6 months after the intervention period. The participation rates in this measurement were 85.9% in the intervention group and 86.1% in the control group. The prevalence of high psychological demands and ERI decreased in the intervention group while no such reduction was observed in the control group. As for health indicators, in the intervention group a modest but significant decrease in mean systolic BP (2.2 mmHg, $p < 0.01$; ➲ Fig. 18.5) was observed. A similar pattern was observed for diastolic blood pressure (➲ Fig. 18.6). No significant decrease was observed in the control group. The beneficial effect of the intervention was significant for both systolic and diastolic BP.

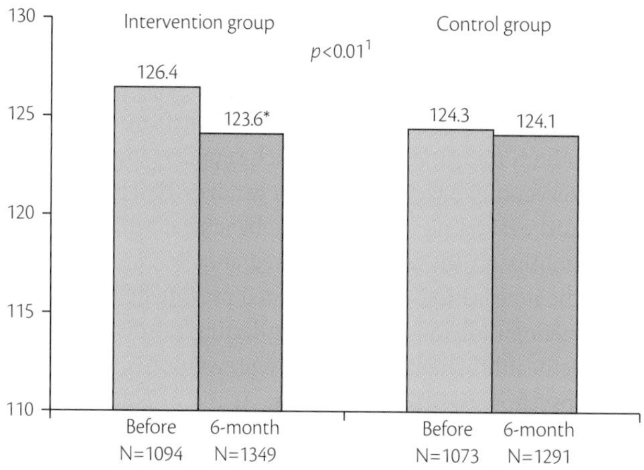

Fig. 18.5 Systolic mean blood pressure (mmHg) before and 6 months after the intervention in the intervention and control groups. Generalized estimating equation analysis controlled for age, gender, education, stressful life events that occurred during the past 12 months, domestic load, smoking status, body mass index and sedentary behaviours, alcohol consumption, family history of cardiovascular disease, and medication for hypertension. [1]The p-value for interaction indicates whether the evolution from before to 6 months is different between the intervention and control groups. *$p \leq 0.05$.

This intervention study has important strengths. A quasi-experimental design including a large number of workers was used. Pre- and post-intervention ambulatory BP measures were measured in each worker every 15 minutes during an entire working day. The intervention was designed to improve precise adverse

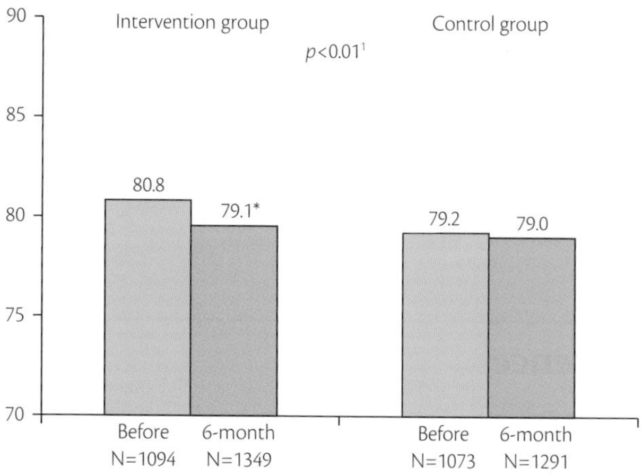

Fig. 18.6 Diastolic mean blood pressure (mmHg) before and 6 months after the intervention in the intervention and control groups. Generalized estimating equation analysis controlled for age, gender, education, stressful life events that occurred during the past 12 months, domestic load, smoking status, body mass index and sedentary behaviours, alcohol consumption, family history of cardiovascular disease, and medication for hypertension. [1]The p-value for interaction indicates whether the evolution from before to 6 months is different between the intervention and control groups. *$p \leq 0.05$.

psychosocial factors at work based on two well-grounded theoretical models and assessed with validated scales. The participation rates at both measurements were very good, which limits the likelihood of selection bias. The beneficial effects on BP were observed in both men and women, which supports the consistency of the intervention effects across both genders. Finally, the results of the third evaluation show that the beneficial effects observed after 6 months on BP were maintained after 30 months [75]. In light of the non-lasting effects presented previously for interventions targeting individuals, these long-lasting results suggest better public health benefits for primary prevention which reduces adverse psychosocial factors at work. At the population level, a 2 mmHg reduction in systolic BP would lead to a reduction of middle-age mortality from CHD and stroke of about 7% and 10%, respectively [75].

In conclusion, there is some previous evidence that primary prevention by interventions that reduce exposure to psychosocial factors at work lead to favourable changes in cardiovascular indicators [71–73]. In addition, results from a recent large prospective intervention study of men and women using a quasi-experimental design with a control group show that reducing exposure to job strain and ERI leads to modest but significant and long-lasting improvement in workers' ambulatory BP [75, 76].

Case resolution

The case illustrates several of the points made in this chapter:

1. The clinical importance of self-monitoring of BP for patients with unstable BP.
2. The deterioration of psychosocial working conditions due to increasing financial constraints leading to increased psychological demands and decreased influence over working conditions with poor support from superiors as well as a poor balance between effort and reward.
3. The interplay between psychosocial working conditions and individual efforts to cope—in current theory often referred to as 'over-commitment'.
4. Both primary and secondary prevention aspects: primary prevention because improved regulation of BP could be seen as primary prevention of CVD, and secondary prevention because this patient had suffered a stroke and secondary prevention aimed at reducing the risk of recurrence.

The advice to this woman was to change her job. She left her job and re-trained. After this she obtained a post as an administrator and her clinical condition improved. However, as described in this chapter, the patient would have benefited from both individual stress management training and an improved work situation and work organization.

Further reading

Chandola T, Brunner E, Marmot M. Chronic stress at work and the metabolic syndrome: prospective study. *Br Med J* 2006; **332**: 521–5.

Gulliksson M, Burell G, Vessby B, et al. Randomized controlled trial of cognitive behavioral therapy vs. standard treatment to prevent recurrent cardiovascular events in patients; 1; with coronary heart disease. *Arch Intern Med* 2011; **171**: 134–40.

Karasek RA, Theorell T. *Healthy work: stress, productivity and the reconstruction of working life*, 1990. New York: Basic Books.

Kivimäki M, Nyberg ST, Batty GD, et al. Job strain as a risk factor for future coronary heart disease: Collaborative metaanalysis of 2358 events in 197,473 men and women. *Lancet*, 2012; **380**: 1491–7.

Nyberg A, Alfredsson L, Theorell T, et al. Managerial leadership and ischaemic heart disease among employees: the Swedish WOLF study. *Occup Environ Med* 2009; **66**: 51–5.

Orth-Gomer K, Wamala SP, Horsten M, et al. Marital stress worsens prognosis in women with coronary heart disease: the Stockholm female coronary risk study. *J Am Med Assoc* 2000; **284**: 3008–14.

Schneiderman N, Orth-Gomér K. Randomized clinical trials. Psychosocial-behavioral interventions for cardiovascular disease. *Handbook of health psychology*, 2nd edn, 2012. New York: Psychology Press, Taylor and Francis.

Siegrist J. Adverse health effects of high-effort/low-reward conditions. *J Occup Health Psychol* 1996; **1**: 27–41.

Williams R, Schneiderman N, Relman A, et al. Resolved: psychosocial interventions can improve clinical outcomes in organic disease-rebuttals and closing arguments. *Psychosom Med* 2002; **64**: 564–7.

References

1 Williams R, Schneiderman N, Relman A, et al. Resolved: psychosocial interventions can improve clinical outcomes in organic disease—rebuttals and closing arguments. *Psychosom Med* 2002; **64**: 564–7.

2 Markovitz JH, Matthews KA, Whooley M, et al. Increases in job strain are associated with incident hypertension in the CARDIA Study. *Ann Behav Med* 2004; **28**: 4–9.

3 Groeschel M, Braam B. Connecting chronic and recurrent stress to vascular dysfunction: no relaxed role for the renin-angiotensin system. *Am J Physiol Renal Physiol* 2011; **300**: F1–F10.

4 Lu XT, Zhao YX, Zhang Y, et al. Psychological stress, vascular inflammation and atherogenesis: potential roles of circulating cytokines. *J Cardiovasc Pharmacol* 2013; **62**: 6–12.

5 Fisher JP, Paton JF. The sympathetic nervous system and blood pressure in humans: implications for hypertension. *J Hum Hypertens* 2012; **26**: 463–75.

6 Shufelt C, Bretsky P, Almeida CM, et al. DHEA-S levels and cardiovascular disease mortality in postmenopausal women: results from the National Institutes of Health—National Heart, Lung, and Blood Institute (NHLBI)-sponsored Women's Ischemia Syndrome Evaluation (WISE). *J Clin Endocrinol Metab* 2010; **95**: 4985–92.

7 De Couck M, Mravec B, Gidron Y. You may need the vagus nerve to understand pathophysiology and to treat diseases. *Clin Sci (Lond)* 2012; **122**: 323–8.

8 Kivimäki M, Nyberg ST, Batty GD, et al. Job strain as a risk factor for future coronary heart disease: collaborative metaanalysis of 2358 events in 197,473 men and women. *Lancet* 2012; **380**: 1491–7.
9 Coyne JC: Improving coping research: Raze the slum before any more building? *J Health Psychol* 1997; **2**: 153–72.
10 Rosenman R, Brand RJ, Scholtz RI, et al. Multivariate prediction of coronary heart disease during 8.5 year follow-up in the Western Collaborative Group Study. *Am J Cardiol* 1976; **37**: 903–10.
11 Chida Y, Steptoe A. The association of anger and hostility with future coronary heart disease—a meta-analytic review of prospective evidence. *J Am Coll Cardiol* 2009; **53**: 936–46.
12 Rugulies R. Depression as a predictor for coronary heart disease. A review and meta-analysis. *Am J Prev Med* 2002; **23**: 51–61.
13 Denollet J. Type D personality. A potential risk factor refined. *J Psychosom Res* 2000; **49**: 255–66.
14 Leineweber C, Westerlund H, Theorell T, et al. Covert coping with unfair treatment at work risk of incident myocardial infarction and cardiac death among men: prospective cohort study. *J Epidemiol Commun Health* 2011; **65**: 420–5.
15 Theorell T, Westerlund H, Alfredsson L, et al. Coping with critical life events and lack of control—the exertion of control. *Psychoneuroendocrinology* 2005; **30**: 1027–32.
16 Berkman LF, Blumenthal J, Burg M, et al. (Enhancing Recovery in Coronary Heart Disease Patients investigators). Effects of treating depression and low perceived social support on clinical events after myocardial infarction: the Enhancing Recovery in Coronary Heart Disease Patients (ENRICHD) randomized trial. *J Am Med Assoc* 2003; **289**: 3106–16.
17 Rosengren A, Wilhelmsen L, Orth-Gomér K. Coronary disease in relation to social support and social class in Swedish men. A 15 year follow-up in the study of men born in 1933. *Eur Heart J* 2004; **25**: 56–63.
18 Blom M, Janszky I, Balog P, et al. Social relations in women with coronary heart disease: the effects of work and marital stress. *J Cardiovasc Risk* 2003; **10**: 201–6.
19 Wang HX, Leineweber C, Kirkeeide R, et al. Psychosocial stress and atherosclerosis: family and work stress accelerate progression of coronary disease in women. The Stockholm Female Coronary Angiography Study. *J Intern Med* 2007; **261**: 245–54.
20 Orth-Gomér K, Schneiderman N, Wang H, et al. Stress reduction prolongs life in women with coronary disease: the Stockholm Women's Intervention Trial for Coronary Heart Disease (SWITCHD). *Circulation: Cardiovasc Qual Outcomes* 2009; **2**: 25–32.
21 Spence JD, Barnett PA, Linden W, et al. Lifestyle modifications to prevent and control hypertension. 7. Recommendations on stress management. Canadian Hypertension Society, Canadian Coalition for High Blood Pressure Prevention and Control, Laboratory Centre for Disease Control at Health Canada, Heart and Stroke Foundation of Canada. *Can Med Assoc J* 1999; **160**: 46–50.
22 Hasson D, Anderberg UM, Theorell T, et al. Psychophysiological effects of a web-based stress management system: a prospective, randomized controlled intervention study of IT and media workers. *BMC Publ Health* 2005; **5**: 78.
23 Schneiderman N, Orth-Gomér K. Randomized clinical trials. Psychosocial-behavioral interventions for cardiovascular disease. *Handbook of health psychology*, 2nd edn, 2012. New York: Psychology Press, Taylor and Francis.
24 Friedman M, Thoresen CE, Gill JJ, et al. Alteration of type A behavior and its effect on cardiac recurrences in post myocardial infarction patients: summary results of the Recurrent Coronary Prevention Project. *Am Heart J* 1986; **112**: 653–65.
25 Gulliksson M, Burell G, Vessby B, et al. Randomized controlled trial of cognitive behavioral therapy vs. standard treatment to prevent recurrent cardiovascular events in patients with coronary heart disease. *Arch Intern Med* 2011; **171**: 134–40.
26 Jones DA, West RR. Psychological rehabilitation after myocardial infarction: multicentre randomized controlled trial. *Br Med J* 1996; **313**: 1517–21.
27 Frasure-Smith N, Lespérance E, Prince RH, et al. Randomised trial of home-based psychosocial nursing intervention for patients recovering from myocardial infarction. *Lancet* 1997; **350**: 473–9.
28 Bureau of Labor Statistics. *Employment, hours, and earnings from the current employment statistics survey (national)*, 2009. Washington, DC: United States Department of Labor. URL: <http://www.bls.gov>
29 European Foundation for the Improvement of Living and Working Conditions. *Fourth European working conditions survey*, 2006. Dublin: Publications of the European Foundation for Improvement of Living and Working Conditions.
30 Karasek RA, Theorell T. *Healthy work: stress, productivity and the reconstruction of working life*, 1990. New York: Basic Books.
31 Siegrist J. Adverse health effects of high-effort/low-reward conditions. *J Occup Health Psychol* 1996; **1**: 27–41.
32 Johnson JV, Hall EM, Theorell T. Combined effects of job strain and social isolation on cardiovascular disease morbidity and mortality in a random sample of the Swedish male working population. *Scand J Work Environ Health* 1989; **15**: 271–9.
33 Weyers S, Peter R, Boggild, et al. Psychosocial work stress is associated with poor self-rated health in Danish nurses: a test of the effort-reward imbalance model. *Scand J Caring Sci* 2006; **20**: 26–34.
34 American Heart Association. *Heart disease and stroke statistics 2009 update: a report from the American Heart Association Statistics Committee and Stroke Statistics Subcommittee*, 2009. Dallas, TX: American Heart Association.
35 Backe EM, Seidler A, Latza U, et al. The role of psychosocial stress at work for the development of cardiovascular diseases: a systematic review. *Int Arch Occ Env Health* 2012; **85**: 67–79.
36 Belkic KL, Landsbergis PA, Schnall PL, et al. Is job strain a major source of cardiovascular disease risk? *Scand J Work Environ Health* 2004; **30**: 85–128.
37 Kivimaki M, Virtanen M, Elovainio M, et al. Work stress in the etiology of coronary heart disease—a meta-analysis. *Scand J Work Environ Health* 2006; **32**: 431–42.
38 Schwartz JE, Pieper CF, Karasek RA. A procedure for linking psychosocial job characteristics data to health surveys. *Am J Public Health* 1988; **78**: 904–9.
39 Yusuf S, Hawken S, Ounpuu S, et al. Effect of potentially modifiable risk factors associated with myocardial infarction in 52 countries (the INTERHEART study): case-control study. *Lancet* 2004; **364**: 937–52.
40 Rothman KJ, Greenland S, Last TL. *Modern epidemiology*, 3rd edn, 2008. Philadelphia: Wolters Kluwer, Lippincott Williams & Wilkins.
41 Aboa-Eboule C, Brisson C, Maunsell E, et al. Effort-reward imbalance at work and recurrent coronary heart disease events: a 4-year prospective study of post-myocardial infarction patients. *Psychosom Med* 2011; **73**: 436–47.
42 Eller NH, Netterstrom B, Gyntelberg F, et al. Work-related psychosocial factors and the development of ischemic heart disease: a systematic review. *Cardiol Rev* 2009; **17**: 83–97.
43 Hemingway H, Marmot M. Evidence based cardiology: psychosocial factors in the aetiology and prognosis of coronary heart disease: systematic review of prospective cohort studies. *Br Med J* 1999; **318**: 1460–7.
44 Brisson C. Women, work and cardiovascular disease. *The workplace and cardiovascular disease. Occupational Medicine state of the art reviews*, Vol. 5, 2000, pp. 49–57. Philadelphia: Hanley & Belfus.
45 Orth-Gomer K, Wamala SP, Horsten M, et al. Marital stress worsens prognosis in women with coronary heart disease: the Stockholm Female Coronary Risk Study. *J Am Med Assoc* 2000; **284**: 3008–14.
46 Marmot M, Wilkinson RG. *Social determinants of health*, 1999. Oxford: Oxford University Press.

47 Siegrist J, Theorell T. Socio-economic position and health: the role of work and employment. In: Siegrist J, Marmot M. (eds) *Social inequalities in health: new evidence and policy implications*, 2006, pp. 73–100. Oxford: Oxford University Press.

48 Kuper H, Singh-Manoux A, Siegrist J, et al. When reciprocity fails: effort-reward imbalance in relation to coronary heart disease and health functioning within the Whitehall II study. *Occup Environ Med* 2002; **59**: 777–84.

49 Kivimaki M, Leino-Arjas P, Luukkonen R, et al. Work stress and risk of cardiovascular mortality: prospective cohort study of industrial employees. *Br Med J* 2002; **325**: 857–60.

50 Bosma H, Peter R, Siegrist J, et al. Two alternative job stress models and the risk of coronary heart disease. *Am J Public Health* 1998; **88**: 68–74.

51 Wege N, Dragano N, Erbel R, et al. When does work stress hurt? Testing the interaction with socioeconomic position in the Heinz Nixdorf Recall Study. *J Epidemiol Commun Health* 2008; **62**: 338–41.

52 Siegrist J, Peter R, Junge A, et al. Low status control, high effort at work and ischemic heart disease: prospective evidence from blue-collar men. *Soc Sci Med* 1990; **31**: 1127–34.

53 Rosenthal T, Alter A. Occupational stress and hypertension. *J Am Soc Hypertens* 2012; **6**: 2–22.

54 Gilbert-Ouimet M, Trudel X, Brisson C, et al. Adverse effect of psychosocial work factors on blood pressure: A systematic review of studies on the demand-control-support and the effort-reward imbalance models. *Scand J Work Environ Health* 2014; **40**: 109–32.

55 Laflamme N, Brisson C, Moisan J, et al. Job strain and ambulatory blood pressure among female white-collar workers. *Scand J Work Environ Health* 1998; **24**: 334–43.

56 Landsbergis PA, Schnall PL, Warren K, et al. Association between ambulatory blood pressure and alternative formulations of job strain. *Scand J Work Environ Health* 1994; **20**: 349–63.

57 Riese H, Van Doornen LJ, Houtman IL, et al. Job strain in relation to ambulatory blood pressure, heart rate, and heart rate variability among female nurses. *Scand J Work Environ Health* 2004; **30**: 477–85.

58 Chandola T, Brunner E, Marmot M. Chronic stress at work and the metabolic syndrome: prospective study. *Br Med J* 2006; **332**: 521–5.

59 Ishizaki M, Nakagawa H, Morikawa Y, et al. Influence of job strain on changes in body mass index and waist circumference—6-year longitudinal study. *Scand J Work Environ Health* 2008; **34**: 288–96.

60 Block JP, He Y, Zaslavsky AM, et al. Psychosocial stress and change in weight among US adults. *Am J Epidemiol* 2009; **170**: 181–92.

61 Kivimaki M, Head J, Ferrie JE, et al. Work stress, weight gain and weight loss: evidence for bidirectional effects of job strain on body mass index in the Whitehall II Study. *Int J Obes (Lond)*. 2006; **30**: 982–7.

62 Berset M, Semmer NK, Elfering A, et al. Does stress at work make you gain weight? A two-year longitudinal study. *Scand J Work Environ Health* 2011; **37**: 45–53.

63 Eek F, Östergren PO. Factors associated with BMI change over five years in a Swedish adult population. Results from the Scania Public Health Cohort Study. *Scand J Public Health* 2009; **37**: 532–44.

64 Brunner EJ, Chandola T, Marmot MG. Prospective effect of job strain on general and central obesity in the Whitehall II Study. *Am J Epidemiol* 2007; **165**: 828–37.

65 Moorman R. Relationship between organizational justice and organizational citizenship behavior: do fairness perceptions influence employee citizenship? *J Appl Psychol* 1991; **76**: 845–55.

66 Nyberg A. *The impact of managerial leadership on stress and health among employees*, 2009. Stockholm: Jarolinska Institutet.

67 Ndjaboue R, Brisson C, Vézina M. Occupational justice and mental health: a systematic review of prospective studies. *Occup Environ Med* 2012; **69**: 694–700.

68 Nyberg A, Alfredsson L, Theorell T, et al. Managerial leadership and ischaemic heart disease among employees: the Swedish WOLF study. *Occup Environ Med* 2009; **66**: 51–5.

69 Theorell T, Emdad R, Arnetz B, et al. Employee effects of an educational program for managers at an insurance company. *Psychosom Med* 2001; **63**: 724–33.

70 Romanowska J, Larsson G, Eriksson M, et al. Health effects on leaders and co-workers of an art-based leadership development program. *Psychother Psychosom* 2011; **80**: 78–87.

71 Rydstedt LW, Johansson G, Evans GW. The human side of the road: Improving the working conditions of urban bus drivers. *J Occup Health Psychol* 1998; **3**: 161–71.

72 Melin B, Lundberg U, Söderlund J, et al. Psychological and physiological stress reactions of male and female assembly workers: a comparison between two different forms of work organizations. *J Organiz Behav* 1999; **20**: 47–61.

73 Orth-Gomer K, Eriksson I, Moser V, et al. Lipid lowering through work stress reduction. *Int J Behav Med* 1994; **1**: 204–14.

74 Gilbert-Ouimet M, Baril-Gingras G, Brisson C, et al. Changes implemented during a workplace psychosocial intervention and their consistency with intervention priorities. *Journal of Occupational and Environmental Medicine*. In press 2015.

75 Trudel X, Milot A, Brisson C, et al. Blood pressure reduction following intervention on psychosocial work factors: a longitudinal study. *J Hypertens* 2011; 29, suppl A e 118.

76 Brisson C, Cantin V, Larocque B. Intervention research on work organization factors and health: research design and preliminary results on mental health. *Can J Commun Ment Health* 2006; **25**: 241–59.

77 Tsutsumi A, Kayaba K, Kario K, et al. Prospective study on occupational stress and risk of stroke. *Arch Intern Med* 2009; **169**: 56–61.

78 Kivimaki M, Theorell T, Westerlund H, et al. Job strain and ischaemic disease: does the inclusion of older employees in the cohort dilute the association? The WOLF Stockholm Study. *J Epidemiol Commun Health* 2008; **62**: 372–4.

79 Tsutsumi A, Kayaba K, Hirokawa K, et al. Psychosocial job characteristics and risk of mortality in a Japanese community-based working population: the Jichi Medical School Cohort Study. *Soc Sci Med* 2006; **63**: 1276–88.

80 Kornitzer M, deSmet P, Sans S, et al. Job stress and major coronary events: results from the Job Stress, Absenteeism and Coronary Heart Disease in Europe study. *Eur J Cardiovasc Prev Rehabil* 2006; **13**: 695–704.

81 Kuper H, Marmot M. Job strain, job demands, decision latitude, and risk of coronary heart disease within the Whitehall II study. *J Epidemiol Commun Health* 2003; **57**: 147–53.

82 Netterstrom B, Kristensen TS, Sjol A. Psychological job demands increase the risk of ischaemic heart disease: a 14-year cohort study of employed Danish men. *Eur J Cardiovasc Prev Rehabil* 2006; **13**: 414–20.

83 Uchiyama S, Kurasawa T, Sekizawa T, et al. Job strain and risk of cardiovascular events in treated hypertensive Japanese workers: hypertension follow-up group study. *J Occup Health* 2005; **47**: 102–11.

84 De Bacquer D, Pelfrene E, Clays E, et al. Perceived job stress and incidence of coronary events: 3-year follow-up of the Belgian Job Stress Project cohort. *Am J Epidemiol* 2005; **161**: 434–41.

85 Alfredsson L, Spetz C-L, Theorell T. Type of occupation and near-future hospitalization for myocardial infarction and some other diagnoses. *Int J Epidemiol* 1985; **14**: 378–88.

CHAPTER 19

Cardioprotective drugs

Johan De Sutter, Miguel Mendes, and Oscar H. Franco

Contents

Summary

Cardioprotective drugs are important in the treatment of patients at risk for or with documented cardiovascular disease (CVD). Beta-blockers are indicated for a wide range of patients with cardiac pathologies, including acute coronary syndrome, stable coronary artery disease, heart failure, and arrhythmias. Most evidence on cardiovascular morbidity and mortality is available for patients post-myocardial infarction (MI) and those with chronic systolic heart failure. Ivabradine is a specific heart-rate-lowering agent which acts on the sinoatrial node cells by selectively and specifically inhibiting the pacemaker I_f current. It can be used for the symptomatic treatment of chronic stable angina pectoris in patients with coronary artery disease (CAD) in sinus rhythm and a heart rate remaining at 70 or more beats/min. Accordingly, in systolic heart failure it reduces the risk of hospitalization for heart failure in patients in sinus rhythm with a heart rate remaining at 70 or more beats/min and persisting symptoms. Angiotensin-converting enzyme inhibitors (ACEi), together with other drugs like beta-blockers, statins, and antiplatelets, are one of the cornerstones of CVD prevention in congestive heart failure, stable angina, and post-acute MI and in secondary prevention after any event or revascularization procedure in CAD. They are also the first-line medication in hypertension, namely in the presence of renal dysfunction, diabetes, or diabetes nephropathy. Angiotensin receptor blockers (ARBs) are mainly alternative drugs for the same indications in case of intolerance to ACEi. ACEi and ARBs should not be used together, except in rare situations, due to the risk of deterioration of renal function and hyperkalaemia. The aldosterone antagonists (AAs) spironolactone and eplerenone are indicated in patients with New York Heart Association class III–IV heart failure or acute MI with impaired left ventricular function, and may also have a role in hypertension. Aliskiren, a direct renin inhibitor (DRi), belongs to the most recent and less studied renin–angiotensin–aldosterone (RAAS) receptor blocker group. For the moment it only has a clinical indication for hypertension. Calcium channel blockers (CCBs) are first-line medication in patients with isolated systolic hypertension, black people, and during pregnancy, in the presence of intermittent claudication, asymptomatic atherosclerosis, or metabolic syndrome. They can be used together with diuretics, ACEi, ARBs, or beta-blockers, with the aim of reaching the guideline-recommended blood pressure targets, improving the surrogate end-points, and limiting side effects. CCBs have also shown clinical efficacy in angina pectoris, alone or in combination with beta-blockers and/or with long-acting nitrates. The non-dihydropyridines verapamil and diltiazem are an alternative to beta-blockers in stable CAD, and can be used alone

(continued)

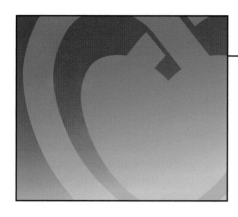

or in association with other drugs to control the ventricular rate in atrial fibrillation or flutter or to prevent some supraventricular tachycardias. Despite great advances in the prevention and treatment of CVD, it remains one of the main causes of mortality and morbidity. Under the principle that a large preventive effect for CVD would require intervention on everyone at increased risk irrespective of their risk factors levels, modifying several risk factors together, and reducing these by as much as possible, in 2003 Wald and Law proposed the polypill concept. A polypill is a pill in which multiple medications effective in the prevention of CVD (e.g. statins, antihypertensives, and aspirin) are combined in a single pill. The concept also includes the strategy of giving this combination pill to everyone over 55 years of age and all those with existing CVD irrespective of age, and stopping all efforts focused on measuring risk factors and screening for CVD. Since the introduction of the concept, much debate has been generated regarding the potential role of a polypill in CVD prevention and treatment, and multiple efforts have focused on developing and testing polypills. Further evaluation on the safety and long-term efficacy of polypills is required, but initial reports are promising and polypills could soon play a crucial role in the treatment and prevention of CVD.

Clinical case

A 63-year-old man with a history of smoking and chronic obstructive pulmonary disease was admitted for a ST-segment elevation myocardial infarction that was treated in the acute phase with primary percutaneous coronary intervention and stenting of the proximal left anterior descending coronary artery. At discharge his echocardiography showed a left ventricular ejection fraction of 45% due to apical hypokinesia without arguments for elevated filling pressures or significant valvular heart disease. He was discharged with a statin, dual antiplatelet therapy, carvedilol 25 mg/day, and lisinopril 10 mg/day.

Two weeks later he is seen for his first out-patient consultation before the start of a cardiac rehabilitation programme. He has no angina and has stopped smoking. However, he mentions complaints of dyspnoea and wheezing. Physical examination shows no signs of fluid retention, but lung auscultation reveals mild wheezing and a prolonged expirium. His blood pressure is 150/90 mmHg and his electrocardiogram shows a regular sinus rhythm 80 beats/min and Q waves in leads V1–V4. The exercise test was stopped because of dyspnoea but no clinical or electrocardiographic signs of ischaemia were noted. His maximal blood pressure was 220/100 mmHg.

Is this patient on an optimal drug treatment? How long should his beta-blocker and angiotensin-converting enzyme inhibitor be continued?

Introduction

This chapter will discuss the important role of beta-blockers, ivabradine, angiotensin-converting enzyme inhibitors (ACEi), angiotensin-receptor blockers (ARBs), and calcium antagonists for either the primary or secondary prevention of cardiovascular disease (CVD). Also the concept of the polypill will be explained as well as our current knowledge on its efficacy, side effects, and cost-effectiveness. Drugs used to prevent thrombosis or for the management of risk factors such as dyslipidaemias, elevated blood pressure, or type 2 diabetes are discussed in ➲ Chapters 17, 15, 14, and 16, respectively. Vitamins, omega-3 fatty acids or other 'nutriceuticals' are dealt with in ➲ Chapter 11.

Beta-blockers

Mechanisms and cardiovascular effects

Beta-adrenergic antagonists, or beta-blockers, bind selectively to beta-adrenoreceptors, resulting in competitive and reversible antagonism of the effect of beta-adrenergic stimuli on various organs. Their prevention of the cardiotoxic effects of catecholamines plays a central role in the treatment of different CVDs [1]. Their anti-ischaemic actions are a result of a decrease in myocardial oxygen demand due to the reduction in heart rate, cardiac contractility, and systolic pressure. They may also increase myocardial perfusion by prolongation of diastole caused by the reduction in heart rate. Their antihypertensive action is a result of inhibition of the release of renin and production of angiotensin II, blockade of pre-synaptic alpha-adrenoreceptors that increase the release of norepinephrine from sympathetic nerve terminals, and decrease of central vasomotor activity and peripheral vasodilator activity mediated via alpha-1 adrenoreceptor blockade (e.g. with carvedilol and labetalol). Many additional myocardial effects have been described, such as improvement of myocardial energetics by inhibition of catecholamine-induced release of free fatty acids from adipose tissue, reduction of myocardial oxidative stress, inhibition of cardiac apoptosis, and substantial improvement of cardiac remodelling. Beta-blockers also have anti-arrhythmic effects as a result of their reduction of heart rate, decrease of spontaneous firing of ectopic pacemakers, slowing of conduction, and increase of the refractory period of the atrioventricular (AV) node [2].

Beta-blockers can be classified into non-selective agents (combined beta-1 and beta-2 blockers), cardioselective beta-1 antagonists, and beta-blockers with vasodilatory properties through direct [possibly nitric oxide (NO)-mediated] vasodilation and added alpha-1 adrenergic blockade. Some beta-blockers, such as pindolol and acebutolol, show a weak agonist response (intrinsic sympathicomimetic activity) and can stimulate and block the beta-adrenoreceptor. However, they are used less frequently today. All beta-blockers have anti-arrhythmic properties by their class II activity. Sotalol is an unique long-acting non-selective

Table 19.1 Types and typical dosages of the most frequently used beta-blockers

	ISA	Lipid solubility	Peripheral vasodilation	Average daily oral dose
Non-selective antagonists:				
Pindolol	++	+	0	10–40 mg twice a day
Propranolol	0	+++	0	40–160 mg twice a day
Sotalol*	0	0	0	80–160 mg twice a day
Timolol	0	+	0	5–40 mg twice a day
Selective beta-1 antagonists:				
Atenolol	0	0	0	25–100 mg once a day
Bisoprolol	0	+	0	2.5–10 mg once a day
Celiprolol	+	+	+	200–600 mg once a day
Esmolol	0	0	0	IV only
Metoprolol-SR	0	+	0	50–200 mg once/twice a day
Nebivolol	0	+++	+	2.5–10 mg once a day
Alpha-1 and beta antagonists:				
Carvedilol				
Labetalol	0	+	+	3.125–50 mg twice a day
	+	+++	+	200–800 mg twice a day

0, no effect; +, mild effect; ++, moderate effect; +++, strong effect.

ISA, intrinsic sympathicomimetic activity; IV, intravenous administration possible; SR, slow release.

*For ventricular arrhythmias and atrial fibrillation.

Source: data from Lopez-Sandon J, Swedberg K, McMurray J, Tamargo J, Maggioni A, Dargie H, Tendera M, Waagstein F, Kjekshus J, Lechat P, Torp-Pedersen C. Expert consensus document on β-adrenergic receptor blockers. The Task Force on Beta-Blockers of the European Society of Cardiology. *Eur Heart J* 2004; **25**: 1341–1362 and Opie LH and Gersh BJ. *Drugs for the heart*, 7th Edition, 2009. Chapter 1, pages 1–37. Saunders, Elsevier Inc.

beta-blocker with added class III anti-arrhythmic activity that is specifically used for the treatment of arrhythmias. Types and typical dosages of the most frequently used beta-blockers for patients with coronary artery disease and heart failure are summarized in ➲ Table 19.1 [1,2].

Indications

The indications for beta-blockers are summarized in ➲ Boxes 19.1 and 19.2. Beta-blockers are indicated for a wide range of patients with cardiac pathologies, including acute coronary syndrome (ACS), stable coronary artery disease (CAD), heart failure, and arrhythmias. Their place in the treatment of hypertension is discussed in ➲ Chapter 14.

Acute coronary syndrome

Several trials and meta-analyses have demonstrated that beta-blockers reduce mortality and reinfarction by 20–25% in those who have recovered from an infarction. The best studied beta-blockers for this indication are propranolol, metoprolol, carvedilol, and timolol, of which only carvedilol has been studied in the reperfusion era [2]. The European Society of Cardiology (ESC) ST-segment elevation myocardial infarction (STEMI) guidelines [3] state that beta-blockers should be used indefinitely in all patients who have recovered from a STEMI, especially in the presence of left ventricular (LV) dysfunction. Accordingly, the ESC non-STEMI guidelines [4] advocate the use of beta-blockers in all patients with reduced systolic function [left ventricular ejection

Box 19.1 Practical tips and tricks for the use of beta-blockers in daily practice

- Beta-blockers can be used in a variety of cardiovascular problems and are very effective for the symptomatic treatment of patients with effort angina or arrhythmias
- Most evidence for reduction of cardiovascular events by beta-blockers is available for patients after ACS, especially in the presence of LV dysfunction and patients with heart failure and reduced ejection fraction
- Absolute contraindications include asthma and high-degree AV block (if no pacemaker)
- COPD is not a contraindication—use a cardioselective beta-blocker
- Start low and go slow in the elderly, in COPD, and in patients with heart failure
- The most frequent side effects include: hypotension (bradycardia); bronchospasm (cold extremities); central effects (fatigue, headache, sleep disturbances, vivid dreams, etc.), and increased insulin resistance (new onset diabetes—not with carvedilol and nebivolol)

Box 19.2 Practical tips and tricks for the use of beta-blockers in patients with heart failure

- Use evidence-based beta-blockers (carvedilol, bisoprolol, metoprolol, nebivolol)
- In case of an episode of exacerbation of heart failure, start only after clinical stabilization
- Start low and go slow (up-titration after a minimum of 2 weeks)
- In case of symptomatic hypotension (<90 mmHg):
  - evaluate the need for other blood pressure-lowering drugs (nitrates, calcium antagonists, other vasodilators)
  - if no signs of congestion, first reduce the diuretic dose
  - if persistent: reduce dose of beta-blockers and get specialist advice
- In case of bradycardia (<50 beats/min):
  - evaluate the need for other heart rate-lowering drugs (digoxine, amiodarone, ivabradine)
  - if symptomatic bradycardia: reduce dose of beta-blockers
  - if persistent: further reduce/stop beta-blocker, ECG, specialist advice
- In case of increase of heart failure signs or symptoms:
  - if increased signs of congestion increase the dose of diuretics and, if needed, reduce the dose of beta-blocker
  - if more complaints of fatigue: decrease the dose of beta-blocker—re-evaluate after 1–2 weeks and specialist advice
  - if severe clinical deterioration: reduce dose or stop beta-blocker and seek specialist advice

fraction (LVEF) ≤ 40%] with or without symptoms of heart failure. They may be useful in other patients, but evidence for their long-term benefit is not established.

Stable coronary artery disease

Beta-blockade is a very effective symptomatic treatment, alone or combined with another drug, in the majority of patients with classic effort angina [2,5]. It has been extrapolated from the post-infarction trials that beta-blockers may also reduce major outcomes in patients with stable CAD. However, this has not been proven in a placebo-controlled trial.

An analysis of the ACTION trial showed no mortality benefit of beta-blocker treatment for patients with stable angina pectoris [6]. Data from the Reduction of Atherothrombosis for Continued Health (REACH) Registry showed that in the CAD-without-myocardial infarction (MI) group, rates of the primary end-point (composite of cardiovascular death, non-fatal MI, or non-fatal stroke) were not significantly different in patients with versus those without beta-blockers [12.9% versus 13.6%; hazard ratio (HR) 0.92, $p = 0.31$]. In fact, for the secondary end-point (primary outcome plus hospitalization for atherothrombotic events or a revascularization procedure), outcomes were actually worse among those who used beta-blockers compared with those who did not [30.6% versus 27,8%, odds ratio (OR) 1.14, $p = 0.01$] [7]. The latest American Heart Association (AHA)/American College of Cardiology Foundation (ACCF) secondary prevention guidelines also stress the fact that evidence supporting the use of beta-blockers is greatest among patients with recent MI (<3 years) and/or left ventricular systolic dysfunction (LVEF ≤ 40%). For patients without these class I indications, beta-blocker therapy is considered optional (class IIa or IIb) [8]. In this era of modern medical and reperfusion therapy there is clearly a need for randomized trials to actually define which patients with stable CAD are best suited to beta-blocker therapy and to identify the optimal duration of treatment.

Larger studies (including APSIS and TIBET) comparing beta-blockers with calcium antagonists for stable angina have shown that treatment with a calcium antagonist such as verapamil SR or nifedipine SR resulted in similar cardiovascular event rates compared with treatment with metoprolol CR or atenolol [5,9,10].

Finally, only one randomized controlled trial has examined the use of beta-blockers in a general post-coronary artery bypass graft (CABG) population; it found no differences in cardiovascular outcomes at 2-year follow-up [11]. Therefore, in the absence of a history of MI or heart failure, there is little evidence to suggest that beta-blockers should be used routinely after CABG [12].

Heart failure

Several randomized trials with bisoprolol [13], carvedilol [14], and metoprolol CR/XL [15] in patients with mild to severely symptomatic heart failure and reduced ejection fraction have shown that treatment with beta-blockers reduces mortality (relative risk (RR) reduction ~ 34% in each trial) and heart failure hospitalizations (RR reduction 28–36%) within about a year of starting treatment. These findings are supported by the SENIORS study in which elderly patients with heart failure (≥70 years, 36% with a LVEF > 35%) were randomized to nebivolol versus placebo [16]. This trial showed a reduction in the RR of 14% in the primary composite end-point of death or cardiovascular hospitalization, but did not reduce mortality. However, bucindolol, a beta-blocker with partial agonist properties, did not show a significant reduction in mortality and short-acting metoprolol tartrate (different from the long-acting succinate formulation used in the MERIT-HF trial) was inferior to carvedilol for increasing survival [17]. The 2012 ESC guidelines for heart failure [18] recommend a beta-blocker in addition to an ACEi (or ARB if ACEi is not tolerated) for all patients with a LVEF ≤ 40% to reduce the risk of heart failure hospitalization and of premature death. They should usually be initiated in stable patients starting with a low dose and up-titrated over several weeks.

No treatment has yet been shown to significantly reduce morbidity and mortality in patients with heart failure and preserved ejection fraction (diastolic heart failure). In these patients beta-blockers may be used to control the ventricular rate of atrial fibrillation or improve myocardial ischaemia.

Arrhythmia

Beta-blockers can be used to slow the heart rate in different arrhythmias including sinus tachycardia, supraventricular tachycardias, and atrial flutter or atrial fibrillation [1,19] Beta-blockers are also effective in the control of ventricular arrhythmias related to sympathetic activation, ACS, and heart failure, including the prevention of sudden cardiac death [1,3,4,18].

Other indications

Beta-blockers can have a place in the treatment of other clinical entities such as aortic dissection, hypertrophic cardiomyopathy, and vasovagal syncope [1]. In the setting of non-cardiac surgery they are recommended in patients scheduled for high-risk surgery (such as vascular surgery) and in some patients scheduled for intermediate-risk surgery. In these patients, treatment should be initiated optimally between 30 days and at least 1 week before surgery, with a target heart rate of 60–70 beats/min and a systolic blood pressure > 100 mmHg [20].

Finally, for patients with only risk factors for CAD, data from the REACH Registry showed that the rates of the primary end-point (composite of cardiovascular death, non-fatal MI, or non-fatal stroke) were actually higher in patients taking beta-blockers with versus those without (14.2.% versus 12.1%; HR 1.18, $p = 0.02$) [7]. Therefore, beta-blockers cannot be routinely recommended for such patients.

Contraindications and side effects

Treatment with beta-blockers may result in adverse events, especially when they are used in large doses (➲ see Boxes 19.1 and 19.2). The most important cardiovascular adverse effects are extreme bradycardia and AV block (especially in patients with impaired sinus node or AV node function) as well as hypotension with dizziness or fatigue. Cold extremities and Raynaud's phenomenon may also occur, although this is less pronounced with cardioselective agents [1,2]. In patients with heart failure, continuation during an episode of heart failure exacerbation has been shown to be safe, although dose reduction may be necessary. Temporal discontinuation is advised in shocked or severely hypoperfused patients. Reinstitution of treatment should be attempted before discharge [18].

Increased insulin resistance and a higher incidence of new-onset diabetes were reported in early trials with beta-blockers, although newer agents such as bisoprolol and carvedilol have no negative effects on glucose metabolism [2]. In patients with insulin-dependent diabetes some warning symptoms of hypoglycaemia (tremor, tachycardia) may be masked by non-selective beta-blockers, and therefore cardioselective agents are preferred [1]. Importantly, ESC guidelines recommend treatment with beta-blockers for all diabetic patients with ACS, post-MI, and heart failure [21].

Beta-blockers can lead to a life-threatening increase in airway resistance, and are therefore contraindicated in patients with asthma. However, chronic obstructive pulmonary disease (COPD) in which airway obstruction is irreversible is not a contraindication. There is evidence from randomized controlled trials that beta-blockers reduce mortality by 15–43% in patients with coexistent COPD and CAD [22,23]. In these patients beta-1-selective beta-blockers should be started at a low dose and up-titrated slowly. As asthma and COPD may coexist, lung function should be monitored. Mild deterioration in pulmonary function and symptoms should not lead to prompt discontinuation, but if symptoms worsen a reduction of the dosage or withdrawal may be necessary [24].

Central effects of beta-blockers include fatigue, headache, sleep disturbances, vivid dreams, and depression. Beta-blockers may also cause or aggravate impotence and loss of libido. However, some studies suggest that erectile dysfunction is no more common with beta-blockers than with other drugs prescribed for heart failure or hypertension and that the anxiety of knowing that beta-blockers may cause erectile dysfunction may be enough to produce this supposed side effect [24].

Ivabradine

Mechanisms and cardiovascular effects

Ivabradine is a specific heart-rate-lowering agent which acts on the sinoatrial node cells by selectively and specifically inhibiting the pacemaker I_f current in a dose-dependent manner. As a result, it reduces heart rate while preserving the force of contraction, cardiac conduction, and blood pressure [25]. Heart rate reduction with ivabradine reduces angina symptoms and improves exercise tolerance [26], and these effects were at least comparable (and even better for exercise tolerance) to treatment with atenolol [27]. The ASSOCIATE trial showed that these beneficial effects persisted on top of atenolol (50 mg) [28].

The prognostic value of ivabradine in patients with CAD was evaluated in the BEAUTIFUL study, a randomized, double-blind, parallel-group trial carried out in 10 917 patients with documented stable CAD, LVEF < 40% and a resting heart rate ≥ 60 beats/min. Patients were randomized to either ivabradine or matching placebo on top of optimal preventive therapy and were followed up for 19 months. There was no measurable effect of treatment on the primary end-point in the overall population, but in patients with elevated heart rate (≥70 beats/min) ivabradine reduced the risk of fatal and non-fatal MI by 36% ($p = 0.001$) and coronary revascularization by 30% ($p = 0.016$) [29]. A post hoc subgroup analysis in 1507 patients in the BEAUTIFUL study with limiting angina at baseline confirmed a 24% reduction of the primary end-point in patients randomized to ivabradine [30]. The on-going SIGNIFY trial is testing the hypothesis that ivabradine improves the prognosis of patients with CAD and normal LV function with a heart rate ≥ 70 beats/min [31].

The SHIFT trial evaluated the prognostic value of ivabradine in patients with systolic heart failure. In this randomized, double-blind, placebo-controlled, parallel-group trial, 6558 patients with symptomatic heart failure, LVEF ≤ 35%, sinus rhythm with a heart rate ≥ 70 beats/min, and a stable background treatment including a beta-blocker if tolerated were randomized between ivabradine and placebo. After a median follow-up of 23 months, there was an 18% ($p < 0.0001$) reduction in the primary end-point (composite of cardiovascular death or hospital admission for worsening heart failure) in the ivabradine group. The effects were mainly driven by hospital admissions for worsening heart failure and deaths due to heart failure [32].

Indications

Based on the studies mentioned in 'Mechanisms and cardiovascular effects', the European Medicines Agency (EMA) stated in 2012 that ivabradine is indicated for symptomatic treatment of chronic stable angina pectoris in CAD patients with normal sinus rhythm, in patients unable to tolerate or with a contraindication to the use of beta-blockers, and in combination with beta-blockers in patients who are inadequately controlled with an optimal dose of beta-blockers and whose heart rate is > 60 beats/min.

The 2012 ESC guidelines for chronic heart failure [18] state that ivabradine should be considered to reduce the risk of heart failure hospitalization in patients in sinus rhythm with a LVEF ≤ 35%, a heart rate remaining at 70 or more beats/min, and persisting symptoms (NYHA class II–IV) despite optimal medical treatment including beta-blockers (class IIa, level of evidence B). In patients who are unable to tolerate a beta-blocker, it may be considered to reduce the risk of heart failure hospitalization in patients in sinus rhythm, with a LVEF ≤ 35% and a heart rate remaining at 70 beats/min or more (class IIb, level of evidence C).

Contraindications and side effects

The most common side effects with ivabradine are visual side effects or 'phosphenes' (a temporary brightness in the field of vision). Ivabradine must not be used in patients who have a resting heart rate below 60 beats/min, very low blood pressure, various types of heart disorder (including cardiogenic shock, rhythm disorders, heart attack, acute heart failure, and unstable angina), or severe liver problems.

Renin–angiotensin–aldosterone receptor blockers (ACEi, ARBs, renin blockers, and aldosterone antagonists)

Mechanisms and cardiovascular effects

There are four classes of RAAS receptor blockers: ACEi, ARBs, aldosterone antagonists (AAs), and direct renin inhibitors (DRi) [33,34] (➲ see Table 19.2).

ACEi, the most used and studied type of RAAS blocker, have a class I indication in the ESC guidelines in hypertension [35], diabetes mellitus [21], heart failure [18], secondary prevention for stable CAD [36], and in the acute phase and post-MI [37–39]. The benefits of ACEi are due to their vasodilating, anti-inflammatory, plaque-stabilizing, antithrombotic, and antiproliferative effects [33].

ARBs have similar properties to ACEi, but with a better tolerability profile. Since they are more expensive and appeared later they are usually considered as an alternative for patients intolerant to ACEi due to non-productive cough or any other reason. They share most of the indications and contraindications for ACEi.

DRi (e.g. aliskiren) are the most recent class and are not so well studied; for the moment they only have a clinical indication in hypertension. Aliskiren has not been studied in heart failure, secondary prevention after myocardial infarction, stroke, or stable angina.

AAs (e.g. spironolactone and eplerenone) have a good evidence of benefits in heart failure in acute MI.

ACEi, ARBs, and DRi act by blockade of the RAAS, with beneficial effects through the cardiovascular risk continuum, either in the presence of only cardiovascular risk factors (hypertension, hypercholesterolaemia, diabetes, and chronic kidney disease) or in the context of clinical entities such as acute MI, stroke, and heart failure.

The end result of the activation of the RAAS is the production of angiotensin II at the renal level, which in the short term results in vasoconstriction, retention of sodium and water, and increased arterial pressure and myocardial contractility with the aim of preserving blood pressure. Vascular smooth muscle and cardiac

Table 19.2 RAAS blockers

Class	Drug	Usual daily dose	
		Heart failure	Hypertension
ACEi	Captopril	6.25–50 mg, t.i.d.	12.5–50 mg, t.i.d.
	Zofenopril	7.5–30 mg, b.i.d.	30 mg, b.i.d. or 60 mg, o.d.
	Benazepril	–	10–40 mg, o.d. or b.i.d.
	Enalapril	2.5–20 mg, b.i.d.	2.5–20 mg, b.i.d.
	Lisinopril	2.5–40 mg, b.i.d.	2.5–40 mg, b.i.d.
	Perindopril	2–16 mg, o.d.	4–16 mg, o.d.
	Quinapril	5–20 mg, b.i.d.	10–40 mg, o.d.
	Ramipril	1.25–10 mg, o.d.	2.5–20 mg, o.d.
	Fosinopril	10–40 mg, o.d.	10–80 mg, o.d.
ARB	Candesartan	4–32 mg, o.d.	8–32 mg, o.d.
	Eprosartan	–	400–800 mg, o.d.
	Irbesartan	–	150–300 mg, o.d.
	Losartan	–	25–100 mg, o.d.
	Olmesartan	–	20–40 mg, o.d.
	Telmisartan	–	20–80 mg, o.d.
DRi	Aliskiren	–	150–300 mg, o.d.
AA	Spironolactone	12.5–50 mg, o.d.	25–50 mg, o.d. or b.i.d.
	Eplerenone	25–50 mg, o.d.	50–100 mg, o.d.; 50 mg, b.i.d.

RAAS, renin–angiotensin–aldosterone system; ACEi, angiotensin-converting enzyme inhibitors; ARB, angiotensin receptor blocker; AA, aldosterone antagonist; DRi, direct renin inhibitors; t.i.d., three times a day; b.i.d., twice a day; o.d., once a day.

hypertrophy and fibrosis are deleterious effects found with long term use.

Renin production, the first step in this chain of reactions, occurs at the level of the juxtaglomerular apparatus when its perfusion decreases. Renin catalyses the conversion of angiotensinogen to angiotensin I, which is hydrolysed by angiotensin-converting enzyme (ACE) into angiotensin II. At the end of the process angiotensin II will act at the suprarenal cortex releasing aldosterone, which is a potent vasoconstrictor and will increase the circulating volume by retention of salt and water. Should an increase in perfusion occur at the juxtaglomerular apparatus, the release of renin will be inhibited by a negative feedback mechanism.

ACEi act by inhibiting the transformation of angiotensin I into angiotensin II, ARBs by blocking the angiotensin II receptor subtype 1, and AAs antagonize the effects of aldosterone.

There are also alternative pathways, the so-called non-ACE pathways, to convert angiotensinogen into angiotensin II, through tissue plasminogen activator, cathepsin, and tonin, and angiotensin I to angiotensin II by chymase and cathepsin, explaining the so-called 'angiotensin II escape' to ACEi.

As well as the already described classical RAAS pathway in the circulation it also exists at the tissue level and works in a complementary manner to the former by paracrine or autocrine activity.

Indications

➲ Table 19.3 shows the recommendations for RAAS blockers in the ESC guidelines.

High-risk individuals and patients with diabetes

The HOPE trial [40] (ramipril versus placebo) studied 9297 high-risk patients (with vascular disease or diabetes plus at least one more risk factor) and demonstrated reductions of 26% for cardiovascular death, 20% for MI, 32% for stroke, and 33% for heart failure with even better results in the diabetes cohort [41].

ACEi also proved to be beneficial in hypertension, reducing mortality (HYVET [42]) and/or cardiovascular events (HYVET-Pilot [43], HYVET [42]), although some trials like CAPP [44] (captopril versus diuretics or beta-blockers) and STOP 2 [45] [diuretic or beta-blockers versus ACEi or calcium channel blockers (CCBs)] did not show any benefit regarding the comparator regime. ACEi are also recognized as one of the best pharmacological groups for diminishing LV hypertrophy [46], a parameter implicated in cardiovascular risk.

Regarding ARBs, losartan showed superiority versus atenolol in the LIFE study [47], by reducing the risk of cardiovascular death, stroke, or acute MI, while decreasing blood pressure and LV hypertrophy. In the VALUE trial [48], valsartan was compared with amlodipine in hypertensive or high-risk patients and

Table 19.3 Class of recommendation for RAAS blockers in the ESC guidelines

	ESC guideline			
Class	**Prevention, 2012 [36]**	**Acute MI with ST-elevation, 2008 [3]**	**ACS without ST-elevation, 2011 [4]**	**Acute and chronic HF, 2012 [18]**
ACEi	IA: Recommended for the initiation and maintenance of antihypertensive treatment, especially in diabetics	IA: In all patients without contraindication	IB: In all patients, to prevent recurrence of ischaemic episodes IA: Within 24 hours in all patients with LVEF ≤ 40% and HF, diabetes, hypertension or CKD, unless contraindicated	IA: To reduce hospitalizations and premature death in addition to a beta-blocker
ARB	IA: Recommended for the initiation and maintenance of antihypertensive treatment, especially in diabetics	IB: In all patients without contraindications who do not tolerate ACEi	IB: For patients intolerant to ACEi	IA: To reduce hospitalizations and premature death in addition to a beta-blocker, in patients intolerant to an ACEi or AA
DRi	No indication	No indication	No indication	No indication
AA	No indication	IB: If LVEF ≤ 40% and signs of heart failure or diabetes if creatinine is <2.5 mg/dl in men and <2.0 mg/dl in women and potassium is <5.0 mEq/L	No indication	IA: To reduce hospitalizations and premature death to all patients with persisting symptoms

ACEi, angiotensin-converting enzyme inhibitors; ARB, angiotensin receptor blocker; AA, aldosterone antagonist; DRi, direct renin inhibitors; LVEF, left ventricular ejection fraction; HF, heart failure; CKD, chronic kidney disease; IA, general agreement that the treatment is beneficial/useful/effective, based on data derived from multiple randomized clinical trials or meta-analysis; IB, general agreement that the treatment is beneficial/useful/effective, based on data derived from a single randomized clinical trial or large non-randomized studies.

demonstrated to be equivalent in lowering cardiac mortality and morbidity. In both the LIFE and VALUE studies, ARBs showed a lower incidence of new cases of diabetes.

In the ONTARGET study [49], which enrolled high-risk cardiovascular patients, telmisartan showed similar cardioprotection when compared with ramipril with the advantage of being better tolerated. In a meta-analysis published in 2012 by McAlister et al. [50] it was shown that ACEi or ARBs are beneficial in patients with, or at an increased risk for, atherosclerotic disease even if their systolic pressure is <130 mmHg before treatment.

The cardiovascular benefits of ACEi and ARBs seem to be related to their ability to reduce blood pressure and insulin resistance and to provide renal protection. Insulin resistance was decreased in HOPE [40] and CHARM [51], respectively, by ramipril and candesartan.

In summary, ACEi or ARBs are widely used in the presence of hypertension, diabetes, or chronic kidney disease to prevent cardiovascular events and progression of nephropathy.

Aliskiren, a DRi, was tested in several hypertension trials alone or in association with an ACEi or an ARB and showed clinical efficacy by itself, which increased when in combination with ramipril or valsartan. Aliskiren was also used in the AVOID study [52] in combination with losartan in patients with diabetes, hypertension, and proteinuria and reduced the albumin/creatinine ratio by 20% compared with losartan alone.

In resistant hypertension, spironolactone, as part of a combination therapy, may provide further reductions in blood pressure as shown in the ASCOT study [53].

Coronary artery disease

The EUROPA study [54] randomized stable CAD patients for perindopril versus placebo. The composite end-point of non-fatal acute MI, cardiovascular death, and resuscitated cardiac arrest was modestly lower. PEACE [55] and ACCOMPLISH [56] both demonstrated similar results.

The mid 1990s saw the first generation of trials in acute MI using an ACEi in unselected patients, for example ISIS-4 [57], (captopril versus placebo) and GISSI-3 [58] (lisinopril versus open control), where unequivocal but mild mortality benefits were obtained. In a second generation of trials on LV dysfunction or overt congestive heart failure, like SAVE [59] (captopril versus placebo), AIRE [60] (ramipril versus placebo), and TRACE [61] (trandolapril versus placebo), larger benefits were detected on mortality, hospitalization, and CHF progression.

In summary, interesting reductions in mortality and cardiovascular events were demonstrated with the use of ACEi in post-acute MI patients, with or without LV dysfunction, with or without overt congestive heart failure, probably due to their anti-LV remodelling and anti-atherosclerotic effects.

ARBs are less studied in the post-acute MI setting. In the OPTIMAAL trial [62], which enrolled patients with congestive heart failure, losartan demonstrated similar outcomes to captopril, although it was slightly better tolerated. In the VALIANT trial [63], valsartan was compared with captopril and showed similar mortality.

Heart failure

The benefits of ACEi in heart failure were demonstrated in several randomized controlled trials using enalapril (CONSENSUS [64], V-HeFT II [65], and SOLVD prevention [66] and treatment [67]), which showed improvement in clinical symptoms and reductions in mortality and hospitalizations.

ARBs were compared with ACEi in patients with heart failure, alone or in combination. In ELITE I [68] losartan was similar to captopril in terms of mortality and renal dysfunction, and in HEAAL [69] it was shown that a higher dose of 150 mg provided larger reductions in mortality and readmissions compared with a lower dose (50 mg). In CHARM, candesartan was studied alone [51] and as an alternative [70] to ACEi: a 30% reduction in cardiovascular death or heart failure hospitalizations was demonstrated. Lee et al. [71] found in a meta-analysis that ARBs reduce mortality and heart failure hospitalizations in patients with congestive heart failure by a similar magnitude to ACEi.

Aliskiren, a DRi, was tested versus placebo in the ALOFT trial [72], a surrogate end-points study, and was shown to lower N-terminal pro-brain natriuretic peptide, brain natriuretic peptide, and urinary aldosterone more than placebo.

The AAs spirolactone and eplerenone are useful complements in patients with heart failure to the RAAS blockade provided by ACEi or ARBs. They provide additional protection because they counteract the so-called 'angiotensin II escape' and block the direct effect of aldosterone, which has additional deleterious effects to angiotensin II on the heart. Spironolactone was used in RALES [73], a trial in patients having NYHA class III and IV heart failure, and produced a 30% reduction in RR of death over 2 years, with a decreased number of readmissions and improvement in NYHA class. Eplerenone, a drug similar to spironolactone, was tested in EPHESUS [74] in patients with acute MI and also reduced mortality at 1 year.

Other indications

ACEi and ARBs were evaluated in some small trials for other indications like prevention of new onset and recurrence of atrial fibrillation, in association with amiodarone for maintenance of sinus rhythm after electrical cardioversion, with the rationale that they could counteract atrial remodelling, but the scientific evidence at present is not fully conclusive.

With regard to stroke prevention, there is much evidence in favour of ACEi used alone or in combination with a diuretic or a CCB, after trials like HOPE [40] where ramipril reduced the RR (32% for any stroke and 61% for fatal stroke) and PROGRESS [75] (perindopril ± indapamide versus placebo), in patients with a previous stroke or transient ischaemic attack, which showed a 28% (for perindopril alone) and 43% (perindopril ± indapamide) reduction of recurrent stroke.

ARBs have also been studied in primary and secondary prevention trials like LIFE [47] (losartan), SCOPE [76] (candesartan), MOSES [77] (eprosartan), TRANSCEND [78], and ONTARGET [79] (telmisartan) for stroke prevention and demonstrated important reductions in RR for stroke and acute MI. Besides these unquestionable benefits, there is some evidence after the PRoFESS

Box 19.3 Practical tips and tricks for RAAS blockers in daily practice

Indications for ACEi/ARBs

- Arterial hypertension (alone or in combination with a diuretic, CCB, or beta-blocker):
  - metabolic syndrome
  - diabetes or diabetic nephropathy
  - renal dysfunction or proteinuria or microalbuminuria
  - LV hypertrophy
  - angina pectoris
  - previous ACS, with or without ST-elevation
  - heart failure and LV dysfunction
- Coronary artery disease:
  - angina pectoris
  - acute phase or post-ACS, with or without ST-elevation
- Heart failure

Contraindications for ACEi/ARBs

- Severe aortic stenosis
- Angio-oedema
- Bilateral renal artery stenosis
- Hypotension
- Hyperkalaemia
- Pregnancy

Most frequent important side effects for ACEi/ARBs

- Dry cough (specially with ACEi, rare with ARBs)
- Hypotension
- Deterioration of renal function
- Hyperkalaemia

Other points

- Aldosterone antagonists (spironolactone and eplerenone) proved to be beneficial in heart failure related or not to acute MI.
- The DRi aliskiren is for the moment only indicated for hypertension.
- Special precautions: in the presence of high-dose diuretic therapy, hyponatraemia, hypotension, and in the elderly, start all RAAS blockers at low doses and increase slowly (not before 2 weeks) until the target recommended dose in ESC guidelines is achieved. Monitor renal function and serum potassium closely.

[49] trial that ARBs should be considered as an alternative in ACEi-intolerant patients for stroke prevention, but not as first choice medication.

Contraindications and side effects

➲ Box 19.3 lists practical tips and tricks for RAAS blockers in daily practice.

Contraindications

ACEi and ARBs are formally contraindicated in previous severe aortic stenosis, angio-oedema, or bilateral renal artery stenosis. ACEi can also produce teratogenic effects, which implicates their interruption in pregnancy.

Moderate renal insufficiency (serum creatinine < 3 mg/dl), mild hyperkalaemia ($K^+ < 6.0$ mEq/L), and asymptomatic low blood pressure are not formal contraindications to ACEi or ARBs, but in these cases they must be started at low doses, small dosage increases must be performed, and renal function closely monitored. If potassium rises to over 6.0 mEq/L or creatinine increases by more the 50% over the baseline value or exceeds 3 mg/dl the drugs must be stopped.

Side effects

Non-productive cough is the most frequent side effect related to ACEi, being present in 5–10% of patients, starting a week to several months after drug initiation. It is frequently unnoticed by patients. It may be related to increased levels of bradykinin and/or substance P in the lungs due to ACE inhibition. This side effect is not dose dependent and disappears in 1 or 2 weeks after drug interruption. The alternative use of ARBs to an ACEi is mainly justified by their lower incidence of this side effect.

Angio-oedema is a rare but potentially life-threatening side effect of ACEi. It is easy to recognize in the presence of severe dyspnoea due to oedema of the larynx, but it can be more difficult to recognize if it becomes overt by mild gastrointestinal symptoms, like nausea, vomiting, diarrhoea, and colic.

ACEi and ARBs may have other important side effects like hypotension, deterioration of renal function, and hyperkalaemia. Hypotension and acute impairment of renal function occur more frequently after the first dose, due to angiotensin II withdrawal in salt- and volume-depleted patients (e.g. patients under high doses of diuretics) or patients with congestive heart failure who have high plasma renin activity. Deterioration of renal function occurs in the same type of patients (hyponatraemic or elderly). Usually, if significant renal dysfunction is found upon starting an ACEi or an ARB the presence of bilateral renal artery stenosis or single kidney artery stenosis must be ruled out. Renal dysfunction normalizes a few days after drug interruption in almost all patients.

Hyperkalaemia, due to a decrease in aldosterone secretion secondary to an ACEi, an ARB, or an AA, typically occurs in patients with some degree of renal or hepatic dysfunction and can be relatively common in patients with congestive heart failure, the elderly, or diabetic patients, especially if they are under potassium supplements, any combination of AA/ACEi/ARB, or a non-steroidal anti-inflammatory drug (NSAID).

ACEi can produce some degree of proteinuria. The presence of proteinuria previously to starting an ACEi or an ARB is not a contraindication.

High doses of captopril have been related to cutaneous rash, neutropenia, taste abnormalities, and nephrotic syndrome. These manifestations were presumed to be due to the sulphydryl group of captopril and are much rarer with daily doses below 100–150 mg.

AAs can induce oligomenorrhoea in women and men can experience gynaecomastia, breast pain, or impotence (more common with spironolactone then with eplerenone). Special caution must be taken in the presence of increased levels of potassium (>5 mEq/L) or creatinine, namely in type 2 diabetic patients with hypertension and microalbuminuria, due to the risk of hyperkalaemia.

After ONTARGET [79] the double or triple drug combination regime of ACEi/ARBs/AAs is not indicated due to the risk of severe hyperkalaemia and renal dysfunction. The only exception, cited in the ESC 2012 heart failure guidelines [36] is symptomatic heart failure after optimal medical treatment, taking into consideration the mild reduction in mortality (11%, $p = 0.086$) found in Val-HeFT [80] and CHARM-Added [81].

Calcium antagonists

Mechanisms and cardiovascular effects

CCBs are a heterogeneous group of drugs that have in common the ability to produce vasodilatation in coronary and peripheral arteries, where they can markedly lower peripheral resistance. This property makes them very useful in hypertension and CAD, namely in stable angina pectoris and vasospasm angina [82,83].

CCBs can be divided in two main classes of drugs: dihydropyridines (DHPs) and non-dihydropyridines (non-DHPs), subdivided into benzothiazepines (e.g. diltiazem) and phenylethylamines (e.g. verapamil).

DHPs (e.g. nifedipine, amlodipine, felodipine, isradipine, lacidipine, lercanidipine, and nisoldipine) are almost pure vasodilators without any significant effect on LVEF or the heart conduction system. The last five have increased arteriolar selectivity compared with nifedipine and amlodipine.

The non-DHPs (diltiazem and verapamil), although not so potent as vasodilators, can slow heart rate and AV conduction and decrease myocardial contractility, similarly to beta-blockers to which they are an alternative in management of angina pectoris or supraventricular arrhythmias in case of contraindication such as asthma.

The main indication for CCBs is in the treatment of arterial hypertension, where they have been shown to decrease LV hypertrophy, stroke incidence, and progression of atherosclerosis and ameliorate endothelial dysfunction. CCBs are neutral regarding metabolic cardiovascular risk factors such as diabetes and hypercholesterolaemia.

In the context of stable CAD, CCBs can be used to control angina when the classical drug regime involving a beta-blocker and a long-acting nitrate fails. They are also specifically indicated in the presence of uncontrolled hypertension, intermittent claudication, or Raynaud's phenomenon.

Indications

➲ Tables 19.4 and 19.5 show the indications/magnitude of effect by pharmacological class and dosages, respectively, for CCBs.

Table 19.4 Calcium channel blockers: indications/magnitude of effect by pharmacological class

Indication	Class of calcium channel blocker		
	Phenylethylamines (verapamil)	Benzothiazepines (diltiazem)	Dihydropyridines (amlodipine)
Hypertension	+ +	+	+ + +
Angina (vasospasm or effort)	+ + +	+ + +	+ + +
Paroxysmal supraventricular tachycardia	+ + +	+ +	–
Atrial flutter and fibrillation	+ +	+ +	–
Hypertrophic cardiomyopathy	+ +	–	–
Raynaud's syndrome	+ +	+ +	+ +

–, no effect/not indicated; +, mild effect/efficacy; + +, moderate effect/efficacy; + + +, intense effect/efficacy.

Table 19.5 Calcium channel blocker (CCB) drug dosing

CCB class	Drug	Form, dose, and frequency	
		Short acting	Long acting
Phenylethylamines	Verapamil	40–80 mg, t.i.d.	120–480 mg, o.d.
Benzothiazepines	Diltiazem	60–90 mg, t.i.d.	120–480 mg, o.d.
Dihydropyridines	Amlodipine	2.5–10 mg, o.d.	
	Felodipine		2.5–20 mg, o.d.
	Isradipine	2.5–10 mg, b.i.d.	5–20 mg, o.d.
	Lacidipine	2–4 mg, o.d.	
	Lercanidipine	10–20 mg, o.d.	
	Nicardipine	20–40 mg, t.i.d.	30–120 mg, o.d.
	Nifedipine	5–10 mg, t.i.d.	30–120 mg, o.d.
	Nisoldipine		10–40 mg, b.i.d.

o.d., once a day; b.i.d., twice a day; t.i.d., three times a day.

High-risk individuals and patients with diabetes

DHP-type CCBs are relatively well tolerated and can be combined with other antihypertensive drugs, they can be used in the presence of end-stage chronic kidney disease, and they do not have any serious side effects. Like other groups of antihypertensive drugs, they reduce LV hypertrophy, an important risk factor for cardiovascular events in the context of hypertension. Nifedipine reduced progression of asymptomatic atherosclerosis in the INTACT trial [84] and improved endothelial function in the ENCORE II study [85].

CCBs are especially indicated for the treatment of isolated systolic hypertension, hypertension in black people, and high blood pressure during pregnancy [86]. They do not have any limitation in chronic kidney disease, even in end-stage disease or in patients under haemodialysis.

Unlike diuretics and beta-blockers, CCBs are neutral in terms of cardiovascular metabolic risk factors, which make them very useful in the setting of diabetes, metabolic syndrome, hypercholesterolaemia, and gout [87].

CCBs act synergistically with the other drugs like ACEi or ARBs, or less frequently with diuretics and beta-blockers, in treatment of hypertension. Their efficacy is increased and the secondary effects reduced.

Several large randomized controlled trials like ALLHAT [88], ASCOT [89], ACCOMPLISH [90], and VALUE [91], showed consistent results to support amlodipine, the most used DHP in the field of hypertension, as a safe and efficacious drug alone or in combination with an ACEi (perindopril in ASCOT and benazepril in ACCOMPLISH) or an ARB (valsartan in VALUE). The amlodipine groups showed significantly reduced mortality and major cardiovascular events like stroke against the comparator groups.

CAFÉ [92], a sub-study of ASCOT, showed that the amlodipine + perindopril regimen lowered central aortic blood pressure to a greater extent than the atenolol/thiazide regimen (by 4 mmHg systolic). Central pressure was related to cardiovascular and renal outcomes, and in another sub-study it was shown that the combination of amlodipine + perindopril was associated with lower variability in blood pressure then the other regime [93,94]. Both mechanisms, lower central blood pressure and lower variability, may explain the better results of the amlodipine + perindopril combination.

The most recent European Society of Hypertension/ESC guidelines for the management of arterial hypertension recommend an association of two drugs as initiating therapy when blood pressure is beyond 20 mmHg of the systolic goal or 10 mmHg above diastolic target, or in milder degrees if multiple risk factors, subclinical organ damage, diabetes, renal disease, or CAD are present. Knowing that doubling the dose of a DHP CCB (amlodipine) is more efficacious than doubling the dose of an ACEi or ARB, it is recommended to increase the CCB first.

Non-DHPs are recommended in patients who are intolerant to beta-blockers and DHP and are an alternative to ACEi and ARBs in patients with severe renal failure or at risk of hyperkalaemia. It has been advocated to use a combination of CCBs, including a non-DHP (like verapamil or diltiazem) and a DHP (like amlodipine) to lower blood pressure, but no outcome data or long-term safety data are available. Unlike diuretics, ACEi, and ARBs, CCBs do not lose their effect by concomitant therapy with NSAIDs—frequently used by elderly hypertensive patients [95,96].

Coronary artery disease

The main indication for CCBs in patients with CAD is control of angina in stable or vasospasm angina when beta-blockers and nitrates fail [97,98]. Non-DHP proved to have a similar efficacy to beta-blockers to release symptoms in stable angina [99]. DHP and non-DHP drugs have similar efficacy in vasospasm angina [100,101].

Although CCBs have been shown to delay progression of atherosclerosis and improve endothelial function in small mechanistic studies, in the ACTION trial [102], a multicentre, randomized controlled trial with long-acting nifedipine (60 mg, once a day) compared with placebo in patients with CAD, no positive effects could be demonstrated for CCBs as secondary prevention drugs (unlike ACEi or ARBs).

The DAVIT-I and DAVIT-II studies taken together demonstrated that verapamil has positive effects in non-ST elevation ACS [103] in patients with preserved LV function, showing significant reductions in sudden death, reinfarction, and total mortality [38]. Moss et al. described similar results for diltiazem in the Multicenter Diltiazem Postinfarction Trial [104].

CCBs have not been shown to be useful in ST elevation ACS. On the contrary, in the HINT trial (nifedipine versus metoprolol) an excess rate of reinfarction was found in the nifedipine group, necessitating premature stoppage of the trial [105].

Heart failure

CCBs are not recommended in the ESC heart failure guidelines, probably as a consequence of the negative inotropism of non-DHPs and the lack of a specific indication for non-DHPs [18,106]. In the PRAISE [107] and V-HeFT III [108] trials, amlodipine and felodipine, respectively, were shown to cause no harm to patients with heart failure if there is still a requirement to treat hypertension or angina after the use of ACE/ARBs and diuretics for hypertension or a beta-blocker with a long-acting nitrate for angina pectoris.

Other indications

Nifedipine has proved to be useful in hypertension during pregnancy without causing teratogenic effects or complications of the peripartum [109]. Nifedipine and diltiazem have been shown to improve symptoms in pulmonary arterial hypertension in some cases when vasoreactivity is still present [110].

Due to their peripheral vasodilatation properties, CCBs can be used in intermittent claudication and Raynaud's syndrome. They may be chosen as a first-line drug or as an alternative to beta-blockers, which frequently worsen the complaints.

Non-DHPs like verapamil and diltiazem have been shown to be an alternative to beta-blockers in the setting of hypertrophic cardiomyopathy [111,112]. They are also useful for controlling the ventricular rate in the setting of multifocal atrial tachycardia, atrial flutter, or fibrillation [113,114], alone or in combination with digoxin or a beta-blocker due to their property of slowing conduction and prolonging refractoriness in the AV node. In paroxysmal supraventricular tachycardia verapamil and diltiazem can be used intravenously to abort the tachycardia or orally to prevent the recurrence of arrhythmia. They should not be used in unstable patients with supraventricular tachycardia due to the risk of hypotension or in wide QRS complex tachycardia (which can have ventricular origin), and are contraindicated in tachycardia related to pre-excitation.

Box 19.4 Practical tips and tricks for the use of CCBs in daily practice

Indications

- Arterial hypertension alone or as a second- or third-line drug, in combination with a diuretic, ACEi, ARB, or beta-blocker. Specific indications in hypertension are:
  - isolated systolic hypertension
  - hypertension in black people
  - hypertension in pregnancy (nifedipine)
  - patients with CAD (angina pectoris)
- Angina pectoris (vasospasm or effort):
  - a DHP can be added to a beta-blocker and/or a nitrate
  - a non-DHP can be an alternative to a beta-blocker
- Supraventricular arrhythmia:
  - rate control on atrial fibrillation or flutter (a non-DHP)
  - prevention of paroxysmal supraventricular tachycardia (a non-DHP)
- Others:
  - Raynaud's syndrome
  - intermittent claudication
  - hypertrophic cardiomyopathy (a non-DHP)

Contraindications

- Severe aortic stenosis
- Grade II or III AV block, for non-DHP
- Heart failure (except amlodipine and felodipine for blood pressure or angina)
- The association of a non-DHP with a beta-blocker, amiodarone, or digoxin

Most frequent side effects

- DHPs (especially with immediate release formulations or high doses): facial flush, headache, dizziness or light-headedness, tachycardia, angina, and pedal oedema
- Verapamil: constipation

Contraindications and side effects

➲ Box 19.4 lists practical tips and tricks for the use of CCBs in daily practice.

Contraindications

CCBs are contraindicated in the presence of heart failure and severe aortic stenosis. The non-DHP compounds are contraindicated in the presence of sick sinus disease and AV block grade II or III due to AV conduction increase, in the absence of a pacemaker. They should not be used added to beta-blockers, amiodarone, or digoxin, especially if there is any degree of AV block.

With the exception of nifedipine and verapamil, CCBs are contraindicated during pregnancy or breast feeding [109].

Side effects

The main side effects of DHPs are facial flush, headache, dizziness or light-headedness, tachycardia angina, and pedal oedema present in 10–20% of patients. These side effects are more frequent with immediate release formulations at high doses [115]. Pedal oedema is minimized by combining the CCB with an ACEi or an ARB. Verapamil is associated with constipation in 10–25% of patients.

Worsening or induction of AV block can be expected with non-DHP drugs. They should be used with great caution in the presence of grade I AV block and their use is not recommended in combination with other dromotropic negative drugs, like beta-blockers, amiodarone, or digoxin.

Polypills

The polypill concept

Changes in the twentieth century characterized by technological advances combined to increase food availability; this, together with subsequent deteriorations in levels of physical activity, has increased the prevalence of risk factors for CVD [116]. Consequently, in an increasing number of populations there is a high level of the risk factors for CVD, especially for many of those living in high-income countries [116]. Although effective therapy for treating CVD is available, due to high costs, low compliance, and poor identification of those at risk many individuals who could benefit from treatment remain untreated or inadequately treated. It seems evident that new and innovative strategies will be indispensable for controlling the global epidemic of heart disease. With this in mind, Wald and Law [116] proposed the concept of the polypill as a population CVD prevention strategy based on mass treatment. The concept proposes a radical approach based on the principle that high risk is common and a large preventive effect for CVD would require intervention in everyone at increased risk irrespective of their risk factor levels, modifying several risk factors together and reducing these risk factors by as much as possible. The authors wrote: 'it is time to discard the view that risk factors need to be measured and treated individually if found to be abnormal' [116]. A polypill is a theoretical combination of six pharmacological compounds that, together, could modify four different risk factors for CVD (cholesterol modification with statins, lowering of blood pressure with three different antihypertensives, antiplatelet aggregation with aspirin, and reduction of hyperhomocysteinaemia with folic acid) and theoretically reduce CVD by more than 80% [116].

The specific components of the originally proposed polypill included: one statin (e.g. atorvastatin 10 mg/day, or simvastatin or lovastatin 40 mg/day taken in the evening or 80 mg/day taken in the morning), three different classes of antihypertensives at half standard dose, folic acid (0.8 mg/day), and aspirin (75 mg/day) [116]. The concept also includes the strategy of giving this combination pill to everyone over 55 years of age and all those with existing CVD irrespective of age, hence stopping all efforts focused on the measurement of risk factors and screening for CVD. Since the introduction of the concept, much debate has been generated regarding the potential role of a polypill in CVD prevention and treatment, and multiple efforts have focused on developing and testing potential polypills.

Strengths, limitations, and efficacy

The proposed polypill could have multiple advantages [116,117]. Among these, one of the most relevant is facilitating the delivery of effective medications for the prevention and treatment of CVD. Having multiple medications combined in a single pill could dramatically improve adherence to medication and improved compliance could greatly contribute to a reduction in CVD events. Other strengths of the polypill include: facilitation of prescription and dose titration, reduction of costs by combining generic components, and provision of a platform for other widespread CVD prevention approaches (e.g. lifestyle advice) [117]. This is further supported given that such a combination pill appears to have high levels of tolerability, bioavailability, and no pharmacokinetic drug–drug interactions among the individual components [118]. Considering these combined strengths, a polypill could in theory provide great gains in terms of prevention of cardiovascular events, even among those free from CVD (➲ see Fig. 19.1).

The polypill concept is still under evaluation and these potential advantages require further investigation. Besides the lack of evidence (given that this is still a concept in the process of development and testing), adverse effects and the costs of medicalizing large proportions of the population could limit the prospects of a future polypill era in CVD prevention. Also it is still unclear whether a polypill would be a safe alternative to individual drugs, and the optimal combination to be included in a polypill is still under debate [117]. Furthermore, after the key medications to be incorporated in a polypill have been identified its registration could also pose a challenge, particularly so for primary prevention as the efficacy of the combination still requires demonstration. Finally, a major concern remains regarding the effect of the availability of a polypill on the communication and implementation of healthy lifestyles (individuals might rely on a polypill to be effective and abandon healthy lifestyle habits).

Despite the uncertainties, the prospects are promising. A polypill could theoretically prevent over 80% of CVD and increase by more than 11 years the CVD-free life expectancy of people aged over 55 taking a polypill daily [116]. If a polypill was to be given to all US adults aged over 55 and those with a history of CVD it could contribute to the prevention of 4 million coronary heart disease events and more than 2 million stroke events over 10 years of treatment [119].

Since the original polypill publication, different combination pills have been developed [117]. A combination of amlodipine 2.5 mg, losartan 25 mg, hydrochlorothiazide 12.5 mg, and simvastatin 40 mg in a polypill was tested among individuals aged over 50 who were free from CVD and compared with placebo on a crossover trial [120]. This polypill effectively reduced systolic blood pressure by 17.9 mmHg (12% reduction), diastolic blood pressure by 9.8 mmHg (11% reduction), and low-density lipoprotein (LDL) cholesterol by 1.4 mmol/L (39% reduction), effects which were very similar to those originally predicted [116,120].

Another proposed polypill is the polycap, which was tested in the Indian Polycap Study (TIPS) [121]. TIPS was a phase II double-blind randomized trial conducted among 2053 individuals in India aged 45–80 years and without CVD, in which the efficacy of the polycap (a combination of thiazide 12.5 mg, atenolol 50 mg, ramipril 5 mg, simvastatin 20 mg, and aspirin 100 mg) was tested against its individual components and specific combinations of antihypertensives. The polycap had similar effects on risk factors and was tolerated in a similar way to the individual components, with a potential combined effect of a 62% reduction in coronary heart disease events and a 48% reduction in stroke events [126]. Although below the originally expected level of CVD reduction of 80%, the effects calculated are still substantial [1,6].

In TIPS-2 (the second Indian Polycap Study) 8 weeks' treatment with a low-dose polycap (one capsule per day) versus full-dose polycap treatment (two capsules per day) with potassium supplementation was tested among 518 individuals at high risk of CVD [122]. The two formulations had similar tolerability while the full-dose polycap was more effective in reducing blood pressure and LDL cholesterol [122].

New evidence and new studies are required to confirm the efficacy and safety of the polypill in preventing hard events (MI and stroke) for both the primary and secondary prevention of CVD.

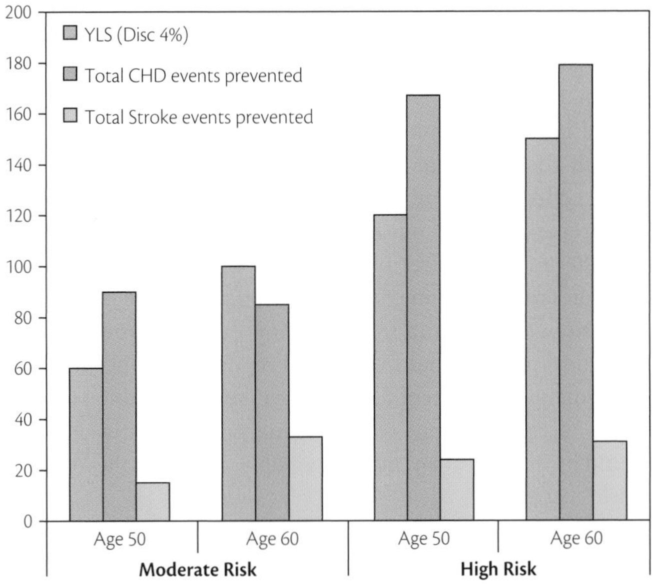

Fig. 19.1 Effects of 10 years of intervention with a polypill. Number of events prevented per 1000 people treated. Moderate risk refers to a 10–20% risk of coronary heart disease (CHD) in 10 years according to the Framingham risk score. High risk refers to a 10-year risk of CHD of ≥20%. YLS (Disc 4%), years of life saved discounted at 4%.

Side effects and cost-effectiveness

Although a polypill could be effective, medicalizing a large proportion of the population could have a great impact in terms of costs and side effects.

Despite the prevalence of participants in randomized trials reporting symptoms attributable to the polypill components being low (ranging from less than 0.1% for some antihypertensives to 3.9% for aspirin), it could be expected that up to 15% of those taking the polypill would experience an adverse effect, and these could be sufficient for permanent discontinuation in up to 2% [116]. Side effects of a polypill would depend on the individual components selected, among which aspirin could generate the most serious adverse effects including haemorrhagic stroke, extracranial haemorrhage, upper abdominal discomfort, and gastrointestinal bleeding. The specific probabilities of experiencing adverse effects while taking a polypill remain unknown, and studies with longer periods of polypill treatment will be necessary to obtain a better estimate. The levels of adverse effects would play a key role in the level of adherence to a polypill as well as in the cost-effectiveness of this treatment.

The potential costs of a polypill have been estimated to be rather low, given that the combination will include only generic components. The costs could range from $1 a day in developed countries to even less than 20 cents a day in developing countries [117]. However, since a polypill is not yet commercially available actual costs are still unknown and will depend on multiple factors, including levels of adverse effects, the cost of the ingredients to be included in the combination, costs of packaging and commercializing, and the costs of research, development, registration, marketing, and distribution, and profit margins for the manufacturers [117]. Given that the costs are unknown, the existing calculations on the cost-effectiveness of a polypill are only speculative; however, since all the individual components have proven to be cost-effective in multiple populations no major differences would be expected for a polypill. The first evaluation of the cost-effectiveness of a polypill calculated how much it should cost in order to be cost-effective for the primary prevention of CVD among men aged 50 years or above [123]. To be cost-effective in populations having levels of 10-year coronary heart disease risk over 20%, the annual cost of a polypill should not exceed €300, taking into account the costs of the medication and costs of care for prescription, evaluation, titration, and treatment of adverse effects [123]. For populations at lower levels of risk this cost should not be above €100 a year for a polypill to be considered cost-effective, at a threshold for cost-effectiveness of €20 000 per year of life saved (➲ see Fig. 19.2). More recently, using the Dutch primary healthcare setting, different potential polypill combinations were tested and found to be cost-effective compared with usual care [124]. The levels of cost-effectiveness ranged between €7900 and €12 300 per quality-adjusted life year (QALY) [124]. The best levels of cost-effectiveness were found for polypill combinations without aspirin and with a double dose of statins [124].

Although these initial reports indicate that it is very probable that a polypill will be cost-effective for the secondary prevention of CVD, the actual costs of a polypill once it becomes available and its cost-effectiveness for the primary prevention of CVD need further evaluation.

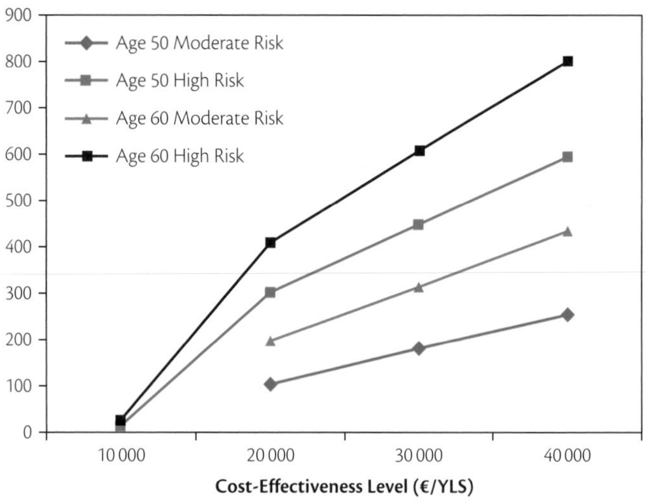

Fig. 19.2 Maximum annual cost of a polypill for primary prevention of CVD at different levels of cost-effectiveness. Annual drug costs are presented in Euros (€). Moderate risk refers to a 10–20% risk of CHD in 10 years according to the Framingham risk score. High risk refers to a 10-year risk of CHD of ≥20%. YLS, years of life saved.

Whether a polypill could be a safe and cost-effective alternative to current methods of preventing CVD remains unknown, and is one of the key challenges for its implementation for the prevention of CVD.

Future prospects

The polypill is a promising concept that has the potential to dramatically change and improve current strategies for preventing CVD. Questions remain regarding its long-term efficacy, safety, tolerability, and cost-effectiveness, especially for primary prevention of CVD. In addition, the impact that the availability of a 'super-pill' on people's willingness to follow a healthy lifestyle and the consequences of medicalizing large proportions of the population remain under debate.

Multiple trials aiming to clarify the role that a polypill could have in the treatment and prevention of CVD are currently being conducted. One of these, TIPS-3, will evaluate a polycap preparation without aspirin versus placebo over 5 years in 5000 individuals free from CVD in China and India [117]. It might take some time before sufficient evidence is accumulated to permit the full incorporation of the polypill concept in clinical practice, but from initial reports the concept seems a promising and potentially effective and affordable solution to the current epidemic of CVD: 'No other preventive method would have so great an impact on public health in the Western world' [116].

Once a polypill becomes available, instead of replacing a healthy lifestyle it should be combined with adequate levels of physical activity, smoking cessation, and an optimal diet to further reduce the levels of CVD.

Solution for the clinical case

The problem of dyspnoea and wheezing of this patient does not seem to be related to heart failure/elevated filling pressures or ischaemia. It is probably caused by his COPD and current intake of a non-selective beta-blocker. His blood pressure is also still too high.

In this case the non-selective beta-blocker should be replaced by a selective beta-blocker (e.g. bisoprolol 5 mg/day up-titrated to 10 mg/day). If beta-blockers are not tolerated at all, ivabradine may be considered.

For his hypertension problem, the dose of the ACEi is still suboptimal and can be increased to 20 mg/day. If the blood pressure is still above 140/90 mmHg, amlodipine 5 mg/day could be added. The combination of an ACEi with an ARB is not recommended in this patient in addition to the treatment with aliskiren.

Both the treatment with the ACEi and the beta-blocker should be continued as the patient suffered from a significant MI with left ventricular dysfunction.

Further reading

Beta-blockers

Erdmann E. Safety and tolerability of beta-blockers: prejudices and reality. *Eur Heart J* 2009; **11** (Suppl. A): A21–A25. [An excellent and critical overview of the absolute and relative contra-indications for beta-blockers in daily practice. The subchapters on asthma/COPD and impotence are especially worth reading.]

Lopez-Sandon J, Swedberg K, McMurray J, et al. Expert consensus document on β-adrenergic receptor blockers. The Task Force on Beta-Blockers of the European Society of Cardiology. *Eur Heart J* 2004; **25**: 1341–62. [This expert consensus document provides detailed information for the different indications for β-blocker treatment.]

McMurray JJ, Adamopoulos S, Anker SD, et al. ESC guidelines for the diagnosis and treatment of acute and chronic heart failure 2012. The Task Force for the Diagnosis and Treatment of Acute and Chronic Heart Failure 2012 of the European Society of Cardiology. *Eur Heart J* 2012; **33**: 1787–847. [These latest ESC guidelines on heart failure describe the place and the practical use of beta-blockers for patients with heart failure.]

Opie LH, Gersh BJ. *Drugs for the heart*, 7th edn, 2009. Philadelphia, PA: Saunders Elsevier, pp. 1–37. [Excellent textbook on cardiovascular drugs. The chapter on beta-blockers provides a detailed description on the pharmacology, types of beta-blockers, indications, and contraindications.]

Ivabradine

Fox K, Ford I, Steg PG, et al. Ivabradine for patients with stable coronary artery disease and left-ventricular systolic dysfunction (BEAUTIFUL): a randomised, double-blind, placebo-controlled trial. *Lancet* 2008; **372**: 807–16. [Landmark study on the effect of ivabradine in patients with stable coronary artery disease and left-ventricular systolic dysfunction.]

McMurray JJ, Adamopoulos S, Anker SD, et al. ESC guidelines for the diagnosis and treatment of acute and chronic heart failure 2012. The Task Force for the Diagnosis and Treatment of Acute and Chronic Heart Failure 2012 of the European Society of Cardiology. *Eur Heart J* 2012; **33**: 1787–847. [These latest ESC guidelines on heart failure describe the place and the practical use of ivabradine for patients with heart failure.]

Swedberg K, Komajda M, Böhm M, et al. SHIFT investigators. Ivabradine and outcomes in chronic heart failure (SHIFT): a randomised placebo-controlled study. *Lancet* 2010; **376**: 875–85. [Landmark study on the effect of ivabradine in patients with chronic systolic heart failure.]

RAAS blockers

Abdulla J, Barlera S, Latini R, et al. A systematic review: effect of angiotensin converting enzyme inhibition on left ventricular volumes and ejection fraction in patients with a myocardial infarction and in patients with left ventricular dysfunction. *Eur J Heart Fail* 2007; **9**: 129–35.

Abdulla J, Pogue J, Abildstrøm SZ, et al. Effect of angiotensin-converting enzyme inhibition on functional class in patients with left ventricular systolic dysfunction—a meta-analysis. *Eur J Heart Fail* 2006; **8**: 90–6.

Anand IS, Bishu K, Rector TS, et al. Proteinuria, chronic kidney disease, and the effect of an angiotensin receptor blocker in addition to an angiotensin-converting enzyme inhibitor in patients with moderate to severe heart failure. *Circulation* 2009; **120**: 1577–84.

Brugts JJ, Ninomiya T, Boersma E, et al. The consistency of the treatment effect of an ACE-inhibitor based treatment regimen in patients with vascular disease or high risk of vascular disease: a combined analysis of individual data of ADVANCE, EUROPA, and PROGRESS trials. *Eur Heart J* 2009; **30**: 1385–94.

Calhoun DA. Aldosterone and cardiovascular disease. *Circulation* 2006; **114**: 2572–4.

Desai A. Hyperkalemia associated with inhibitors of the renin-angiotensin-aldosterone system. *Circulation* 2008; **118**: 1609–11.

Leopold JA. Aldosterone, mineralocorticoid receptor activation, and cardiovascular remodeling. *Circulation* 2011; **124**: e466–e468.

Maron BA, Leopold JA. Aldosterone receptor antagonists. *Circulation* 2010; **121**: 934–9.

van Vark LC, Bertrand M, Akkerhuis KM, et al. Angiotensin-converting enzyme inhibitors reduce mortality in hypertension: a meta-analysis of randomized clinical trials of renin-angiotensin-aldosterone system inhibitors involving 158 998 patients. *Eur Heart J* 2012; **33**: 2088–97.

Calcium antagonists

Collier DJ, Poulter NR, Dahlof B, et al. Impact of amlodipine-based therapy among older and younger patients in the Anglo-Scandinavian Cardiac Outcomes Trial-Blood Pressure Lowering Arm (ASCOT-BPLA). *J Hypertens* 2011; **29**: 583–91.

Epstein M. *Calcium antagonists in clinical medicine*, 2nd edn, 1998. Philadelphia, PA: Hanley & Helfus, pp. 1–26.

Jerums G, Allen TJ, Campbell DJ, et al. Long-term renoprotection by perindopril or nifedipine in non-hypertensive patients with Type 2 diabetes and microalbuminuria. *Diabet Med* 2004; **21**: 1192–9.

The polypill

Indian Polycap Study (TIPS), Yusuf S, Pais P, Afzal R, et al. Effects of a polypill (Polycap) on risk factors in middle-aged individuals without cardiovascular disease (TIPS): a phase II, double-blind, randomised trial. *Lancet* 2009; **373**: 1341–51.

Lonn E, Bosch J, Teo KK, et al. The polypill in the prevention of cardiovascular diseases: key concepts, current status, challenges, and future directions. *Circulation* 2010; **122**: 2078–88.

Wald NJ, Law MR. A strategy to reduce cardiovascular disease by more than 80%. *Br Med J* 2003; **326**: 1419.

References

1 Lopez-Sandon J, Swedberg K, McMurray J, et al. Expert consensus document on β-adrenergic receptor blockers. The Task Force on Beta-Blockers of the European Society of Cardiology. *Eur Heart J* 2004; **25**: 1341–62.

2 Opie LH, Gersh BJ. *Drugs for the heart*, 7th edn, 2009. Philadelphia, PA: Saunders Elsevier, pp. 1–37.

3 Van de Werf F, Bax J, Betriu A, et al. Management of acute myocardial infarction in patients presenting with persistent ST-segment elevation: the Task Force on the Management of ST-Segment Elevation Acute Myocardial Infarction of the European Society of Cardiology. *Eur Heart J* 2008; **29**: 2909–45.

4 Hamm CW, Bassand JP, Agewall S, et al. ESC guidelines for the management of acute coronary syndromes in patients presenting without persistent ST-segment elevation. The Task Force for the Management of Acute Coronary Syndromes (ACS) in Patients Presenting Without Persistent ST-segment Elevation of the European Society of Cardiology (ESC). *Eur Heart J* 2011; **32**: 2909–3054.

5 Messerli FH, Mancia G, Conti CR, et al. Guidelines on the management of stable angina pectoris: executive summary: the Task Force on the Management of Stable Angina Pectoris of the European Society of Cardiology. *Eur Heart J* 2006; **27**: 2902–3.

6 Voko Z, de Brouwer S, Lubsen J, et al. Long-term impact of secondary preventive treatments in patients with stable angina. *Eur J Epidemiol* 2011; **26**: 375–83.

7 Bangalore S, Steg G, Deedwania P, et al. B-blocker use and clinical outcomes in stable outpatients with and without coronary artery disease. *J Am Med Assoc* 2012; **308**: 1340–9.

8 Smith S, Benjamin E, Bonow R, et al. AHA/ACCF secondary prevention and risk reduction therapy for patients with coronary and other atherosclerotic vascular disease: 2011 update: a guideline from the American Heart Association and American College of Cardiology Foundation. *Circulation* 2011; **124**: 2458–73.

9 Rehnqvist N, Hjemdahl P, Billing E, et al. Treatment of stable angina pectoris with calcium antagonist and beta-blockers. The APSIS study, angina prognosis in Stockholm. *Cardiologia* 1995; **40** (Suppl. 1): 301.

10 Dargie HJ, Ford I, Fox KM.Total ischaemic burden European trial (TIBET). Effects of ischaemia and treatment with atenolol, nifedipine SR and their combination on outcome in patients with chronic stable angina. The TIBET Study Group. *Eur Heart J* 1996; **17**: 104–12.

11 MACB Study Group. Effect of metoprolol on death and cardiac events during a 2-year period after coronary artery bypass grafting. *Eur Heart J* 1995; **16**: 1825–32.

12 Okrainec K, Platt R, Pilote L, et al. Cardiac medical therapy in patients after undergoing coronary artery bypass graft surgery. *J Am Coll Cardiol* 2005; **45**: 177–84.

13 The Cardiac Insufficiency Bisoprolol Study II (CIBIS-II): a randomized trial. *Lancet* 1999; **353**: 9–13.

14 Packer M, Coats AJ, Fowler MB, et al. Effect of carvedilol on survival in severe chronic heart failure. *N Engl J Med* 2001; **344**: 1651–8.

15 Effect of metoprolol CR/XL in chronic heart failure: metoprolol CR/XL. Randomised Intervention Trial in Congestive Heart Failure (MERIT-HF). *Lancet* 1999; **353**: 2001–7.

16 Flather MD, Shibata MC, Coats AJ, et al. Randomized trial to determine the effect of nebivolol on mortality and cardiovascular hospital admission in elderly patients with heart failure (SENIORS). *Eur Heart J* 2005; **26**: 215–25.

17 Beta-Blocker Evaluation of Survival Trial Investigators. A trial of the beta-blocker bucindolol in patients with advanced chronic heart failure. *N Engl J Med* 2001; **344**: 1659–67.

18 McMurray JJ, Adamopoulos S, Anker SD, et al. ESC guidelines for the diagnosis and treatment of acute and chronic heart failure 2012. The Task Force for the Diagnosis and Treatment of Acute and Chronic Heart Failure 2012 of the European Society of Cardiology. *Eur Heart J* 2012; **33**: 1787–847

19 Camm AJ, Kirchhof P, Lip GY, et al. Guidelines for the management of atrial fibrillation: the Task Force for the Management of Atrial Fibrillation of the European Society of Cardiology (ESC). European Heart Rhythm Association; European Association for Cardio-Thoracic Surgery. *Eur Heart J* 2010; **31**: 2369–429.

20 Poldermans D, Bax JJ, Boersma E, et al. Guidelines for pre-operative cardiac risk assessment and perioperative cardiac management in non-cardiac surgery. Task Force for Preoperative Cardiac Risk Assessment and Perioperative Cardiac Management in Non-cardiac Surgery; European Society of Cardiology (ESC). *Eur Heart J* 2009; **30**: 2769–812.

21 Ryden L, Standl E, Bartnik M, et al. Guidelines on diabetes, pre-diabetes and cardiovascular diseases: executive summary. The Task Force on Diabetes and Cardiovascular Diseases of the European Society of Cardiology (ESC) and of the European Association for the study of Diabetes (EASD). *Eur Heart J* 2007; **28**: 88–136.

22 Andrus MR, Hollday KP, Clark DB. Use of beta-blockers in patients with COPD. *Ann Pharmacother* 2004; **38**: 142–5.

23 Gottlieb SS, McCarter RJ, Vogel RA. Effect of beta-blockade on mortality among high-risk and low-risk patients after myocardial infarction. *N Engl J Med* 1998; **339**: 489–97.

24 Erdmann E. Safety and tolerability of beta-blockers: prejudices and reality. *Eur Heart J* 2009; **11** (Suppl. A): A21–A25.

25 Pinto FJ. Coronary artery disease management with ivabradine in clinical practice. *Eur Heart J* 2011; **13** (Suppl. C): C25–C29.

26 Borer JS, Fox K, Jaillon P, et al. Antianginal and anti-ischemic effect of ivabradine an I_f inhibitor in stable angina. A randomized, double-blind, multicentered, placebo controlled trial. *Circulation* 2003; **107**: 817–23.

27 Tardiff JC, Ford I, Tendera M, et al. Anti-anginal and anti-ischemic efficacy of the I_f current inhibitor ivabradine vs. atenolol in stable angina. A 4-month randomized, double-blind, multicenter trial. *Eur Heart J* 2005; **26**: 2529–37.

28 Tardiff JC, Ponikowski P, Kahan T. Efficacy of the I_f current inhibitor ivabradine in patients with chronic stable angina receiving beta-blocker therapy: a 4 month, randomized, placebo-controlled trial. *Eur Heart J* 2009; **30**: 540–8.

and irregular dosing in the CAPE II trial. *J Am Coll Cardiol* 2002; **40**: 917–25.

100 Theroux P, Taeymans Y, Morissette D, et al. A randomized study comparing propranolol and diltiazem in the treatment of unstable angina. *J Am Coll Cardiol* 1985; **5**: 717–22.

101 Parodi O, Simonetti I, Michelassi C, et al. Comparison of verapamil and propranolol therapy for angina pectoris at rest: a randomized, multiple-crossover, controlled trial in the coronary care unit. *Am J Cardiol* 1986; **57**: 899–906.

102 Poole-Wilson PA, Kirwan BA, Voko Z, et al. Safety of nifedipine GITS in stable angina: the ACTION trial. *Cardiovasc Drugs Ther* 2006; **20**: 45–54.

103 Hamm CW, Bassand JP, Agewall S, et al. ESC guidelines for the management of acute coronary syndromes in patients presenting without persistent ST-segment elevation: The Task Force for the Management of Acute Coronary Syndromes (ACS) in Patients Presenting Without Persistent ST-segment Elevation of the European Society of Cardiology (ESC). *Eur Heart J* 2011; **32**: 2999–3054.

104 Moss AJ, Oakes D, Rubison M, et al. Effects of diltiazem on long-term outcome after acute myocardial infarction in patients with and without a history of systemic hypertension. The Multicenter Diltiazem Postinfarction Trial Research Group. *Am J Cardiol* 1991; **68**: 429–33.

105 Sleight P. Calcium antagonists during and after myocardial infarction. *Drugs* 1996; **51**: 216–25.

106 de Vries RJ, van Veldhuisen DJ, Dunselman PH. Efficacy and safety of calcium channel blockers in heart failure: focus on recent trials with second-generation dihydropyridines. *Am Heart J* 2000; **139**: 185–94.

107 O'Connor CM, Carson PE, Miller AB, et al. Effect of amlodipine on mode of death among patients with advanced heart failure in the PRAISE trial. Prospective Randomized Amlodipine Survival Evaluation. *Am J Cardiol* 1998; **82**: 881–7.

108 Cohn JN, Ziesche S, Smith R, et al. Effect of the calcium antagonist felodipine as supplementary vasodilator therapy in patients with chronic heart failure treated with enalapril: V-HeFT III. Vasodilator-Heart Failure Trial (V-HeFT) Study Group. *Circulation* 1997; **96**: 856–63.

109 Regitz-Zagrosek V, Blomstrom Lundqvist C, Borghi C, et al. ESC guidelines on the management of cardiovascular diseases during pregnancy. *Eur Heart J* 2011; **32**: 3147–97.

110 Galie N, Torbicki A, Barst R, et al. Guidelines on diagnosis and treatment of pulmonary arterial hypertension. The Task Force on Diagnosis and Treatment of Pulmonary Arterial Hypertension of the European Society of Cardiology. *Eur Heart J* 2004; **25**: 2243–78.

111 Maron BJ, McKenna WJ, Danielson GK, et al. American College of Cardiology/European Society of Cardiology Clinical Expert Consensus Document on Hypertrophic Cardiomyopathy. A report of the American College of Cardiology Foundation Task Force on Clinical Expert Consensus Documents and the European Society of Cardiology Committee for Practice Guidelines. *Eur Heart J* 2003; **24**: 1965–91.

112 Gersh BJ, Maron BJ, Bonow RO, et al. 2011 ACCF/AHA guideline for the diagnosis and treatment of hypertrophic cardiomyopathy: executive summary: a report of the American College of Cardiology Foundation/American Heart Association Task Force on Practice Guidelines. *Circulation* 2011; **124**: 2761–96.

113 European Heart Rhythm Association; European Association for Cardio-Thoracic Surgery, Camm AJ, Kirchhof P, Lip GYH, et al. Guidelines for the management of atrial fibrillation. *Eur Heart J* 2010; **31**: 2369–429.

114 Blomström-Lundqvist C, Scheinman MM, Aliot EM, et al. ACC/AHA/ESC guidelines for the management of patients with supraventricular arrhythmias—executive summary. *Eur Heart J* 2003; **24**: 1857–97.

115 Messerli FH, Grossman E. Pedal edema—not all dihydropyridine calcium antagonists are created equal. *Am J Hypertens* 2002; **15**: 1019–20.

116 Wald NJ, Law MR. A strategy to reduce cardiovascular disease by more than 80%. *Br Med J* 2003; **326**: 1419.

117 Lonn E, Bosch J, Teo KK, et al. The polypill in the prevention of cardiovascular diseases: key concepts, current status, challenges, and future directions. *Circulation* 2010; **122**: 2078–88.

118 Patel A, Shah T, Shah G, et al. Preservation of bioavailability of ingredients and lack of drug-drug interactions in a novel five-ingredient polypill (polycap): a five-arm phase I crossover trial in healthy volunteers. *Am J Cardiovasc Drugs* 2010; **10**: 95–103.

119 Muntner P, Mann D, Wildman RP, et al. Projected impact of polypill use among US adults: medication use, cardiovascular risk reduction, and side effects. *Am Heart J* 2011; **161**: 719–25.

120 Wald DS, Morris JK, Wald NJ. Randomized polypill crossover trial in people aged 50 and over. *PLoS ONE* 2012; **7**: e41297.

121 Indian Polycap Study (TIPS), Yusuf S, Pais P, Afzal R, et al. Effects of a polypill (Polycap) on risk factors in middle-aged individuals without cardiovascular disease (TIPS): a phase II, double-blind, randomised trial. *Lancet* 2009; **373**: 1341–51.

122 Yusuf S, Pais P, Sigamani A, et al. Comparison of risk factor reduction and tolerability of a full-dose polypill (with potassium) versus low-dose polypill (polycap) in individuals at high risk of cardiovascular diseases: the Second Indian Polycap Study (TIPS-2) Investigators. *Circ Cardiovasc Qual Outcomes* 2012; **5**: 463–71.

123 Franco OH, Steyerberg EW, de Laet C. The polypill: at what price would it become cost effective? *J Epidemiol Community Health* 2006; **60**: 213–17. [Erratum in *J Epidemiol Community Health* 2006; **60**: 735.]

124 van Gils PF, Over EA, Hamberg-van Reenen HH, et al. The polypill in the primary prevention of cardiovascular disease: cost-effectiveness in the Dutch population. *Br Med J Open* 2011; **1**: e000363.

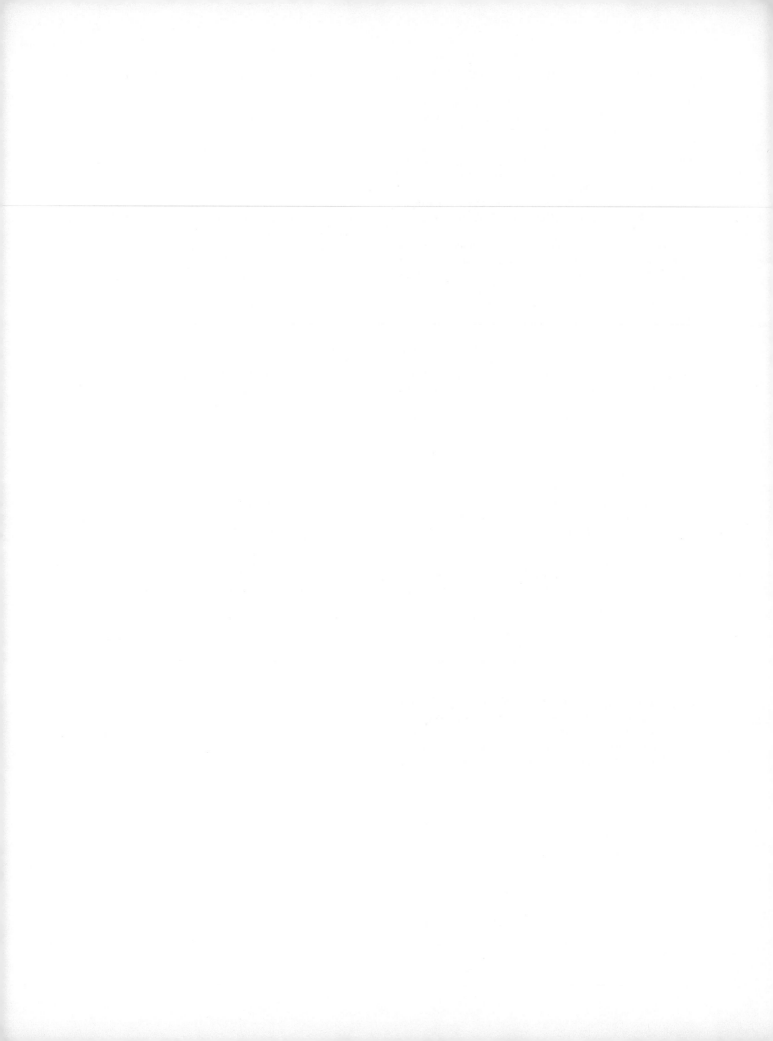

PART 4

Setting and delivery of preventive cardiology

CHAPTER 20

General remarks

Pantaleo Giannuzzi

Contents

Summary

Cardiac patients should be advised about and have the opportunity to access a comprehensive cardiovascular prevention and rehabilitation programme, addressing all aspects of lifestyle—smoking cessation, healthy eating, and being physically active—together with more effective management of blood pressure, lipids, and glucose. To achieve the clinical benefits of a multidisciplinary and multifactorial prevention programme we need to integrate professional lifestyle interventions with effective risk factor management and evidence-based drug therapies, appropriately adapted to the medical, cultural, and economic setting of a country. The challenge is to engage and motivate cardiologists, physicians, and health professionals to routinely practise high-quality preventive cardiology and promote a healthcare system which invests in prevention.

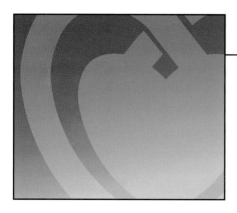

Introduction

Non-communicable diseases (NCDs) are the leading cause of death world-wide, killing more people each year than all other causes combined. Of the 57 million deaths that occurred globally in 2008, 36 million, or almost two thirds, were due to NCDs, mainly cardiovascular diseases (CVD), cancers, diabetes, and chronic lung diseases. About a quarter of global deaths from NCDs occur before the age of 60, and the combined burden of these diseases is rising fastest in lower-income countries, populations, and communities, where they impose large, avoidable human, social, and economic costs. NCDs are caused, to a large extent, by four behavioural risk factors that are pervasive aspects of economic transition, rapid urbanization, and twenty-first-century lifestyles: namely tobacco use, an unhealthy diet, insufficient physical activity, and the harmful use of alcohol. Together these behavioural risk factors are strongly associated with other major cardiovascular (CV) risk factors including hypertension, diabetes, obesity, and metabolic syndrome [1].

Interventions to prevent NCDs on a population-wide basis are not only achievable but also cost-effective. The level of income of a country or population is not a barrier to success. Low-cost solutions can work anywhere to reduce the major risk factors for NCDs.

Currently, the main focus of healthcare for NCDs in many low- and middle-income countries is hospital-centred acute care. Patients with NCDs present at hospitals with CVD, cancer, diabetes, and chronic respiratory diseases that have reached the point of acute events or long-term complications. This is a very expensive approach that will not contribute to a significant reduction in the burden of NCDs. It also denies people the health benefits of taking care of their conditions at an early stage.

Evidence from high-income countries shows that a comprehensive focus on prevention and improved treatment following CV events can lead to dramatic declines in mortality rates. Similarly, progress in cancer treatment combined with early detection and screening interventions have improved survival rates for many cancers in high-income countries. Survival rates in low- and middle-income countries, however, remain very low. A combination of population-wide and individual interventions can reproduce successes in many more countries through cost-effective initiatives that strengthen health systems [2,3].

Strategies for preventive cardiology: healthcare systems for CV prevention

A strategic objective in the fight against the CVD epidemic must be to ensure early detection and care using cost-effective and sustainable healthcare interventions.

High-risk individuals and those with established CVD can be treated with regimens of low-cost generic medicines that significantly reduce the likelihood of death or CV events. A regimen of aspirin, statins, and blood pressure-lowering agents could significantly reduce vascular events in people at high CV risk and is considered a 'best buy'. When coupled with preventive measures such as smoking cessation the therapeutic benefits can be profound. Another best buy is the administration of aspirin to people who develop a myocardial infarction (MI). In all countries these best buys need to be scaled up and delivered through a primary healthcare approach [4].

What is needed are high levels of commitment, good planning, community mobilization, and an intense focus on a small range of critical actions. With these, quick gains will be achieved in reducing the major behavioural risk factors, namely tobacco use, harmful use of alcohol, unhealthy diet, and physical inactivity, together with key risk factors for cancer, notably some chronic infections.

Notable interventions with an evident impact include: increases in tobacco taxes and restrictions on smoking in public places and workplaces; increases in alcohol taxes and restriction of sales; mandatory and voluntary reduction of salt in foods; and improved access to places for physical activities such as walking.

In addressing CVD, the population-wide approach to prevention has great potential to decrease the burden of disease but it does not provide an adequate response to the need to strengthen healthcare for people with CVD. The burden of disease can be reduced considerably in the short to medium term if the population-wide approach is complemented by healthcare interventions for individuals who either already have CVD or those who are at high risk. CVD can best be addressed by a combination of primary prevention interventions targeting whole populations, measures that target high-risk individuals, and improved access to essential healthcare interventions for people with CVD [4–7].

For primary prevention of coronary heart disease (CHD) and stroke, individual healthcare interventions can be targeted to those at high total CV risk or those with levels of a single risk factor above traditional thresholds, such as hypertension and hypercholesterolaemia [4]. The former approach is more cost-effective than the latter and has the potential to substantially reduce CV events [1,4,6]. Furthermore, application of this approach is also feasible in primary care in low-resource settings, including by non-physician health workers [8,9]. It has been estimated that a regimen of aspirin, statin, and blood pressure-lowering agents may significantly reduce the risk of death from CVD in people at high CV risk (people with a 10-year CV risk equal to or above 15% and those who have suffered a previous CV event). It has been estimated that providing such a regimen to those eligible between the ages of 40 and 79 could avert about a fifth of CV deaths in the next 10 years, with 56% of deaths averted in people younger than 70 years [4].

For secondary prevention (SP) of CVD (prevention of recurrences and complications in those with established disease), aspirin, beta-blockers, angiotensin-converting enzyme inhibitors, and lipid-lowering therapies reduce the risk of recurrent CV events, including in those with diabetes. The benefits of these interventions are largely independent, so that when used together with smoking cessation about three-quarters of recurrent vascular events may be prevented [5].

Currently there are major gaps in the implementation of SP interventions that can be delivered in primary care settings [6,7]. General practitioners are critical to the implementation and success of CVD prevention programmes. In most countries, they deliver the majority of consultations and provide most public health medicine (preventive care, disease screening, chronic disease monitoring, and follow-up). In the case of CVD prevention they have a unique role in identifying individuals at risk of but without established CVD and assessing their eligibility for intervention based on their profile. Thus, the physician in general practice is the key person to initiate, coordinate, and provide long-term follow-up for CVD prevention, while the practising cardiologist should be the advisor in cases where there is uncertainty over the use of preventive medication or when usual preventive options are difficult to apply [6,7].

Nurse-coordinated prevention programmes are also effective across a variety of practice settings and should be well integrated into healthcare systems. Nurse case management models tested in several randomized trials of SP have shown significant improvements in risk factors, exercise tolerance, glucose control, and appropriate use of medication, along with decreases in cardiac events and mortality, regression of coronary atherosclerosis, and improved patient perception of health compared with usual care. Other studies have demonstrated the effectiveness of nurse-led prevention clinics in primary care compared with usual care, with greater success in secondary as opposed to primary prevention [10,11].

Hospital-based programmes: specialized prevention centres

All patients with CVD should be discharged from hospital with clear guideline-orientated treatment recommendations to minimize the risk of further adverse events. The 2012 ESC guidelines provide a checklist of measures necessary at discharge from hospital to ensure that intense risk factor modification and lifestyle change are implemented in all patients following the diagnosis of an acute coronary syndrome, including recommendation for enrolment in a CV prevention and rehabilitation programme [7].

Secondary preventive efforts within a structured rehabilitation programme have been shown to be particularly important and cost-effective after a CV event. Intensive research in the field of preventive cardiology has led to the spread of cardiac rehabilitation (CR) programmes, once limited to exercise training, to comprehensive SP centres. CR after cardiac events or interventions in a specialized centre helps to maintain long-term adherence to the optimal treatment programme by educating the patient and repeatedly emphasizing the importance of maintaining the prescribed treatments and recommended lifestyle. Data demonstrate that CR/SP programmes reduce CV risk and event rates, foster healthy behaviours, and promote active lifestyles [12–15].

There is compelling scientific evidence that CR is an effective treatment for patients with CHD [7,12–15]. A meta-analysis of 8940 patients from 48 trials of CR showed that a structured service, compared with usual care, was associated with a reduction in all-cause mortality (odds ratio 0.80; 95% CI 0.68–0.93) and cardiac mortality (odds ratio 0.74; 95% CI 0.61–0.96) [16]. Another meta-analysis of the effectiveness of SP programmes from 63 randomized controlled trials including 21 295 patients showed a summary risk ratio for all-cause mortality of 0.85 (95% CI 0.77–0.94) and for recurrent myocardial infarction of 0.83 (95% CI 0.74–0.94) [17]. In a systematic review of trials of SP, multidisciplinary disease management programmes led to a reduction in hospital admissions and recurrent MI [14,15]. So the distinction between 'CR' and 'SP' is artificial, and these meta-analyses demonstrate the overall benefits of an integrated multidisciplinary and comprehensive multifactorial approach to reducing CV risk, CV events, and all-cause mortality.

However, despite the strength of this evidence, CR in Europe continues to be considerably underused with poor referral and a low participation rate. The results of the EUROASPIRE III survey showed inadequate control of lifestyle and risk factors and underuse of CR in Europe. Fewer than half of patients with CHD were advised to follow a CR programme, and just over a third actually participated in some form of CR. Yet, of those who were advised to attend a CR/SP programme, four-fifths did so. These results are similar to those of the EUROASPIRE II survey, which demonstrated that two in five coronary patients reported receiving advice to follow a CR programme and only a third actually attended some form of CR. The comparison between those 13 countries which participated in both the EUROASPIRE II and III surveys demonstrated that the proportion of patients advised to follow a CR programme increased from 44.5 to 55.7% ($p < 0.0001$) and the participation rate also increased from 38.0 to 46.1% ($p < 0.0001$). In EUROASPIRE III, there was considerable variation between European countries in participation in a CR programme, with the highest attendance reported in Lithuania and Ireland, the lowest in Turkey, Cyprus, and the Russian Federation, and virtually no attendance in Greece and Spain. These differences are most likely to reflect the heterogeneity of healthcare systems and the availability of CR/SP services in some regions of Europe [18,19].

Addressing the factors that limit participation is particularly important given recent data that demonstrate an inverse relationship between participation in a CR/SP programme and adverse CV events. The relationship between the number of CR/SP sessions attended and CV outcomes was recently evaluated in an analysis of Medicare claims data including 30 161 patients with CHD (with recent coronary artery bypass surgery, MI, or acute coronary syndrome) who attended at least one CR/SP session [20]. After 4 years of follow-up, patients who attended 36 sessions had a 14% lower risk of death and a 12% lower risk of MI than those who attended 24 sessions; a 22% lower risk of death and a 23% lower risk of MI than those who attended 12 sessions; and a 47% lower risk of death and a 31% lower risk of MI than those who attended one session. However, only 18% of the patients completed the maximum 36 sessions. This dose-dependent improvement further highlights the importance of patient retention in CR/SP programmes. Clinical outcomes following percutaneous coronary intervention were assessed in a retrospective analysis of 2395 patients (40% of whom attended CR). Participation in CR was associated with decreased all-cause mortality (hazard ratio 0.53–0.55, $p < 0.001$), although no effect on cardiac death or MI was noted [21].

These important and recent findings further support the recommendations provided in clinical guidelines, and also the reimbursement policy instituted in many countries.

CR/SP programmes are based on long-established models involving hospital, ambulatory, community, or home-based programmes, according to local and national traditions. However, most of the CR programmes rely mainly on short-term interventions and are not adequately implemented in the long term. Short-term interventions are unlikely to bring in long-term benefits with regard to lifestyle and risk factor management, improve quality of life, or decrease morbidity and mortality. Recent studies as EUROACTION and GOSPEL provided scientific evidence for a beneficial long-term effect and improved prognosis in patients with CHD [22,23]. The EUROACTION model of a nurse-led preventive cardiology programme in patients with CHD is an example of what a comprehensive approach to reducing total CV risk can achieve. This cluster randomized controlled trial demonstrated improved lifestyle and risk factor outcomes compared with usual care. Over 1 year EUROACTION prevented smoking relapse, increased fruit and vegetable consumption and physical activity with a corresponding reduction in weight and waist circumference, improved blood pressure and lipid control, and increased prescribing of angiotensin-converting enzyme inhibitors and statins [22]. The GOSPEL study was a multicentre, randomized controlled trial that compared a long-term multifactorial educational and behavioural intervention coordinated by a cardiologist versus usual care after a standard CR programme following MI [23]. At 3 years all the clinical end-points were reduced by the intensive intervention: CV mortality, non-fatal MI, and stroke by 33% and cardiac death plus non-fatal MI by 36%, total stroke by 32%, and total mortality by 21%. So there is considerable potential to further reduce the risk of CVD in existing CR/SP programmes.

Different patterns of rehabilitative care are currently delivered by specialized hospital-based teams: residential CR for more complicated, disabled patients and outpatient CR for more independent, low-risk, and clinically stable patients requiring less supervision. Whereas the core components and goals of CR/SP are standardized and documented in position papers, the structure and type of CR units vary in different countries [14,15]. While the objectives are identical to those of the outpatient CR programmes, residential rehabilitation programmes are specifically structured to provide more intensive and/or complex interventions, and have the advantage of being able to start early after the acute event, to include more complicated high-risk or clinically unstable patients, to include more severely incapacitated and/or elderly patients (especially those with comorbidity), and thus to facilitate the transition from the hospital phase to a more stable clinical condition which may allow the maintenance of an independent life at home. One major disadvantage of residential programmes is the relatively short duration of intervention with regard to risk factor management and lifestyle changes. Therefore, residential CR programmes should be followed up by a long-term outpatient risk reduction and SP programme, with appropriate clinical and functional monitoring. Home-based rehabilitation programmes directed by physicians and coordinated by nurses have also been developed as a way of expanding the delivery of SP services.

Conclusions

All coronary patients should be advised about and have the opportunity to access a comprehensive CV prevention and rehabilitation programme, addressing all aspects of lifestyle—smoking cessation, healthy eating, and being physically active—together with more effective management of blood pressure, lipids, and glucose. To achieve the clinical benefits of a multidisciplinary and multifactorial prevention programme we need to integrate professional lifestyle interventions with effective risk factor management, and evidence-based drug therapies, appropriately adapted to the medical, cultural, and economic setting of a country. The challenge is to engage and motivate cardiologists, physicians, and health professionals to routinely practise high-quality preventive cardiology and a healthcare system which invests in prevention.

Further reading

Giannuzzi P, Saner H, Björnstad H, et al. Secondary prevention through cardiac rehabilitation: position paper of the working group on cardiac rehabilitation and exercise physiology of the European Society of Cardiology. *Eur Heart J* 2003; **24**: 1273–8.

Graham I, Atar D, Borch-Johnsen K, et al. European guidelines on cardiovascular disease prevention in clinical practice: full text. Fourth Joint Task Force of the European Society of Cardiology and Other Societies on Cardiovascular Disease Prevention in Clinical Prevention in Clinical Practice (constituted by representatives of nine societies and by invited experts). *Eur J Cardiovasc Prev Rehabil* 2007; **14** (Suppl. 2): S1–S113.

Perk J, De Backer G, Golhke H, et al. European guidelines on cardiovascular disease prevention in clinical practice (version 2012): Fifth Joint Task Force of the European Society of Cardiology and Other Societies on Cardiovascular Disease Prevention in Clinical Prevention in Clinical Practice (constituted by representatives of nine societies and by invited experts). *Eur Heart J* 2012; **33**: 1635–701.

Piepoli MF, Corrà U, Benzer W, et al. Secondary prevention through cardiac rehabilitation: from knowledge to implementation. A position paper from the Cardiac Rehabilitation Section of the European Association of Cardiovascular Prevention and Rehabilitation. *Eur J Cardiovasc Prev Rehabil* 2010; **17**: 1–17.

Piepoli MF, Corrà U, Adamopoulos S, et al. Secondary prevention in the clinical management of patients with cardiovascular diseases. Core components, standards and outcome measures for referral and delivery: a policy statement from the Cardiac Rehabilitation Section of the European Association for Cardiovascular Prevention and Rehabilitation. Endorsed by the Committee for Practice Guidelines of the European Society of Cardiology. *Eur J Prev Cardiol* 2012; **21**: 664–81.

References

1 World Health Organization. *Global status report on noncommunicable disease, 2010*, 2011. Geneva: World Health Organization.

2 World Health Organization. *Global strategy for the prevention and control of noncommunicable diseases*, 2000. Geneva: World Health Organization.

3 World Health Organization. *Prevention of cardiovascular disease: guidelines for assessment and management of total cardiovascular risk*, 2007. Geneva: World Health Organization.

4 Lim SS, Gaziano TA, Gakidou E, et al. Prevention of cardiovascular disease in high-risk individuals in low-income and middle-income countries: health effects and costs. *Lancet* 2007; **370**: 2054–62.

5 Yusuf S. Two decades of progress in preventing vascular disease. *Lancet* 2002; **360**: 2–3.

6 Graham I, Atar D, Borch-Johnsen K, et al. European guidelines on cardiovascular disease prevention in clinical practice: full text. Fourth Joint Task Force of the European Society of Cardiology and Other Societies on Cardiovascular Disease Prevention in Clinical Prevention in Clinical Practice (constituted by representatives of nine societies and by invited experts). *Eur J Cardiovasc Prev Rehabil* 2007; 14 (Suppl. 2): S1–S113.

7 Perk J, De Backer G, Golhke H, et al. European guidelines on cardiovascular disease prevention in clinical practice (version 2012): Fifth Joint Task Force of the European Society of Cardiology and Other Societies on Cardiovascular Disease Prevention in Clinical Prevention in Clinical Practice (constituted by representatives of nine societies and by invited experts). *Eur Heart J* 2012; **33**: 1635–701.

8 World Health Organization. *Package of essential noncommunicable disease interventions for primary healthcare in low-resource setting*, 2010. Geneva: World Health Organization.
9 Abegunde DO, Shengelia B, Luyten A, et al. Can non-physician healthcare workers assess and manage cardiovascular risk in primary care? *Bull World Health Organ* 2007; **85**: 432–40.
10 Berra K, Fletcher BJ, Hayman LL, et al. Global cardiovascular disease prevention: a call to action for nursing: the global burden of cardiovascular disease. *J Cardiovasc Nurs* 2011; **26**: S1–S2.
11 Koelewijn-van Loon MS, van der Weijden T, Ronda G, et al. Improving lifestyle and risk perception through patient involvement in nurse-led cardiovascular risk management: a cluster-randomized controlled trial in primary care. *Prev Med* 2010; **50**: 35–44.
12 Giannuzzi P, Saner H, Björnstad H, et al. Secondary prevention through cardiac rehabilitation: position paper of the working group on cardiac rehabilitation and exercise physiology of the European Society of Cardiology. *Eur Heart J* 2003; **24**: 1273–8.
13 Piepoli MF, Corrà U, Benzer W, et al. Secondary prevention through cardiac rehabilitation: from knowledge to implementation. A position paper from the Cardiac Rehabilitation Section of the European Association of Cardiovascular Prevention and Rehabilitation. *Eur J Cardiovasc Prev Rehabil* 2010; **17**: 1–17.
14 Balady GJ, Ades PA, Bittner VA, et al. Referral, enrolment, and delivery of cardiac rehabilitation/secondary prevention programs at clinical centers and beyond: a presidential advisory from the American Heart Association. *Circulation* 2011; **124**: 2951–60.
15 Piepoli MF, Corrà U, Adamopoulos S, et al. Secondary prevention in the clinical management of patients with cardiovascular diseases. Core components, standards and outcome measures for referral and delivery: a policy statement from the Cardiac Rehabilitation Section of the European Association for Cardiovascular Prevention and Rehabilitation. Endorsed by the Committee for Practice Guidelines of the European Society of Cardiology. *Eur J Prev Cardiol* 2012; **21**: 664–81.
16 Taylor RS, Brown A, Ebrahim S, et al. Exercise-based rehabilitation for patients with coronary heart disease: systematic review and meta-analysis of randomized controlled trials. *Am J Med* 2004; **116**: 782–92.
17 Clark AM, Hartling L, Vandermeer B, et al. Meta-analysis: secondary prevention programs for patients with coronary artery disease. *Ann Intern Med* 2005; **143**: 659–72.
18 Kotseva K, Wood D, De Backer G, et al; on behalf of EUROASPIRE Study Group. Cardiovascular prevention guidelines—the clinical reality: a comparison of EUROASPIRE I, II and III surveys in 8 European countries. *Lancet* 2009; **372**: 929–40.
19 Kotseva K, Wood D, De Backer G, et al; on behalf of EUROASPIRE Study Group. EUROASPIRE III: a survey on the lifestyle, risk factors and use of cardioprotective drug therapies in coronary patients from twenty two European countries. *Eur J Cardiovasc Prev Rehabil* 2009; **16**: 121–37.
20 Hammill BG, Curtis LH, Schulman KA, et al. Relationship between cardiac rehabilitation and long-term risks of death and myocardial infarction among elderly Medicare beneficiaries. *Circulation* 2010; **121**: 63–70.
21 Goel K, Lennon RJ, Tilbury RT, et al. Impact of cardiac rehabilitation on mortality and cardiovascular events after percutaneous coronary intervention in the community. *Circulation* 2011; **123**: 2344–52.
22 Wood DA, Kotseva K, Connolly S, et al; on behalf of the EUROACTION Study Group. EUROACTION: a European Society of Cardiology demonstration project in preventive cardiology. A paired cluster randomised controlled trial of a multi-disciplinary family based preventive cardiology programme for coronary patients and asymptomatic high risk individuals. *Lancet* 2008; **371**: 1999–2012.
23 Giannuzzi P, Temporelli PL, Marchioli R, et al Global secondary prevention strategies to limit event recurrence after myocardial infarction: results of the GOSPEL study, a multicenter, randomized controlled trial from the Italian Cardiac Rehabilitation Network. *Arch Intern Med* 2008; **168**: 2194–204.

CHAPTER 21

Acute care, immediate secondary prevention, and referral

Ugo Corrà and Bernhard Rauch

Contents

Summary

Preventive cardiology (PC), as performed in various cardiac rehabilitation (CR) settings, is effective in reducing recurrent cardiovascular events after both acute coronary syndromes and myocardial revascularization. However, the need for newly structured PC programmes and processes to provide a continuum of care and surveillance from acute to post-acute phases is still evident. Phase I CR is becoming more and more important, serving as a bridge between acute therapeutic interventions and phase II CR. After clinical stabilization, phase I CR ideally involves multifaceted and multidisciplinary interventions, including post-acute clinical evaluation and risk assessment, general counselling, supportive counselling, early mobilization, discharge planning, and referral to phase II CR. All these interventions are important and contribute equally to achievement of the preventive target, which is to effectively reduce lifelong cardiovascular risk and guarantee an individual full participation in social activities. All the interventions within phase I CR should be supervised and provided in a comprehensive manner involving several healthcare professionals. For explanatory purposes, these components are analysed and described separately.

Introduction

Despite remarkable progress in diagnosis and therapy, acute events such as coronary syndromes (ACS), decompensated heart failure, and major arrhythmia, still pose a huge challenge in cardiovascular medicine. Whereas in-hospital mortality of patients has markedly decreased since 1990, medium- and long-term prognosis strongly depends on the risk constellation, including age, left ventricular function, persistent ventricular arrhythmias, diabetes, and other risk factors and comorbidities. In a German survey, 1-year mortality after acute myocardial infarction (MI) was as low as 3.2% in a low-risk population but increased to as much as 25% in high-risk patients [1]. Individual risk management therefore remains a major challenge, and this chapter will concentrate on the first steps to be considered during the early days in hospital after surviving an ACS and/or after a myocardial revascularization (MR) intervention. The basic items described here should be considered in the post-acute management of all cardiovascular patients.

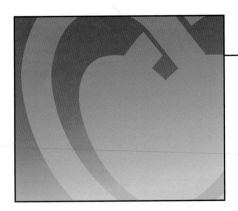

Preventive cardiology and cardiac rehabilitation in the acute setting

Improvements in diagnostic and therapeutic procedures as well as increasing economic pressure and competition have led to a continuous shortening of the in-hospital stay after an acute event. By contrast, there are a growing number of old, increasingly frail patients with multiple morbidities who require intense clinical supervision and care. Optimal coordination between inpatient and outpatient care is an increasing challenge for healthcare providers. Furthermore, the long-term success of any acute or elective cardiac intervention strongly depends on the sustained implementation of preventive measures. Accordingly cardiac rehabilitation (CR) plays a major role as a bridge between the acute treatment and outpatient care.

Recent scientific data have demonstrated that preventive cardiology (PC) as performed in various CR settings is effective in reducing recurrent cardiovascular events after both ACS and MR [2–13]:

- Phase I CR (described in this chapter) represents the earliest preventive intervention beginning right after the acute event during the hospital stay.
- Phase II CR is a structured and comprehensive therapeutic intervention starting early after hospital discharge. It may be performed in various settings (outpatient, inpatient, centre-based, or home-based) depending on clinical, administrative, or logistic circumstances (see ➲ Chapters 22 and 23).
- Phase III CR represents the long-term outpatient supervision of patients' adherence to prescribed risk control measures and is usually the responsibility of general practitioners and cardiologists. Special phase III prevention programmes have been established in some countries to support long-term secondary prevention [7,14]

This classification may not represent clinical practice in all European countries as implementation, organization, and structure differ considerably for various reasons [14]. In the future phase I and phase II CR may become merged because of the need for newly structured cardiovascular prevention programmes that are able to provide a continuum of care and surveillance from the acute to the post-acute phase.

In-hospital phase I rehabilitation: core components

Inpatient phase I rehabilitation should begin as soon as possible after clinical stabilization of the patient [15]. It comprises a complex, multifaceted, and multidisciplinary intervention. (➲ Box 21.1). All these interventions are important and make an equal contribution to achievement of the preventive target [16]. In-hospital phase I CR is therefore the first step in the lifelong programme of preventive cardiology and should be regarded as a bridge to phase II rehabilitation programmes.

Box 21.1 Core components of phase I rehabilitation after acute coronary event or myocardial revascularization

- Post-acute clinical evaluation and risk assessment
- General counselling: basic information and reassurance
- Supportive counselling (i.e. psychological support)
- Early mobilization
- Discharge planning, including referral to outpatient care
- Referral to phase II cardiac rehabilitation

For logistical reasons, in clinical practice not all in-hospital phase I CR components outlined in ➲ Box 21.1 can be delivered to all patients. However, this form of intervention represents a major component of in-hospital care, and provides safe access to a phase II CR programme for all eligible patients.

Post-acute clinical evaluation and risk assessment

The post-acute clinical evaluation and risk assessment should be based not only on the available information about the coronary anatomy but mainly on a careful examination of the acute medical and/or surgical records. It should include a review of the clinical history, the level of physical activity before the acute event, the actual clinical signs and symptoms, physical and functional examination, as well as results of technical diagnostic tests such as electrocardiogram (ECG) and ECG monitoring, echocardiography, and laboratory examinations [16,17]. In this way the severity of coronary artery disease, myocardial damage, arrhythmic burden, comorbidities, and potential frailty are evaluated to assess the individual cardiovascular risk burden and prognosis and to determine subsequent short- and long-term evidence-based treatment [18].

Importantly, every member of the therapeutic team should be well informed about the clinical status and all risk factors. This is a prerequisite for a complete counselling intervention and adequate prescription of a physical activity and exercise programme. A detailed description of clinical evaluation and risk assessment is outlined in Chapter 5.

General counselling

Patients with ACS or after MR differ in their desire for information, including advice about their illness, its causes, and prognosis, treatment options, potential lifestyle changes, activity levels, and disease management in daily life. In addition, individual beliefs and attitudes as well as psychosocial factors may influence the coping process. Negative emotions (denial, fear, anger) may affect compliance, and patients' adherence should be addressed during CR.

Interventions correcting misconceptions are important to improve knowledge and reduce emotional stress in patients, partners, and family members. Of note, patients' needs are both diverse and specific, depending on issues such as age, gender, ethnicity, and educational and social level [19]. Thus, the approach should be tailored to the patient, as a unique person. Moreover, patients often have difficulties in understanding and accepting detailed and complicated information, and their receptivity and understanding may be limited by physical illness and psychological or cognitive barriers. Information should therefore be provided in a clear and simple way, based on a patient's personal characteristics and needs. Reassurance, individual support, and empathy should underpin all discussions.

General counselling is based on detailed knowledge of all members of the healthcare team about the individual patient's risk profile as well as social background. All members of the team should have regular meetings to discuss clinical cases and to coordinate therapeutic interventions. Counselling of patients by a team member should be restricted to his or her speciality; medical aspects, as well as summarizing information and advice, is the responsibility of the cardiologist. Medical and social aspects are always interrelated and influence one another to a considerable extent. It is not generally sufficient to prescribe medication and lifestyle changes without knowing the potential promoters and barriers in the patient's social life.

Thus, during phase I CR, counselling should be initiated after a careful consideration of the patient's pre-existing knowledge and individual needs (➲ Box 21.2). This could be accompanied by general information on the nature of cardiovascular disease and risk factor management using audio or video resources. Post-discharge telephone counselling may reinforce patients' adherence to medication and lifestyle changes. However, these interventions do not confer sustained emotional or physical benefit, rather they help to increase patients' and family members' knowledge and involvement as a bridge to phase II CR.

Box 21.2 General counselling during in-hospital cardiac rehabilitation: suggested topics to discuss during hospital stay and at discharge

- Offer reassurance and explanation of cardiac condition, treatment, and procedures
- Give general and individualized information on coronary artery disease and acute myocardial infarction and its consequences
- Provide information on how to recognize and interpret signs and symptoms of ischaemia, heart failure, and arrhythmias
- Develop an action plan with the patient and the caregiver to ensure early response to warning symptoms
- Advise on acute and chronic treatment and type and doses of medications, highlighting the importance of compliance and adherence
- Reinforce the role of cardiovascular prevention: the identification and modification of risk factors should be addressed in general and focused on the individual's needs
- Explain the inpatient activity programme, its advantages, related risks, warning symptoms, and monitoring
- Give initial information on the resumption of physical, sexual, and daily living activities (including driving and return to work)
- Address the potential consequences for social life, like family and personal relationships and social support/isolation
- Provide potential means for social support
- Provide information on phase II cardiac rehabilitation and its components (i.e. more educational activity and intense and individualized risk factor management)

Psychological and social support

As well as the risk of premature death, many patients may experience a significant loss of independence and a decline in physical function during the first year following an acute cardiovascular event.

In addition, after ACS or MR patients are in a clinically and psychologically critical condition and experience difficulties in understanding and accepting the 'new' situation and the potential consequences for their future and life expectancy. Life-threatening situations may have occurred and survival of the acute phase is considered the primary goal, whereas efforts for long-term cardiovascular prevention and lifestyle changes may be felt to be secondary at this stage. Patients therefore need to be supported to cope with their situation. Early mobilization to regain physical independence and individual self confidence is a prerequisite for coping, but clear medical information about the causes and consequences of the disease and psychological support also are required.

During the acute hospital stay structured psychological interventions are not feasible in most cases, but may be started within phase II CR. In addition, hospital discharge is too early in most cases to provide sufficient social and vocational counselling. Social counselling during phase I CR should therefore reinforce patients' participation in phase II CR, which, apart from implementation of secondary prevention, supports vocational and social reintegration.

Recommendations for counselling on mobilization and physical activity

In-hospital phase I CR is the first step in regaining physical independence and individual self-confidence. The risks and complications of prolonged immobilization affect almost all organ systems and may have severe psychological consequences (➲ Table 21.1). The primary purpose of early mobilization is to prevent such complications. Additional goals are to regain cardiovascular fitness and functional abilities and to increase comfort and psychological well-being. Early remobilization is therefore now common practice in the care of hospitalized patients and may be implemented through a broad range of activities as outlined in ➲ Box 21.3. The following limitations, however, should be considered:

- Scientific data on early remobilization are rare, and there are no evidence-based guidelines on how to perform early remobilization most effectively in clinical practice. A systematic review of experimental data from studies conducted in the 1970s and 1980s showed a trend towards an increased survival of ACS patients receiving early mobilization relative to those who did not [20]. More research is necessary to determine the minimum standards for safe and effective remobilization.

Table 21.1 Risks and complications of immobility.

Respiratory	Retention of secretions and decreased respiratory excursions Atelectasis and pneumonia
Cardiovascular	Orthostatic hypotension Hypovolaemia Deep-vein thrombosis, local and systemic embolism
Musculoskeletal	Muscle mass reduction and wasting Joint contractures Bone demineralization (osteoporosis) Heterotopic ossification
Gastrointestinal	Decreased motility Constipation
Neurological	Polyneuropathy
Endocrine	Hyperglycaemia with insulin resistance Catabolism
Genitourinary	Urinary stasis Renal calculi
Psychological	Depression Delirium

Source: Amidei C, Mobilization in critical care: a concept analysis. *Intensive and Critical Care Nursing* 2012; **28**: 73–81.

- The scientific uncertainty may translate into clinical practice and lead to unjustified delays in remobilization of patients. Some of these uncertainties concern safety and monitoring issues as well as the correct adjustment of the programme intensity. Cardiovascular risks like recurrent ischaemia, heart failure, and arrhythmias have to be taken into account as well as comorbidities, puncture sites, and wound healing or Dressler's syndrome after heart surgery.
- Underuse of a structured early remobilization may also be the result of economic pressure and time constraints. Patients with multiple morbidities, advanced obesity, and/or frailty may be particularly affected by those restrictions.

Box 21.3 Physical activities in early mobilization

- Positioning prone or side to side in bed
- Use of continuous lateral rotating therapy beds
- Breathing exercises
- Passive and active range of motion
- Dangling
- Moving out of bed to a chair
- Movement in the bed to an upright position
- Ambulation using aids
- Ambulation using a staircase
- Tilting on a table
- Use of active resistive exercise
- Use of electrical muscle stimulation

Amidei C, Mobilization in critical care: a concept analysis. *Intensive and Critical Care Nursing* 2012; **28**: 73–81.

Box 21.4 Recommendations on how to handle early remobilization in clinical practice

- Prescribe early mobilization, specifying the type and dosage (intensity, duration, frequency)
- Individually adjust mobilization and the physical activity intervention according to the patient's clinical condition and response to exercise
- Adopt a stepwise increase in the dosage in an individualized fashion and include additional types of interventions and exercise programmes
- Regularly monitor heart rate, breathing rate, and blood pressure, as well as signs and symptoms of ischaemia, heart failure, and arrhythmias
- Use a multidisciplinary approach with frequent interaction between healthcare providers (physician, nurse, physiotherapist, etc.)

Amidei C, Mobilization in critical care: a concept analysis. *Intensive and Critical Care Nursing* 2012; **28**: 73–81.

Despites these limitations and potential restrictions, a few recommendations on how to handle early remobilization in clinical practice are available [21] (➲ Box 21.4).

Discharge planning

Transitions of care are defined as 'a set of actions designed to ensure the coordination and continuity of healthcare as patients transfer between different locations or different levels of care in the same location' [22]. Correctly performed care transitions are associated with significant reductions in readmissions and total healthcare costs [23]. Patients and medical institutions taking over care therefore have to be informed and instructed in a very clear way about long-term medication and the individual's most important lifestyle changes. The importance of these instructions has been highlighted by the following studies:

- Among 5353 patients post-MI, those on optimal medication (including five guideline recommended drugs; 46%) had a significantly lower risk of death after 1 year compared with those taking no drugs or one drug only (adjusted OR 0.260, 95% CI 0.179–0.379, $p < 0.001$) [24].
- Among 18 835 patients in 41 countries post-ACS, those who reported persistent smoking and non-adherence to diet and exercise had a 3.8-fold (95% CI 2.5–5.9) increased risk of a cardiovascular event (myocardial infarction, stroke, or death) compared with those who never smoked and who modified their diet and exercise [18].

The importance of starting patients on appropriate secondary prevention at the time of hospital discharge cannot be over-emphasized, as secondary prevention treatment tends to decrease rather than increase after hospitalization [25,26]. In the EUROASPIRE III survey of secondary prevention in 22 countries, 95% of patients were on antiplatelet drugs at the time of discharge, 82.5% on beta-blockers, and 81% on statins, but these proportions had decreased within 6–36 months after discharge. After this time period less than half of the patients were meeting risk factor targets such as for blood pressure (44%) and lipid (48.5%) control [27]. Attending CR, however, was associated with an increased likelihood of meeting risk factor targets [28].

The core components of discharge planning are given in ➲ Box 21.5. It is important to involve the patient and relatives/caregivers in discharge planning as soon as possible, including the core components of outpatient care and subsequent phase II CR. While discharge policies, protocols, and practices have to consider the individual's needs and be sensitive to different requirements, standardized discharge protocols should be developed to promote consistency of clinical practice between specialists and general practitioners and to reinforce the appropriate use of clinic resources. A structured and comprehensive discharge letter can be regarded as a prerequisite for an effective continuation of healthcare and to guarantee consistency within an individual's care. Standardized templates for discharge letters and other communications are available to promote efficiency and consistency of clinical practice—an example is given in ➲ Box 21.6.

Box 21.5 Components of the discharge planning process: topics to be discussed before discharge

- Early on identify and assess patients requiring assistance with discharge planning
- Collaborate with the patient, family, and healthcare team to facilitate discharge planning
- Coach secondary prevention recommendations and strategies
- Recommend options for continuing outpatient care by general practitioners and the cardiologist; strongly recommend participation in cardiac rehabilitation
- Communicate and coordinate with community agencies and care facilities to promote patient access and to address gaps in service; this also may be done during phase II cardiac rehabilitation
- Provide a detailed discharge letter

Adapted from CADPACC (1995) [33].

Referral to phase II cardiac rehabilitation

Referral to phase II CR should be a primary aim for all patients recovering from acute cardiovascular disease [16]. Participating in a CR programme yields well-established benefits (reduction in cardiac and non-cardiac mortality as well as reduced morbidity and cardiac risk factors). CR plays a crucial role in secondary prevention, helping individuals to return to a productive and satisfying life.

Box 21.6 Example of a structured discharge letter

DATE OF ADMISSION:
DATE OF DISCHARGE:
DIAGNOSIS:

1. Admitting diagnosis: ____________
2. Secondary diagnosis: ____________

PATIENT MEDICAL HISTORY:

- Family history: ____________
- Social history: ____________
- Allergies: ____________
- Brief medical history: ____________
- History of present illness: ____________

HOSPITAL STAY:

- Physical examination at admission: ____________
- Diagnostic procedures performed: ____________
- Consults obtained: ____________
- Hospital course and treatment: ____________
- Counselling/advising: ____________

DISCHARGE:

- Condition on discharge and remaining active problems (if appropriate): ____________
- Functional status at discharge: ____________
- Discharge medications: ____________

DISCHARGE INSTRUCTIONS:

- Discharge diet (if appropriate): ____________
- Discharge physical activity recommendation: ____________

PREVENTIVE GOALS:

Non-diabetics

- Stop smoking
- Total cholesterol < 175 mg/dl
- LDL cholesterol < 100 mg/dl
- Blood pressure < 140/90 mmHg
- Ideal body weight: ____kg
- Waist circumference < 102 cm (male) or < 88 cm (female)

Diabetics

- Stop smoking
- Total cholesterol < 175 mg/dl
- LDL cholesterol < 100 mg/dl
- Blood pressure < 130/80 mmHg
- Glycated haemoglobin < 7%
- Ideal body weight: ____kg
- Waist circumference < 102 cm (male) or < 88 cm (female)

REFERRAL AND FOLLOW-UP:

Inpatient, phase II cardiac rehabilitation:

- Why ____________
- When ____________
- Where ____________

Outpatient, phase II cardiac rehabilitation:

- Why ____________
- When ____________
- Where ____________

Regrettably, referral to phase II CR is unsatisfactory in most European countries, with patchy distribution and large disparities in staffing and uptake. The low service uptake depends on environmental factors like the availability of CR centres and/or support from the healthcare system, as well as on patient characteristics like age, gender and ethnicity, social factors, clinical conditions (i.e. comorbidities), and psychological factors [9,29–31].

In addition, lack of information and support from physicians and other healthcare professionals during the hospital stay can have a negative impact on participation in CR [32]. Physicians themselves therefore need to be better educated about the benefits of CR.

The patient's perspectives and attitudes are also important. As already mentioned, an increasing number of patients with ACS only experience a short hospital stay. For this reason patients often do not feel that they are suffering from a serious disease. Participation in CR may therefore be felt to be unnecessary. Moreover, entering a CR programme may make the situation seem more serious, which is difficult for some patients to accept.

Automatic referral to phase II CR using electronic patient records or standard discharge orders in combination with individual and personal information and reinforcement appears to be the best way to get a high admission rate to phase II CR [33,34].

Conclusions

In patients after ACS or MR, phase I CR during the hospital stay serves as a bridge between the acute therapeutic interventions and a fully comprehensive secondary prevention intervention such as phase II CR. Ideally phase I CR is structured and follows an evidence-based programme, including psychological support, individual information, structured physiotherapeutic programmes, and early supervised exercise training. During phase I CR, patients should be informed about the importance and the contents of secondary prevention with respect to cardiovascular risk reduction and social reintegration. On the basis of this information patients should automatically be referred to phase II CR, ideally with a choice about the most appropriate rehabilitation setting for them.

Further reading

Balady GJ, Ades PA, Bittner VA, et al. Referral, enrollment, and delivery of cardiac rehabilitation/secondary prevention programs at clinical centers and beyond: a presidential advisory from the American Heart Association. *Circulation* 2011; **124**: 2951–60.

Bjarnason-Wehrens B, McGee H, Zwisler AD, et al. Cardiac rehabilitation in Europe: results from the European Cardiac Rehabilitation Inventory Survey. *Eur J Cardiovasc Prev Rehabil* 2010; **17**: 410–18.

Goel K, Lennon R, Tilbury R, et al. Impact of cardiac rehabilitation on mortality and cardiovascular events after percutaneous coronary intervention in the community. *Circulation* 2011; **123**: 2344–52.

Grace SL, Chessex C, Arthur H, et al. Systematizing inpatient referral to cardiac rehabilitation 2010: Canadian Association of Cardiac Rehabilitation and Canadian Cardiovascular Society joint position paper endorsed by the Cardiac Care Network of Ontario. *Can J Cardiol* 2011; **27**: 192–9.

Hammill B, Curtis L, Schulman K, et al. Relationship between cardiac rehabilitation and long-term risks of death and myocardial infarction among elderly Medicare beneficiaries. *Circulation* 2010; **121**: 63–70.

Giannuzzi P, Temporelli L, Marchioli R, et al.; for the GOSPEL Investigators. Global secondary prevention strategies to limit event recurrence after myocardial infarction. *Arch Intern Med* 2008; **168**: 2194–204.

Piepoli M, Corrà U, Benzer W, et al. Secondary prevention through cardiac rehabilitation: from knowledge to implementation. A position paper from the Cardiac Rehabilitation Section of the European Association of Cardiovascular Prevention and Rehabilitation. *Eur J Cardiovasc Prev Rehabil* 2010; **17**: 1–17.

Piepoli MF, Corrà U, Adamopoulos S, et al. Secondary prevention in the clinical management of patients with cardiovascular diseases. Core components, standards and outcome measures for referral and delivery. *Eur J Prev Cardiol* 2012; **21**: 664–81.

Rauch B, Riemer T, Schwaab B, et al.; for the OMEGA study group. Short-term comprehensive cardiac rehabilitation after AMI is associated with reduced 1-year mortality: results from the OMEGA study. *Eur J Prev Cardiol* 2014; **21**: 1060–9.

References

1 Lorenz H, Jünger C, Seidl K, et al. Do statins influence the prognostic impact of non-sustained ventricular tachycardia after ST-elevation myocardial infarction? *Eur Heart J* 2005; **26**: 1078–85.

2 Taylor R, Brown A, Ebrahim S, et al. Exercise-based rehabilitation for patients with coronary heart disease: systematic review and meta-analysis of randomized controlled trials. *Am J Med* 2004; **116**: 682–92.

3 Clark A, Hartling L, Vandermeer B, et al. Meta-analysis: secondary prevention programs for patients with coronary artery disease. *Ann Intern Med* 2005; **143**: 659–72.

4 Heran B, Chen J, Ebrahim S, et al. Exercise-based cardiac rehabilitation for coronary heart disease. *Cochrane Database Syst Rev* 2011; (7): CD001800.

5 Dendale P, Berger J, Hansen D, et al. Cardiac rehabilitation reduces the rate of major adverse cardiac events after percutaneous coronary intervention. *Eur J Cardiovasc Nurs* 2005; **4**: 113–16.

6 Suaya JA, Shepard DS, Normand SLT, et al. Use of cardiac rehabilitation by Medicare beneficiaries after myocardial infarction or coronary bypass surgery. *Circulation* 2007; **116**: 1653–62.

7 Giannuzzi P, Temporelli L, Marchioli R, et al.; for the GOSPEL Investigators. Global secondary prevention strategies to limit event recurrence after myocardial infarction. *Arch Intern Med* 2008; **168**: 2194–204.

8 Hammill B, Curtis L, Schulman K, et al. Relationship between cardiac rehabilitation and long-term risks of death and myocardial infarction among elderly Medicare beneficiaries. *Circulation* 2010; **121**: 63–70.

9 Jünger C, Rauch B, Schneider S, et al. Effect of early short-time cardiac rehabilitation after acute ST-elevation and non-ST-elevation myocardial infarction on 1-year mortality. *Curr Med Res Opin* 2010; **26**: 803–11.

10 Schwaab B, Waldmann A, Katalinic A, et al. In-patient cardiac rehabilitation versus medical care - a prospective multicentre controlled 12 months follow-up in patients with coronary heart disease. *Eur J Cardiovasc Prev Rehabil* 2011; **18**: 581–6.

11 Goel K, Lennon R, Tilbury R, et al. Impact of cardiac rehabilitation on mortality and cardiovascular events after percutaneous coronary intervention in the community. *Circulation* 2011; **123**: 2344–52.

12 Martin BJ, Hauer T, Arena R, et al. Cardiac rehabilitation attendance and outcomes in coronary artery disease patients. *Circulation* 2012; **126**: 677–87.

13 Rauch B, Riemer T, Schwaab B, et al.; for the OMEGA study group. Short-term comprehensive cardiac rehabilitation after AMI is associated with reduced 1-year mortality: results from the OMEGA study. *Eur J Prev Cardiol* 2014; **21**: 1060–9.

14 Bjarnason-Wehrens B, McGee H, Zwisler AD, et al. Cardiac rehabilitation in Europe: results from the European Cardiac Rehabilitation Inventory Survey. *Eur J Cardiovasc Prev Rehabil* 2010: **17**: 410–18.

15 Piepoli MF, Corrà U, Abreu A, et al. Challenges in secondary prevention of cardiovascular diseases. A review of the current practice. *Int J Cardiol* 2014, doi: 10.1016/j.ijcard.2014.11.107

16 Piepoli M, Corrà U, Benzer W, et al. Secondary prevention through cardiac rehabilitation: from knowledge to implementation. A position paper from the Cardiac Rehabilitation Section of the European Association of Cardiovascular Prevention and Rehabilitation. *Eur J Cardiovasc Prev Rehabil* 2010; **17**: 1–17.

17 Piepoli MF, Corrà U, Adamopoulos S, et al. Secondary prevention in the clinical management of patients with cardiovascular diseases. Core components, standards and outcome measures for referral and delivery. *Eur J Prev Cardiol* 2012; **21**: 664–81.

18 Chow CK, Jolly S, Rao-Melacini P, et al. Association of diet, exercise, and smoking modification with risk of early cardiovascular events after acute coronary syndromes. *Circulation* 2010; **121**: 750–8.

19 Scott IA. Determinants of quality of in-hospital care for patients with acute coronary syndromes. *Dis Manag Health Outcomes* 2003; **11**: 801–16.

20 Cortes OL, Villar JC, Devereaux PJ, et al. Early mobilisation for patients following acute myocardial infarction: a systematic review and meta-analysis of experimental studies. *Int J Nurs Stud* 2009; **4**: 1496–500.

21 Amidei C. Mobilization in critical care: a concept analysis. *Intens Crit Care Nurs* 2012; **28**: 73–81.

22 Coleman EA, Berenson RA. Lost in transition: challenges and opportunities for improving the quality of transitional care. *Ann Intern Med* 2004; **141**: 533–6.

23 Lambrinou E, Kalogirou F, Lamnisos D, et al. Effectiveness of heart failure management programmes with nurse-led discharge planning in reducing re-admissions: a systematic review and meta-analysis. *Int J Nurs Stud* 2012; **49**: 610–24.

24 Bramlage P, Messer C, Bitterlich N, et al. The effect of optimal medical therapy on 1-year mortality after acute myocardial infarction. *Heart* 2010; **96**: 604–10.

25 Andrikopoulos G, Tzeis S, Nikas N, et al. Short-term outcome and attainment of secondary prevention goals in patients with acute coronary syndrome—results from the countrywide TARGET study. *Int J Cardiol* 2013; **168**: 922–7.

26 Zeymer U, James S, Berkenboom G, et al.; on behalf of APTOR Investigators. Differences in the use of guideline recommended therapies among 14 European countries in patients with acute coronary syndromes undergoing PCI. *Eur J Prev Cardiol* 2012; **20**: 218–28.

27 Kotseva K, Wood D, De Backer G, et al.; on behalf of the EUROASPIRE Study Group. EUROASPIRE III: a survey on the lifestyle, risk factors and use of cardioprotective drug therapies in coronary patients from 22 European countries. *Eur J Cardiovasc Prev Rehabil* 2009; **16**: 121–37.

28 Cooney MT, Kotseva K, Dudina A, et al.; on behalf of the EUROASPIRE Investigators. Determinants of risk factor control in subjects with coronary heart disease: a report from the EUROASPIRE III investigators. *Eur J Prev Cardiol* 2012; **20**: 686–91.

29 Balady GJ, Ades PA, Bittner VA, et al. Referral, enrollment, and delivery of cardiac rehabilitation/secondary prevention programs at clinical centers and beyond: a presidential advisory from the American Heart Association. *Circulation* 2011; **124**: 2951–60.

30 Fernandez RS, Salamonson Y, Griffiths R, et al. Sociodemographic predictors and reasons for participation in an outpatient cardiac rehabilitation programme following percutaneous coronary intervention. *Int J Nurs Pract* 2008; **14**: 237–42.

31 Fernandez RS, Davidson P, Griffiths R. Cardiac rehabilitation coordinators' perception of patient-related barriers to implementing cardiac evidence-based guidelines. *J Cardiovasc Nurs* 2008; **23**: 449–57.

32 Parkosewich JA. Cardiac rehabilitation barriers and opportunities among women with cardiovascular disease. *Cardiol Rev* 2008; **16**: 36–52.

33 Grace SL, Chessex C, Arthur H, et al. Systematizing inpatient referral to cardiac rehabilitation 2010: Canadian Association of Cardiac Rehabilitation and Canadian Cardiovascular Society joint position paper endorsed by the Cardiac Care Network of Ontario. *Can J Cardiol* 2011; **27**: 192–9.

34 Grace SL, Leung YW, Reid R, et al.; CRCARE Investigators. The role of systematic inpatient cardiac rehabilitation referral in increasing equitable access and utilization. *J Cardiopul Rehabil Prev* 2012; **32**: 41–7.

CHAPTER 22

Hospital-based rehabilitation units

Heinz Völler, Rona Reibis, Bernhard Schwaab, and Jean-Paul Schmid

Contents

Summary

Inpatient rehabilitation is a transition phase and a component of integrated healthcare for high-risk patients with different cardiovascular diseases. Therefore its main focus is on functional and structural evaluation and risk stratification for the rehabilitation process and post-discharge period. An exercise electrocardiogram, echocardiography, and a 6-minute walk test should be considered in all patients, at admission as well as at discharge. Particular attention should be given to specific conditions such as diabetes mellitus, myocarditis, patients with cardiac devices, and/or after heart valve interventions. Variables of frailty should be considered, particularly in the elderly. Because cognitive decline complicates early recovery after heart interventions, a cognition test may be needed.

Introduction

Inpatient cardiac rehabilitation (CR) was established in Europe in the late 1960s for patients who had suffered from an acute myocardial infarction with a long hospital stay and—in the time before thrombolysis or percutaneous coronary intervention (PCI)—often with significant structural damage and a low exercise capacity. Today patients are revascularized early and have a shorter length of stay. However, the procedures are often complex and are carried out in elderly patients, usually with end stage diseases (e.g. ischaemic cardiomyopathy and heart failure), with some requiring an implantable cardioverter defibrillator (ICD) or cardiac resynchronization therapy (CRT) or a left ventricular assist device (LVAD) as a bridge to transplantation. With rapid technical progress frailer patients are being treated, and not only those with coronary artery disease (CAD) but also heart valve diseases, predominantly aortic stenosis, and after transcatheter aortic valve implantation (TAVI).

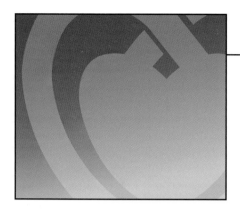

Hospital-based rehabilitation units should be considered as a transition phase and as a part of integrated healthcare for high-risk patients with different cardiovascular diseases. This chapter focuses on how to care for patients in the early phase after the index cardiac event or after a long and complicated stay for patients with several comorbidities.

Clinical assessment

Laboratory

Beyond cardiovascular risk factors (cholesterol, triglycerides, glucose) special attention must be given to inflammation (red and white blood cell count, C-reactive protein), renal function (creatinine/glomerular filtration rate), and electrolytes. Thyroid function should be checked, because of the risk of hyperthyroidism after angiography or a PCI.

If diarrhoea develops after in-hospital treatment with antibiotics, *Clostridium difficile* must be ruled out [1,2]. After heart valve replacement patients must have laboratory tests for anticoagulation (international normalized ratio, INR) and intravascular haemolysis (lactate dehydrogenase).

Wound healing

After cardiac surgery clinical risk assessment should include physical examination of the chest and legs. Because more than 5% of patients at the start of inpatient rehabilitation have wound infections, standardized procedures should be followed [1]. After performing a wound smear to build up an antibiogram (to test the sensitivity of an isolated bacterial strain to different antibiotics), treatment with antibiotics must be initiated together with consultation by wound nurse and laboratory measurement of inflammation.

Testing

All patients referred to CR should be investigated clinically and should undergo two-dimensional echocardiography and resting and exercise ECG at admission and, if possible, at discharge. The main focus is on functional and structural evaluation, and thus on risk stratification for the rehabilitation process and the post-discharge period [3].

Exercise ECG/Holter ECG/6-minute walk test

A symptom-limited exercise ECG is helpful for determining individual exercise capacity and training heart rate. It has been shown to be safe and reliable even in the early phase of recovery from acute myocardial infarction and following myocardial revascularization without any adverse effect on left ventricular (LV) function [3]. The duration and watt load depends on age, gender, previous exercise capacity, the main diagnosis, comorbidities, type of intervention (after PCI, post-cardiac surgery, surgery of the great arteries), and post-operative complications (post-cardiotomy syndrome, wound infection, post-operative atrial fibrillation, renal failure). Even in patients with an expected low overall capacity (i.e. frail, older, or deconditioned patients), exercise ECG is useful for estimating resilience and haemodynamic behaviour as well as potential rhythm disorders. In high-risk patients (those with severe in-hospital complications, persistent clinical instability, advanced heart failure) a submaximal exercise test should be considered only after stabilization.

A symptom-limited or submaximal exercise ECG can be performed on a bicycle ergometer or a treadmill [4]. A stepwise or ramp stress protocol, starting with 10 to 50 W, followed by 10–25 W incremental steps every 1–2 minutes until exhaustion should be adjusted to the patient's characteristics. During the test, a three-lead ECG should be recorded continuously for ST segment analysis and rhythm disorders. Blood pressure should be assessed indirectly by arm cuff sphygmomanometry every 2 minutes during the load period, and three times during the recovery period. Standard ECG and clinical criteria for termination should be employed. An abnormal ECG or the development of angina with ECG abnormalities during the test will require further investigation. Improvement in the submaximal work load can be documented by comparing the submaximal and maximal work loads on admission and at discharge.

The cardiopulmonary exercise test includes analysis of ventilator gas exchange (peak VO_2 uptake and breathing pattern) and should be considered in specific subgroups of patients (in chronic heart failure or patients with resynchronization devices) for an objective estimation of working capability. It has also been proposed as a valuable tool in several cardiac conditions (such as risk stratification after acute coronary syndrome, myocardial revascularization, or to evaluate patients before correction of valve diseases) [5–7].

To stratify the risk of sudden cardiac death and registration of post-operative asymptomatic atrial fibrillation, a three-channel Holter ECG, including pacemaker analysis if required, should be considered. As a measurement of autonomic activity, the heart rate variability (SDNN) can be calculated.

At the start and at the end of a CR programme, a standardized 6-minute walk test based on a distance measuring device should be considered. Before starting the test, the patient should be familiarized with the procedure to be followed and their environment. The 6-minute walk test is a well-recognized measure of physical performance, even in elderly patients, and can be performed in 75% of patients shortly after the index event [1].

Echocardiography

Immediately after admission, all patients should undergo two-dimensional echocardiography by an experienced investigator to define global and regional LV systolic and diastolic function, LV end-diastolic and end-systolic diameter, the morphology and function of native valves, and measurement of systolic pulmonary artery pressure. Following valve replacement or reconstruction, the transvalvular gradient, calculated orifice area, and para- or trans-valvular regurgitation should be evaluated. In patients after coronary artery bypass grafting (CABG) attention should be drawn particularly to regional left and right ventricular function to exclude silent perioperative myocardial infarction or graft dysfunction.

The incidence of pericardiotomy syndrome has been reported in up to 30% of patients after cardiac surgery and must be excluded [8]. Inflammation of the pleura, pericardium, and pulmonary parenchyma has been described early after thoracotomy, and also as a result of cardiac injury after radiofrequency catheter ablation [9] or PCI intervention [10]—the indication to perform a pleural or pericardial puncture depends entirely on the clinical condition of the patient. In any case, frequent echocardiographic follow-ups should be considered.

Table 22.1 Geriatric baseline examination

Instruments	Impairment	Score
Cognitive function: MMSE (Mini Mental State Exam)	≥21 to <27 points <21	1 2
Gait function: Timed up and go test	≥20 seconds	
Nutritional status (Mini Nutritional Assessment Short Form [71])	≤12 points	1
Activity of daily living: Basic activities of daily living Instrumental activities of daily living	One limitation One limitation	1 1
Frailty (Clinical Frailty Scale [72])		≥3

Reproduced from Schoenenberger AW, Stortecky S, Neumann S, Moser A, Jüni P, Carrel T, Huber C, Gandon M, Bischoff S, Schoenenberger CM, Stuck AE, Windecker S, Wenaweser P. Predictors of functional decline in elderly patients undergoing transcatheter aortic valve implantation (TAVI). *Eur Heart J* 2013; **34**: 684–92.

In addition to QRS width criteria for patients after cardiac resynchronization therapy the first echocardiographic-guided optimization with individual determination of interventricular delay can be performed during inpatient stay [11]. If incomplete interventional revascularization was performed, dynamic or pharmacological stress echocardiography may be considered before considering further interventions in asymptomatic patients.

Cognition/frailty

Cognitive decline starts in the general population in middle age, but it is more pronounced in patients affected by CAD and/or heart failure [12–14]. Cognitive decline often complicates early recovery after CABG (in almost 50% of patients) and after prolonged hospital stay (peri-procedural stroke or resuscitation). Even though it is so frequent, no specific studies have been performed in patients with this clinical disorder referred for CR. Therefore a cognition test should be performed at the start of CR [15–17]. Sensitive and practical tests with sufficient reliability are the Mini Mental State Examination and the Montreal Cognition Assessment [18].

Beyond cognitive decline, other variables of frailty, such as vulnerability to poor resolution of homeostasis after a cardiac event and the consequent cumulative decline in many physiological systems, should be assessed. Mobility [the 'Timed up and go' (TUG) test or the handgrip strength test] [19], nutritional state (mini nutritional assessment), and activities of daily living (basic and instrumental activities of daily living) should be assessed [20]. A high frailty index not only has prognostic implications but also represents a greater burden on the rehabilitation programme (➲ Table 22.1). In these patients, sessions to enhance postural control and strength should be as important as exercise training.

Special conditions

Implanted devices

A growing proportion of patients referred to CR have implanted electrical devices, including single- and dual-chamber pacemakers, defibrillators (ICDs), and resynchronization pacemakers without (CRT-P) or with defibrillators (CRT-D). While ICDs may reduce the risk of sudden death [22], CRT has been demonstrated to improve functional and prognostic parameters in selected groups of patients with congestive heart failure [23].

Inpatient rehabilitation enables maximization of patient care by close observation of clinical behaviour and also allows reliable rhythm monitoring at rest, during routine daily activities, and under different types and intensities of exercise.

Patients with an implantable device require a multimodal approach in specialized rehabilitation units. After device implantation, wound healing is only completed after about 3 weeks, while internal lead fixation takes on average 6–8 weeks. During this time the main focus is on prevention of local infections and early lead dislocation. Nevertheless, immediately after device implantation participation in a rehabilitation programme is feasible, as long as the rehabilitation clinic maintains close supervision and observes medical precautions.

Complete follow-up (including controls of the lead threshold, potential and impedance testing, and battery capacity) should be routinely performed in every patient with an implantable device during CR. Thus, rehabilitation clinics should be provided with state-of-the-art programmers for devices from all the main manufacturers. The majority of modern devices are equipped for telemetric transmission of technical data via an integrated system. During CR the automatic remote monitoring system can be used [24]. The Holter ECG recording at rest and during exercise on a bike or a treadmill is a useful way to detect possible lead malfunctions (over- and under-sensing, far-field sensing, cross-talk, etc.) or concomitant significant arrhythmias (atrial fibrillation, non-sustained ventricular tachycardias) [25]. If there are persistent inappropriate ICD shocks (lead malfunction, supraventricular tachycardia including fast atrial fibrillation), a magnet placed over the ICD deactivates the detection algorithms and stops the therapy delivery.

The interpretation of a Holter ECG and exercise ECGs, as well as optimization of the device programming, is the task of a specialist physician. Since interpretation of the ECG during different stimulation modalities may be difficult, experienced physicians in this field should be on site, or readily available, to set optimal programming. For lead or device malfunction, contact with and rapid referral to the implantation centre is essential.

Exercise rehabilitation has been considered to potentially increase the risk of both appropriate and inappropriate device shocks, but it also improves functional capacity in patients with ICD or CRT devices [26]. The prescription of exercise for patients with an ICD depends on the underlying disease, and LV function, primary rhythm disorders, revascularization status, functional status, comorbidities, and age must all be considered [27]. Furthermore, the ICD activation threshold for anti-tachycardia pacing (ATP) and shock delivery should be included in the training setting to avoid unintended ICD shocks. Recent European recommendations [28] suggest that peak target heart rates should remain 10 to 20 beats below the ICD activation threshold, but there are no specific indications regarding the optimal modality of exercise rehabilitation (intensity, frequency, or duration).

To avoid electromagnetic interference, electrical devices for therapeutic applications are generally contraindicated in this population during the rehabilitation programme; however, exposure to microwaves and ultrasound is considered safe [29].

Patients with ICDs often complain of psychological problems during their daily activities. A multidisciplinary CR programme should include psychosocial support and assistance, with vocational counselling and job analysis in younger employees in particular. Counselling and education targeted at reducing depression and anxiety have been shown to improve device and disease acceptance [30]. In 2009 the European Heart Rhythm Association published detailed recommendations for driving by ICD patients [31].

In conclusion, each patient should be assessed individually, according to the specific indication for device implantation (primary or secondary prevention), the period of haemodynamic stability, and the type/frequency of ventricular arrhythmias.

Myocarditis

Myocarditis is an inflammatory disease of the heart and is an important cause of dilated cardiomyopathy. Because of the broad spectrum of symptoms, the clinical manifestation varies from asymptomatic to presentation with signs of myocardial infarction or life-threatening end stage heart failure. Therefore diagnosis of myocarditis based on the clinical presentation alone is not usually possible. The ECG is widely used as a screening tool despite low sensitivity. Biomarkers lack specificity, but may help to confirm the diagnosis of myocarditis [32]. The diagnostic value of virus serology in comparison to endomyocardial biopsy (EMB) is low, because patients are often referred for diagnosis with a significant delay from the onset of the initial infection and most viruses involved in the pathogenesis of myocarditis are widely prevalent in the general population. Echocardiography can also reveal nonspecific features of myocarditis and, importantly, it evaluates systolic and diastolic function, cardiac chamber sizes, and wall thickness. It is one of the important investigations for ruling out other causes of heart failure.

Cardiac magnetic resonance imaging (MRI) is becoming the only non-invasive test for the confirmation of myocarditis [33], but no detailed information about the degree of inflammation or the presence and type of virus is available [34]. Therefore, the gold standard in the diagnosis of myocarditis is still EMB. Beyond the Dallas criteria, only EMB-based immunohistological methods and molecular biological detection of cardiotropic viruses can be used to try and differentiate the acute phase of virus-induced injury (this takes only a few days) and the subacute phase which is characterized by autoimmune reactions and takes a few weeks to several months. Because of the limited availability of specialized facilities and experience in histological interpretation, EMB is infrequently used to diagnose myocarditis.

Therefore in patients who are referred to CR, myocarditis is often an underdiagnosed cause of heart failure or the diagnosis of myocarditis is unproven. These shortcomings have important clinical implication: myocarditis is a cause of sudden death in young adults and additional physical activity in someone with myocarditis may result in ventricular tachycardia/fibrillation [35–37].

While there is no direct evidence for CR in patients with myocarditis, avoidance of aerobic physical activity in the acute phase is recommended [38]. Thereafter, depending on improvement in clinical symptoms and stabilization of the patient (with disappearance of immunohistological evidence of inflammatory infiltrations) physical activity at low to moderate intensity is allowed [39–41]. However, physicians must be aware that the same rehabilitation programmes offered to patients with CAD should not be prescribed for myocarditis patients. Athletes with myocarditis should be withdrawn from all competitive sports for at least 6 months and may return to training and competition if LV function and cardiac dimensions have returned to normal and there are no clinically relevant arrhythmias on the Holter ECG [40]. Physical exercise is recommended for patients with stable heart failure and a previous history of myocarditis [42].

Based on expert opinion, the following advice should be considered for prescription of CR in patients with myocarditis:

- In the acute phase of myocarditis (EMB based) or when the diagnosis is presumed based on clinical presentation (reduced LV function, pericardial effusion, or rhythm disturbances) patients should not be referred to an exercise training programme but should be carefully monitored and appropriately treated in a hospital setting.
- In the subacute phase (EMB based), if LV function and cardiac dimensions have returned to normal and if there are no clinically relevant arrhythmias, CR-based exercise training could be initiated at a low level of physical activity (level 6–8 on the Borg scale). Only slow and gradual increases in heart rate should be considered and low-intensity continuous, or interval, training should be preferred.
- When inflammation is resolved in the EMB and cardiac function and ECG findings return to normal, symptom-limited exercise testing should be performed to guide exercise training [43].

However, patients are usually referred to CR without an EMB-proven diagnosis of myocarditis. If the above-mentioned non-invasive determinations reveal only mild functional or structural deterioration, a symptom-limited exercise stress test is a pre-requisite to starting training. Aerobic exercise could be safely prescribed based on a previously performed cardiopulmonary exercise test (determining the anaerobic threshold which should be avoided). Training must be guided by a physician and monitored by ECG, with frequent control of the LV function with two-dimensional echocardiography as well as determination of biomarkers (brain natriuretic peptide).

Patients who have suffered from myocarditis are often middle aged and have experienced a long deconditioning period. Therefore the implementation of exercise recommendations depends on the interaction between physician and patient. It will usually be necessary for clinicians to individualize exercise prescription for particular patients, balancing their clinical status with the proposed level of physical activity. Patients with myocarditis need psychosocial support from the interdisciplinary team to enhance their return to work.

Diabetes mellitus

CR requires a multilayered diagnostic and therapeutic approach, particularly for complicated high-risk patients (the obese, those with an inactive lifestyle or with manifest end-organ damage) [46]. Thus, diabetic patients should be interviewed, examined, educated, and treated in a multidisciplinary fashion.

Medical history is of particular importance and should include:

- year of initial diagnosis of diabetes
- history of anti-diabetic medication
- concomitant cardiovascular risk factors (dyslipidaemia, arterial hypertension, smoking behaviour, obesity, sedentary habits, family history of cardiovascular diseases)
- previous cardiovascular events (coronary artery disease (CAD(?)), heart failure, stroke)
- clinical signs of peripheral artery disease (intermittent claudication)
- neuropathic pain (burning, cold pain, electric shocks)
- renal insufficiency and degree of severity
- sleeping behaviour (sleep apnoea)

Patients with diabetes are at increased risk of multiple diabetic complications (➲ Table 22.2). Thus, clinical investigation plays a key role in assessing progression of the disease. Physicians should be aware that clinical symptoms in diabetic patients are often atypical.

Table 22.2 Complications associated with diabetes mellitus

Complications	Diagnostics
Hypo- and hyperglycaemia (including perception disorders)	Fasting plasma glucose level, HbA1c, regular self-testing
Retinopathy	Ophthalmoscopy (microaneurysms, exudates, haemorrhages)
Nephropathy	Abdominal ultrasound (nephrosclerosis, renal artery stenosis), creatinine clearance, microalbuminuria ≥ 30 mg/L in a spot urine sample, proteinuria
Coronary artery disease	Resting and stress ECG, stress imaging testing
Diabetic diastolic heart failure	Clinical investigation (signs of heart failure), two-dimensional echocardiography with tissue Doppler, NT proBNP
Peripheral sensory neuropathy	Vibration perception, Achilles tendon and patellar tendon reflex
Diabetic PAD	Arterial pulse status, auscultation, ankle–brachial index (<0.9 possible PAD, >1.3 possible media sclerosis)
Diabetic foot syndrome	Inspection (wounds, ulcer), X-ray (bone deformity), presence of infection (antibiogram)
Autonomic neuropathy	24-hour blood pressure, Holter ECG (SDNN), pupillary dysfunction
Erectile dysfunction	Exploration of sexual behaviour

HbA1c, glycated haemoglobin; NT proBNP, N-terminal pro-brain natriuretic peptide; PAD, peripheral arterial disease; SDNN, Standard Deviation of Normal to Normal.

The oral glucose tolerance test (OGTT) will detect impaired glucose tolerance in a quarter of patients without a previously established glucometabolic disorder [47]. Thus, the goal in every cardiac patient should be the formal evaluation of pathological glucose metabolism using a routinely performed OGTT during CR. This is a class I recommendation in the 2013 European Association for the Study of Diabetes (EASD) guidelines [48].

Comprehensive education, dietary counselling, individualized antidiabetic treatment, and a training programme are all important aspects of care. Physical stress should be avoided in the period of maximum insulin effect and during the evening (to prevent nocturnal hypoglycaemia). In the first days after initiation of an exercise programme plasma glucose levels should be measured by self-testing at the beginning and 1–2 hours after finishing sports. If blood glucose is not decreasing at 1–2 hours the stress intensity should be reduced. Cardiopulmonary exercise testing may be advisable to determine an individual's aerobic training modality (intensity and frequency). In patients treated with insulin or sulphonylurea/meglitinide a dose reduction might be appropriate during physical training. If the glucose level is <100 mg/dl (<5.6 mmol/L) at the start of exercise, an additional intake of carbohydrates can be beneficial. If the glucose level is >250 mg/dl (>13.8 mmol/L) exercise training is still possible as long as the patient is feeling comfortable and has no signs of ketonuria.

Return to work might be complicated by metabolic imbalance (hyper- or hypoglycaemia), leading to loss of fitness to drive, prohibition of night shifts, and in rare cases to a ban on employment. The organizational structure of modern rehabilitation clinics enables consultation with social services, ambulatory experts on diabetes, and employers to help patients pass the period of instability and to complete the restoration of capability.

Heart valve intervention

There is little direct evidence concerning rehabilitation of patients after valve repair or replacement, in comparison with that for patients with CAD [49]. It has been demonstrated that CR after heart valve surgery increases exercise capacity, quality of life, and the proportion of patients returning to work [50]. After a 3-week inpatient CR programme in patients after mitral surgery, a 22% increase in VO_2 max has been described [51,52].

Ischaemic cardiomyopathy is frequently associated with relative insufficiency of the mitral valve due to annulus dilatation, papillary muscle dysfunction, or rupture of the chordae. If regurgitation is haemodynamically relevant, patients usually undergo either valve reconstruction with plastic reduction and ring implantation or complete valve replacement. In rehabilitation settings, and for cases of ischaemic cardiomyopathy and concomitant valve surgery, the patient's management should be mainly focused on the underlying disease (CAD) with additional specific recommendations for treatment of the heart valve [53].

In the elderly the percentage of patients with CAD and concomitant aortic stenosis is increasing. This population is characterized by a high perioperative risk due to many comorbidities (e.g. heart and/or renal failure, lung diseases, peripheral and/or cerebrovascular arteriosclerosis) and frailty [54–56]. In Europe

TAVI is being increasingly used to treat this group. TAVI patients benefit from inpatient rehabilitation to the same degree as patients after surgical heart valve replacement [57]. Physicians in hospital-based rehabilitation units must be aware of the possible complications associated with TAVI. The most common are heart block, vascular complications, and renal failure, and systolic as well as diastolic heart failure [57,62]. Therefore the patient's weight must be recorded every day.

Baseline echocardiography should be performed in all patients at admission and at discharge from CR to assess the presence of transvalvular gradients, prosthesis para- or transvalvular regurgitation, systolic and diastolic LV function, and systolic pulmonary artery pressure [58]. If fever of unknown origin occurs, blood cultures and trans-oesophageal echocardiography should be performed to exclude endocarditis of a prosthetic valve [53].

Oral anticoagulation is necessary in patients after heart valve replacement—for 3 months after biological valve replacement or lifelong after mechanical prosthesis [53,59]. Atrial fibrillation is a common post-operative complication, particularly in patients after valve replacement, with an incidence of 40% in isolated valve surgery and up to 50% if valve surgery and CABG are combined [60]. Thus, heart rate should be monitored during exercise. Patients should be educated about INR self-management, pharmacological interactions, lifestyle, and nutrition [61]. Physically active patients on oral anticoagulation should be educated to choose low-risk sports to avoid bleeding complications.

Furthermore, depending on the pattern of recovery, an individualized aerobic exercise programme must be initiated during in-hospital CR. In patients with preserved LV function and uncomplicated post-operative follow-up a submaximal exercise test can be performed about 2 weeks after surgery to define the training programme. After conventional valve replacement with median sternotomy any movement involving lateral force should be progressively increased slowly to avoid sternal disruption [63].

Social medicine

Due to the high burden of morbidity and mortality, patients with cardiovascular diseases and their relatives require interdisciplinary support. As well as treatment of the event leading to referral to CR, inpatient rehabilitation offers the opportunity to support aspects of social medicine including disability, employment, psychosocial, and gender-related factors as well as the economic circumstances of patients.

The association between socioeconomic status and health is widely understood [64]. The impact of unemployment on the incidence of cardiovascular disease is still a matter of debate [65,66], but its impact on the incidence of cardiovascular risk factors is regarded as scientifically proven [67,68]. Imminent unemployment, particularly in younger patients during their early working life, can provoke anxiety, uncertainty and overall negative effects on social life and psychological behaviour [69].

During the rehabilitation period physicians are urged to estimate the working abilities of patients of working age. To assess their overall capacity, patients should undergo pre-discharge echocardiography, cardiopulmonary exercise testing, and a Holter ECG to detect relevant arrhythmias. Physicians are often requested to provide an expert opinion in case of any reduction in earning capacity or insurance conflicts.

Patients with CAD are often concerned about their physical capacity, which can lead to avoidance behaviour including fear of moving, sexual dysfunction, reduced motivation, and personal disengagement [70]. Besides education and qualified psychological supervision it can be necessary to offer organizational social support before returning patients to normal life.

After an acute cardiovascular event older retired patients often require high-level, long-term care.

Outlook

Hospital-based rehabilitation units are a cornerstone of integrated healthcare for high-risk patients. Inpatient rehabilitation should be considered as a transition phase to starting a comprehensive residential or ambulatory rehabilitation programme. Because these units are highly specialized and are staff- and cost-intensive the facilities should be reserved for the patients at highest risk and with the most complicated problems. Inpatient rehabilitation should be focused on those who are most likely to benefit, representing cost-effective use of limited resources.

Further reading

Almeida OP, Garrido GJ, Beer C, et al. Cognitive and brain changes associated with ischaemic heart disease and heart failure. *Eur Heart J* 2012; **33**: 1769–76.

Clegg A, Young J, Iliffe S, et al. Frailty in elderly people. *Lancet* 2013; **381**: 752–62.

Haennel RG. Exercise rehabilitation for chronic heart failure patients with cardiac device implants. *Cardiopulm Phys Ther J* 2012; **23**: 23–8.

Kamke W, Dovifat C, Schranz M, et al. Cardiac rehabilitation in patients with implantable defibrillators. Feasibility and complications. *Z Kardiol* 2003; **92**: 869–75.

Kindermann I, Barth C, Mahfoud F, et al. Update on myocarditis. *J Am Coll Cardiol* 2012; **59**: 779–92.

Kindermann I, Kindermann M, Kandolf R, et al. Predictors of outcome in patients with suspected myocarditis. *Circulation* 2008; **118**: 639–48.

Meurin P, Iliou MC, Ben Driss A, et al.; Working Group of Cardiac Rehabilitation of the French Society of Cardiology. Early exercise training after mitral valve repair: a multicentric prospective French study. *Chest* 2005; **128**: 1638–44.

Nombela-Franco L, Webb JG, de Jaegere PP, et al. Timing, predictive factors, and prognostic value of cerebrovascular events in a large cohort of patients undergoing transcatheter aortic valve implantation. *Circulation* 2012; **126**: 3041–51.

Piepoli MF, Conraads V, Corrà U, et al. Exercise training in heart failure: from theory to practice. A consensus document of the Heart Failure Association and the European Association for Cardiovascular Prevention and Rehabilitation. *Eur J Heart Fail* 2011; **13**: 347–57.

Pelliccia A, Corrado D, Bjørnstad HH, et al. Recommendations for participation in competitive sport and leisure-time physical activity in individuals with cardiomyopathies, myocarditis and pericarditis. *Eur J Cardiovasc Prev Rehabil* 2006; **13**: 876–85.

Reibis R, Treszl A, Bestehorn K, et al. Comparable short term prognosis in diabetic and non-diabetic patients with acute coronary syndrome after cardiac rehabilitation. *Eur J Cardiovasc Prev Rehabil* 2011; **19**: 15–22.

Rodés-Cabau J, Webb JG, Cheung A, et al. Long-term outcomes after transcatheter aortic valve implantation: insights on prognostic factors and valve durability from the Canadian multicenter experience. *J Am Coll Cardiol* 2012; **60**: 1864–75.

Salzwedel A, Nosper M, Roehrig B, et al. Outcome quality of in-patient cardiac rehabilitation in elderly patients—identification of relevant parameters. *Eur J Prev Cardiol* 2014; **21**: 172–80.

Schoenenberger AW, Stortecky S, Neumann S, et al. Predictors of functional decline in elderly patients undergoing transcatheter aortic valve implantation (TAVI). *Eur Heart J* 2013; **34**: 684–92.

Völler H, Kamke W, Klein H, et al. Clinical practice of defibrillator implantation after myocardial infarction: impact of implant time: results from the PreSCD II Registry. *Europace* 2011; **13**: 499–508.

References

1 Salzwedel A, Nosper M, Roehrig B, et al. Outcome quality of in-patient cardiac rehabilitation in elderly patients—identification of relevant parameters. *Eur J Prev Cardiol* 2014; **21**: 172–80.

2 Horstkotte D, Lengyel M, Mistiaen WP, et al. Recommendations for post-discharge patient follow up after cardiac valve interventions: a position paper. *J Heart Valve Dis* 2007; **16**: 575–89.

3 Kim C, Kim DY, Lee DW. The impact of early regular cardiac rehabilitation program on myocardial function after acute myocardial infarction. *Ann Rehabil Med* 2011; **35**: 535–40.

4 Piepoli MF, Corrà U, Benzer W, et al. Secondary prevention through cardiac rehabilitation: from knowledge to implementation. A position paper from the Cardiac Rehabilitation Section of the European Association of Cardiovascular Prevention and Rehabilitation. *Eur J Cardiovasc Prev Rehabil* 2010; **17**: 1–17.

5 Adamas J, Roberts J, Simms K, et al. Measurement of functional capacity requirements to aid in development of an occupation-specific rehabilitation training program to help firefighters with cardiac disease safely return to work. *Am J Cardiol* 2009; **103**: 762–5.

6 Bensimhon DR, Leifer ES, Ellis SJ, et al.; HF-ACTION Trial Investigators. Reproducibility of peak oxygen uptake and other cardiopulmonary exercise testing parameters in patients with heart failure (from the Heart Failure and A Controlled Trial Investigating Outcomes of exercise TraiNing). *Am J Cardiol* 2008; **102**: 712–17.

7 Fitchet A, Doherty PJ, Bundy C, et al. Comprehensive cardiac rehabilitation programme for implantable cardioverter-defibrillator patients: a randomised controlled trial. *Heart* 2003; **89**: 155–60.

8 Light RW. Pleural effusions following cardiac injury and coronary artery bypass graft surgery. *Semin Respir Crit Care Med* 2001; **22**: 657–64.

9 Wood MA, Ellenboggen KA, Hall J, et al. Post-pericardiotomy syndrome following linear left atrial radiofrequency ablation. *J Interv Card Electrophysiol* 2003; **9**: 55–7.

10 Velander M, Grip L, Mogensen L. The postcardiac injury syndrome following percutaneous transluminal coronary angioplasty. *Clin Cardiol* 1993; **16**: 353–4.

11 Vidal B, Sitgens, M, Marigliano A, et al. Optimizing the programation of cardiac resynchronization therapy devices in patients with heart failure and left bundle branch block. *Am J Cardiol* 2007; **100**: 1002–6.

12 Singh-Manoux A, Kivimaki M, Glymour MM, et al. Timing of onset of cognitive decline: results from Whitehall II prospective cohort study. *Br Med J* 2012; **344**: d7622.

13 Almeida OP, Garrido GJ, Beer C, et al. Cognitive and brain changes associated with ischaemic heart disease and heart failure. *Eur Heart J* 2012; **33**: 1769–76.

14 Jefferson AL, Himali JJ, Beiser AS, et al. Cardiac index is associated with brain aging: the Framingham Heart Study. *Circulation* 2010; **122**: 690–7.

15 Roach GW, Kanchuger M, Mangano CM, et al. Adverse cerebral outcomes after coronary bypass surgery. Multicenter Study of Perioperative Ischemia Research Group and the Ischemia Research and Education Foundation Investigators. *N Engl J Med* 1996; **335**: 1857–62.

16 Newman MF, Kirchner JL, Phillips-Bute B, et al. Longitudinal assessment of neurocognitive function after coronary-artery bypass surgery. *N Engl J Med* 2001; **344**: 395–401.

17 Sun X, Lindsay J, Monsein LH, et al. Silent brain injury after cardiac surgery: a review: cognitive dysfunction and magnetic resonance imaging diffusion-weighted imaging findings. *J Am Coll Cardiol* 2012; **60**: 791–7.

18 Nasreddine ZS, Phillips NA, Bédirian V, et al. The Montreal Cognitive Assessment, MoCA: a brief screening tool for mild cognitive impairment. *J Am Geriatr Soc* 2005; **53**: 695–9.

19 Clegg A, Young J, Iliffe S, et al. Frailty in elderly people. *Lancet* 2013; **381**: 752–62.

20 Schoenenberger AW, Stortecky S, Neumann S, et al. Predictors of functional decline in elderly patients undergoing transcatheter aortic valve implantation (TAVI). *Eur Heart J* 2013; **34**: 684–92.

21 Völler H, Kamke W, Klein HU, et al. Clinical practice of defibrillator implantation after myocardial infarction: impact of implant time: results from the PreSCD II Registry. *Europace* 2011; **13**: 499–508.

22 Bardy GH, Lee KL, Mark DB, et al.; Sudden Cardiac Death in Heart Failure Trial (SCD-HeFT) Investigators. Amiodarone or an implantable cardioverter-defibrillator for congestive heart failure. *N Engl J Med* 2005; **352**: 225–37.

23 Tang AS, Wells GA, Talajic M, et al. Resynchronization-Defibrillation for Ambulatory Heart Failure Trial Investigators. Cardiac-resynchronization therapy for mild-to-moderate heart failure. *N Engl J Med* 2010; **363**: 2385–95.

24 Zartner PA, Toussaint-Goetz N, Photiadis J, et al. Telemonitoring with implantable electronic devices in young patients with congenital heart diseases. *Europace* 2012; **14**: 1030–7.

25 Kamke W, Dovifat C, Schranz M, et al. Cardiac rehabilitation in patients with implantable defibrillators. Feasibility and complications. *Z Kardiol* 2003; **92**: 869–75.

26 Isaksen K, Morken IM, Munk PS, et al. Exercise training and cardiac rehabilitation in patients with implantable cardioverter defibrillators: a review of current literature focusing on safety, effects of exercise training and the psychological impact of programme participation. *Eur J Prev Cardiol* 2012; **19**; 804–12.

27 Haennel RG. Exercise rehabilitation for chronic heart failure patients with cardiac device implants. *Cardiopulm Phys Ther J* 2012; **23**: 23–8.

28 Piepoli MF, Conraads V, Corrà U, et al. Exercise training in heart failure: from theory to practice. A consensus document of the Heart Failure Association and the European Association for Cardiovascular Prevention and Rehabilitation. *Eur J Heart Fail* 2011; **13**: 347–57.

29 Reibis RK. Rehabilitation of patients with cardiac pacemakers and implanted cardioverter-defibrillators: recommendations for training, physiotherapeutic procedures and re-employment. *Dtsch Med Wochenschr* 2010; **135**: 759–64.

30 Vazquez LD, Conti, JB, Sears SF. Female-specific education, management, and lifestyle enhancement for implantable cardioverter defibrillator patients: the FEMALE-ICD study. *Pacing Clin Electrophysiol* 2010; **33**: 1131–40.

31 Task Force members, Vijgen J, Botto G, Camm J, et al. Consensus statement of the European Heart Rhythm Association: updated recommendations for driving by patients with implantable cardioverter defibrillators. *Europace* 2009; **11**: 1097–107.

32 Cooper LT Jr. Myocarditis. *N Engl J Med* 2009; **360**: 1526–38.

33 Hundley WG, Bluemke DA, Finn JP, et al. ACCF/ACR/AHA/NASCI/SCMR 2010 expert consensus document on cardiovascular magnetic resonance: a report of the American College of Cardiology Foundation Task Force on Expert Consensus Documents. *Circulation* 2010; **121**: 2462–508.

34 Kindermann I, Barth C, Mahfoud F, et al. Update on myocarditis. *J Am Coll Cardiol* 2012; **59**: 779–92.

35 Fabre A, Sheppard MN. Sudden adult death syndrome and other non-ischaemic causes of sudden cardiac death. *Heart* 2006; **92**: 316–20.

36 Alter P, Grimm W, Herzum M, et al. Physical activity and sports in heart failure due to myocarditis and dilated cardiomyopathy. *Herz* 2004; **29**: 391–400.

37 Maron BJ. Sudden death in young athletes. *N Engl J Med* 2003; **349**: 1064–75.

38 Piepoli MF, Guazzi M, Boriani G, et al. Exercise intolerance in chronic heart failure: mechanisms and therapies. Part I. *Eur J Cardiovasc Prev Rehabil* 2010; **17**: 637–42.

39 Wike J, Kernan M. Sudden cardiac death in the active adult. *Curr Sports Med Rep* 2005; **4**: 76–82.

40 Maron BJ, Ackerman MJ, Nishimura RA, et al. Task Force 4: HCM and other cardiomyopathies, mitral valve prolapse, myocarditis, and Marfan syndrome. *J Am Coll Cardiol* 2005; **45**: 1340–5.

41 Kindermann I, Kindermann M, Kandolf R, et al. Predictors of outcome in patients with suspected myocarditis. *Circulation* 2008; **118**: 639–48.

42 Pelliccia A, Corrado D, Bjørnstad HH, et al. Recommendations for participation in competitive sport and leisure-time physical activity in individuals with cardiomyopathies, myocarditis and pericarditis. *Eur J Cardiovasc Prev Rehabil* 2006; **13**: 876–85.

43 Fletcher GF, Balady GJ, Amsterdam EA, et al. Exercise standards for testing and training: a statement for healthcare professionals from the American Heart Association. *Circulation* 2001; **104**: 1694–740.

44 Ford ES, Ajani UA, Croft JB, et al. Explaining the decrease in U.S. deaths from coronary disease, 1980–2000. *N Engl J Med* 2007; **356**: 2388–98.

45 Preis SR, Hwang SJ, Coady S, et al. Trends in all-cause and cardiovascular disease mortality among women and men with and without diabetes mellitus in the Framingham Heart Study, 1950 to 2005. *Circulation* 2009; **119**: 1728–35.

46 Reibis R, Treszl A, Bestehorn K, et al. Comparable short term prognosis in diabetic and non-diabetic patients with acute coronary syndrome after cardiac rehabilitation. *Eur J Cardiovasc Prev Rehabil* 2011; **19**: 15–22.

47 Ettefagh L, Maleki M, Panahi A, et al. The prevalence of impaired glucose metabolism in patients referred to cardiac rehabilitation. *J Cardiopulm Rehabil Prev* 2013; **33**: 42–6.

48 Rydén L, Grant PJ, Anker SD, et al. ESC guidelines on diabetes, pre-diabetes, and cardiovascular diseases developed in collaboration with the EASD Task Force on diabetes, pre-diabetes, and cardiovascular diseases of the European Society of Cardiology (ESC) and developed in collaboration with the European Association for the Study of Diabetes (EASD). *Eur Heart J* 2013; **34**: 3035–87.

49 Kiel M. Cardiac rehabilitation after heart valve surgery. *PM R* 2011; **3**: 962–7.

50 Gohlke-Bärwolf C, Roskamm H. [Results of heart valve replacement. Prognosis—occupational and general disability—occupational rehabilitation]. *Versicherungsmedizin* 1992; **44**: 163–8.

51 Meurin P, Iliou MC, Ben Driss A, et al.; Working Group of Cardiac Rehabilitation of the French Society of Cardiology. Early exercise training after mitral valve repair: a multicentric prospective French study. *Chest* 2005; **128**: 1638–44.

52 Gohlke-Bärwolf C, Gohlke H, Samek L, et al. Exercise tolerance and working capacity after valve replacement. *J Heart Valve Dis* 1992; **1**: 189–95.

53 Butchart EG, Gohlke-Bärwolf C, Antunes MJ, et al.; Working Groups on Valvular Heart Disease, Thrombosis, and Cardiac Rehabilitation and Exercise Physiology, European Society of Cardiology. Recommendations for the management of patients after heart valve surgery. *Eur Heart J* 2005; **26**: 2463–71.

54 Nombela-Franco L, Webb JG, de Jaegere PP, et al. Timing, predictive factors, and prognostic value of cerebrovascular events in a large cohort of patients undergoing transcatheter aortic valve implantation. *Circulation* 2012; **126**: 3041–51.

55 Rodés-Cabau J, Webb JG, Cheung A, et al. Long-term outcomes after transcatheter aortic valve implantation: insights on prognostic factors and valve durability from the Canadian multicenter experience. *J Am Coll Cardiol* 2012; **60**: 1864–75.

56 Makkar RR, Fontana GP, Jilaihawi H, et al.; PARTNER Trial Investigators. Transcatheter aortic-valve replacement for inoperable severe aortic stenosis. *N Engl J Med* 2012; **366**: 1696–704.

57 Nitardy A, Salzwedel A, Wegscheider K, et al. Effect of cardiac rehabilitation on functional and emotional status in patients after transcatheter aortic-valve replacement. *Circulation* 2012; **126**: A12981.

58 ACC/AHA Task Force on Practice Guidelines. ACC/AHA guidelines for the management of patients with valvular heart disease. *J Am Coll Cardiol* 1998; **32**: 1486–88.

59 Fitzmaurice DA, Machin SJ, on behalf of the British Society of Haematology Task Force for Haemostasis and Thrombosis: recommendations for patients undertaking self management of oral anticoagulation. *Br Med J* 2001; **323**: 985–9.

60 Mitchell LB, Exner DV, Wyse DG, et al. Prophylactic oral amiodarone for the prevention of arrhythmias that begin early after revascularization, valve replacement or repair. *J Am Med Assoc* 2005; **294**: 3093–100.

61 Heneghan C, Ward A, Perera R; Self-Monitoring Trialist Collaboration, Bankhead C, Fuller A, Stevens R, et al. Self-monitoring of oral anticoagulation: systematic review and meta-analysis of individual patient data. *Lancet* 2012; **379**: 322–34.

62 Khatri PJ, Webb JG, Rodés-Cabau J, et al. Adverse effects associated with transcatheter aortic valve implantation: a meta-analysis of contemporary studies. *Ann Intern Med* 2013; **158**: 35–46.

63 Robicsek F, Fokin A, Cook J, et al. Sternal instability after midline sternotomy. *Thorac Cardiov Surg* 2000; **48**: 1–8.

64 Elovainio M, Ferrie JE, Singh-Manoux A, et al. Socioeconomic differences in cardiometabolic factors: social causation or health-related selection; Evidence from the Whitehall II Cohort Study 1991–2004. *Am J Epidemiol* 2011; **174**: 779–89.

65 Weber A, Schmid K, Scharf B, et al. Cardiovascular diseases caused by unemployment? An analysis from the viewpoint of social medicine. *Wien Klin Wochenschr* 1997; **109**: 202–10.

66 Weber A, Lehnert G. Unemployment and cardiovascular diseases: a causal relationship? *Int Arch Occup Environ Health* 1997; **70**: 153–60.

67 Henriksson KM, Lindblad U, Agren B, et al. Associations between unemployment and cardiovascular risk factors varies with the unemployment rate: the Cardiovascular Risk Factor Study in Southern Sweden (CRISS). *Scand J Public Health* 2003; **31**: 305–11.

68 Janlert U, Asplund K, Weinehall L. Unemployment and cardiovascular risk indicators. Data from the MONICA survey in northern Sweden. *Scand J Soc Med* 1992; **20**: 14–18.

69 Backhans MC, Hemmingsson T. Unemployment and mental health—who is (not) affected? *Eur J Public Health* 2012; **22**: 429–33.

70 Bäck, M, Jansson B, Cider A, et al. Validation of a questionnaire to detect kinesiophobia (fear of movement) in patients with coronary artery disease. *J Rehabil Med* 2012; **44**: 363–9.

71 Kaiser MJ, Bauer JM, Ramsch C, et al.; MNA-International Group. Validation of the Mini Nutritional Assessment short-form (MNA-SF): a practical tool for identification of nutritional status. *J Nutr Health Aging* 2009; **13**: 782–8.

72 Rockwood K, Song X, Macknight C, et al. A global clinical measure of fitness and frailty in elderly people. *Can Med Assoc J* 2005; **173**: 489–95.

CHAPTER 23

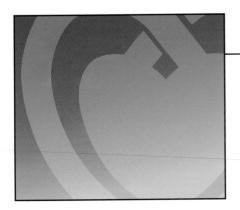

Ambulatory preventive care: outpatient clinics and primary care

Jean-Paul Schmid and Hugo Saner

Contents

Summary

Cardiac rehabilitation (CR) services aim to restore the physical, psychosocial, and vocational status of cardiac patients. In recent times, the role of these services has evolved due to the progress of interventional cardiology with its prompt and effective treatment of acute coronary syndromes. The focus has moved from the restoration of a patient's health following an acute event towards a more pronounced long-term targeted secondary prevention intervention. As a consequence, CR services have also expanded their indication in order to include not just patients after myocardial infarction or surgery, but also a variety of 'non-acute' cardiovascular disease (CVD) states like stable coronary heart disease and peripheral obstructive artery disease as well as asymptomatic patients with no history of CVD but with a constellation of cardiovascular risk factors, especially metabolic syndrome or diabetes mellitus. The biggest challenge for CR in building on its achievements to date is to ensure the highest standards of comprehensive evidence-based preventive and rehabilitative care. The personnel for a CR programme should comprise professionals who are able to provide an effective CR and secondary prevention service and undergo continuing professional development through regular refresher courses. Furthermore, the clinic facilities must provide a safe and functional environment. The most important part of organizing a CR service is probably recruiting all eligible patients and overcoming barriers to their participation. Patient assessment at the beginning of a CR programme is essential. It serves to identify the cardiovascular risk profile, to set the goals which should be achieved during rehabilitation, to estimate the patient's risk, and to determine exercise capacity and training intensity. Recording data prospectively on the process and outcomes of the CR programme allows for continuous monitoring of the programme's efficacy and safety and serves as a tool for bench-marking against national standards. Finally, regular audit is needed for quality control, both locally and as part of a national audit programme for CR. It demonstrates what programmes are achieving in relation to defined clinical outcomes, and enables local results to be compared with national outcomes.

The role of outpatient clinics in preventive cardiology: introduction

As stated by WHO in 1964, in their definition of cardiac rehabilitation (CR) for patients with cardiovascular disease (CVD) [1], CR services aim to restore the physical, psychosocial, and vocational status of cardiac patients. The first structured physical activity programme for patients after an acute myocardial infarction was set up in 1952 by Newman et al. in a fixed in-hospital setting in the United States [2], and countries with a tradition of spa resorts or mountain sanatoria (Germany, Austria, Italy, and some other southern and eastern European countries) adopted this residential rehabilitation centre approach, usually involving short-duration, intensive CR (3–4 weeks). In most other parts of the world, in particular the Anglo-Saxon countries, ambulatory services developed with either a centre- or home-based approach.

A typical and well-approved centre-based outpatient format today corresponds to an 8–12 week programme, offering 36 training and information sessions. However, many other programme variants, differing in duration, content, and intensity have been developed [3]. Although the approach to CR delivery varies between European countries, depending on their healthcare system, cultural traditions, and social norms, all have the same aims:

- to improve the patient's functional capacity
- to prepare for a return to work and to maintain an independent lifestyle as long as possible
- to support psychological adaptation to the chronic disease process
- to motivate the patient for long-term behavioural and lifestyle changes
- to reduce morbidity and enhance long-term prognosis.

In recent years, the role of CR clinics, in particular as far as the outpatient setting is concerned, has changed. It has moved from the restoration of a patient's health following an acute event to being a more pronounced long-term targeted secondary prevention intervention. This implies that patient care is not restricted solely to patients after a myocardial infarction, cardiac surgery, or decompensated heart failure, but now includes a variety of 'non-acute' CVD states like stable coronary heart disease and peripheral obstructive artery disease as well as asymptomatic patients with no history of CVD but with a constellation of cardiovascular risk factors, especially metabolic syndrome or diabetes mellitus.

Compared with usual care alone, exercise-based CR improves the cardiovascular risk factor profile, exercise tolerance, and health-related quality of life and reduces mortality in patients with coronary heart disease [4]. The long-term benefit of CR is thereby driven by successful achievement of healthy behavioural changes. This is acknowledged in the most recent European guidelines on CVD prevention in clinical practice, where multimodal interventions, integrating education on healthy lifestyle with medical resources, exercise training, stress management, and counselling on psychosocial risk factors, are recommended (class I, level of evidence A) in individuals at very high risk of CVD [5]. However, the initiation of behavioural changes is often difficult and principles for effective communication have been recommended (➲ Box 23.1) [5].

Box 23.1 Principles of effective communication to facilitate behavioural change

- Spend enough time with the individual to create a therapeutic relationship—even a few more minutes can make a difference.
- Acknowledge the individual's personal view of his/her disease and contributing factors.
- Encourage expression of worries and anxieties, concerns, and self-evaluation of motivation for behaviour change and chances of success.
- Speak to the individual in his/her own language and be supportive of every improvement in lifestyle.
- Ask questions to check that the individual has understood the advice and has any support they require to follow it.
- Acknowledge that changing lifelong habits can be difficult and that gradual change that is sustained is often more permanent than a rapid change.
- Accept that individuals may need support for a long time and that repeated efforts to encourage and maintain lifestyle change may be necessary in many individuals.
- Make sure that all health professionals involved provide consistent information.

Source: data from Perk J, De Backer G, Gohlke H, et al. European guidelines on cardiovascular disease prevention in clinical practice (version 2012). The Fifth Joint Task Force of the European Society of Cardiology and Other Societies on Cardiovascular Disease Prevention in Clinical Practice (constituted by representatives of nine societies and by invited experts). *Eur Heart J* 2012; **33**: 1635–701.

CR in the era of modern cardiology has become more challenging with the advent of primary angioplasty for acute coronary syndromes and early discharge from hospital, and programmes need to evolve with changing trends in acute management of coronary and other vascular diseases and increasing demands for these services. The biggest challenge for CR in building on its achievements to date is to ensure the highest standards of comprehensive evidence-based preventive and rehabilitative care. Continuing education of all healthcare professionals involved in CR (e.g. how to facilitate behavioural changes) as well as reporting and evaluating of programme outcome data are essential.

Indications for outpatient cardiovascular rehabilitation

The 2011 American Heart Association/American College of Cardiology Foundation update on secondary prevention and risk reduction therapy for patients with coronary and other atherosclerotic vascular disease [6] states that all eligible patients with an acute coronary syndrome or immediately after coronary artery bypass surgery or a percutaneous coronary intervention (PCI)

Table 23.1 Indications for outpatient CR (a) and conditions favouring a residential CR programme if available (b)

(a) Indications for outpatient CR

Risk profile	Indications
Low risk	Multiple cardiovascular risk factors in need of an intervention, especially diabetes mellitus or metabolic syndrome
	Condition after elective percutaneous coronary intervention
	Young patients (<45 years of age) with uncomplicated heart surgery (heart valves, congenital heart disease without relevant systemic impairment)
Medium risk	Condition after acute coronary syndrome (NSTEMI or STEMI)
	Patients > 45 years after CABG, heart valve surgery, or vascular surgery (aorta or large peripheral vessels) with an uncomplicated course
	Patients with peripheral artery disease
High risk	Patients with first diagnosis of heart failure (systolic or diastolic dysfunction)
	Patients after heart transplantation
	Condition of cardiopulmonary decompensation of any origin
	Any heart or vascular surgery with complicated course
	Patients with complex congenital heart disease
	Patients with pulmonary arterial hypertension
	Condition after aortic dissection

NSTEMI, non-ST-segment elevation myocardial infarction; STEMI, ST-segment elevation myocardial infarction; CABG, coronary artery bypass graft.

(b) Conditions favouring a residential CR programme

The need for intensive nursing and medical supervision
Unreasonable distance of CR centre from home (e.g. commuting distance > 1 hour)
Pronounced frailty/multimorbidity which impairs mobility
Need for temporary relief and/or distance from social environment (professional and private)

Source: data for (a) and (b) from Karoff M, Held K, Bjarnason-Wehrens B. Cardiac rehabilitation in Germany. *Eur J Cardiovasc Prev Rehabil* 2007; **14**: 18–27.

should be referred to a comprehensive outpatient cardiovascular rehabilitation programme (class I, level of evidence A). However, data also support CR for stable coronary artery disease [7] and for patients with heart failure [8,9], peripheral artery disease [10], and diabetes mellitus [11]. A wide range of other disease states have also been recognized as indications for both outpatient and residential cardiovascular rehabilitation programmes. ➲ Table 23.1 summarizes one example of the indications for CR as applied in Switzerland and Germany.

In general, the indications for referring patients to a CR programme, either alone or in combination, are:

- a recent medico-surgical intervention
- reduced exercise capacity
- presence of unsatisfactorily controlled cardiovascular risk factors.

After recent hospitalization CR should be started early after discharge or during the first follow-up office visit. There is solid evidence that CR starting within 2 weeks of either discharge or diagnosis is safe, feasible, and more clinically effective [13] and improves programme uptake and adherence [14]. Patients with staged PCI do not need to wait until revascularization is complete. The initial medical assessment will determine the ischaemic threshold of the patient and whether any remaining coronary stenosis is still clinically relevant. Training below the ischaemic threshold is safe, provided that the threshold is beyond an exercise capacity of 50 W during an ergometer stress test [15].

Organization of an outpatient clinic

Personnel

The personnel for a CR programme should comprise professionals who are able to provide an effective CR and secondary prevention service (see ➲ Fig. 23.1) [16], for example:

- a programme director—any member of the team, with good organizational, management, and interpersonal skills able to ensure proper organization, policies, and procedures that are consistent with evidence-based guidelines
- a medical director (who could be the programme director) who is a specialist in cardiology and oversees the CR programme policies and medical care
- trained and well-instructed personnel immediately available to respond to medical emergencies
- a multidisciplinary team consisting of cardiologists, physiotherapists, nurses, psychologist, dietician, exercise physiologists, occupational therapist, and social services worker
- consultant professionals, i.e. internist, neurologist, diabetologist, cardiac surgeon, and general physician.

Each team member must have certified qualifications for their given areas of expertise and training. The personnel involved in the CR process should undergo continuing professional development through regular refresher courses providing updates and continuing post-graduate education, including in cardiopulmonary resuscitation skills.

Infrastructure

The clinic facilities must provide a safe and functional environment. Setting this up comprises planning the utilization of space, the acquisition of equipment and its maintenance, the reduction and control of environmental hazards and risks, the maintenance of safe conditions (emergency access to all patient areas), and climate control (adequate temperature and humidity).

The following should constitute the *basic facilities* for CR services:

- a dedicated consultation area for medical and psychological assessment
- appropriate rooms for education and counselling (for individual or group interventions)
- an examination room (e.g. echocardiography)
- an exercise testing laboratory

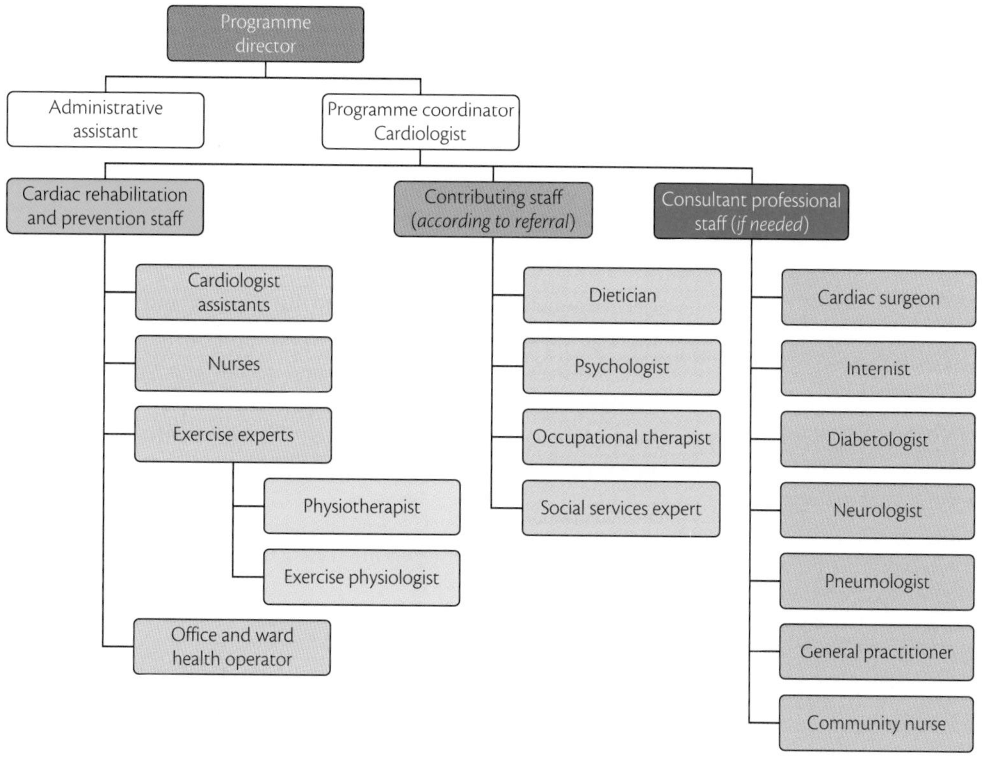

Fig. 23.1 Organization chart of personnel involved in a cardiac rehabilitation and secondary prevention programme.

- an exercise (training) room—the space must meet the requirements for the activities and services being offered and the unique needs of patients (approximately 4 m^2 per patient is recommended)
- resting/dressing room with separate toilets and shower facilities.

The specific selection of equipment depends on the preferences of the individual programme, the available space, and budget limitations. All equipment should be commercial grade with stringent maintenance guidelines to ensure patient safety. Staff should be thoroughly trained in the use of all equipment and information for its correct use and calibration, and reference standards should be readily available. A chair and an examination table, suitable for supine or recumbent positions, should be available in all patient areas. The minimum equipment requirement for a CR centre is summarized in ➲ Table 23.2 [16].

Patient recruitment

One of the most important parts of organizing a CR service is recruiting all eligible patients and overcoming barriers to their participation. No eligible patient should be missed, but patients who may not benefit from CR, for physical, psychosocial, or other reasons, should not be offered a place on a programme if the risk of premature discontinuation is high.

The main barriers to professionals referring patients for CR include insufficient knowledge or scepticism about patient benefits, an over-reliance on physicians as gatekeepers, and value judgements that patients are not likely to participate. Systems factors are related to territory, remuneration, and insufficient time and staff capacity. Patients may also have limited knowledge of programmes and find that the process of obtaining a referral is sometimes confusing and challenging [18].

Patient assessment

Patient assessment at the beginning of a CR programme is essential. It serves to identify the cardiovascular risk profile, to set the

Table 23.2 Minimum equipment requirements for a cardiac rehabilitation centre

Function	Equipment
Assessment of clinical status	Stethoscope and sphygmomanometer Weighing scale Chemistry analysis Urine analysis ECG
Assessment of left ventricular function*	Echocardiography equipment
Assessment of arrhythmias	Ambulatory ECG Holter monitoring apparatus
Assessment of functional capacity*	Treadmill or ergometer for exercise stress test Respiratory gas analyser for spiroergometry Equipment/facilities for 6-minute walk or shuttle walk test
Assessment of psychosocial status	Licensed tests and screening instruments (ideally computerized)
Equipment for conducting an exercise training programme (it is possible to conduct CR exercise programmes with minimal equipment)	Stethoscope and sphygmomanometer ECG monitoring equipment/telemetry system Exercise equipment (gymnastic tools, Thera bands®, weight training machines, treadmills, ergometers, arm ergometer)
Emergency equipment [17]	Written emergency instructions are required, together with ready access to a telephone to summon assistance

*Depending on circumstances and type of patients.

Table 23.3 Key points for patient assessment at CR entry

Clinical history	Screening for cardiovascular risk factors, comorbidities, and disabilities
Symptoms	NYHA class for dyspnoea and CCS class for angina
Adherence	To the medical regime and self-monitoring (weight, blood pressure, symptoms)
Physical examination	General health status, heart failure signs, cardiac and carotid murmurs, blood pressure control, extremities for presence of arterial pulses and orthopaedic pathology, cardiovascular accidents with/without neurological sequelae
ECG	Heart rate, rhythm, repolarization
Cardiac imaging	Two-dimensional and Doppler echocardiography: in particular ventricular function and heart valve diseases
Blood testing	Routine biochemical assay, fasting blood glucose (HbA1c if fasting blood glucose is elevated), total cholesterol, LDL-C, HDL-C, triglycerides
Physical activity level	Domestic, occupational, and recreational needs, activities relevant to age, gender, and daily life, readiness to change behaviour, self-confidence, barriers to increased physical activity, and social support in making positive changes
Peak exercise capacity	Symptom-limited exercise testing, either on a bicycle ergometer or a treadmill
Education	Clear, comprehensible information on the basic purpose of the CR programme and the role of each component
Expected outcomes	Formulation of 'tailored', patient-specific, objectives of the CR programme, eventually also involving family members

NYHA, New York Heart Association; CCS, Canadian Cardiovascular Society; HbA1c, glycated haemoglobin; LDL-C, low-density lipoprotein cholesterol; HDL-C, high-density lipoprotein cholesterol.

Source: data from Piepoli MF, Corrà U, Benzer W, et al. Secondary prevention through cardiac rehabilitation: from knowledge to implementation. A position paper from the Cardiac Rehabilitation Section of the European Association of Cardiovascular Prevention and Rehabilitation. *Eur J Cardiovasc Prev Rehabil* 2010; **17**: 1–17.

goals which should be achieve during rehabilitation, to estimate the patient's risk, and to determine exercise capacity and training intensity. The key points are enumerated in ➲ Table 23.3.

Delivering a comprehensive CR programme: minimum standards and core components

The achievements of CR so far may be compromised by CR programmes which do not comply with the required minimum standards and/or core components of a comprehensive CR programme [20]. The British Association for Cardiovascular Prevention and Rehabilitation (BACPR) has defined seven standards and seven core components for CVD prevention and rehabilitation (for details see [21]).

The seven core components of a modern cardiovascular prevention and rehabilitation programme consist of:

1. health behaviour change and education
2. lifestyle risk factor management: physical activity and exercise, diet, and smoking cessation
3. psychosocial health
4. medical risk factor management
5. cardioprotective therapies
6. long-term management
7. audit and evaluation.

Outcome measures and audit

Recording data prospectively on the process and outcomes of the CR programme allows for continuous monitoring of the programme's efficacy and safety and serves as a tool for benchmarking against national standards. Patient data should be collected at programme entry and at the end of the programme. Recording of the following variables is recommended:

- exercise capacity
- health-related quality of life (one generic and one disease specific questionnaire)
- smoking status
- complications (cardiovascular and non-cardiovascular)
- attendance rate and rate of discontinuation
- patient satisfaction.

Regular audit is essential for quality control, both locally and as part of a national audit programme for CR. It demonstrates what programmes are achieving in relation to defined clinical outcomes, and enables local results to be compared with national outcomes. Therefore outcome data from each individual centre should be entered onto a national database.

The role of primary care in preventive cardiology: introduction

Primary care physicians have a pivotal role in the successful implementation of primary and secondary prevention guidelines for both population and high-risk approaches to reduce the burden of CVD. Increasingly, in this era of health cost containment, the primary care physician is recognized as: (1) the main and sometimes the only source of healthcare for a large number of individuals; (2) an affordable physician; and (3) the gatekeeper for referral to medical specialists. Although the majority of primary care physicians intuitively support the concept of preventive cardiology and generally have a high level of knowledge of cardiovascular risk factors, a significant gap remains between physician knowledge and attitudes and the actual practice of preventive cardiology. For patients with suspected or overt CVD, the cardiologist in clinical practice takes over the task of identifying particular risk factors to define targets for treatment and to help to motivate patients to maintain a healthy lifestyle and to be compliant with drug treatment. In some countries, primary care physicians and clinical cardiologists are supported by nurse specialists with special training in CVD prevention measures.

Cardiovascular disease prevention in general practice

The following key points underlie the basis of cardiovascular disease prevention in general practice:

- Risk factor screening, including the lipid profile, may be considered in adult men ≥40 years old and in women ≥50 years old of age or who are post-menopausal [22].
- The physician in general practice is the key person to initiate, coordinate, and provide long-term follow-up for CVD prevention [23]. This includes lifestyle interventions and medication for primary and secondary prevention.
- Aspirin, statins, and antihypertensive agents have class I indications in patients with established atherosclerosis.
- Fewer than 50% of patients are fully adherent with these medications and non-adherence is associated with worse outcomes.
- Starting these medications is associated with a lowering of risk, whereas stopping these medications is associated with an elevation of risk; not taking them at all is associated with the highest risk.

Primary care physicians are a critical professional group for the successful implementation of CVD prevention programmes in Europe. In most countries they deliver more than 90% of consultations and provide the vast majority of preventive care, disease screening, chronic disease monitoring, and follow-up. The general practitioner is in many instances the main, and sometimes the only, source of healthcare for a large number of individuals, and usually the gatekeeper for referral to medical specialists. The majority of primary care physicians intuitively support the concept of preventive cardiology and generally have a high level of knowledge about cardiovascular risk factors. However, a significant gap remains between physician knowledge and attitudes and the actual practice of preventive cardiology. Despite the enormous burden of CVD, many patients at high risk remain undiagnosed and untreated. General practitioners perform a unique role in CVD prevention by identifying individuals at risk of developing CVD and assessing their eligibility for intervention based on their cardiovascular risk profile.

A major task of the general practitioner is to identify high-risk individuals. However, despite the enormous burden of CVD many patients at high risk remain undiagnosed and untreated. Even among patients with established disease there are substantial treatment gaps: among patients receiving lipid-modifying therapy, 43% do not achieve total cholesterol targets [<4.5 mmol/L (175 mg/dl) in Europe] [24] whereas 64% failed to reach low-density lipoprotein cholesterol targets in the United States [25]. There has also been little improvement over time in the management of other CVD risk factors such as smoking, obesity, and diabetes [26]. Another challenge for primary care physicians is the adoption of risk calculators for predicting those at greatest risk of developing CVD who may particularly benefit from interventions. A number of studies have investigated the use of prediction rules and risk calculators by primary care physicians. A European Society of Cardiology (ESC) survey conducted in six European countries showed that physicians largely rely on their own expertise for the prevention and treatment of CVD: although most cardiologists and physicians (85%) knew they should base CVD risk assessment on the combination of all CVD risk factors, 62% of physicians used subjective methods to gauge risk rather than using risk calculators [27]. The most common barriers to guideline implementation were government or local health policy (40%), patient compliance (36%), and lack of time (23%). Suggestions proposed to improve implementation included the development of clear, easy to use, and simple guidelines (46% prompted; 23% unprompted) and financial incentives (24% unprompted).

The most important aspects of risk stratification and risk assessment in clinical practice are described in detail in Chapter 5. The key messages are: (1) risk factor management unequivocally reduces morbidity and mortality; (2) in apparently healthy people CVD risk is most frequently the result of multiple interacting risk factors; (3) a risk estimation system such as SCORE can assist in making logical management decisions, and may help to avoid both under- and over-treatment; and (4) all risk estimation systems are relatively crude, and attention to qualifying statements is required. In this regard, the total risk approach allows flexibility: if perfection cannot be achieved with one risk factor, trying harder with others can still reduce overall risk.

There are a number of barriers to implementing routine risk assessment. A survey among general practitioners and internists working in clinical practice in two Swiss regions [28] revealed that 74% rarely or never used CVD prediction rules due to fears of oversimplification of risk assessment (58%) or overuse of medical therapy (54%). More than half of the physicians (57%) believed that the numerical information resulting from prediction rules is frequently unhelpful for clinical decision-making [28]. A Dutch qualitative study of the use of risk tables as a key component of risk assessment for primary prevention reported that physicians' knowledge of the risk tables, and their ability to communicate that knowledge to patients, influenced their implementation [29]. The most important barrier to conduction of risk assessment by general practitioners in a routine patient consultation is the fact that there is little time for discussion [29,30].

There is also great concern among general practitioners about overestimating risk in national populations, which may lead to overuse of medical therapy [29,30]. The results of a Norwegian study suggest that using the European SCORE assessment would double the number of individuals who need drugs for primary prevention of CVD [31]. Providing medication to increasing numbers of patients may result in higher healthcare costs. However, modelling strategies to make more efficient use of resources and to identify most of the CVD burden have shown conflicting results. Finally, application of risk scoring in general practice versus individual risk factor treatment has not been shown to reduce cardiovascular events. The use of risk scoring based on electronic patient records is promising, but needs to be tested in a general practice setting.

Patients with established atherosclerosis, namely coronary, cerebrovascular, and peripheral artery disease, constitute a high-risk

Box 23.2 Proposed list of priorities for CVD prevention

1. Patients with established CVD, peripheral artery disease, and cerebrovascular atherosclerotic disease.
2. Asymptomatic individuals who are at high risk of developing atherosclerotic CVD.
3. First-degree relatives of patients with early onset CVD (defined as men aged <55 years and women aged <65 years).
4. First-degree relatives of asymptomatic individuals at high risk.
5. Other individuals met in connection with ordinary clinical practice.

group and have a highly elevated risk of future ischaemic events. The mainstay of management in these patients is the appropriate use of evidence-based secondary prevention measures, including lifestyle interventions and medication such as antiplatelet, lipid-lowering, and antihypertensive agents. However, the number of patients with established CVD, and of otherwise healthy individuals who are at high risk of developing CVD, is large and this presents a considerable challenge to the medical community—the tasks of CVD prevention are difficult to accomplish in the context of the daily patient workload. Therefore it is useful to define priorities for CVD prevention. The Fifth Joint European Society's Task Force on CVD Prevention in Clinical Practice [5] has developed guidelines proposing the order in which preventive action should be taken, because with limited resources full-scale action directed to all groups potentially needing preventive advice may not be feasible in the national healthcare structure (➲ Box 23.2). The highest priority is given to patients with established CVD, the lowest to the general population met in clinical practice.

Cardiovascular disease prevention in primary care

The role of the cardiologist

The following key points underlie the role of the cardiologist in cardiovascular disease prevention in primary care:

- The practising cardiologist should be the advisor in cases where there is uncertainty over the use of preventive medication or when the usual preventive options are difficult to apply [32–34].
- The practising cardiologist should regularly review the hospital discharge recommendations after a cardiac event or intervention [32–34].
- The practising cardiologist is critical to the implementation of primary and secondary CVD prevention based on CVD prevention guidelines.
- The cardiologist working in primary care is crucial for the referral of eligible patients to CR services and to overcome the barriers to participation.

Cardiologists working out of hospital have an essential role in CVD prevention by acting as consultants to general practitioners and general internists. Another pivotal role of the practising cardiologist consists of the evaluation of patients with cardiovascular problems who are referred from the primary care physician. A thorough examination by a practising cardiologist will often include assessment of exercise capacity, measurement of the ankle–brachial index, assessment of pre-clinical atherosclerosis by vascular ultrasound, and evaluation of cardiac structure and function by echocardiography. The results of these interventions in many patients with perceived low risk will often change the perception of risk profoundly. Although the identification and basic treatment of risk factors and advice about lifestyle modification is the task of the general practitioner or the general internist, the practising cardiologist needs to advise in cases where there is uncertainty about preventive drug therapy or when the usual preventive modalities are difficult to apply (e.g. nicotine addiction, resistant obesity, side effects, or insufficient efficacy of medication). In women, the advice of a cardiologist is often requested when balancing hormone replacement therapy with symptoms and total cardiovascular risk. Cardiologists give important advice on treatment with antiplatelets and oral anticoagulation in various cardiovascular conditions, with or without previous interventional therapy.

The cardiologist also plays a central role in the implementation of evidence-based medicine in patients following an acute coronary event or intervention. The hospital discharge recommendations are reviewed with the patient, and the cardiologist recommends a future treatment strategy. The cardiologist's recommendations are also crucial for patient compliance with the treatment. Giving written information and ensuring that, at set intervals, treatment goals have been reached has a significant impact on mid-term prognosis [33,35].

The impact of the practising cardiologist on CVD prevention may be enhanced by the use of electronic medical records. The ability to systematically identify all patients with risk factors, address and document their barriers to care, and control of implementation of risk reduction at pre-determined intervals should result in better outcomes.

The role of nurses

The following key point underlies the role of nurses in cardiovascular disease prevention in primary care:

- Nurse-led clinics or nurse-coordinated multidisciplinary prevention programmes are more effective than usual care in reducing cardiovascular risk in a variety of healthcare settings.

Several randomized trials of comprehensive CR programmes have shown significant improvements in risk factors, exercise tolerance, glucose control, and appropriate use of medication, along with decreases in cardiac events and mortality, regression of coronary atherosclerosis, and improved patient perception of health compared with usual care [16,17]. Other studies have demonstrated the effectiveness of nurse-led prevention clinics in primary care compared with usual care, with greater success in secondary as opposed to primary prevention [38–40].

Differences are found in the degree of effectiveness of various nurse-led programmes, which could reflect an inadequate dose of the intervention, inconsistencies in the components of the intervention, or a lack of specific expertise, as well as the inherent difficulty of achieving meaningful change in multiple factors. Models of nurse case management which were more intensive with more sustained contact have shown the most successful outcomes, including regression of atherosclerosis and decreased cardiac events [41]. The EUROACTION trial consisted of eight visits with a multidisciplinary team, attendance at a group workshop, and supervised exercise class over a 16-week period [42]; other studies have evaluated interventions of shorter durations. A common conclusion from all these prevention programmes is the need for sustained contact to maintain positive lifestyle changes. However, further research is needed to determine the optimal format of interventions necessary to achieve sustained risk reduction, and how this can be titrated and adapted for people with different risks and healthcare needs in a variety of healthcare and community settings.

Further reading

Perk J, Mathes P, Gohlke H, et al. *Cardiovascular prevention and rehabilitation*, 2007. London: Springer.

References

1 WHO Expert Committee. *Rehabilitation of patients with cardiovascular disease*. WHO Technical Report Series no. 270, 1964. Geneva: World Health Organization.
2 Newman LB, Andrews MF, Koblish MO, et al. Physical medicine and rehabilitation in acute myocardial infarction. *AMA Arch Intern Med* 1952; **89**: 552–61.
3 Bjarnason-Wehrens B, McGee H, Zwisler AD, et al. Cardiac rehabilitation in Europe: results from the European Cardiac Rehabilitation Inventory Survey. *Eur J Cardiovasc Prev Rehabil* 2010; **17**: 410–18.
4 Heran BS, Chen JM, Ebrahim S, et al. Exercise-based cardiac rehabilitation for coronary heart disease. *Cochrane Database Syst Rev* 2011; (7): CD001800.
5 Perk J, De Backer G, Gohlke H, et al. European guidelines on cardiovascular disease prevention in clinical practice (version 2012). The Fifth Joint Task Force of the European Society of Cardiology and Other Societies on Cardiovascular Disease Prevention in Clinical Practice (constituted by representatives of nine societies and by invited experts). *Eur Heart J* 2012; **33**: 1635–701.
6 Smith SC Jr, Benjamin EJ, Bonow RO, et al. AHA/ACCF secondary prevention and risk reduction therapy for patients with coronary and other atherosclerotic vascular disease: 2011 update: a guideline from the American Heart Association and American College of Cardiology Foundation endorsed by the World Heart Federation and the Preventive Cardiovascular Nurses Association. *J Am Coll Cardiol* 2011; **58**: 2432–46.
7 Goel K, Lennon RJ, Tilbury RT, et al. Impact of cardiac rehabilitation on mortality and cardiovascular events after percutaneous coronary intervention in the community. *Circulation* 2011; **123**: 2344–52.
8 Haykowsky MJ, Liang Y, Pechter D, et al. A meta-analysis of the effect of exercise training on left ventricular remodeling in heart failure patients: the benefit depends on the type of training performed. *J Am Coll Cardiol* 2007; **49**: 2329–36.
9 Piepoli MF, Davos C, Francis DP, et al. Exercise training meta-analysis of trials in patients with chronic heart failure (ExTraMATCH). *Br Med J* 2004; **328**: 189.
10 Tendera M, Aboyans V, Bartelink ML, et al. ESC guidelines on the diagnosis and treatment of peripheral artery diseases: document covering atherosclerotic disease of extracranial carotid and vertebral, mesenteric, renal, upper and lower extremity arteries: the Task Force on the Diagnosis and Treatment of Peripheral Artery Diseases of the European Society of Cardiology (ESC). *Eur Heart J* 2011; **32**: 2851–906.
11 Umpierre D, Ribeiro PA, Kramer CK, et al. Physical activity advice only or structured exercise training and association with HbA1c levels in type 2 diabetes: a systematic review and meta-analysis. *J Am Med Assoc* 2011; **305**: 1790–9.
12 Karoff M, Held K, Bjarnason-Wehrens B. Cardiac rehabilitation in Germany. *Eur J Cardiovasc Prev Rehabil* 2007; **14**: 18–27.
13 Haykowsky M, Scott J, Esch B, et al. A meta-analysis of the effects of exercise training on left ventricular remodeling following myocardial infarction: start early and go longer for greatest exercise benefits on remodeling. *Trials* 2011; **12**: 92.
14 Parker K, Stone JA, Arena R, et al. An early cardiac access clinic significantly improves cardiac rehabilitation participation and completion rates in low-risk ST-elevation myocardial infarction patients. *Can J Cardiol* 2011; **27**: 619–27.
15 Hambrecht R, Walther C, Mobius-Winkler S, et al. Percutaneous coronary angioplasty compared with exercise training in patients with stable coronary artery disease: a randomized trial. *Circulation* 2004; **109**: 1371–8.
16 Piepoli MF, Corrà U, Adamopoulos S, et al. Secondary prevention in the clinical management of patients with cardiovascular diseases. Core components, standards and outcome measures for referral and delivery. A Policy Statement from the Cardiac Rehabilitation Section of the European Association for Cardiovascular Prevention and Rehabilitation. Endorsed by the Committee for Practice Guidelines of the European Society of Cardiology. *Eur J Prev Cardiol* 2012; **21**: 664–81.
17 Field JM, Hazinski MF, Sayre MR, et al. Part 1: executive summary: 2010 American Heart Association Guidelines for Cardiopulmonary Resuscitation and Emergency Cardiovascular Care. *Circulation* 2010; **122**: S640–S656.
18 Clark AM, King-Shier KM, Duncan A, et al. Factors influencing referral to cardiac rehabilitation and secondary prevention programs: a systematic review. *Eur J Prev Cardiol* 2013; **20**: 692–700.
19 Piepoli MF, Corrà U, Benzer W, et al. Secondary prevention through cardiac rehabilitation: from knowledge to implementation. A position paper from the Cardiac Rehabilitation Section of the European Association of Cardiovascular Prevention and Rehabilitation. *Eur J Cardiovasc Prev Rehabil* 2010; **17**: 1–17.
20 Doherty P, Lewin R. The RAMIT trial, a pragmatic RCT of cardiac rehabilitation versus usual care: what does it tell us? *Heart* 2012; **98**: 605–6.
21 BACPR. *The BACPR standards and core components for cardiovascular disease prevention and rehabilitation 2012*. URL: <http://www.bacpr.com/resources/46C_BACPR_Standards_and_Core_Components_2012.pdf>

22 Reiner Z, Catapano AL, De Backer G, et al. ESC/EAS guidelines for the management of dyslipidaemias: the Task Force for the management of dyslipidaemias of the European Society of Cardiology (ESC) and the European Atherosclerosis Society (EAS). *Eur Heart J* 2011; **32**: 1769–818.

23 Zhao L, Kolm P, Borger MA, et al. Comparison of recovery after mitral valve repair and replacement. *J Thorac Cardiovasc Surg* 2007; **133**: 1257–63.

24 Ghandehari H, Kamal-Bahl S, Wong ND. Prevalence and extent of dyslipidemia and recommended lipid levels in US adults with and without cardiovascular comorbidities: the National Health and Nutrition Examination Survey 2003–2004. *Am Heart J* 2008; **156**: 112–19.

25 Kotseva K, Wood D, De Backer G, et al. Cardiovascular prevention guidelines in daily practice: a comparison of EUROASPIRE I, II, and III surveys in eight European countries. *Lancet* 2009; **373**: 929–40.

26 Kotseva K, Wood D, De Backer G, et al.; on behalf of the EUROASPIRE Study Group. EUROASPIRE III: a survey on the lifestyle, risk factors and use of cardioprotective drug therapies in coronary patients from twenty two European countries. *Eur J Cardiovasc Prev Rehabil* 2009; **16**: 121–37.

27 Graham IM, Stewart M, Hertog MG. Factors impeding the implementation of cardiovascular prevention guidelines: findings from a survey conducted by the European Society of Cardiology. *Eur J Cardiovasc Prev Rehabil* 2006; **13**: 839–45.

28 Eichler K, Zoller M, Tschudi P, et al. Barriers to apply cardiovascular prediction rules in primary care: a postal survey. *BMC Fam Pract* 2007; **8**: 1.

29 van Steenkiste B, van der Weijden T, Stoffers HE, et al. Barriers to implementing cardiovascular risk tables in routine general practice. *Scand J Prim Healthcare* 2004; **22**: 32–7.

30 Marshall T. Estimating the value of information in strategies for identifying patients at high risk of cardiovascular disease. *Inform Prim Care* 2006; **14**: 85–92.

31 Hartz I, Njolstad I, Eggen AE. Does implementation of the European guidelines based on the SCORE model double the number of Norwegian adults who need cardiovascular drugs for primary prevention? The Tromso study 2001. *Eur Heart J* 2005; **26**: 2673–80.

32 Mosca L, Benjamin EJ, Berra K, et al. Effectiveness-based guidelines for the prevention of cardiovascular disease in women—2011 update: a guideline from the American Heart Association. *Circulation* 2011; **123**: 1243–62.

33 Heidenreich PA, Trogdon JG, Khavjou OA, et al. Forecasting the future of cardiovascular disease in the United States: a policy statement from the American Heart Association. *Circulation* 2011; **123**: 933–44.

34 Redberg RF, Benjamin EJ, Bittner V, et al. AHA/ACCF [corrected] 2009 performance measures for primary prevention of cardiovascular disease in adults: a report of the American College of Cardiology Foundation/American Heart Association Task Force on performance measures (writing committee to develop performance measures for primary prevention of cardiovascular disease): developed in collaboration with the American Academy of Family Physicians; American Association of Cardiovascular and Pulmonary Rehabilitation; and Preventive Cardiovascular Nurses Association: endorsed by the American College of Preventive Medicine, American College of Sports Medicine, and Society for Women's Health Research. *Circulation* 2009; **120**: 1296–336.

35 Chow CK, Jolly S, Rao-Melacini P, et al. Association of diet, exercise, and smoking modification with risk of early cardiovascular events after acute coronary syndromes. *Circulation* 2010; **121**: 750–8.

36 Berra K, Miller NH, Fair JM. Cardiovascular disease prevention and disease management: a critical role for nursing. *J Cardiopulm Rehabil* 2006; **26**: 197–206.

37 Berra K, Fletcher BJ, Hayman LL, et al. Global cardiovascular disease prevention: a call to action for nursing: the global burden of cardiovascular disease. *J Cardiovasc Nurs* 2011; **26**: S1–S2.

38 Voogdt-Pruis HR, Beusmans GH, Gorgels AP, et al. Effectiveness of nurse-delivered cardiovascular risk management in primary care: a randomized trial. *Br J Gen Pract* 2010; **60**: 40–6.

39 Campbell NC, Ritchie LD, Thain J, et al. Secondary prevention in coronary heart disease: a randomised trial of nurse led clinics in primary care. *Heart* 1998; **80**: 447–52.

40 Koelewijn-van Loon MS, van der Weijden T, Ronda G, et al. Improving lifestyle and risk perception through patient involvement in nurse-led cardiovascular risk management: a cluster randomized controlled trial in primary care. *Prev Med* 2010; **50**: 35–44.

41 Haskell WL, Alderman EL, Fair JM, et al. Effects of intensive multiple risk factor reduction on coronary atherosclerosis and clinical cardiac events in men and women with coronary artery disease. The Stanford Coronary Risk Intervention Project (SCRIP). *Circulation* 1994; **89**: 975–90.

42 Wood DA, Kotseva K, Connolly S, et al. Nurse-coordinated multidisciplinary, family-based cardiovascular disease prevention programme (EUROACTION) for patients with coronary heart disease and asymptomatic individuals at high risk of cardiovascular disease: a paired, cluster-randomised controlled trial. *Lancet* 2008; **371**: 1999–2012.

CHAPTER 24

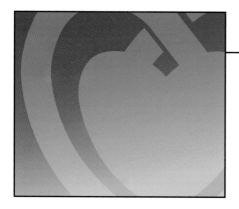

Health promotion to improve cardiovascular health in the general population

Emer Shelley and Margaret E. Cupples

Contents

Summary

Prevention of cardiovascular disease (CVD) requires a consideration of the extent to which the social, physical, and fiscal environment facilitates heart-healthy lifestyles. Health promotion encompasses the actions of governments and other agencies to enable citizens to 'make the healthier choice the easier choice'. It may involve 'health proofing' public policy, the creation of supportive environments, the activities of community organizations, health education to develop personal skills, and prioritization of prevention by the health services. The high-risk strategy for prevention offers major benefits for those with diagnosed CVD and those known to be at increased risk compared with their peers. From a population health perspective, strategies to reduce risk in the majority not known to be at high risk are potentially of much greater benefit. Disadvantaged social groups are at increased risk of CVD compared with those who are better off, yet they may be unable to follow advice due to circumstances beyond their control. Prevention programmes to improve CVD risk in communities should tailor objectives and programme design, including evaluation, to the resources available. Baseline information is required on knowledge, attitudes, and behaviours, as well as risk factors and morbidity, in order to raise awareness of needs, support programmes appropriately, and help reduce inequalities. Responsibility for changing behaviour rests with the individual but preventive services can provide support and involve partners and family members. Healthcare settings can take a lead, for example by providing healthy food menus and smoke-free environments, and professionals can be powerful advocates for national prevention policies.

Introduction: health promotion—concept and practice

The concluding paragraph of the 2012 European guidelines on cardiovascular disease (CVD) prevention [1] recognizes the broader context in which patients live and professionals practise, and the importance of health promotion as complementary to the prevention of cardiovascular disease in the clinical arena. Specifically, the authors hope for:

> a real partnership among politicians, physicians, allied health personnel, scientific associations, heart foundations, voluntary organizations, and consumers' associations to foster both health

promotion at the population level and primary and cardiovascular prevention at the clinical level, using the complete spectrum of evidence in medicine from experimental trials to observations in populations [1]

At the World Health Organization (WHO) conference which adopted the Ottawa Charter in 1986, health promotion was defined as 'activities of government and other agencies, including health services, to enable communities and individuals to increase control over and to improve their health' [2]. Five areas for action were identified:

- build healthy public policy
- create supportive environments
- strengthen community action
- support the development of personal skills
- reorientate health services.

Nurturing health is recognized to be not just the responsibility of the individual and the health services. Planners in all sectors of society should take account of the impact of local and national initiatives on people's health. Effective health promotion may depend on policies relating to environmental planning, transport, economics, education, and legislation as well as to health and social care. While there have been notable successful initiatives, such as the implementation of smoke-free public places in many countries, the increasing prevalence of obesity, physical inactivity, diabetes, and other non-communicable diseases has heightened awareness of the need for sustained, multisectoral engagement to improve population health.

Health education, involving communication to impart knowledge, influence attitudes, and impact on behaviour so as to maintain health, is one component of health promotion. However, the general population are unlikely to implement health education messages aimed at promoting cardiovascular health if they are not supported in doing so. Likewise, patients may find it difficult or impossible to follow advice from health professionals unless their physical, social, and economic environment facilitates heart-healthy options. The aim of health promotion can be summed up as 'making the healthy choice the easier choice'. Addressing environmental and other factors which impact on health is key to preventing non-communicable diseases, including CVD [3,4]:

> Good health requires a universal, comprehensive, equitable, effective, responsive and accessible quality health system. But it is also dependent on the involvement of and dialogue with other sectors and actors, as their performance has significant health impacts. Collaboration in coordinated and intersectoral policy actions has proven to be effective. [4]

The WHO conference on health promotion in Adelaide in 2010 identified strategies to integrate health into policies across all sectors and levels of government, including interministerial and interdepartmental committees, community consultations, cross-sector action teams, health impact assessments, and legislative frameworks [5]. Guidance on the role of the health sector includes providing support to 'champions'—people who are respected in the community for their work, wisdom, and, often, their personal example of engaging in health-promoting behaviours (see ➲ Box 24.1). In accordance with this guidance, cardiologists in many countries have been prominent in advocating for policies and practices to maintain cardiovascular health.

Box 24.1 Partnership between health and other sectors: Adelaide statement on Health in All Policies [5]

New role for the health sector

To advance Health in All Policies the health sector must learn to work in partnership with other sectors. Jointly exploring policy innovation, novel mechanisms and instruments, as well as better regulatory frameworks will be imperative. This requires a health sector that is outward oriented, open to others, and equipped with the necessary knowledge, skills, and mandate. This also means improving coordination and supporting champions within the health sector itself.

New responsibilities of health departments in support of a Health in All Policies approach will need to include:

- understanding the political agendas and administrative imperatives of other sectors
- building the knowledge and evidence base of policy options and strategies
- assessing comparative health consequences of options within the policy development process
- creating regular platforms for dialogue and problem solving with other sectors
- evaluating the effectiveness of intersectoral work and integrated policy-making
- building capacity through better mechanisms, resources, agency support, and skilled and dedicated staff
- working with other arms of government to achieve their goals and in so doing advance health and well-being.

Source: World Health Organization. Adelaide Statement on Health in All Policies: moving towards a shared governance for health and well-being. WHO, Government of South Australia, Adelaide 2010. <http://www.who.int/social_determinants/hiap_statement_who_sa_final.pdf>

Health promotion should be considered in the context of a comprehensive approach to behaviour change (➲ Fig. 24.1) [6]. In addition to interventions delivered at the level of the individual or the whole community, many health promotion programmes focus on a setting such as the workplace or social groups at high risk, for example local communities in areas with high levels of deprivation [7]. Some initiatives alter the physical environment 'to make the healthy choice the easier choice' [2], while others address a topic across a range of groups and settings, for example promoting healthy eating through the education, retail, catering, and health sectors in a particular geographical area, supported by sustained coverage in local media.

Most population-based interventions for health improvement aim to alter health behaviour, either as a primary objective or as an intermediate objective towards changing risk factors and impacting on morbidity and mortality. The challenges involved should not be underestimated:

> However, health promotion activities—and mass public health campaigns in particular—have often failed to have the desired effect in

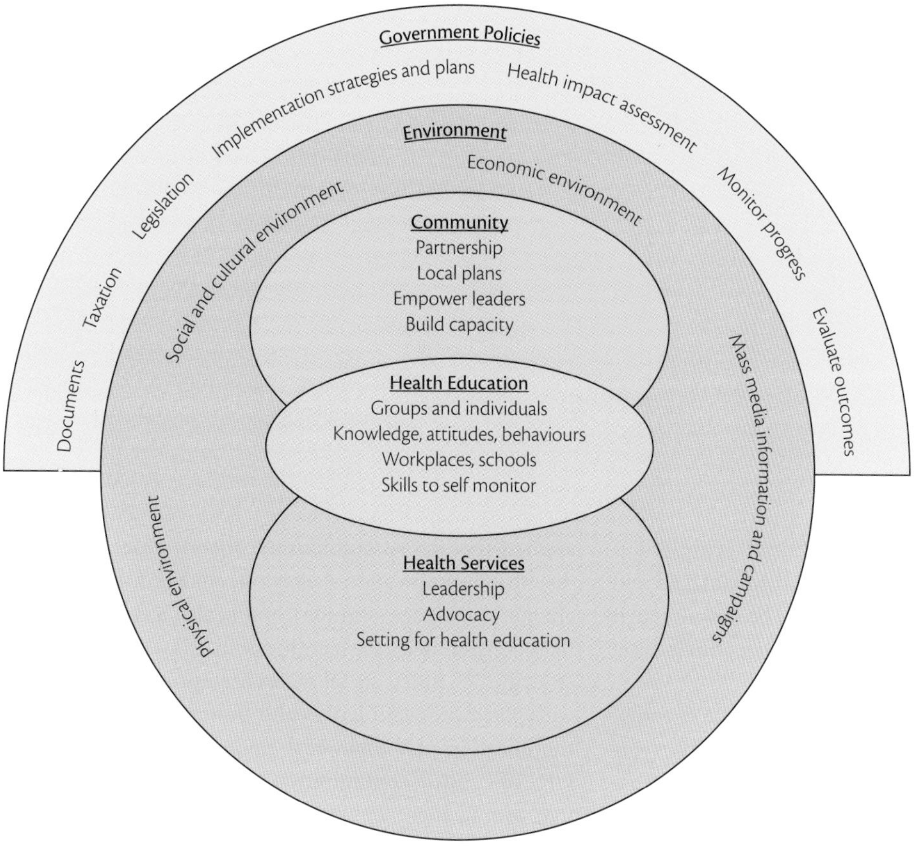

Fig. 24.1 Components of a comprehensive, multisectoral approach to health promotion derived from theories of health promotion and evidence of effective interventions for behaviour change and maintenance of healthy lifestyles [2,5,6].

terms of reducing disease incidence and burden, simply because compliance with the message, in the form of the intended behaviour change, is harder to achieve than its precursors of raising awareness, providing knowledge and altering attitudes. [6]

The case for health promotion in the general population

Geoffrey Rose [8] identified that the 'high-risk strategy', that is, targeting preventive care at those who have the greatest risk of an adverse event, delivers large benefits for those with symptomatic disease or known to be at the upper end of the risk distribution. However, most events occur in the much larger number of people with moderately elevated levels of risk factors. Rose concluded that even modest benefits from a population strategy for prevention could result in large reductions in cardiovascular events.

The importance of reducing risk factors in the population has been illustrated by the IMPACT model. This was developed to estimate the contribution to reductions in CVD mortality of changes to risk factors in the population and of treatments, including secondary prevention, in those with CVD [9]. There is substantial evidence that approximately half of the decrease in CVD mortality in many countries in recent decades can be attributed to risk factor reduction, including lifestyle changes; in most countries the proportion of the decrease in CVD mortality that is attributable to risk factor reduction is higher than that attributable to improvements in medication and other cardiac interventions (➲ Fig. 24.2) [10]. However, the model also highlights that in many countries some lifestyle risk factors such as obesity and physical inactivity are increasing, emphasizing the ongoing need for effective health promotion.

Lower mortality from acute coronary syndromes has been associated with an increased prevalence of heart failure and other non-communicable diseases in ageing populations. Thus, as the number of survivors of these diseases increases, there is an increasing need for population-level efforts to promote health and well-being. The case for health promotion in the general population is strengthened by the parallel effect of some lifestyle risk factors on cardiovascular health and the prevention of other chronic diseases. For example, initiatives which lead to a decrease in the prevalence of smoking will not only have an important impact on CVD but will also reduce cases of lung cancer and chronic obstructive pulmonary disease.

There are important socioeconomic differentials in risk factors for CVD [11]. Those who are better off and better educated may access information and make personal choices concerning healthier lifestyles. Those who are less well off may be unable to make such choices even if they wish to do so. The impact of this may extend across generations: there is evidence that some individuals are at increased risk of CVD from a very young age, even *in utero*, and as they get older they are likely to retain that higher risk compared with their peers [12,13]. Health promotion policies have the potential to benefit the whole population, but should particularly aim to support those groups in society which are at the highest risk and are most disadvantaged in order to avoid the

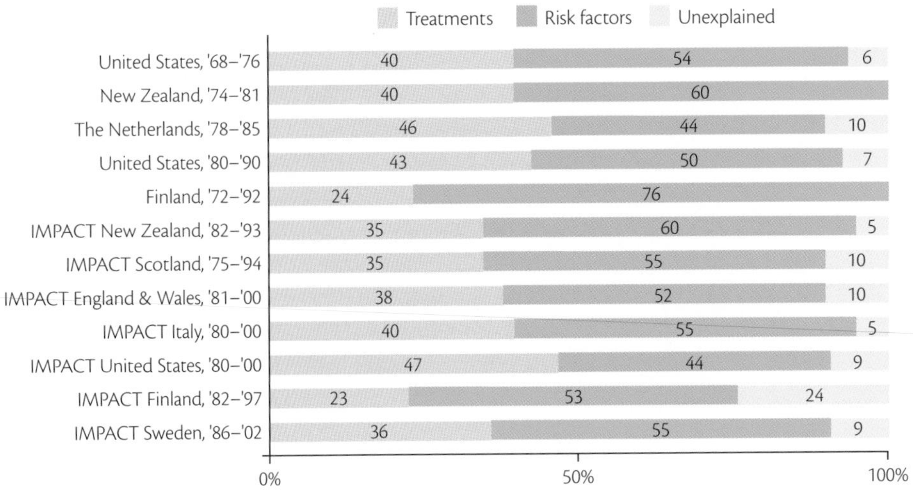

Fig. 24.2 Percentage of the decrease in deaths from coronary heart disease attributed to treatments and risk factor changes in different populations.
Reproduced from Perk J, De Backer G, Gohlke H, Graham L, Reiner Z, Verschuren M and The Fifth Joint Task Force of the European Society of Cardiology and Other Societies on Cardiovascular Disease Prevention in Clinical Practice. European guidelines on cardiovascular disease prevention in clinical practice. *Eur Heart J* 2012; **33**: 1635–1701. doi:10.1093/eurheartj/ehs092

potential outcome of increasing health inequalities. It is important to identify the specific needs of those who are disadvantaged and how best to provide support for them in adopting behaviours such as stopping smoking, eating more healthily, and becoming more physically active.

There is also a growing awareness of the importance of translating knowledge about promoting heart-healthy lifestyles for implementation in minority communities and preventing the escalation of CVD risk factors in emerging economies with different cultural contexts. For example, a large survey of adults in China in 2007 and 2008 found a low prevalence of CVD; however, 28% had at least three risk factors, predicting an increasing prevalence of CVD in the near future unless urgent action is taken to implement interventions to reduce risk factors and actively engage the population in health promotion [14].

Community CVD prevention programmes

The first comprehensive health promotion programme for cardiovascular health was the North Karelia Project in Finland, launched in 1972 [15]. It involved a wide range of prevention initiatives, including health and education services, the media, food producers, supermarkets, and voluntary and community organizations. Population-based registers and surveys showed a subsequent decrease in previously high levels of CVD risk factors and mortality to levels pertaining in the rest of Finland. The project had an impact on health behaviours and lifestyles, and the associated changes in CVD mortality occurred within a relatively short time frame. It was considered that the project, supported by government policies, contributed to the continued downward trends in CVD mortality in Finland.

In the 1980s demonstration programmes for community CVD prevention included the Minnesota Heart Health Program, the Stanford Five-City Project, and the Pawtucket Heart Health Program supported by the National Heart Lung and Blood Institute (NHLBI) in the United States [16]. These programmes applied theories of community organization for health and the 'health communication–behaviour change' formulation, aiming to change knowledge, attitudes, and health behaviours, improve risk factors, and decrease cardiovascular events [17]. Intervention strategies included social marketing, programmes in schools and workplaces, education of health professionals and the public, and modification of the physical environment [18]. A review of the NHLBI-funded community CVD prevention studies concluded that overall there was limited evidence of additional risk factor reduction in intervention compared with comparison communities, although there were some benefits, with evidence of improved health behaviours in specific settings such as schools and workplaces [19].

Thirty-six community studies reporting from 1970 to mid 2008 were included in a systematic review of evaluated programmes for primary prevention of CVD [20]. The interventions studied were multifaceted and most were evaluated using controlled before–after studies. A minority of studies reported changes in CVD and/or total mortality, mainly showing greater decreases in the intervention community although these were not statistically significant. Similarly, many of the studies reporting changes in CVD risk factors found positive trends in favour of the community interventions. Although it was not possible to do a meta-analysis, the authors calculated an average net reduction in 10-year CVD risk of 0.65%. They estimated a number needed to treat of 154 to avoid one case of CVD over 10 years which, if realized over the whole population has a potentially important impact on people's health.

Many of the studies included in that review [20] were carried out in the 1970s and 1980s when knowledge and attitudes, risk factors, disease prevalence, and treatments were quite different from those now pertaining in most developed countries. It is possible that a well-planned, focused intervention programme would now yield greater benefits than studies done when epidemiological and clinical knowledge about risk factors was much less. The potential for benefit from modern programmes is supported by the results of the Cardiovascular Health Awareness Program (CHAP) in Canada, a community cluster randomized trial which focused on residents aged 65 and over [21]. Community health professionals, supported by volunteers, undertook risk assessment and education sessions. When the year before the introduction of CHAP was compared with the year after, statistically significant reductions were reported in the intervention communities in relation to hospital admissions for acute myocardial infarction and heart failure.

Many programmes have demonstrated the feasibility of implementing community-based CVD prevention strategies. However, the resources required to influence behaviour in communities and populations should not be underestimated [22]. Formative evaluation and community analysis are essential for developing and updating effective health messages: 'the core of a successful program is the community organization process' [18]. Planning should include 'social diagnosis', using multiple sources of information and involving the community, to learn about attitudes and readiness to change [7]. In addition to gathering information about risk factors and health behaviours, information should also be collected about aspects of the environment which are relevant to behaviour change and about local organizations which may hinder or facilitate programme implementation.

Large-scale community interventions acquire information regarding the population burden of CVD, risk factors, and unhealthy behaviours from population surveys and CVD registers. This information may be used to strengthen the case for international and national policies to support heart-healthy behaviour. It may also be used to raise awareness of heart health in communities targeted for interventions, but in so doing the messages may also reach control or comparator communities. Overlapping media coverage between the control and intervention communities is one reason that has been suggested for why community CVD programmes have not shown greater net benefits [20]. Other possible reasons for programmes not showing greater effects include methodological issues such as statistical power and study design [19,20]. The challenges of programme design and outcome evaluation should not be underestimated, particularly when reference populations are undergoing secular changes which may impact favourably on CVD risk [19].

Despite the acknowledged challenges and limitations, evidence of benefit was considered sufficient to warrant community interventions being included as an essential component of a strategic approach to CVD control in the United States [23]. Health professionals working within the community were recommended to:

> 'apply established theory and prior experience in community studies and test interventions involving modern forms of health communication, environmental change, and policy';
>
> 'design community interventions with shorter durations and intermediate end points for widespread implementation; these should include smaller, high-risk population subgroups, as defined by race/ethnicity, socioeconomic status, or geography' [23]

Such community interventions were considered complementary to services in primary care relating to primary and secondary prevention and cardiac rehabilitation [23]. From a health promotion perspective, a comprehensive integrated approach to CVD prevention would incorporate policies supported by legislation and public education with population based socioenvironmental approaches and integrated healthcare delivery systems [24]. Mindful of that broader context, lessons from CVD prevention programmes and from interventions on other issues, such as HIV, can be applied to the current and serious threats to the population's cardiovascular health [19].

Planning and evaluating health promotion programmes

The prospect of becoming involved in health promotion for the whole population may be daunting, and its feasibility and the openness of the target audience to change are key initial considerations. There may also be a need to reflect on the balance between potential benefits in the short term, such as working with families of recently diagnosed cases of CVD, versus longer-term investment, for example contributing to health promotion in youth organizations.

In addition to reviewing evidence of the effectiveness of previous interventions, an essential initial step in programme planning, reviews recommend that plans for evaluation should be incorporated from the outset as an integral component of a health promotion programme, tailored to the complexity of the intervention [25]. Evidence of the cost-effectiveness of health promotion interventions, including those focused on heart health, may be found in a wide range of parameters relating to patients, their families, and the general population [26]. Such parameters include quality of life, measures of morbidity and mortality, use of healthcare services, and, in the wider economy, levels of productivity and absence from work. In addition, attention should be given to the effect of interventions on health inequalities. Where an intervention is not supported by evidence, a key issue is whether there is potential for harm. Negative impacts include the opportunity costs of diverting resources from potentially more beneficial programmes.

Feasibility may be facilitated by dividing possible interventions into different settings and target audiences. Health promotion initiatives in schools may be delivered in the context of health education. Voluntary groups working with older people can be powerful allies for action in the community. Groups with the lowest level of education are a priority, and it is a particular challenge to engage them in interventions aiming to change their behaviour. Voluntary and state-funded organizations may be available and willing to support health promotion in disadvantaged communities.

A key issue in planning is that interventions are sustainable. One-off standalone events consume considerable effort and are likely to be of limited benefit. However, such events can make useful contributions to a longer-term health promotion programme. Thus, 'heart health weeks' or similar events organized by heart foundations gain media attention for their health education messages as well as providing opportunities for community events. In the context of a longer-term programme, such annual events can contribute to maintaining and improving population health.

Table 24.1 Planning and implementation phases of health promotion programmes, based on the precede–proceed model [7]

Phase	Purpose	Examples of methods
1. Social diagnosis	To place planning and implementation in the context of people's assessment of their quality of life and their relationship with their community	Multiple sources of information: interviews, surveys, and focus groups. Assess feasibility and use interactions to engage target audience in programme planning
2. Epidemiological, behavioural, and environmental diagnosis	To collect baseline data on the extent of the health problem, on underlying lifestyles and behaviours, and on the extent to which the environment facilitates healthier choices	Analysis of demography and health statistics; health behaviour surveys; analysis of the social and physical environment of factors beyond the control of individuals and the community
3. Educational and ecological diagnosis	Having identified interventions, to select personal and environmental factors which if modified are most likely to result in sustained change in targeted behaviours	Study knowledge, attitudes, and beliefs about the chosen behaviours in more depth; database of facilities and services to enable change; identify motivators to initiate and sustain more healthy behaviour
4. Administrative and policy diagnosis	To plan how the programme will be implemented	Quantify resources and describe how the programme will be administered, including compatibility with governance requirements of parent organization(s); specify arrangements for cooperation with other organizations
5. Programme implementation	To deliver the programme to the target audience	Detailed plan to communicate messages and provide opportunities for target audience to engage with programme messages; incorporate findings from baseline and process evaluation into plans for further roll-out
6. Process evaluation	To detail how the programme is being delivered	Quantify how the programme is delivered; blueprint delivery against plans; adapt plans to incorporate lessons from process evaluation

Having considered the scope of a proposed programme, it is important to take a structured approach to planning, incorporating evaluation from the outset. The 'precede–proceed' model includes eight phases, four of which relate to planning in advance of implementation, as well as process evaluation during intervention (➲ Table 24.1) [7]. The remaining phases relate to impact and outcome evaluation, referring to intermediate and overall objectives, respectively. In practice there is overlap between the initial phases, and there are frequently pressures to commence intervention before planning details have been completed. While it is essential at baseline to consider the overall design, including evaluation, implementation can commence before all the planning data have been fully assessed.

At the outset it is important to have information about the knowledge, attitudes, and behaviours of the target audience, as well as about the policy and environmental factors which impact on behaviour. This information can be used to tailor efforts to raise awareness of the issue and to disseminate information about the programme. The reviews, surveys, and focus groups which inform programme planning also provide baseline data for evaluation. Process evaluation occurs while the intervention is under way, to inform further development.

A well-resourced programme may aim to change risk factors and affect morbidity and mortality by using a complex design and including detailed implementation monitoring and disease surveillance. A project with goodwill and enthusiasm but limited resources may aim to alter attitudes and increase awareness and knowledge, tailoring evaluation in proportion to the scale of the project. Having defined and measured the objectives at baseline, 'impact evaluation' measures the extent to which the programme meets its intermediate objectives, such as social and environmental factors which affect behaviour [25]. 'Outcome evaluation' quantifies changes in measurements of the overall objectives identified at the outset.

Smaller health promotion interventions can use the conclusions from their evaluation to inform further projects. With more complex designs, for example incorporating reference communities or stepwise entry of communities into a study, it may be possible to separate the effects of the programme from secular change. These larger programmes may test hypotheses and be able to attribute change to the intervention, i.e. they can demonstrate internal validity [25]. If the programme is built on a sound theoretical base, it may also demonstrate external validity and provide evidence that the findings may apply in other settings or populations.

The evidence about planning and evaluation of effective health promotion programmes was summarized by a WHO report [6] as follows:

> Finally, most behavioural interventions may need to be piloted on a small scale and over a very limited time frame before they are scaled up to the broader community, provincial, regional or national levels. A built-in monitoring and evaluation scheme, with continuous data collection and analysis for both formative (on-going) and summative (ex-post) evaluation, is essential, as are the prior definition of anticipated primary and secondary outcomes and the establishment of benchmarks for proper assessment of programme effectiveness.

These conclusions are consistent with those of reviews by the National Institute for Health and Care Excellence (NICE) in the UK on the application of theories of behaviour change in populations, and on working effectively with communities [26,27].

Cardiovascular health promotion and the health professional

A shared responsibility?

Successful health promotion initiatives are based on population interventions, with underpinning frameworks based on theoretical models of behaviour change. Health promotion requires the collaborative working of various sectors of government and the wider community to support individuals to make healthy lifestyle choices. It must also be recognized that individuals have a personal responsibility for their own health but the value of support provided by family and friends and by clinicians needs to be acknowledged. Such sources of personal support can make an impact, both directly, for example in ensuring that the individual is not alone in declining to smoke, avoiding unhealthy food, or taking physical activity, and indirectly, by advocating the implementation of environmental, cultural, and policy changes so that healthy lifestyle choices are easier for individuals to make and to maintain. Provision of user-friendly community facilities with support that is relevant to the culture and context of local people can make health-related information that was already publicly available more accessible to individuals and encourage their involvement in health-promoting community activities. Where individuals share healthy lifestyle goals with significant others in their lives, healthy lifestyle behaviours are more likely to be sustained, with a 'ripple' effect on other family members, encouraging the wider adoption of these behaviours in the community in which they live.

In clinical practice

Those who deliver healthcare are trusted sources of information about health. Health service settings provide special opportunities for health promotion, as in the Health Promoting Hospitals (HPH) network, of which WHO Europe is a partner [28]. The aim of this network is to achieve health gain by improving the quality of healthcare and of the relationship between hospitals, health services, the community, and the environment. Its standards relate to patients and their relatives, and to staff.

Hospitals are obviously not the main agents in health promotion, but health promotion is a core dimension of quality in their services, along with patient safety and clinical effectiveness. As institutions with a large number of workers and service users they can set examples which can reach a large section of the population and influence both lifestyle behaviour and professional practice in other settings. Awareness of their role within health promotion for the general population is important. For example, options for healthy eating need to be incorporated in the food being served to patients in the coronary care unit; banning smoking in and around medical facilities can support similar actions being taken in other institutions and workplaces; and supporting staff to engage in physical activity initiatives can help others recognize that there is value in increasing their own levels of activity.

Clinicians, through personal interactions with patients, can also influence levels of participation in health promotion and prevention services. Evidence shows how patients who are invited to participate in cardiac rehabilitation are more likely to attend if invited by a clinician, and if they perceive that the person making such a referral believes that the programme will make a worthwhile improvement to their future health [29].

General practice also provides important opportunities for health promotion. It is estimated that in many countries two in three people consult their general practitioner at least once a year (rates vary with level of income of different countries and depending on consultation charges). Patients view general practitioners as reliable sources of advice and Lobelo et al. [30] in a review article highlight how health professionals' own behaviours can influence that of their patients. Those who are more active are more likely to educate their patients about physical activity, and patients are more likely to follow the advice of such individuals. Thus doctor–patient encounters in primary care present a major opportunity to prevent disease and to promote healthy lifestyles.

Within society

Professionals providing clinical care may also provide leadership by making the case for policy development and creation of an environment which supports heart health (➲ Box 24.2). Policy is essential for some aspects of intervention, for example creating safe spaces for physical activity or to improve access to healthy food options. In this context professionals can become involved in heart foundations and similar organizations which can be powerful advocates for national prevention policies.

Influenced by such health professionals, the government in the Republic of Ireland was the first to introduce legislation to ban smoking in workplaces in 2004. The first city in the world to ban indoor smoking in all public places was San Luis Obispo, California, in 1990, and the success of this legislation encouraged other cities and states to follow suit. There is growing evidence of health benefits from reduced exposure to second-hand smoke; a meta-analysis in 2012 concluded that implementation of smoke-free legislation was associated with a lower risk of smoking-related cardiac, cerebrovascular, and respiratory disease [31]. However whilst some sectors of the population and policymakers have approved and supported the extension of such actions, others have not, claiming that it was 'an improper intrusion of government into people's lives' [32]. Health professionals and researchers need to lobby to influence key decision makers within society and to clearly present the arguments for population health benefits that may be derived from supporting

Box 24.2 The role of health professionals in influencing policy

1. Providing evidence on health issues
2. Harnessing public opinion—trusted authority
3. Lobbying politicians for legislative support
4. Leadership and advocacy

people in their decisions to adopt and maintain health promoting behaviours.

Geoffrey Rose [8] in setting out the theory of the population and high-risk strategies, identified the strengths of the population strategy as being radical, powerful, and appropriate. However, he also identified limitations and problems associated with it, including acceptability, feasibility, costs, and safety. While being mindful of those disadvantages, and of the ethics associated with population health interventions, health professionals can play a very powerful role as advocates within society for heart health (➲ Box 24.3).

In conclusion, to maximize the effectiveness of efforts to prevent CVD it is imperative that these are set within the context of health promotion for the whole population and that this concept is supported at all levels—from individuals to governments. As highlighted in the 2012 European guidelines on prevention of cardiovascular disease in clinical practice, partnership working between politicians, health professionals, statutory agencies, voluntary organizations, and individuals is the key to success in reducing cardiovascular morbidity and mortality and improving health outcomes [1].

Box 24.3 Guidelines to improve the effectiveness of population-based behaviour change interventions [6]

- Strong leadership, ownership of and commitment to programme objectives, and resoluteness during implementation are crucial
- Multi-pronged interventions covering legislation, regulation, public education, counselling, etc., are more likely to be effective than single-target interventions
- Multilevel interventions including policies, programmatic and organizational changes, and a built-in intelligence scheme are more successful than stand-alone initiatives
- Timing, or a 'window of opportunity', is crucial in securing buy-in by programme leaders, service providers, stakeholders, and, above all, potential beneficiaries
- Without adequate financing, most programmes are likely to fail regardless of how solid the underlying theory is
- It is imperative to make a thorough assessment of the (dis) incentives and cues for action, in order to influence the behaviour of service providers and beneficiaries

Further reading

Connolly S, Holden A, Turner E, et al. MyAction: an innovative approach to the prevention of cardiovascular disease in the community. *Br J Cardiol* 2011; **18**: 171–6.

European Heart Network. *Diet, physical activity and cardiovascular disease prevention in Europe*, 2011. Brussels: European Heart Network. URL: < http://www.ehnheart.org/ >

Karwalajtys T, Kaczorowski J. An integrated approach to preventing cardiovascular disease: community-based approaches, health system initiatives, and public health policy. *Risk Manage Healthcare Policy* 2010; **3**: 39–48.

Pennant M, Davenport C, Bayliss S, et al. Community programs for the prevention of cardiovascular disease: a systematic review. *Am J Epidemiol* 2010; **172**: 501–16.

Scholes S, Bajekal M, Love H, et al. Persistent socioeconomic inequalities in cardiovascular risk factors in England over 1994-2008: A time-trend analysis of repeated crosssectional data. *BMC Public Health* 2012; **12**: 129.

World Health Organization. *Adelaide statement on health in all policies: moving towards a shared governance for health and well-being*, 2010. Adelaide: WHO, Government of South Australia. URL: < http://www.who.int/social_determinants/hiap_statement_who_sa_final.pdf >

References

1 Perk J, De Backer G, Gohlke H, et al; and The Fifth Joint Task Force of the European Society of Cardiology and Other Societies on Cardiovascular Disease Prevention in Clinical Practice. European guidelines on cardiovascular disease prevention in clinical practice. *Eur Heart J* 2012; **33**: 1635–701.

2 World Health Organization. *Ottawa Charter for Health Promotion. First International Conference on Health Promotion, Ottawa, 21 November 1986*. URL: < http://www.who.int/healthpromotion/conferences/previous/ottawa/en >

3 Rasanathan K, Krech R. Action on social determinants of health is essential to tackle noncommunicable diseases. *Bull World Health Organ* 2011; **89**: 775–6.

4 World Health Organization. *Rio political declaration on social determinants of Health. Rio de Janeiro, Brazil 21 October 2011*. Geneva: World Health Organization. URL: < http://www.who.int/sdhconference/declaration/Rio_political_declaration.pdf >

5 World Health Organization. *Adelaide statement on health in all policies: moving towards a shared governance for health and well-being*, 2010. Adelaide: WHO, Government of South Australia. URL: < http://www.who.int/social_determinants/hiap_statement_who_sa_final.pdf >

6 World Health Organization. *Behaviour change strategies and health: the role of health systems. Regional Committee for Europe, Fifty-eighth session*. Copenhagen: WHO Europe. URL: < http://www.euro.who.int/__data/assets/pdf_file/0003/70185/RC58_edoc10.pdf >

7 Green L, Kreuter M. *Health program planning: an educational and ecological approach*, 4th edn, 2005. New York: McGraw-Hill.

8 Rose G. *The strategy of preventive medicine*, 1992. Oxford: Oxford University Press.

9 Unal B, Critchley JA, Capewell S. Modelling the decline in coronary heart disease deaths in England and Wales, 1981-2000: comparing contributions from primary prevention and secondary prevention. *Br Med J* 2005; **331**: 614.

10 Di Chiara A, Vanuzzo D. Does surveillance impact on cardiovascular prevention? *Eur Heart J* 2009; **30**: 1027–9.
11 Scholes S, Bajekal M, Love H, et al. Persistent socioeconomic inequalities in cardiovascular risk factors in England over 1994-2008: A time-trend analysis of repeated crosssectional data. *BMC Public Health* 2012; **12**: 129.
12 Painter RC, de Rooij SR, Bossuyt PM, et al. Early onset of coronary artery disease after prenatal exposure to the Dutch famine. *Am J Clin Nutr* 2006; **84**: 322–7.
13 Vos LE, Oren A, Uiterwaal C, et al. Adolescent blood pressure and blood pressure tracking into young adulthood are related to subclinical atherosclerosis: the Atherosclerosis Risk in Young Adults (ARYA) study. *Am J Hypertens* 2003; **16**: 549–55.
14 Yang Z-J, Liu J, Ge J-P, et al. Prevalence of cardiovascular disease risk factor in the Chinese population: the 2007–2008 China National Diabetes and Metabolic Disorders Study. China National Diabetes and Metabolic Disorders Study Group. *Eur Heart J* 2012; **33**: 213–20.
15 Puska P. Successful prevention of con-communicable diseases: 25 year experiences with North Karelia Project in Finland. *Public Health Med* 2002; **4**: 5–7.
16 Pirie PL, Stone EJ, Assaf AR, et al. Program evaluation strategies for community-based health promotion programs: perspectives from the cardiovascular disease community research and demonstration studies. *Health Educ Res* 1994; **9**: 23–36.
17 Farquhar JW, Maccoby N, Wood PD. Education and communication studies. In: Holland WW, Detels R, Knox G (eds) *Oxford textbook of public health*, Vol 3, 1985, pp. 207–21. Oxford: Oxford University Press.
18 Mittelmark MB, Hunt MK, Heath GW, et al. Realistic outcomes: lessons from community-based research and demonstration programs for the prevention of cardiovascular diseases. *J Public Health Policy* 1993: **14**: 437–62.
19 Merzel C, D'Afflitti J. Reconsidering community-based health promotion: promise, performance, and potential. *Am J Public Health* 2003; **93**: 557–74.
20 Pennant M, Davenport C, Bayliss S, et al. Community programs for the prevention of cardiovascular disease: a systematic review. *Am J Epidemiol* 2010; **172**: 501–16.
21 Kaczorowski J, Chambers LW, Dolovich L, et al. Improving cardiovascular health at population level: 39 community cluster randomised trial of Cardiovascular Health Awareness Program (CHAP). *Br Med J* 2011; **342**: d442.
22 Kraemer HC, Winkleby MA. Do we ask too much from community-level interventions or from intervention researchers? *Am J Public Health* 1997; **87**: 1727.
23 Cooper R, Cutler J, Desvigne-Nickens P, et al. Trends and disparities in coronary heart disease, stroke, and other cardiovascular disease in the United States: findings of the National Conference on Cardiovascular Disease Prevention. *Circulation* 2000; **102**: 3137–47.
24 Karwalajtys T, Kaczorowski J. An integrated approach to preventing cardiovascular disease: community-based approaches, health system initiatives, and public health policy. *Risk Manage Healthcare Policy* 2010; **3**: 39–48.
25 Windsor R, Clark N, Boyd NR, et al. Evaluation of health promotion, health education, disease prevention programs, 3rd edn, 2004. New York: McGraw Hill.
26 Programme Development Group, NICE Project Team and external contractors. *Behaviour change at population, community and individual levels*, 2007. London: National Institute for Health and Care Excellence.
27 National Institute for Health and Care Excellence. *Community engagement to improve health*, 2008. London: National Institute for Health and Care Excellence.
28 World Health Organization/Europe. *Health promoting hospitals network (HHN)*. URL: < http://www.euro.who.int/en/what-we-do/health-topics/Health-systems/public-health-services/activities/health-promoting-hospitals-network-hph > (accessed 1 November 2012).
29 McCorry NK, Corrigan M, Tully MA, et al. Perceptions of exercise among people who have not attended cardiac rehabilitation following myocardial infarction. *J Health Psychol* 2009; **14**: 924–32.
30 Lobelo F, Duperly J, Frank E. Physical activity habits of doctors and medical students influence their counselling practices. *Br J Sports Med* 2009; **43**: 89–92.
31 Tan CE, Glantz SA. Association between smoke-free legislation and hospitalizations for cardiac, cerebrovascular, and respiratory diseases: a meta-analysis. *Circulation* 2012; **126**: 2177–83.
32 McGreevy, P. Gov. vetoes smoking ban at state parks and beaches. *Los Angeles Times*, 4 May 2010. URL: < http://articles.latimes.com/2010/may/04/local/la-me-0504-smoking-20100504 >

CHAPTER 25

Community-based prevention centres

Susan Connolly and Margaret E. Cupples

Contents

Summary

The need for a new approach to cardiovascular disease prevention, both secondary and primary, that is different from traditional health service provision through hospital cardiac rehabilitation services and general practice is evident. The targets set in the cardiovascular prevention guidelines for modifiable cardiovascular risk factors—smoking, diet and physical activity, weight and its distribution, blood pressure, lipids and diabetes—are not being adequately achieved for either coronary or other vascular patients or for those at high multifactorial risk of developing CVD. There is also evidence of increasing disparity in levels of risk between different community groups, largely attributable to social determinants of health. Community-based prevention centres provide a novel approach to reducing cardiovascular risk, in which there is shared working between professionals and the public and a shared understanding of the barriers individuals experience in their attempts to engage in effective measures for both secondary and primary prevention.

Rationale for community services

Concept of community

A clear understanding of the concept of community-based services is dependent on a definition of 'community'. In some contexts 'community' may be perceived as meaning a specific locality, people belonging to an institution, or individuals who have a common interest though they may be disparate in location [1]. The concept on which community-based prevention centres is based comprises ecological, demographic, and cultural factors. Thus, they are designed for use by people who share social interaction, facilities, and services within a geographical area, including all age groups, and who have common normative beliefs, interests, and values. The idea of a shared relationship is of major importance to ensure that these centres are relevant to the people for whose benefit they are intended.

Benefits of a community setting

People's preference for attending prevention programmes which are based outside a hospital setting was shown by Dalal and Evans [2]. They reported that, after myocardial infarction, people who were given the option were more likely to choose home-based rather than hospital-based cardiac rehabilitation and, of those who did, more (87% vs. 49%, respectively) completed the programme. Those who were older and self-employed tended to prefer a home-based programme—distance from hospital and parking problems were cited as reasons for people choosing this option.

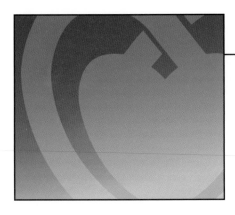

Community settings, with a location close to home and good facilities for car parking [3], can often be more flexible with timing of appointments than can hospital-based services and can minimize barriers to people's participation in prevention programmes, not only for those who are self-employed but also others, including those with family and caring responsibilities. The importance of recognizing these issues is indicated by a Cochrane review [4], which found that the main reasons people give for not accepting an invitation to attend hospital centre-based cardiac rehabilitation services include work or domestic commitments as well as accessibility and parking.

A community-based setting which is easily accessible and located in familiar surroundings can provide, especially for older people, a level of confidence in their process of engagement with health professionals that may be absent in an unfamiliar hospital setting. A systematic review of qualitative factors affecting participation in cardiac rehabilitation [5] highlighted that as well as considering system-level barriers it is important to consider personal patient-level barriers, such as embarrassment, when planning prevention programmes. A patient's health beliefs concerning illness perceptions and approaches to treatment and prevention may be more easily identified within a community context than in other settings. Addressing these beliefs provides maximal opportunities for behaviour change [6].

Moving prevention programmes from the context of hospital, a focus for illness, to the context of a community where there is more focus on well-being can help with adherence to a healthier lifestyle. The role of 'important others' in social relationships is recognized: they act as 'subjective norms' in influencing intentions to engage in specific health behaviours and contribute to increasing self-efficacy [7,8].

There is a need to provide both social and professional support to communicate effectively the health benefits of prevention programmes and, in relation to physical activity, convey a belief that enjoyable and regular physical activities that are sustained are valuable and important for well-being [9]. The 'behaviour change wheel' is a framework which describes the intricate relationship of multiple components involved in behavioural change [10]. It acknowledges both external influences and personal agency, recognizing how physical and social opportunities may work for or against motivational factors and how interventions and policies may need to be changed in order to promote behavioural change. A community base is the ideal setting in which to implement this approach in that it best facilitates identification of the conditions in an individual's social and physical environment which need to be in place for a specified behavioural target to be achieved.

Furthermore, a key component of a community-based centre is the concept that information about its facilities and services is disseminated through a shared communication network within families and between friends. This should ensure the cultural appropriateness of the message in respect of its language and its implications for the community's social norms of lifestyle behaviour.

Models of community-based prevention programmes

Primary prevention

The literature contains many examples of successful community-level interventions for cardiovascular disease (CVD) prevention but the majority of such interventions to date have been at a population level (i.e. health promotion). Examples include screening for risk factors, mass media campaigns, collaboration with local restaurants, and provision of accessible areas for safe recreation [11] based within a diverse array of community settings including schools, worksites, religious organizations, and healthcare facilities. Other community-based prevention strategies have focused on a more individual approach (via self-selection), for example work-based walking programmes or smoking cessation services located in local pharmacies [12,13]. Such health promotion approaches have usually resulted in small changes in risk factors for individuals but have the advantage of having a wide impact.

However, whilst small changes in blood pressure (BP) or cholesterol will have a significant impact at a population level, these measures will be of insufficient benefit in those at high CVD risk, and such individuals will require a more intensive individualized approach. For reasons already discussed, the community may provide the ideal location for a prevention programme caring for such high-risk individuals. To date, the concept of community-based prevention centres for individuals at high CVD risk has been explored mostly in the areas of diabetes prevention and reducing racial disparities in health.

Diabetes prevention

The DEPLOY Pilot study [14] was a randomized controlled trial that evaluated the effectiveness of an intensive lifestyle intervention based on that of the Diabetes Prevention Program (DPP) [15] but which was delivered by wellness instructors in YMCA community facilities rather than case managers. The participants were individuals at risk for diabetes mellitus (principally obese older women) and the intervention consisted of weekly group-based education sessions delivered over 16 weeks. At the end of 6 months and 1 year there was evidence of sustained weight loss (6% of total body weight), which was similar to that achieved in the DPP, and there were also significant reductions in total cholesterol.

However, in contrast to the DPP this study did not report any improvement in glycaemic control (glycated haemoglobin, HbA1c). The HELP PD Project [16] also examined the effectiveness of a DPP-type intensive lifestyle intervention in a similar at risk group for diabetes mellitus, again in a community setting. The intervention, this time delivered by dieticians and community health workers (CHWs), consisted of weekly group-based education sessions but also included personalized consultations. Adherence to the programme was relatively high, and similar weight loss to that achieved in DEPLOY was also seen at 6 months and 1 year. In addition, there were significant reductions in blood glucose and improvements in measures of insulin resistance.

Whilst both these studies were small and restricted to single communities, the replication of the weight loss results achieved by the DPP in the second study in less controlled settings is encouraging. An important common theme to both these projects was the use of non-clinical staff (YMCA wellness instructor in DEPLOY; CHWs in HELP PD). The DPP intervention was costly to run, mainly due to its intensity and involvement of professional healthcare staff: the use of non-clinical staff could potentially help to reduce the expense of such effective interventions, which by their nature need to be relatively intensive to achieve behaviour change [17].

Addressing racial disparities

The advantage of using CHWs, such as those in the HELP PD project, is not just related to their lower cost. CHWs are typically indigenous to the community being served and therefore have a unique knowledge of local and cultural factors that may influence uptake and adherence to such a programme. Evidence for the inclusion of CHWs as key resources in delivering preventive interventions is increasing, particularly in the area of reducing racial disparities in health [18].

In developed countries, those from black and minority ethnic groups (e.g. UK South Asians, black Americans, Hispanics) are at substantially higher risk for CVD, partially due to disparities in cardiovascular risk factors but also due to disparities in CVD prevention and treatment [19]. The reasons for this are complex and exist at three levels including that of the institution/system, provider (lack of cultural appropriateness/understanding), and patient (education, poverty, literacy, lack of trust in the healthcare system) [20]. Some of these barriers may be overcome by employing CHWs to deliver preventive services to these individuals in the familiarity of their own communities, and this approach has been used with some success to improve lifestyles in the Hispanic/Latino population [21, 22, 23] and African Americans in the United States [3]. Where the intervention is delivered in the community (i.e. the venue) will vary depending on the needs of the community being addressed. For example, settings as diverse as barber shops [24] and churches [25] have been used to successfully deliver hypertension outreach and diabetes prevention programmes to African Americans.

However, in those at high risk for CVD lifestyle interventions in themselves will not suffice, and appropriate pharmacotherapy for cardiovascular risk factor management (e.g. BP and lipids) is also important. The evidence for nurse-led case management of CVD in both primary and secondary care is already well established and it would seem a logical progression to adapt this model to the community setting [26]. Moreover, combining a nurse-led model with the integration of CHWs is attractive as it potentially facilitates the delivery of not just a more comprehensive multifactorial intervention but one that is also appropriate for that particular community, for the reasons already discussed.

Such an approach has recently been evaluated in the setting of a randomized controlled trial whereby black American adults with a family history of CVD were enrolled to participate in an enhanced primary care (EPC) group or an urban community-based multifactorial CVD risk reduction intervention (CBC) [3]. In the CBC group, the intervention, designed by a community advisory panel, was delivered by a nurse (who oversaw BP, lipids, and pharmacotherapy/compliance) and a CHW (who delivered dietary/exercise counselling and smoking cessation advice) in a non-clinical site in the community. Medications were provided free of charge at local pharmacies and participants were able to attend biweekly sessions led by the CHW at the YMCA for free. Whilst both groups were found to have significant reductions in BP and low-density lipoprotein (LDL) cholesterol at 1 year compared with baseline, the CBC group were twice as likely to achieve their BP and LDL cholesterol targets and also showed evidence of a significant reduction in smoking. A 5-year follow-up demonstrated some attenuation of the difference between the two groups but, compared with baseline measurements, the positive changes were preserved. This integrated approach of clinical (nurse) and CHW therefore is promising and worthy of further investigation.

Secondary prevention/rehabilitation

Basic principles for provision of care

Just like those at high multifactorial risk, people who have established CVD also require clinical management at the level of the individual. There is clear evidence, from a variety of different settings, for the efficacy of secondary prevention initiatives, including cardiac rehabilitation, in reducing morbidity and mortality [27, 28, 29]. However, the implementation of secondary prevention in clinical practice remains sub-optimal [30] and the importance of investing in interventions for lifestyle changes and appropriate pharmacotherapy has been highlighted [29].

A Cochrane review [4] of 12 randomized controlled trials concluded that home- and centre-based forms of cardiac rehabilitation seem to be equally effective in patients with a low risk of further events after myocardial infarction or revascularization. Tailoring provision of care to individuals' personal preferences for home- or hospital-based programmes improved adherence [4] and, in the context of everyday practice, improved the achievement of targets for secondary prevention [2]. Of particular relevance to the provision of care in community-based centres, no significant differences in clinical outcomes were found between traditional cardiac rehabilitation, an intensive nurse-managed physician-supervised programme, and a community-based programme administered by exercise physiologists using a computerized guideline-driven management system [31].

Safety

Whether programmes are provided by hospitals or community-based centres, core standards have been defined to ensure their effective and safe delivery [32,33], including appropriate risk stratification of exercise participants [34], proficiency in cardiopulmonary resuscitation by staff, and ready access to appropriate equipment and assistance.

Models of delivery

Programmes should be tailored to the needs and preferences of local communities within the constraints of local resources, but it is recognized that secondary prevention is more effectively delivered through organized planned reviews rather than on an opportunistic basis [29]. Ongoing support to maintain healthy lifestyles, promote adherence to prescribed medications, and facilitate regular monitoring of risk factors can be provided through community-based prevention centres [31]. Better engagement is found in groups for whom there is easy access to community-based facilities that can be shared with family members, such as described by an urban initiative which provided a comfortable setting, music, a children's play area, flexible timing of appointments, and the option of follow-up by telephone [3]. Consideration of these details can help people overcome barriers to the uptake of preventive care.

Effective promotion of secondary prevention in various healthcare systems has been achieved by nurses in the community engaging with individuals [35, 36, 37] and coordinating multidisciplinary, family-based prevention programmes [38]. However, tailored care, specifically targeting barriers to secondary prevention for individuals within the setting of general practice, was found to be no more effective than usual care in improving lifestyles or risk factor control [39]. In contrast, in a cluster randomized controlled trial the EUROACTION demonstration project in preventive cardiology evaluated a nurse-led multidisciplinary prevention programme in both hospital (coronary patients) and primary care (individuals at high risk of developing CVD), across eight countries in Europe [38]. The EUROACTION programme involved families and multidisciplinary input—nurses, dieticians, physiotherapists, and physicians—in a comprehensive approach to achieving healthier lifestyles and improved risk factor management (➲ Fig. 25.1, ➲ Table 25.1). EUROACTION did achieve improvements in lifestyle (diet and physical activity) and more effective control of risk factors in both patients and their partners in hospital and primary care settings (➲ Figs 25.2, 25.3, 25.4, 25.5). These results are in keeping with earlier conclusions regarding the value of ongoing support [40], with more sustained nurse contact showing the most successful outcomes [38].

Collaborative working

Many different types of secondary prevention programmes exist but multidisciplinary input is fundamental to their success, allowing individuals' needs to be addressed by the most relevant professional, lay health worker, or peer. Awareness of people's social circumstances and family history is relevant to an understanding of their reluctance to engage in secondary prevention and to the identification and provision of appropriate support. Collaborative working of staff involved in community-based centres and other sources of healthcare should ensure efficient service provision, with maximal uptake by patients, their friends, and their families.

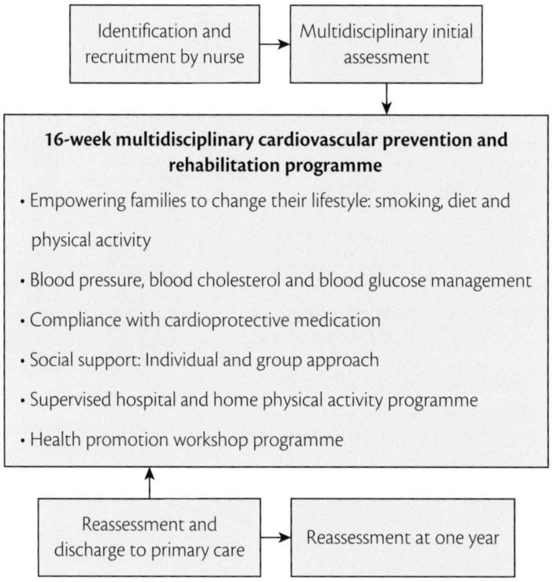

Fig. 25.1 EUROACTION: a European Society of Cardiology demonstration project in preventive cardiology.

Source: data from Wood DA, Kotseva K, Connolly S, Jennings C, Mead A, Jones J, et al. Nurse-coordinated multidisciplinary, family-based cardiovascular disease prevention programme (EUROACTION) for patients with coronary heart disease and asymptomatic individuals at high risk of cardiovascular disease: a paired, cluster-randomised controlled trial. *Lancet* 2008 Jun 14; **371**(9629): 1999–2012.

Integration of primary and secondary prevention

Further evolution of prevention initiatives has led to the concept of integrating primary and secondary preventive care. This approach represents a logical progression, as the distinction between patients with established CVD and those who are at high

Table 25.1 Health promotion workshop topics for a hospital cardiovascular prevention and rehabilitation programme

1. Information about coronary heart disease and cardiac procedures
2. Understanding cardiovascular risk: (i) Adopting healthy lifestyle habits to reduce cardiovascular risk ◆ smoking and cardiovascular disease ◆ healthy eating: choosing the right foods ◆ benefits of physical activity (ii) Other risk factors: blood pressure, blood cholesterol and blood glucose, how lifestyle change and medication help
3. Understanding cardioprotective medications
4. Living with coronary heart disease: (i) Recovering from cardiac events and procedures (ii) Sexual activity and CHD (iii) Returning to work
5. Coping emotionally with coronary heart disease: (i) Managing stress and learning how to relax (ii) Anxiety and depression—positive thinking

Reprinted from *The Lancet*, **371**, DA Wood et al, Nurse-coordinated multidisciplinary, family-based cardiovascular disease prevention programme (EUROACTION) for patients with coronary heart disease and asymptomatic individuals at high risk of cardiovascular disease: a paired, cluster-randomised controlled trial, 1999–2012, 2008, with permission from Elsevier.

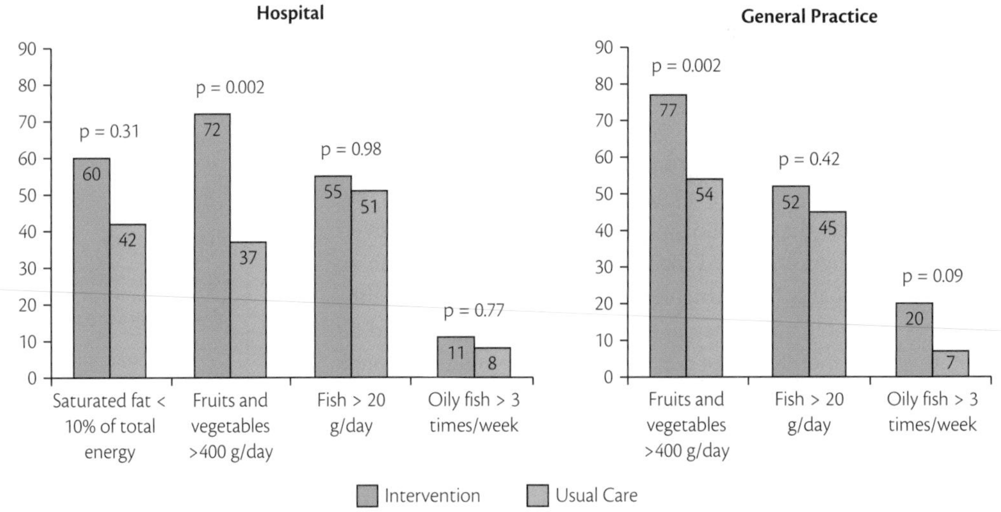

Fig. 25.2 Proportion of patients achieving the European target for a healthy diet.

Source: data from Murphy AW, Cupples ME, Smith SM, Byrne M, Byrne MC, Newell J. Effect of tailored practice and patient care plans on secondary prevention of heart disease in general practice: cluster randomised controlled trial. *BMJ* 2009; **339**: b4220 and Wood DA, Kotseva K, Connolly S, Jennings C, Mead A, Jones J, et al. Nurse-coordinated multidisciplinary, family-based cardiovascular disease prevention programme (EUROACTION) for patients with coronary heart disease and asymptomatic individuals at high risk of cardiovascular disease: a paired, cluster-randomised controlled trial. *Lancet* 2008 Jun 14; **371**(9629): 1999–2012.

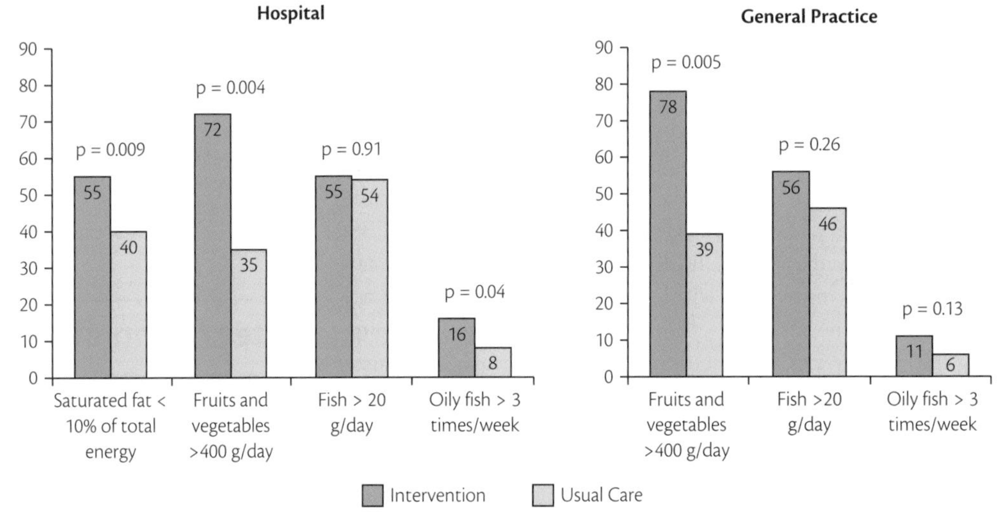

Fig. 25.3 Proportion of partners achieving the European target for a healthy diet.

Source: data from Murphy AW, Cupples ME, Smith SM, Byrne M, Byrne MC, Newell J. Effect of tailored practice and patient care plans on secondary prevention of heart disease in general practice: cluster randomised controlled trial. *BMJ* 2009; **339**: b4220 and Wood DA, Kotseva K, Connolly S, Jennings C, Mead A, Jones J, et al. Nurse-coordinated multidisciplinary, family-based cardiovascular disease prevention programme (EUROACTION) for patients with coronary heart disease and asymptomatic individuals at high risk of cardiovascular disease: a paired, cluster-randomised controlled trial. *Lancet* 2008 Jun 14; **371**(9629): 1999–2012.

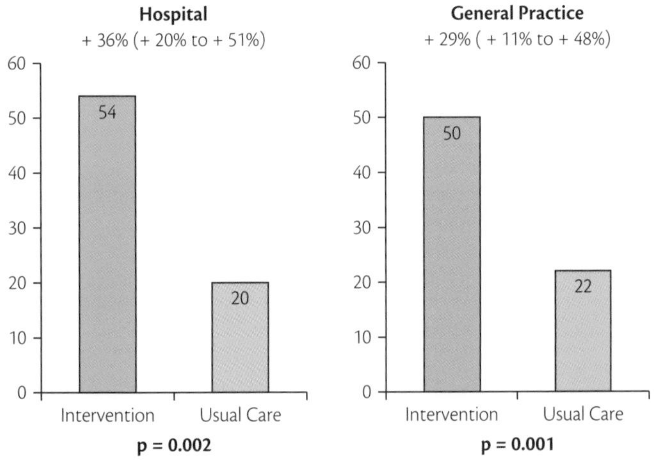

Fig. 25.4 Proportion of patients achieving the European guidelines for physical activity.

Source: data from Murphy AW, Cupples ME, Smith SM, Byrne M, Byrne MC, Newell J. Effect of tailored practice and patient care plans on secondary prevention of heart disease in general practice: cluster randomised controlled trial. *BMJ* 2009; **339**: b4220 and Wood DA, Kotseva K, Connolly S, Jennings C, Mead A, Jones J, et al. Nurse-coordinated multidisciplinary, family-based cardiovascular disease prevention programme (EUROACTION) for patients with coronary heart disease and asymptomatic individuals at high risk of cardiovascular disease: a paired, cluster-randomised controlled trial. *Lancet* 2008 Jun 14; **371**(9629): 1999–2012.

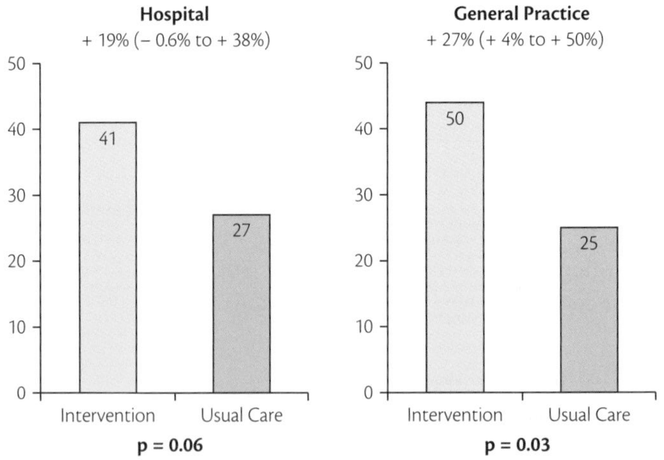

Fig. 25.5 Proportion of partners achieving the European guidelines for physical activity.

Source: data from Murphy AW, Cupples ME, Smith SM, Byrne M, Byrne MC, Newell J. Effect of tailored practice and patient care plans on secondary prevention of heart disease in general practice: cluster randomised controlled trial. *BMJ* 2009; **339**: b4220 and Wood DA, Kotseva K, Connolly S, Jennings C, Mead A, Jones J, et al. Nurse-coordinated multidisciplinary, family-based cardiovascular disease prevention programme (EUROACTION) for patients with coronary heart disease and asymptomatic individuals at high risk of cardiovascular disease: a paired, cluster-randomised controlled trial. *Lancet* 2008 Jun 14; **371**(9629): 1999–2012.

multifactorial risk is somewhat arbitrary. All these patients merit appropriate preventive strategies to help them reduce their cardiovascular risk, including healthy lifestyle change, the medical management of risk factors (e.g. BP, lipids), and the prescription of appropriate cardioprotective medication.

COACH was one of the first studies to evaluate such an integrated approach, targeting underserved populations in a community setting. Eligible patients were either African American or white with prior diagnosed CVD or at high risk for CVD (elevated cholesterol, BP, type 2 diabetes) who were invited to attend a programme delivered by both a nurse practitioner and CHWs in urban community health centres in the United States [41]. The study focused on behavioural interventions to effect therapeutic lifestyle change/adherence as well as prescription/titration of medications. Over 500 patients participated, and at 1 year the intervention group had greater overall improvement in total cholesterol, LDL cholesterol, systolic and diastolic BP, and HbA1c, demonstrating that an integrated approach to primary and secondary prevention in the community was both feasible and efficacious.

Similar to the COACH programme, the MyAction programme in the UK [42] is also a model of integrated primary and secondary preventive care. One-year outcomes in EUROACTION showed that such an approach yielded significant improvements in both lifestyle and medical risk factors for patients with coronary heart disease, high-risk individuals, and partners compared with usual care. In the UK, national health policy has emphasized a shift in the delivery of care from the hospital setting to the community, particularly in the area of chronic disease management. Thus, the EUROACTION investigators developed the MyAction model for the UK National Health Service whereby primary and secondary preventive care was integrated in a community setting. The programme was delivered by a skilled, appropriately trained multidisciplinary team (MDT) [42] which was nurse-led and included dieticians and physical activity specialists and was supported by a psychologist and consultant cardiologist. Coronary patients (with stable and unstable angina) were recruited from the local hospital and patients at high multifactorial risk were referred from primary care. All patients and their partners received the same intervention, which included an extensive individualized baseline assessment by the MDT followed by a 12-week education and supervised exercise programme with a repeat assessment at the end of the programme. The programme successfully recruited and retained the majority of patients referred, together with their partners, and a significant improvement was seen in both lifestyle and medical risk factors, as well as increased use of cardioprotective medication [42].

The initial MyAction pilot was carried out in a principally white, relatively affluent population; it was a descriptive study with no control group, and had a relatively short follow-up period of 16 weeks. However, the programme has since been set up in other communities, starting with Westminster in London where there are substantial areas of social deprivation and a high prevalence of black and minority ethnic (BME) groups. Despite such a culturally and socioeconomically diverse population, the programme has achieved high uptake and adherence in its target group, and clinical outcomes are remarkably similar in both white and BME groups [43] thus extending the evidence for generalizability of the programme. The MyAction programme in Galway, Republic of Ireland, serving a more rural population, has also reported impressive 1-year lifestyle and risk factor outcomes [44].

These outcomes are similar to, and in some cases better than, those achieved in EUROACTION (which was a randomized controlled trial) where the benefits were also still evident at 1 year.

The future

Both the COACH and MyAction models support the concept of integrating primary and secondary preventive care in community-based centres. This is an important concept worthy of further exploration as it would permit streamlining of preventive services for all those at high CVD risk. Such an approach would have the advantage of combating the silos of care that currently exist and which can lead to significant disparities in care delivery. For example in traditional cardiac rehabilitation programmes, patients with exertional angina, peripheral arterial disease, and transient ischaemic attack or minor stroke often do not receive the intensity of preventive interventions delivered to those following myocardial infarction [45,46]. There is no reason why such patients could not also be included in such programmes as they are in MyAction, making them truly pan-vascular prevention programmes. Integrating the care of all vascular patients with those at high risk of developing CVD, including those with diabetes, in community prevention centres will lead to better outcomes for patients and their families. Recruitment and retention of patients will be higher in community centres. The delivery of one comprehensive programme of care for vascular and high-risk patients addressing lifestyle, risk factor control, and use of cardioprotective medications will replace the existing silos of preventive care. The 1-year outcomes of this novel approach to cardiovascular prevention in the community are better than those of traditional hospital-based cardiac rehabilitation and general practice. MyAction is a cost-effective service for prevention of CVD.

Conclusion

Community is characterized by commonality of geography, interests, societal values, and even behaviour. Basing services in the community offers much potential for overcoming existing barriers to preventive healthcare such as distance, unfamiliarity, and fear/distrust of hospitals while also permitting the delivery of a programme that is best placed (i.e. 'tailored') to meet that community's needs, including the use of staff indigenous to that community (e.g. CHWs).

There is now a strong evidence base that encompasses successful community-based models of care in primary prevention, both in terms of health promotion and interventions focused on high-risk individuals, the latter mainly relating to diabetes prevention and tackling racial disparities in health. Furthermore, secondary prevention and rehabilitation in the community has been shown to be safe and as effective as traditional hospital-based care for many patients, with evidence for higher adherence. Key to the successful delivery of all such programmes is the use of a skilled, appropriately trained MDT that works collaboratively with existing community services and user groups.

Integration of primary and secondary preventive care in a community setting has also been shown to be effective and feasible but requires further exploration before adopting this model on a more wider basis. The ideal composition of not just the MDT itself but also the intervention remains to be defined. However, it is likely that there is not a 'one size fits all' approach; rather interventions should ideally be tailored to participants' needs and to those of the local community. In addition, the sustainability and the cost-effectiveness of such programmes remains to be determined.

Further reading

Ackermann RT, Finch EA, Brizendine E, et al. Translating the Diabetes Prevention Program into the community. The DEPLOY Pilot Study. *Am J Prev Med* 2008; **35**: 357–63.

Allen JK, Dennison-Himmelfarb CR, Szanton SL, et al. Community Outreach and Cardiovascular Health (COACH) Trial: a randomized, controlled trial of nurse practitioner/community health worker cardiovascular disease risk reduction in urban community health centers. *Circ Cardiovasc Qual Outcomes* 2011; **4**: 595–602.

Allen JK, Scott LB. Alternative models in the delivery of primary and secondary prevention programs. *J Cardiovasc Nurs* 2003; **18**: 150–6.

Becker DM, Yanek LR, Johnson WR Jr, et al. Impact of a community-based multiple risk factor intervention on cardiovascular risk in black families with a history of premature coronary disease. *Circulation* 2005; **111**: 1298–304.

Commission on Social Determinants of Health. *Closing the gap in a generation: health equity through action on the social determinants of health*, 2008. Final Report of the Commission on Social Determinants of Health. Geneva: World Health Organization.

Cupples ME, McKnight A. Randomised controlled trial of health promotion in general practice for patients at high cardiovascular risk. *Br Med J* 1994; **309**: 993–6.

Gordon NF, English CD, Contractor AS, et al. Effectiveness of three models for comprehensive cardiovascular disease risk reduction. *Am J Cardiol* 2002; **89**: 1263–8.

Katula JA, Vitolins MZ, Rosenberger EL, et al. One-year results of a community-based translation of the Diabetes Prevention Program: Healthy-Living Partnerships to Prevent Diabetes (HELP PD) project. *Diabetes Care* 2011; **34**: 1451–7.

Kotseva K, Wood D, De BG, et al. Cardiovascular prevention guidelines in daily practice: a comparison of EUROASPIRE I, II, and III surveys in eight European countries. *Lancet* 2009; **373**: 929–40.

Michie S, van Stralen MM, West R. The behaviour change wheel: a new method for characterising and designing behaviour change interventions. *Implement Sci* 2011; **6**: 42.

Murphy AW, Cupples ME, Smith SM, et al. Effect of tailored practice and patient care plans on secondary prevention of heart disease in general practice: cluster randomised controlled trial. *Br Med J* 2009; **339**: b4220.

Piepoli MF, Corrà U, Adamopoulos S, et al. Secondary prevention in the clinical management of patients with cardiovascular diseases. Core components, standards and outcome measures for referral and delivery. *Eur J Prev Cardiol* 2012; **21**: 664–81.

Victor RG, Ravenell JE, Freeman A, et al. Effectiveness of a barber-based intervention for improving hypertension control in black men: the BARBER-1 study: a cluster randomized trial. *Arch Intern Med* 2011; **171**: 342–50.

Wood DA, Kotseva K, Connolly S, et al. Nurse-coordinated multidisciplinary, family-based cardiovascular disease prevention programme (EUROACTION) for patients with coronary heart disease and asymptomatic individuals at high risk of cardiovascular disease: a paired, cluster-randomised controlled trial. *Lancet* 2008; **371**: 1999–2012.

References

1 Zagaria P, Flaherty P. *The development of community based services in Minnesota*, 1973. St Paul, MN: Minnesota State Planning Agency.

2 Dalal HM, Evans PH. Achieving national service framework standards for cardiac rehabilitation and secondary prevention. *Br Med J* 2003; **326**: 481–4.

3 Becker DM, Yanek LR, Johnson WR Jr, et al. Impact of a community-based multiple risk factor intervention on cardiovascular risk in black families with a history of premature coronary disease. *Circulation* 2005; **111**: 1298–304.

4 Dalal HM, Zawada A, Jolly K, et al. Home based versus centre based cardiac rehabilitation: Cochrane systematic review and meta-analysis. *Br Med J* 2010; **340**: b5631.

5 Neubeck L, Freedman SB, Clark AM, et al. Participating in cardiac rehabilitation: a systematic review and meta-synthesis of qualitative data. *Eur J Cardiovasc Prev Rehabil* 2012; **19**: 494–503.

6 French D, Maissi E, Marteau TM. The purpose of attributing cause: beliefs about the causes of myocardial infarction. *Soc Sci Med* 2005; **60**: 1411–21.

7 Joekes K, Van ET, Schreurs K. Self-efficacy and overprotection are related to quality of life, psychological well-being and self-management in cardiac patients. *J Health Psychol* 2007; **12**: 4–16.

8 Woodgate J, Brawley LR. Self-efficacy for exercise in cardiac rehabilitation: review and recommendations. *J Health Psychol* 2008; **13**: 366–87.

9 McCorry NK, Corrigan M, Tully MA, et al. Perceptions of exercise among people who have not attended cardiac rehabilitation following myocardial infarction. *J Health Psychol* 2009; **14**: 924–32.

10 Michie S, van Stralen MM, West R. The behaviour change wheel: a new method for characterising and designing behaviour change interventions. *Implement Sci* 2011; **6**: 42.

11 Pearson TA, Wall S, Lewis C, et al. Dissecting the 'black box' of community intervention: lessons from community-wide cardiovascular disease prevention programs in the US and Sweden. *Scand J Public Health Suppl* 2001; **56**: 69–78.

12 Sinclair HK, Bond CM, Stead LF. Community pharmacy personnel interventions for smoking cessation. *Cochrane Database Syst Rev* 2004; (1): CD003698.

13 Haines DJ, Davis L, Rancour P, et al. A pilot intervention to promote walking and wellness and to improve the health of college faculty and staff. *J Am Coll Health* 2007; **55**: 219–25.

14 Ackermann RT, Finch EA, Brizendine E, et al. Translating the Diabetes Prevention Program into the community. The DEPLOY Pilot Study. *Am J Prev Med* 2008; **35**: 357–63.

15 Knowler WC, Barrett-Connor E, Fowler SE, et al. Reduction in the incidence of type 2 diabetes with lifestyle intervention or metformin. *N Engl J Med* 2002; **346**: 393–403.

16 Katula JA, Vitolins MZ, Rosenberger EL, et al. One-year results of a community-based translation of the Diabetes Prevention Program: Healthy-Living Partnerships to Prevent Diabetes (HELP PD) project. *Diabetes Care* 2011; **34**: 1451–7.

17 Moyer VA, US Preventive Services Task Force. Behavioral counseling interventions to promote a healthful diet and physical activity for cardiovascular disease prevention in adults: US Preventive Services Task Force recommendation statement. *Ann Intern Med* 2012; **157**: 367–71.

18 Artinian NT, Fletcher GF, Mozaffarian D, et al. Interventions to promote physical activity and dietary lifestyle changes for cardiovascular risk factor reduction in adults: a scientific statement from the American Heart Association. *Circulation* 2010; **122**: 406–41.

19 Jolly K, Gill P. Ethnicity and cardiovascular disease prevention: practical clinical considerations. *Curr Opin Cardiol* 2008; **23**: 465–70.

20 Stuart-Shor EM, Berra KA, Kamau MW, et al. Behavioral strategies for cardiovascular risk reduction in diverse and underserved racial/ethnic groups. *Circulation* 2012; **125**: 171–84.

21 Balcazar H, Alvarado M, Ortiz G. Salud Para Su Corazon (health for your heart) community health worker model: communityand clinical approaches for addressing cardiovascular disease risk reduction in Hispanics/Latinos. *J Ambul Care Manage* 2011; **34**: 362–72.

22 Hayashi T, Farrell MA, Chaput LA, et al. Lifestyle intervention, behavioral changes, and improvement in cardiovascular risk profiles in the California WISEWOMAN project. *J Womens Health (Larchmt)* 2010; **19**: 1129–38.

23 Staten LK, Scheu LL, Bronson D, et al. Pasos Adelante: the effectiveness of a community-based chronic disease prevention program. *Prev Chronic Dis* 2005; **2**: A18.

24 Victor RG, Ravenell JE, Freeman A, et al. Effectiveness of a barber-based intervention for improving hypertension control in black men: the BARBER-1 study: a cluster randomized trial. *Arch Intern Med* 2011; **171**: 342–50.

25 Davis-Smith YM, Boltri JM, Seale JP, et al. Implementing a diabetes prevention program in a rural African-American church. *J Natl Med Assoc* 2007; **99**: 440–6.

26 Allen JK, Scott LB. Alternative models in the delivery of primary and secondary prevention programs. *J Cardiovasc Nurs* 2003; **18**: 150–6.

27 Clark AM, Hartling L, Vandermeer B, et al. Meta-analysis: secondary prevention programs for patients with coronary artery disease. *Ann Intern Med* 2005; **143**: 659–72.

28 Cole JA, Smith SM, Hart N, et al. Systematic review of the effect of diet and exercise lifestyle interventions in the secondary prevention of coronary heart disease. *Cardiol Res Pract* 2011; **2011**: 232351.

29 Perk J, De BG, Gohlke H, et al. European Guidelines on cardiovascular disease prevention in clinical practice (version 2012). The Fifth Joint Task Force of the European Society of Cardiology and Other Societies on Cardiovascular Disease Prevention in Clinical Practice (constituted by representatives of nine societies and by invited experts). Developed with the special contribution of the European Association for Cardiovascular Prevention and Rehabilitation (EACPR). *Eur Heart J* 2012; **33**: 1635–701.

30 Kotseva K, Wood D, De BG, et al. Cardiovascular prevention guidelines in daily practice: a comparison of EUROASPIRE I, II, and III surveys in eight European countries. *Lancet* 2009; **373**: 929–40.

31 Gordon NF, English CD, Contractor AS, et al. Effectiveness of three models for comprehensive cardiovascular disease risk reduction. *Am J Cardiol* 2002; **89**: 1263–8.

32 BACPR. *The BACPR standards and core components for cardiovascular disease prevention and rehabilitation 2012.* URL:http://www.bacpr.com/resources/46C_BACPR_Standards_and_Core_Components_2012.pdf

33 Piepoli MF, Corrà U, Adamopoulos S, et al. Secondary prevention in the clinical management of patients with cardiovascular diseases. Core components, standards and outcome measures for referral and delivery. *Eur J Prev Cardiol* 2012; **21**: 664–81.

34 Association of Chartered Physiotherapists in Cardiac Rehabilitation. *Competencies for the exercise component of phase III cardiac rehabilitation*, 2008. London: ACPICR.

35 Campbell NC, Ritchie LD, Thain J, et al. Secondary prevention in coronary heart disease: a randomised trial of nurse led clinics in primary care. *Heart* 1998; **80**: 447–52.

36 Campbell NC, Thain J, Deans HG, et al. Secondary prevention clinics for coronary heart disease: randomised trial of effect on health. *Br Med J* 1998; **316**: 1434–7.

37 Cupples ME, McKnight A. Randomised controlled trial of health promotion in general practice for patients at high cardiovascular risk. *Br Med J* 1994; **309**: 993–6.

38 Wood DA, Kotseva K, Connolly S, et al. Nurse-coordinated multidisciplinary, family-based cardiovascular disease prevention programme (EUROACTION) for patients with coronary heart disease and asymptomatic individuals at high risk of cardiovascular disease: a paired, cluster-randomised controlled trial. *Lancet* 2008; **371**: 1999–2012.

39 Murphy AW, Cupples ME, Smith SM, et al. Effect of tailored practice and patient care plans on secondary prevention of heart disease in general practice: cluster randomised controlled trial. *Br Med J* 2009; **339**: b4220.

40 Cupples ME, McKnight A. Five year follow up of patients at high cardiovascular risk who took part in randomised controlled trial of health promotion. *Br Med J* 1999; **319**: 687–8.

41 Allen JK, Dennison-Himmelfarb CR, Szanton SL, et al. Community Outreach and Cardiovascular Health (COACH) Trial: a randomized, controlled trial of nurse practitioner/community health worker cardiovascular disease risk reduction in urban community health centers. *Circ Cardiovasc Qual Outcomes* 2011; **4**: 595–602.

42 Connolly S, Holden A, Turner E, et al. MyAction: an innovative approach to the prevention of cardiovascular disease in the community. *Br J Cardiol* 2011; **18**: 171–6.

43 Connolly S, Kotseva K, Clements SJ, et al. Reducing cardiovascular risk in black and minority ethnic groups. *Eur J Prev Cardiol* 2012; **19**(Suppl. 1): S121.

44 Gibson I, Flaherty G, Cormican S, et al. Translating guidelines to practice: findings from a multidisciplinary preventive cardiology programme in the west of Ireland. *Eur J Prev Cardiol* 2014; **21**: 366–76.

45 Alberts MJ, Bhatt DL, Mas JL, et al. Three-year follow-up and event rates in the international Reduction of Atherothrombosis for Continued Health Registry. *Eur Heart J* 2009; **30**: 2318–26.

46 Mechtouff L, Touze E, Steg PG, et al. Worse blood pressure control in patients with cerebrovascular or peripheral arterial disease compared with coronary artery disease. *J Intern Med* 2010; **267**: 621–33.

PART 5

Evaluation of preventive cardiology

CHAPTER 26

Evaluation of preventive cardiology

Kornelia Kotseva, Neil Oldridge, and Massimo F. Piepoli

Contents

Summary

The Joint European Societies (JES) guidelines on cardiovascular (CVD) prevention published in 1994, 1998, 2003, 2007, and 2012 defined lifestyle and risk factor targets for patients with coronary or other atherosclerotic disease and people at high risk of developing CVD. However, EUROASPIRE and other surveys in Europe and the United States showed inadequate lifestyle and risk factor management and underuse of prophylactic drug therapies in both primary and secondary prevention of CVD. The European Association of Cardiovascular Prevention and Rehabilitation, the American Heart Association (AHA), and the American College of Cardiology Foundation (ACCF) in collaboration with three other associations have developed core components, standards, and outcome measures to evaluate the quality of care and to provide guidelines to healthcare professionals and institutions to identify opportunities for improvement. Optimal control of cardiovascular risk factors is one of the most effective methods for reducing vascular events in patients with atherosclerotic disease or in those at high cardiovascular risk. Improving treatment adherence is a very important step in optimizing cardiovascular risk factor management. Health-related quality of life (HRQL) is considered as an outcome measure in research studies and in clinical practice. HRQL measures can help to improve patient–clinician communication, screening, monitoring, and continuous assessment of quality of care. Further research is needed to investigate the effects of interventions to improve treatment adherence on clinical end-points and the association between assessing HRQL and an improvement in quality of care.

Measuring quality of care

Introduction

Over the last decade it has become increasingly apparent that the quality of medical care, which should be effective, timely, safe, and patient-orientated, has the potential for improvement. In the United States it is estimated that as much as 30–40% of healthcare spending is wasted—through overuse, underuse, misuse, duplication, system failures, unnecessary repetition, poor communication, and inefficiency [1]—suggesting an issue concerning the quality of healthcare. The quality of healthcare is under scrutiny in many countries and various quality-improvement strategies have been proposed.

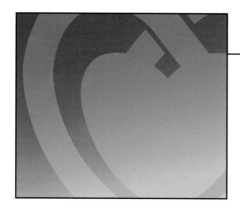

The quality of healthcare is defined as 'the degree to which healthcare services for individuals and populations increase the likelihood of desired health outcomes and are consistent with current professional knowledge' [2]. Thus it has been classified traditionally under three elements [3]:

1. structure (clinician/organization/patient characteristics)
2. process (appropriateness of treatment, patient/clinician interaction), and
3. outcomes (effects of care on the health status of patients).

Clinical audits of lifestyle and risk factor management

Audits of clinical practice provide an objective assessment of clinical outcomes and quantify the extent to which the standards set in the guidelines on cardiovascular disease (CVD) prevention are being implemented in everyday clinical practice. The Joint European Societies (JES) guidelines on cardiovascular (CV) prevention published in 1994, 1998, 2003, 2007, and 2012 defined lifestyle and risk factor goals for both patients with coronary heart disease (CHD) and those at high risk of developing CVD [4–8]. Guideline implementation has been evaluated with three cross-sectional surveys called EUROASPIRE (European Action on Secondary and Primary Prevention through Intervention to Reduce Events) starting in the mid 1990s. They were carried out by the European Society of Cardiology (ESC) Euro Heart Survey Programme in 1995–6 in nine countries, in 1999–2000 in 15 countries, and in 2006–7 in 22 countries [9–14]. The main outcome measures were the proportions of coronary and high risk patients achieving the lifestyle, risk factor, and therapeutic targets for CVD prevention as defined in the current guidelines. Data collection was based on a review of patients' medical notes and a prospective interview and examination at least 6 months after an acute coronary event or procedure (coronary patients) or the start of blood pressure (BP) and/or lipid-lowering and/or glucose-lowering therapy (high-risk individuals), using standardized methods and instruments.

The overall objectives of the EUROASPIRE III survey were:

- To determine in hospitalized coronary patients (acute myocardial infarction and ischaemia and following revascularization by angioplasty or coronary artery surgery) and in high-risk individuals being treated in primary care whether the joint European guidelines on CVD prevention are being followed in everyday clinical practice.
- To determine whether the practice of preventive cardiology in patients with established coronary disease in EUROASPIRE III has improved by comparison with those centres which took part in EUROASPIRE I and II.

A total of 8966 coronary patients (25.3% of whom were women) were interviewed on average 1.2 years following their index event [12]. At interview, 17% of patients smoked cigarettes, with only one in two of those who smoked before the index event having stopped. The prevalence rates of overweight and obesity were alarming in all countries: 35% were obese [body mass index (BMI) ≥30 kg/m^2] and 53% had central obesity (waist circumference ≥ 102 cm in men or ≥ 88 cm in women). The majority of patients (56%) had raised BP (≥140/90 mmHg; ≥130/80 mmHg for patients with diabetes). The prevalence of elevated total cholesterol (≥4.5 mmol/L) and low-density lipoprotein (LDL) cholesterol (≥2.5 mmol/L) was 51% and 55% respectively. Just over a third of patients (35%) had diabetes (self-reported or fasting plasma glucose ≥ 7 mmol/L). The therapeutic control of BP was poor, with only 37% of patients on BP-lowering medication being controlled (BP < 140/90 mmHg; <130/80 mmHg for patients with diabetes). In those on lipid-lowering medication just over a half (55%) had reached the total cholesterol goal of <4.5 mmol/L. Only 10% of patients with self-reported diabetes had fasting plasma glucose of <6.1 mmol/L. The use of cardioprotective medication was as follows: aspirin or other antiplatelet drugs 91%, beta-blockers 80%, angiotensin-converting enzyme (ACE) inhibitors or angiotensin receptor blockers (ARBs) 71%, statins 78%. Furthermore, only a third of patients were referred to and attended prevention and rehabilitation programmes [15].

Comparison between those countries that participated in the three surveys demonstrated a compelling need for more effective lifestyle and risk factor management of patients with CHD [13]. Findings showed a continuing and widening gap between the guidelines and patients' lifestyles in terms of stopping smoking and reducing obesity and central obesity, no improvement in blood pressure control, increase in the prevalence of diabetes, and at the same time a substantial increase in the use of cardioprotective medication. Although lipid management continued to improve, primarily because of statin therapy, almost half of all patients still remained above the recommended lipid targets (➲ Fig. 26.1).

In primary prevention the gap between evidence-based guidelines and clinical practice was even greater than that seen for coronary patients [14]. A total of 4366 patients (58% female) considered to be at high CV risk were interviewed after the start of drug treatment. Overall, 17% smoked cigarettes, 44% were obese (62% centrally obese), 71% had raised blood pressure, 66% had total cholesterol ≥5 mmol/L (≥4.5 mmol/L in people in diabetes), and 39% had diabetes. Risk factor control was very poor, with only 26% of patients using antihypertensive medication achieving the BP goal, and 31% of patients on lipid-lowering medication achieving the total cholesterol goal. Only 9% of patients with self-reported diabetes had fasting plasma glucose <6.1 mmol/L. The use of BP-lowering medication in people with hypertension was: beta-blockers 34%, ACE inhibitors/ARBs 61%, calcium channel blockers 26%, diuretics 37%. Statins were prescribed in 47% of people with hypercholesterolaemia.

The slow incorporation of primary prevention strategies into clinical practice has been reported in similar studies in Europe and the United States. The EURIKA study compared the status of primary prevention among patients with varying degrees of CVD risk according to the 2007 guidelines on CVD prevention [16]. This study was conducted in 2009 in 12 European countries and included 7641 outpatients free of clinical CVD and with at least one major CVD risk factor. Among patients treated for hypertension and dyslipidaemia, only 39% and 41% achieved the BP and lipids (total and LDL cholesterol) targets, respectively. Only a third of patients with diabetes met the goal for glycated haemoglobin

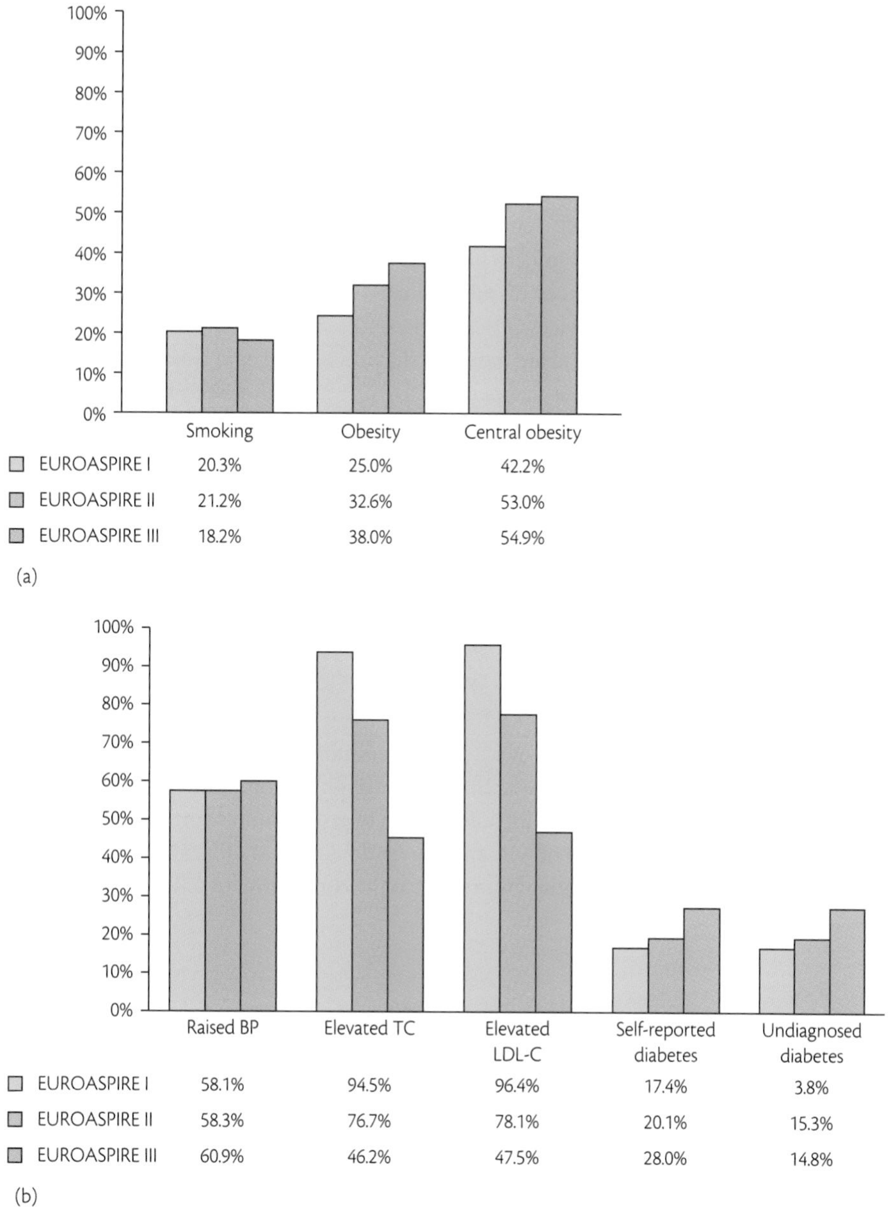

Fig. 26.1 Comparison between the EUROASPIRE I, II, and III surveys. (a) Prevalence of smoking, obesity (body mass index ≥ 30 kg/m^2), and central obesity (waist circumference ≥88 cm for women and ≥102 cm for men). (b) Prevalence of elevated BP (systolic/diastolic BP ≥ 140/90 mmHg for non-diabetics or ≥ 130/80 mmHg for diabetics), total cholesterol (TC; ≥4.5 mmol/L) and LDL cholesterol (LDL-C; ≥2.5 mmol/L), and diabetes mellitus (fasting plasma glucose ≥ 7 mmol/L in patients without a history of diabetes).

(HbA1c). Inadequate lifestyle and risk factor management and underuse of prophylactic drug therapies in both coronary and high-risk patients has also been reported in other national and multinational surveys [17–26]. So, the challenge to improve quality of care is common to many parts of the world.

Outcome measures in primary and secondary prevention of cardiovascular disease

The ability to quantify the quality of CV care critically depends on the translation of recommendations for high-quality care into the measurement of that care. Therefore developing a framework to measure components of the quality of healthcare is of paramount importance. The ESC, the American College of Cardiology (ACC), and the American Heart Association (AHA) have developed a multifaceted strategy to facilitate the process of improving the quality of CV care [27–31]. These documents are designed to provide healthcare professionals and institutions that deliver care with performance measures of the quality of care and to identify opportunities for improvement. The development of performance systems is based on the identification of a set of measures targeting a specific patient population observed over a defined time period.

Quantifying clinical performance is a necessary step in improving the quality of healthcare. Performance and outcome measures are intended as means to measure and improve care, tailored to each clinical condition; their application is designed to allow transparent control of the quality of healthcare. The intention behind the measurement of performance is to allow healthcare providers to learn how systems may be redesigned so that the required processes of care are applied uniformly to patients who are most likely to benefit [28]. Without the ability to quantify quality, the opportunity to identify practices that lead to higher-quality care, and the opportunity to learn how such care was delivered, quality cannot be improved.

Outcome measures in primary prevention

The AHA and American College of Cardiology Foundation (ACCF) in collaboration with three other associations have developed recommendations for performance measures for primary prevention of CVD, providing a detailed specification for each measure, including the numerator, denominator, period of assessment, method of reporting, sources of data, rationale, and challenges to implementation [31]. They are ideally intended for prospective use to enhance the quality improvement process but may also be applied retrospectively. The performance measures recommended in this document are based on processes of care that are expected to produce benefit in primary prevention of CVD. The Writing Committee identified 13 measures to be included in the performance measure set and evaluated the use of each measure for accountability/public reporting (A/PR) and internal quality improvement (IQI). ➲ Table 26.1 summarizes the AHA/ACCF Primary Prevention of Cardiovascular Disease Performance Measurement Set, including measures for lifestyle and medical risk factor management. Two measures (global risk estimation and aspirin use) were designed for IQI only.

The document also provides a detailed description of each performance in terms of screening, lifestyle counselling, and management of weight, BP, and lipids. ➲ Figure 26.2 presents a data collection instrument to aid compliance and measurement. Individual institutions may modify the sample instrument or develop a different tool based on local practice and standards.

Outcome measures in secondary prevention

Quantifying clinical performance is a necessary step for improving the quality of healthcare. The European Association of Cardiovascular Prevention and Rehabilitation have developed a policy statement on the core components, standards, and outcome measures for referral and delivery in the clinical management of patients with CVD [28]. Both structure-based and process-based measures are designed to help healthcare providers identify potentially correctable sources of suboptimal clinical care in cardiac rehabilitation (CR) services. Structure-based measures quantify the infrastructure for CR and are based on the provision of appropriate environment, equipment, and personnel to provide high-quality standards of care.

Process-based measures quantify specific aspects of care and are designed to capture all relevant dimensions of secondary preventive care while outcome measures identify the expected goals of the intervention. The following steps should apply to all clinical conditions:

- Individualized assessment and evaluation of modifiable CVD risk factors.
- Development of individualized risk reduction interventions for identified conditions and coordination of care among all healthcare providers.
- Evidence of a plan to monitor response and document programme effectiveness through ongoing analysis of aggregate data. This includes: a plan to assess completion of the prescribed course of CR, and prevention and a standardized plan to reassess patient outcomes at the completion of CR.

Table 26.1 AHA/ACCF primary prevention of cardiovascular disease performance set

Performance measure name	Measure description	Designation
1. Lifestyle/risk factor screening	Assessment of lifestyles and risk factors for development of CVD	A/PR IQI
2. Dietary intake counselling	Counselling to eat a healthy diet	A/PR
3. Physical activity counselling	Counselling to engage in regular physical activity	A/PR
4. Smoking/tobacco use	Risk assessment for smoking and tobacco use behaviours	A/PR IQI
5. Smoking/tobacco cessation	Cessation intervention for active smoking (tobacco use)	A/PR
6. Weight/adiposity assessment	Measurement of weight and body mass index and/or waist circumference	A/PR
7. Weight management	Counselling to achieve and maintain ideal body weight	A/PR IQI
8. Blood pressure measurement	Measurement of blood pressure in all patients	A/PR
9. Blood pressure control	Effective blood pressure control or combination therapy for patients with hypertension	A/PR IQI
10. Blood lipid measurement	Fasting lipid profile performed	A/PR IQI
11. Blood lipid therapy and control	Proportion of patients who meet current LDL-C treatment targets OR who are prescribed one or more lipid-lowering medications at maximum tolerated dose	A/PR
12. Global risk estimation	Use of a multivariable risk score to estimate a patient's absolute risk for development of coronary heart disease	IQI
13. Aspirin use	Aspirin in patients without clinical evidence of atherosclerotic disease who are at higher CVD risk	IQI

A/PR indicates accountability/public reporting measures (appropriate for all uses, including internal quality improvement, pay for performance, physician ranking, and public reporting); CVD, cardiovascular disease; IQI, internal quality improvement measures (recommended for use in internal quality improvement programmes only; not appropriate for any other use, e.g. pay for performance, physician ranking, or public reporting); LDL-C, low-density lipoprotein cholesterol.

Reproduced from Redberg RF, Benjamin EJ, Bittner V, et al. AHA/ACCF 2009 performance measures for primary prevention in adults: A report of the American College of Cardiology Foundation/American Heart Association Task Force on performance measures (Writing Committee to develop performance measures for primary prevention of cardiovascular disease): Developed in collaboration with the American Academy of Family Physicians; American Association of Cardiovascular and Pulmonary Rehabilitation; and Preventive Cardiovascular Nurses Association. *Circulation* 2009; **120**: 1296–1336.

Sample Prospective Data Collection Flow Sheet

American Heart Association and American College of Cardiology Foundation
Primary Prevention of Cardiovascular Disease Performance Measurement Set

SAMPLE

Today's Date ____/_____/__ Date of last visit _____/_______/_____

Patient Name or Code ____________________ Birth Date _____/______/_____

Medical History

Age: _____ years	***†‡Family History of Premature CHD: ____(Y/N)** (CHD in male first-degree relative <55 years; CHD in female first-degree relative <65 years)	***†‡Diabetes: ____(Y/N)**	**Gender:** ☐ Male ☐ Female
Check below if patient is: ☐ **†Age 45 or older and male** ☐ **†Age 55 or older and female**	**Optional** Chronic renal disease: ______ (Y/N) (Glomerular filtration rate <60 mL/min/1.73 m^2.)	***†‡Hypertension: ____(Y/N)** (Systolic BP of 140 mmHg or greater or a diastolic BP of 90 mmHg or greater on at least three occasions, or both, or taking anti-hypertensive medication.)	**Vascular Disease: ____(Y/N)** (Peripheral arterial disease, carotid artery disease, or abdominal aortic aneurysm)

Lifestyle Factors *(complete for all patients)*

Tobacco Use:

☐ Never smoked
☐ Former smoker
Date quit: ____/_____ (month, if known/year)
☐ ***‡†Current smoker**

Intervention: Complete if patient is current smoker:

☐ Patient was advised to quit smoking
☐ Referred for smoking cessation counselling
☐ Medication prescribed: ______________________
(e.g. bupropion, varenicline, nicotine patches, gum, or lozenges)
☐ Other ______________________

Physical Activity:
(Intensity, frequency, and duration of exercise daily/weekly):
____
____

Goal: At least 30 minutes of moderate-intensity physical activity (such as brisk walking) on most (and preferably all) days of the week.

Patient reports usually meeting the physical activity goal:
☐ Yes
☐ No

If no, was patient advised to increase physical activity to reach goal?
☐ Yes
☐ No

Optional **Exposure to Secondhand and Tobacco Smoke:**
(Someone at home or at work smokes in presence of patient)
☐ Yes
☐ No

Optional **Alcohol Use:**
☐ Never
☐ 1–2 drinks/day
☐ >2 drinks per day
1 drink = 4 oz wine, 2 oz spirits, or 1 beer

Diet Assessment:
☐ Was the patient's usual diet discussed?

Optional **Global Risk Estimation** *(Complete for all men age 35 and over and all women age 45 and over with at least 1 of the risk factors marked with an asterick [*]).*

10-year CHD risk = _____%
(from worksheet in Appendix F) (Also available at: http://www.framinghamheartstudy.org/risk/coronary.html)

Optional **Aspirin** *(Complete if patient is male with 10-year CHD risk of ≥10% **OR** female with 10-year CHD risk of ≥20%)*

☐ Patient advised to use aspirin (preferabley low dose)
☐ Medical or patient reason(s) for not advising aspirin use *(MD, DO, NP, or PA only)*:
____
____

Cardiac Medications (antihypertensives, lipid-lowering medications, and aspirin; smoking cessation medications)

Name	Dosage	When taken	Reason taken (e.g. high blood pressure)

Allergies:

Fig. 26.2 Sample flow chart for prospective data collection.
Reproduced with permission from Redberg RF, Benjamin EJ, Bittner V, et al. AHA/ACCF 2009 performance measures for primary prevention in adults: a report of the American College of Cardiology Foundation/American Heart Association Task Force on performance measures (Writing Committee to develop performance measures for primary prevention of cardiovascular disease): developed in collaboration with the American Academy of Family Physicians; American Association of Cardiovascular and Pulmonary Rehabilitation; and Preventive Cardiovascular Nurses Association. *Circulation* 2009; **120**: 1296–1336.

(continued)

- Assessment and documentation of each patient's risk for adverse events during exercise.
- A process to assess patients for undercurrent changes in symptoms.
- Methodology to document programme effectiveness and initiate quality improvement strategies.

➲ Table 26.2 provides an example of a checklist for monitoring the comprehensiveness and appropriateness of preventive intervention during and after a CR programme: a follow-up programme is included as well other pharmacological and non-pharmacological prescriptions.

Examples of tools for monitoring the responses and document programme effectiveness in the different areas, through detailed individual analysis of the changes in patients' attitudes, are presented in ➲ Tables 26.3 and 26.4.

All these tools are provided as examples and not as endorsed instruments: local health systems are encouraged to develop and

Physical Exam Findings	
Height: ____ inches	Blood Presssure: ____/____ mmHg
Weight: ____ lbs.	Medical or patient reason(s) BP could not be measured *(MD, DO, NP, or PA only)*:
BMI: ____ kg/m² (from table)	*Complete if BP is > 140/90 mmHg:* Two or more antihypertensive medications prescribed? ☐ Yes ☐ No
Waist Circumference: ____ inches	☐ Medical or patient reason(s) no (or only 1) antihypertensive medication ordered *(MD, DO, NP, or PA only)*: ____
Medical or patient reason(s) that height and/or weight and waist circumference could not be measured *(MD, DO, NP, or PA only)*: ____	

Diet Counselling *(Complete for all patients)*	
Goal: An overall healthy eating pattern: ■ Lots of fruits, vegetables ■ Whole grains ■ Low-fat or nonfat dairy products ■ Fish, legumes, poultry, and lean meats ■ Limit salt intake ■ Limit alcohol intake (≤2 drinks/d in men, ≤1 drink/d in women) among those who drink.	☐ Patient was advised to eat a healthy diet ☐ Specific dietary recommendations (e.g., no added salt, decrease saturated fat, diabetic or DASH diet, decreased cholesterol intake): ____ ☐ Referred to nutritionist or dietician ☐ Diet discussed with patient and literature/brochure provided

Weight Management *(Complete if BMI >30 kg/m² OR waist circumference >40 inches in men or >35 inches in women)*

☐ Patient was advised to lose weight

☐ Specific recommendations: ____
(e.g., reducing calorie intake, increasing physical activity)

☐ Referred to weight management specialist or programme e.g., nutritionist or dietician

Medical reason(s) that weight management counselling was not provided *(MD, DO, NP, or PA only)*:

Fasting Lipid Profile *(Complete for all men age 35 and over and all women age 45 and over with at least 1 of the risk factors marked with a ‡* **under medical history in first section***)*

	Results	*Check all that apply:*
Enter date of most recent fasting lipid profile: ___/___/____	Total cholesterol: ____ mg/dL	☐ ***Total cholesterol is 240 mg/dL)***
	LDL-C: ____ mg/dL	☐ **LDL-C is ≥130 mg/dL***
	HDL-C: ____ mg/dL	☐ **HDL-C is <40 mg/dL if patient is male OR <50 mg/dL if patient is female†**

Medical or patient reason(s) that fasting lipid profile was not performed ***(MD, DO, NP, or PA only):***

Blood Lipid Management
(Complete if LDL-C is:

- Greater than or equal to 190 mg/dL (**women**) [and <2 of the risk factors marked with† under medical history above are present or global risk is low (<10%)] **OR**
- Greater than or equal to 160 mg/dL (**men**) [and <2 of the risk factors marked with† under medical history above are present or global risk is low (<10%)] **OR**
- Greater than or equal to 130 mg/dL [and <2 of the risk factors marked with† under medical history above are present or global risk is intermediate (<10% to 20%)] **OR**
- Greater than or equal to 100 mg/dL [and global risk is high (<20%)]

NOTE: Subtract 1 risk factor† if HDL-C ≥60 mg/dL

At leat 1 lipid-lowering medication prescribed at maximum tolerated dose?

☐ Yes

☐ No

☐ Medical or patient reason(s) no lipid-lowering medication was prescribed *(MD, DO, NP, or PA only)*: ____

NOTE: Items marked "optional" are for internal quality improvement only.

Fig. 26.2 *(continued)*

implement systemic tools that are most appropriate and effective for their particular setting.

Adequate communication with a patient's on-going healthcare provider is crucial, with the development of a complete discharge letter for the physician and for the patient, which should underline the risk factors, the relevant targets, and the secondary prevention measures, exercise capacity, and programme in which the patient has been enrolled. This communication should be developed and verified at the end of the different phases of the preventive cardiology process—at hospital discharge at the end of the intensive CR programme.

Assessment of health-related quality of life

Introduction

Outcomes, such as deaths, infections, and objective clinical and physiological laboratory tests, are routinely monitored to improve the quality of care but provide little or no information about the impact of either an illness or its treatment from the patient's own perspective. On the other hand, patient-reported outcomes (PROs) provide direct information about how a patient functions

Table 26.2 Checklist to assess the comprehensiveness of the prevention therapies in a cardiac rehabilitation programme

To be completed by physician, nurse, or other care provider at patient's enrolment and discharge
Admission date: ____________
Discharge date: ____________
Diagnosis: ____________
Check each condition and therapy prescribed or check reason for contraindication
◆ **Full risk assessment**
• Formulation of tailored, patient-specific, counselling with the objectives of a secondary preventive programme
• No, with reason in discharge summary
◆ **Physical activity counselling**
• Made
• No, with reason in discharge summary
◆ **Exercise training prescription**
• Prescription made
• No, with reason in discharge summary
◆ **Diet/nutritional counselling**
• Counselling made
• No, with reason in discharge summary
◆ **Weight control management** (if patient is obese or overweight)
• Made
• No, with reason in discharge summary
◆ **Lipid management**
• Made
• No, with reason in discharge summary
◆ **Blood pressure monitoring**
• Made
• No, with reason in discharge summary
◆ **Smoking cessation** (if patient is a smoker)
• Made
• No, with reason in discharge summary
• Smoking cessation teaching and pharmacological therapy *not required* (patient is non-smoker or former smoker of greater than 1 year)
◆ **Psychosocial management**
• Made
• No, with reason in discharge summary
◆ **Vocational management**
• Made
• No, with reason in discharge summary
◆ **Education on warning signs of instability and self management**
• Made
• No, with reason in discharge summary
◆ **Education on appropriate medical therapy given**
• Made
• No, with reason in discharge summary
◆ **Referral to a phase III or to community programme (Coronary Club)**
• Made
• No, with reason in discharge summary
◆ **Follow-up appointment documented in medical record**
• Date: ____________ Time: ____________ or Call ____________
• No, with reason in discharge summary

Source: data from Piepoli MF, Corrà U, Adamopoulos S, et al. Secondary prevention in the clinical management of patients with cardiovascular diseases. Core components, standards and outcome measures for referral and delivery. *Eur J Prev Cardiol* 2012 Jun 20 [Epub ahead of print] doi: 10.1177/2047487312449597

or feels in relation to a health condition and its therapy without interpretation of the patient's responses by a physician or anyone else [32,33].

Initiatives focusing on a greater use of PRO measures have been established to assess their potential for improving quality of care in the European Union, the UK, and the United States [34–39]. The assessment of health-related quality of life (HRQL) has been suggested as one potential patient-centred care strategy for improving quality of care in patients with cardiovascular disease [40]. This section summarizes the decision-making points that help determine which HRQL measure to consider as an outcome measure in research studies and in clinical practice.

'Quality of life is a vague and ethereal entity, something that many people talk about, but which nobody very clearly knows what to do about' [42] and is affected by various factors including culture, religion, education, finances, and the environment. These factors are seldom the direct focus of healthcare, yet the goal of healthcare is to improve people's quality of life. In order to link clinical variables with quality of life in healthcare, HRQL has become the accepted PRO term when describing the impact of healthcare on a patient's quality of life [43]. While there is no consensus regarding the definition of HRQL, it is generally considered as the patient's perspective of the impact on their health status of either disease or medical care.

Specifically HRQL is the patient's perception of his or her own physical, psychological, and social functioning which is consistent with the definition of a PRO [32,33,43].

Measures of health-related quality of life

Patient-reported HRQL outcomes are valuable in national and international research studies for assessing achievement of health goals and health disparities between population segments, evaluating the effectiveness of healthcare intervention, and making between-diagnosis treatment comparisons. The European Medicines Agency and the US Food and Drug Administration have both provided guidance to standardize the use and interpretation of HRQL PRO measures in randomized clinical trials (RCTs) [44]. In clinical practice, HRQL measures can help in improving shared decision-making (patient–clinician communication), screening (identifying at-risk patients), monitoring (determining disease progression and

(continued)

Table 26.3 Sample data collection tool for the performance and outcome measurements of each component during and after a cardiac rehabilitation programme

	Outcome measures	Initial assessment	Intervention plan and communication	Reassessment prior to completion of programme	Changes in intervention plan and communication
Date:					
Physical activity habits	>30 min, minimum 3–4 days per week	□ Optimal habits □ Suboptimal	□ Intervention plan developed with the patient □ Education completed □ Education suboptimal: please specify	□ Optimal habits □ Suboptimal habits	*Complete only if habits remain suboptimal* □ A new intervention plan is developed with the patient □ Healthcare provider notified
Exercise training/ capacity	Development of an individualized exercise prescription	□ Assessment and exercise prescription completed □ Assessment and exercise prescription not completed	□ Exercise prescription communicated to the patient and healthcare provider	□ Exercise prescription completed □ Exercise prescription not completed	□ Revised exercise prescription communicated to the patient and healthcare provider
Diet/ nutritional counselling	Wide variety of foods; low-salt foods; Mediterranean diet	□ Optimal control □ Suboptimal control	*Applies to all patients with CVD* Education completed: □ Target food goals □ Lifestyle modification	*Complete only if suboptimal control on initial assessment* □ Patient encouraged to contact healthcare provider about reassessment	□ Policy is in place to communicate with healthcare providers as needed
Weight management	Body mass index: 18.5–24.9 kg/m^2 AND Waist circumference: men < 94 cm women < 80 cm	□ At target □ Above target	*Applies to all patients* □ Education completed concerning target goals, diet, change, regular physical activity OR □ Referral to a weight management programme AND □ Healthcare provider notified if above target	□ At target □ Above target	*Complete only if remains above target* □ Additional education completed for target goals, diet, behaviour change, exercise OR □ Referral to a weight management programme AND □ Healthcare provider notified
Lipid control	LDL cholesterol level at target	□ Optimal control □ Suboptimal control	*Applies to all patients with CVD* Education completed: □ Target lipid goals □ Medication compliance □ Lifestyle modification	*Complete only if suboptimal control on initial assessment* □ Patient encouraged to contact healthcare provider about reassessment	□ Policy is in place to communicate with healthcare providers as needed
BP control	Systolic and diastolic values at target	□ Patient with diagnosis of treated or untreated hypertension □ Not hypertensive	*Complete only if patient has a diagnosis of hypertension* Education completed: □ Target BP goal □ Medication compliance □ Lifestyle modification	□ Intermittent monitoring of BP during CR	□ Policy in place concerning communication with healthcare providers, including thresholds for communication
Tobacco use	Complete cessation of tobacco use	□ Never □ Recent (quit less 12 months ago) □ Current	*Complete only if current or recent* □ Individual education and counselling OR □ Referral to a tobacco cessation programme AND □ Healthcare provider notified	□ Abstaining □ Still smoking	*Complete only if still smoking* □ Individual education and counselling OR □ Referral to a tobacco cessation programme AND □ Healthcare provider notified
Psychological distress	Assessment of presence or absence of psychological distress: depression, anxiety, type D personality, HRQL using a valid and reliable screening tool	□ Patient screened for distress/depression □ Patient not screened for distress/depression	*Complete only if screening tool indicates possible distress* □ Results discussed with patient AND □ Healthcare provider notified	□ Patient rescreened for distress □ Patient not rescreened	*Complete only if screening tool indicates possible distress* □ Results discussed with patient AND □ Healthcare provider notified

Table 26.3 (*continued*) Sample data collection tool for the performance and outcome measurements of each component during and after a cardiac rehabilitation programme

	Outcome measures	Initial assessment	Intervention plan and communication	Reassessment prior to completion of programme	Changes in intervention plan and communication
Medications	Adherence to prescribed preventive medications	□ Patient has been prescribed preventive medications by his/her healthcare provider(s)	□ Individual education and counselling about the importance of adherence to appropriate preventive medications OR □ Group education and counselling about the importance of adherence to appropriate preventive medications	□ Individual or group education completed	□ Patient is encouraged to discuss questions or concerns about prescribed preventive medications with his/her healthcare providers

HRQL, health-related quality of life.

Source: data from Piepoli MF, Corrà U, Adamopoulos S, et al. Secondary prevention in the clinical management of patients with cardiovascular diseases. Core components, standards and outcome measures for referral and delivery. *Eur J Prev Cardiol* 2012 Jun 20 doi: 10.1177/2047487312449597.

Table 26.4 Sample data collection tool for the outcome and performance measurements in patients with CVD during and after the CR programme

Outcome measures	1. Stabilize clinical status and/or improve functional capacity 2. Optimize cardiovascular therapy 3. Identify and control clinical or behavioural precipitating factors 4. Increased participation in domestic, occupational, and recreational activities 5. Improved psychosocial well-being, prevention of disability, and enhancement of opportunities for independent self-care 6. Improved aerobic fitness 7. Return to work when possible 8. Formulation of 'tailored', patient-specific, plan or CR programme
Initial assessment: risk stratification tools	1. Clinical history 2. Define severity of disease 3. Response to current and previous therapy 4. Physical examination 5. Blood testing 6. Chest X-ray (optional) 7. ECG 8. Two-dimensional and Doppler echocardiography: additional non-invasive imaging tests (if needed) 9. Exercise tolerance 10. Psychosocial evaluation
Intervention plan and communication	1. Education: provide clear, comprehensible information on the basic purpose of the CR programme and the role of each component 2. Lifestyle approach: patients should initiate and/or maintain lifestyle modifications 3. Weight control management (if needed) 4. Smoking cessation and alcohol restriction 5. Diet/nutritional counselling: fluid and sodium intake, caloric restriction, or self-indulgence (according to severity of disease) 6. Self-care management counselling: to the medical regime and self-monitoring (weight, BP, symptoms) 7. Physical activity counselling 8. Exercise training (if applicable) 9. Psychosocial management (if needed)
Reassessment and surveillance	Timing of lifestyle and clinical reassessment should be defined also according to severity of disease and the response to initial cardiovascular treatments **Reassess lifestyle approach:** 1. Weight management, smoking and alcohol habits 2. Diet/nutritional behaviour 3. Self-care management 4. Exercise prescription 5. Pharmacological adherence **Reassess clinical status:** 1. Suboptimal clinical status with non-optimized CV therapy: modify CV evidence-based regime or drug doses if possible 2. Suboptimal clinical status with optimized CV therapy: consider comorbidities, non-pharmacological therapies (if feasible) 3. Improved clinical status with non-optimized CV therapy: modify/improve CV evidence-based regime or drug doses if possible 4. Improved clinical status with optimized CV therapy: confirm medical evidence-based regime and start updated CV function reassessment

(*continued*)

Table 26.4 (*continued*) Sample data collection tool for the outcome and performance measurements in patients with CVD during and after the CR programme

	Timing: Risk Category according to baseline clinical CVD condition: 1. Low: lifestyle, clinical and functional reassessment <12 months 2. Moderate: lifestyle, clinical and functional reassessment <6 months 3. High: lifestyle, clinical and functional reassessment <3 months (consider remote monitoring if available and/or applicable)
Changes in intervention plan and communication	Complete only if clinical condition remains suboptimal. Go back to 'reassessment and surveillance': review reported items. 1. Promote patients' care within the multidisciplinary team, to ensure optimal pharmacological treatment, self-care management, and to facilitate access to supportive services 2. Evaluate the new intervention plan and target goals with the patient, caregiver, and healthcare provider

Source: data from Piepoli MF, Corrà U, Adamopoulos S, et al. Secondary prevention in the clinical management of patients with cardiovascular diseases. Core components, standards and outcome measures for referral and delivery. *Eur J Prev Cardiol* 2012 Jun 20 doi: 10.1177/2047487312449597.

response to treatment), and continuous assessment of quality of care [45]. It is important to bear in mind that measures developed for research purposes may not be easily used in clinical practice.

In a recent systematic literature review of PRO measures used in 180 double-blind, placebo-controlled trials, only 12 CVD RCTs (7%) were identified with five using a generic and 11 using a disease-specific questionnaire [46]. There is no such thing as a 'best measure' in an absolute sense, only measures which may be best suited to a particular purpose. It is necessary to bear in mind that HRQL is not a surrogate measure but a meaningful outcome of healthcare [43]. To help in making the decision about which HRQL measure to use in studies or clinical practice, certain questions need to be asked about

- the type of measure
- the domains covered
- the population in which the measure was developed and in which it is to be used
- the reliability, validity, and responsiveness of the measure
- how the results will be interpreted

as well as questions about

- who completes the measure

and

- the burden associated with administering the measure.

There are three types of measures of HRQL—generic, specific, and utility measures. For most research studies and clinical practices, the choice of HRQL questionnaire will be a selection between either a generic measure (which permits comparisons with other conditions but is less relevant to a specific disease or condition) or a disease-specific questionnaire (which is obviously more relevant to patients with that disease, e.g. with CHD, and so likely to be more responsive or sensitive to change in health status). For studies in which an economic evaluation, i.e. the cost-effectiveness of an intervention, is the focus, generic health status and utility measures are recommended [47].

Generic measures

The Short Form 36 Survey (SF-36) is a widely used generic measure of HRQL in healthcare [48]. The SF-36 consists of eight scales (vitality, physical functioning, bodily pain, general health perceptions, physical role functioning, emotional role functioning, social role functioning, and mental health); each is scored on a scale of 0–100, which can then be aggregated as two component summary scores, a physical and a mental component score [48]. Another generic HRQL measure, widely used in Europe, is the EuroQoL EQ-5D (EQ-5D; <http://www.euroqol.org/eq-5d.html>).

The EQ-5D (replaced by the EuroQoL-5D-5L) is applicable to a wide range of health conditions and treatments, is self-administered, consists of five dimensions (mobility, self-care, usual activities, pain/discomfort, anxiety/depression). Each is scored on a scale of 1–5, providing a simple descriptive profile and a single index value for health status that can also be used for economic evaluations.

Specific measures

The majority of patients with CHD present with one of the three main diagnoses—angina, myocardial infarction (MI), or heart failure—and specific questionnaires are available to assess HRQL in each of these three diagnoses.

Seattle Angina Questionnaire (SAQ)

The SAQ is a validated and widely used 19-item, self-administered questionnaire designed to measure functional status and HRQL in patients with angina and coronary artery disease [49]. The items are scored on 5- to 6-point Likert scales in five dimensions (physical limitation, angina stability, angina frequency, treatment satisfaction, and quality of life) with higher scores indicating higher levels of functioning and HRQL.

Minnesota Living with Heart Failure Questionnaire (MLHF)

The MLHF is a valid and widely used 21-item questionnaire for patients with heart failure [50]. The MLHF assesses the effects of symptoms, functional limitations, and psychological distress on an individual's HRQL, asking patients to indicate using a 6-point Likert scale to assess how much each of 21 facets prevents them from living as they desire (higher scores indicate poorer HRQL).

MacNew Heart Disease HRQL Questionnaire

The original interviewer-administered version of the English language MacNew for patients with MI [51] was modified and validated as a self-administered 27-item instrument [52]. The MacNew uses a 7-point Likert scale (higher scores indicate higher HRQL) in three domains (physical, emotional, social) with a global score and has been validated in patients with angina, MI, and heart failure in a number of other languages (<http://www.macnew.org/wp/>).

HeartQoL Questionnaire

The HeartQoL, published in 2014, is a validated 14-item instrument developed in an international sample of over 6300 patients with angina, MI, or heart failure [53,54]. There are two domains, physical (10 items) and emotional (four items) HRQL, with a global score; each item is scored on a 4-point Likert scale with lower scores indicative of poorer HRQL.

Core HRQL measures have been used in oncology for about 20 years allowing between-diagnosis comparisons [55,56]. Two of the CHD-specific HRQL questionnaires already described, the MacNew and the HeartQoL, permit between-diagnosis comparisons in patients with CHD, for example comparing patients with MI and heart failure following interventions such as revascularization or CR which are used in both groups. The major advantage of both the MacNew and the HeartQoL questionnaires is that as they have been validated in each of the three major CHD diagnoses only one questionnaire needs to be used when assessing patients with any one of the diagnoses.

Utility measures

The essence of economic evaluation is a comparison of the cost-effectiveness, costs, and consequences of alternative healthcare programs [46]. Recent advances have incorporated HRQL to assess the consequences of interventions and are expressed in terms of patient preferences for alternative health states or outcomes in terms of quality-adjusted life years (QALYs), a utility measure which incorporates both quantity (life years expected) and quality of life during those life years. Utility measures for estimating quality of life for economic evaluations include the time trade-off and standard gamble as well as generic health state classification systems such as the Health Utility Index, the EuroQoL, and the Quality of Well-being [46].

Population in which measures were developed

All of these CHD-specific questionnaires meet the criteria of whether the domains assessed are relevant in that they were all developed in patient populations with one of the three major CHD diagnoses.

It goes without saying that CHD-specific HRQL measures were developed in and designed for use with patients with CHD. However, if the study question is about change in HRQL in patients with angina, the MLHF questionnaire is inappropriate and the SAQ would be the questionnaire to use; if the study question is about differences in HRQL in patients with angina and patients with heart failure, either the MacNew or the HeartQoL would be the questionnaire of choice not the MLHF questionnaire.

Reliability, validity, and responsiveness of measures

Whatever HRQL is the preferred HRQL measure for a given study or clinical practice is, the HRQL questionnaire selected needs to have been shown to be:

- reliable (does the questionnaire produce results that are reproducible and internally consistent?)
- valid (does the questionnaire measure what it claims to measure), and
- responsive (does the questionnaire detect changes over time that matter to patients?).

Each of the CHD-specific measures mentioned in this discussion have been repeatedly demonstrated to be reliable, valid, and responsive in the patient populations for which they were designed, so this is not a problem. A description of CHD-specific questionnaires and representative psychometric statistics are presented in ➲ Table 26.5.

Interpretation of results

The scores obtained in any given questionnaire in any given study or clinical practice are numbers representing the distribution (central tendency; mean, median, mode) and variation (range, standard deviation). These need to be referenced to external data from a larger reference group in order to interpret the findings in a study or in a clinical practice. To be of most value when interpreting results, normative data need to be available for each HRQL questionnaire. Normative scores and ranges for specific groups, for example gender, age, or severity of disease, enhance the interpretation and understanding of the results in a study or clinical practice. Importantly, information about statistical significance should be complemented by information about clinical meaningfulness:

- Do score differences meet a minimal clinically important difference criterion?
- If so, does the change in scores in an individual patient mean a change in treatment is necessary?
- Do differences in mean scores between groups reflect a clinically important difference in the effectiveness of two treatments?

Administration of health-related quality of life measures

PRO measures provide information directly about how a patient functions or feels in relation to a health condition and its therapy without interpretation of the patient's responses by a physician or anyone else [32,33]. It stands to reason, therefore, that whenever possible these measures should be completed by the patient him- or herself as the perceptions of a health professional or a proxy may be different from those held by the patient. Typically this is not a problem when assessing HRQL in patients with CHD but may be an issue when a patient has, for example, a cognitive impairment or communication disorder, and then proxies may provide more useful information. But whenever possible, the patient should have the last word.

How often will patients be asked to complete HRQL measures? If the purpose is to screen patients, then the HRQL questionnaire may need to be administered only once. On the other hand, if the purpose is to monitor the impact of a treatment, procedure, or therapy, then the HRQL questionnaire needs to be administered before and at various times after the treatment, procedure, or therapy. While

Table 26.5 Description of coronary heart disease-specific questionnaires

	SAQ	MLHF	MacNew	HeartQoL
Diagnosis	Angina	Heart failure	CHD; angina; MI; heart failure	CHD; angina; MI; heart failure
No. of items	19	21	27	14
Domains	Physical limitation; angina stability; angina frequency; treatment satisfaction; disease perception	Total; physical; emotional	Global: physical; emotional; social	Global: physical; emotional
Psychometric properties				
Reliability*: CHD, angina, MI, heart failure	Physical limitation: NA, 0.94*, NA, NA	Total: NA, NA, 0.92*, NA	Global: 0.95*, 0.96*, 0.96*, 0.94*	Global: 0.90*, 0.80*, 0.81*, 0.82*
Validity†: CHD, angina, MI, heart failure	Physical limitation: NA, 0.73, NA, NA	Total: NA, NA, NA, 0.74	Physical/emotional: 0.69/0.79, 0.67/0.74, 0.61/0.81, 0.60/0.78	Physical/emotional: 0.60/0.68, 0.64/0.65, 0.62/0.64, 0.60/0.67
Responsiveness: CHD, angina, MI, heart failure	Physical limitation: NA, 0.87‡, NA, NA	Total: NA, NA, NA, 0.89§	Global: 0.81‡, 0.80‡, 0.71‡, 0.72‡	Global: 0.51–0.64‡, 0.74‡, 0.70‡

SAQ, Seattle Angina Questionnaire; MLHF, Minnesota Living with Heart Failure; MacNew, MacNew Heart Disease Health-related Quality of Life; HeartQoL, Heart Disease Health-related Quality of Life; and representative psychometric properties in patients with one of three coronary heart disease (CHD) diagnoses, angina, myocardial infarction (MI), or heart failure.

*Cronbach's alpha (threshold for good internal consistency <0.80; for excellent internal consistency >0.90).

†Convergent validity (threshold for strong >0.50); EQ-5D with reference to SF-12 physical; SAQ, MLHF, MacNew, and HeartQoL with reference to SF-36 physical and emotional.

‡Standardized response mean.

§Effect size.

NA, not applicable.

more frequent assessment means more complete information when monitoring change as a result of an intervention or even time, there is also added burden on both patient and clinic staff.

- How long does it take to complete the questionnaire? There are various modes of administration: in-clinic or out-of-clinic, pen and paper, computer, mail, telephone, or web-based. Each has its own advantages and disadvantages that need to be considered.
- How many questionnaires are needed? Core instruments validated in patients with angina, MI, and heart failure, such as the MacNew and the HeartQoL questionnaires, mean only one questionnaire instead of three diagnosis-specific instruments and would increase efficiency in a busy clinical practice.
- How long does it take to score and interpret the questionnaire? Questionnaires, which can be scored with simple algorithms are more useful in clinical practice, while more complicated scoring systems may be needed for fine-tuning in a research project.

Health-related quality of life measures and quality of care

Assessing PROs such as HRQL has been suggested as one potential research strategy for improving quality of care in patients with CVD [40, 41]. We already discussed how to decide whether or not to assess HRQL as a PRO in CVD research studies and clinical practice and, if the decision is positive, which HRQL measures to consider.

However, whether or not there is an association between assessing HRQL and an improvement in quality of care has not been clarified. In mid January 2015, a PubMed search on 'quality of care', 'quality of life' (as less specific than HRQL), and 'heart disease' (as less specific than CHD) in the last 10 years revealed very little CHD-specific information—3 hits for clinical trials or RCTs in patients with heart disease. As for clinical practice, a similar PubMed search with the following terms, 'quality of care', 'quality of life', 'heart disease', and 'clinical practice' revealed zero hits for clinical trials or RCTs in patients with CVD.

There is limited evidence about the value of PROs in clinical practice and, while there is evidence of a continuing increase in the use and value of PROs in heart disease studies, PROs are 'underused once their relevance to clinical decision making has been taken into account'. [57,58]. Patient-centred strategies, such as providing information on the patient's condition and treatment and information on complaints procedures, may be associated positively with quality improvement in hospitals [35]. However, at this time, the evidence for an association between assessment of HRQL and an improvement in quality of care is limited and uncertain.

Assessment and intervention to improve treatment adherence

Introduction

Drugs don't work in patients who don't take them

C. Everett Koop

Optimal control of CVD risk factors is one of the most effective methods for reducing vascular events in patients with coronary or other atherosclerotic disease or in people at high CV risk. Thus, improving treatment adherence is a very important step in optimizing management of CV risk factors. *Adherence* has been defined as an 'active, voluntary involvement of the patient in the management of his or her disease, by following a mutually agreed course of treatment and sharing responsibility between the patient and healthcare providers' [59].

Treatment adherence usually refers to the extent to which patients take treatments (lifestyle modifications or medications) as prescribed, as well as whether they continue to take prescribed treatments [60]. Treatment adherence has been divided into two main concepts, namely medication adherence and persistence. *Medication adherence* refers to the intensity of drug use during the duration of therapy, and is usually calculated by dividing the number of treatments actually taken by the number of treatments prescribed. *Persistence* refers to the overall duration of time that a patient remains on treatment from the initiation to discontinuation of a prescribed therapy [60–64].

A variety of studies have demonstrated that adherence and persistence in both people at high risk and patients with CVD are low and they drop significantly after the first 6 months of therapy [65–67]. Two-year statin adherence rates were found to be only 40% for patients with acute coronary syndrome, 36% for chronic coronary disease, and 25% for primary prevention [67]. Almost a quarter of patients (23%) did not even fill their cardiac medications prescriptions by day seven of discharge [68]. Among patients discharged with prescriptions for aspirin, statin, and beta-blockers after acute MI, one study found that 34% of patients stopped at least one medication and 12% discontinued use of all three medications within a month of hospital discharge [69]. A longitudinal database study using Medication Event Monitoring System (MEMS) data, demonstrated that about half of the patients who were prescribed an antihypertensive drug had stopped taking it within a year [70].

Association between medication adherence and outcomes

Patients with poor adherence have higher CV event rates and all-cause mortality and increased healthcare costs compared with those with good adherence [8,61,66,71–74]. A meta-analysis of observational studies on the association between adherence to drug therapy and mortality demonstrated that good adherence to drug therapy is associated with positive health outcomes [75]. Moreover, the same association was observed between good adherence to placebo and mortality, which supports the existence of a 'healthy adherer' effect, implying that adherence to drug therapy may be a surrogate marker for overall healthy behaviour. Therefore, measures should be taken to improve adherence and health behaviour in general.

Methodology for assessing medication adherence

There are many different methods for measuring treatment adherence. In general, these methods can be categorized as direct and indirect [60]. *Direct* methods include:

- directly observed therapy
- measurement of the level of medicine or metabolite in the blood, and
- measurement of biological marker in the blood.

These techniques are considered to be more robust than indirect methods but have several limitations as patients may hide pills in their mouths and discard them later. In addition, measurements of the blood concentration of a medication or metabolites, although accurate, require substantial time and expense and are not practical for routine clinical use (➲ Table 26.6).

Indirect methods of adherence assessment include [60]:

- patient questionnaires
- self-reports
- pill counts
- rate of prescription refills
- assessment of the patient's clinical response
- MEMS
- measurement of physiological markers, and
- patient diaries.

Each of these methods has advantages and disadvantages, and the use of a specific method to assess adherence will depend on the clinical scenario and availability of data. In general, pill counts and self-reports are not considered to be reliable because they can be biased by inaccurate patient recall or by patient's overly optimistic estimation of their behaviour in an effort to please their healthcare providers. This bias also affects the ascertainment of patients' adherence to prescribed lifestyle interventions. In outpatient clinical settings there is a need for a valid, reliable, cost-effective tool that is acceptable to both healthcare providers and patients in measuring medication adherence.

The Morisky Medication Adherence Scale (MMAS-4) is a commonly used, validated, self-reported adherence measure that has been shown to be predictive of medication adherence. The four-item questionnaire was originally published in 1986 and modified in 1990 [76]. It is used mainly in the clinical setting, with the clinician directly assessing medication-taking behaviour and providing immediate feedback, either giving suggestions about how to incorporate the behaviour into the patient's lifestyle or reinforcing positive adherence behaviour. In 2008, Morisky published an updated eight-item version of the Medication Adherence Scale (MMAS-8) which has demonstrated a higher level of reliability and higher sensitivity and specificity than the four-item scale. It proved to be reliable, with good concurrent and predictive validity in patients with hypertension, and can be used as a screening test in outpatient settings with other patient groups [77]. Validated translated versions of the MMAS-8 are available in several European, Asian, and South American languages.

The Heart and Soul Study was a prospective cohort study of psychosocial factors and CV outcomes in patients with CHD. The primary predictor variable was a single question about overall medication adherence: 'In the past month, how often did you take your medications as the doctor prescribed?'. Possible responses were: 'All of the time' (100%), 'Nearly all of the time' (90%), 'Most of the time' (75%), 'About half the time' (50%), or 'Less than half the time' (<50%). The results demonstrated that self-reported medication non-adherence was strongly associated with adverse CV events (hazards ratio 2.3; 95% confidence interval, 1.3–4.3; $p = 0.006$) [78].

Table 26.6 Methods for measuring patient medication adherence

Test	Advantages	Disadvantages
Direct methods:		
Directly observed therapy	Most accurate	Patients can hide pills in their mouth and then discard them; impractical for routine use
Measurement of the level of medicine or metabolite in blood	Objective	Variations in metabolism and 'white-coat adherence' can give a false impression of adherence; expensive
Measurement of the biological marker in blood	Objective; in clinical trials can also be used to measure placebo	Requires expensive quantitative assays and collection of bodily fluids
Indirect methods:		
Patient questionnaires, patient self-reports	Simple; inexpensive; the most useful method in the clinical setting	Susceptible to error with increases in time between visits; results are easily distorted by patient
Pill counts	Objective, quantifiable, and easy to perform	Data easily altered by the patient (e.g. pill dumping)
Rates of prescription refills	Objective; easy to obtain data	A prescription refill is not equivalent to ingestion of medication; requires a closed pharmacy system
Assessment of the patient's clinical response	Simple; generally easy to perform	Factors other than medication adherence can affect clinical response
Electronic medication monitors	Precise; results are easily quantified; tracks patterns of taking medication	Expensive; requires return visits and downloading data from medication vials
Measurement of physiological markers (e.g. heart rate in patients taking beta-blockers)	Often easy to perform	Marker may be absent for other reasons (e.g. increased metabolism, poor absorption, lack of response)
Patient diaries	Help to correct for poor recall	Easily altered by the patient
When the patient is a child, questionnaire for caregiver or teacher	Simple; objective	Susceptible to distortion

Electronic monitoring systems are becoming more widely available, and is one of the more frequently used methods in the literature. MEMS assessments are considered to be reliable, although they are expensive and logistically complex. Assessment of medication refill rate is an accurate measure of adherence, especially in a closed pharmacy system. Adherence based on pharmacy refill data has been correlated with a broad range of patient outcomes [71].

Reasons for non-adherence to medication

The reasons for poor adherence are often multifactorial. However, many health professionals believe that patients are solely responsible for their adherence behaviour and do not account for other causes related to socioeconomics or the healthcare system. Non-adherence can be intentional or unintentional.

Intentional non-adherence is an active rational decision process in which the patient weighs risks and benefits of treatment against any adverse effects [79]. *Unintentional* non-adherence is a passive process in which the patient may be careless or forgetful about adhering to the treatment regimen. On the basis of electronic monitoring systems, the patterns for medication adherence can range from: (1) close to perfect adherence; (2) taking nearly all doses with some timing irregularity; (3) missing an occasional single day's dose, and some timing inconsistencies; (4) taking drug holidays three or four times per year; (5) taking drug holidays monthly or more often and with frequent omissions; and (6) taking few or no doses [60,62]. Most deviations in medication adherence are due to omissions of doses or delay in taking medications. In addition, it is known that patients improve their medication adherence shortly before and after an appointment with a physician, known as 'white-coat adherence' [60].

The 2003 World Heart Organization report 'Adherence to long-term therapies: evidence for action' categorized the factors affecting adherence into five groups: patient-related, therapy-related, condition-related, healthcare system, and socioeconomic factors [59]. Although the research on adherence has been focused primarily on patient-related factors, there is increasing evidence that the factors in the other four groups are equally important in understanding and improving adherence (➲ Fig. 26.3).

Demographic characteristics related to medication non-adherence, including younger age, sex, and non-white race, are not strong predictors of patient adherence. In contrast, mental health disorders, depression, stress, anxiety, severe physical (e.g. vision problems or impaired dexterity) or cognitive impairment, and asymptomatic or chronic health conditions requiring long-term therapies are strongly associated with non-adherence. Depression can double the risk for medication non-adherence, even after control for age, ethnicity, education, social support, and measures of severity of cardiac disease.

Patients' knowledge about their heart status and their health beliefs and attitudes, such as low perceived risk of their condition, low perceived need, or benefit from medication, poor understanding of disease state, ineffectiveness, lack of motivation, low

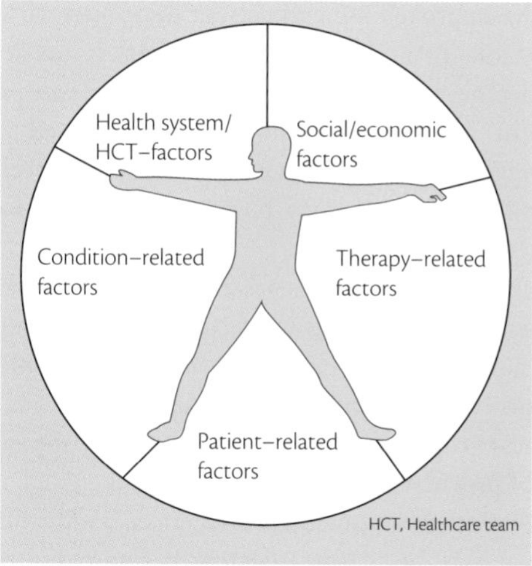

Fig. 26.3 The five dimensions of adherence.
Reproduced with permission from the World Health Organization, 'Adherence to long-term therapies: evidence for action', Geneva, copyright 2003, World Health Organization. Available online at:
<http://www.who.int/chp/knowledge/publications/adherence_full_report.pdf>

self-efficacy, or fear of adverse effects from a treatment often result in poorer adherence. In addition, different degrees of readiness to change, self-management skills, and active participation in their care appear to be strong predictors of patient adherence [61].

On the other hand, *condition-related factors* are also an important component of treatment adherence. Asymptomatic conditions or misperception about CV risk factors can also negatively affect adherence, as patients are more adherent with treatment of symptomatic heart disease. Chronic health conditions requiring long-term therapies can also adversely affect treatment adherence. Adherence is generally worse among patients with chronic asymptomatic conditions such as hypertension and hyperlipidaemia compared with those who have symptomatic disease. A meta-analysis of data from 20 studies assessing adherence using prescription refill frequency showed that about a third of patients who have had an MI and half of those without infarction do not adhere to long-term cardioprotective medication [80].

Therapy-related factors are another major aspect of treatment adherence. Communication barriers, a complex medication schedule, such as frequency of dosing, number of concurrent medications, drug tolerability and side effects, and changes in medications can have a significant impact on patients' motivation and willingness to adhere to treatments. Increasing numbers of single doses were directly associated with dramatically decreasing adherence. [81]. There is evidence that simplifying medication regimens increase the likelihood of adherence.

Factors, associated with the *healthcare system* can also positively or negatively affect treatment adherence. The actions of healthcare providers that can have a negative impact on treatment adherence include poor provider–patient therapeutic relationship, poor knowledge on medication and/or low acceptance of guidelines, poor communication (e.g. limited or confusing advice for how long to take medication, frequency or timing of dosing), prescription of complex drug regimens, the failure to explain the benefits and possible adverse effects of treatments, the failure to consider the patient's lifestyle or the affordability of medications, lack of continuity of care, and lack of access to healthcare. A variety of studies found that fewer than 50% of patients leave the hospital or the office not being able to list their medications or did not know their purpose and how to take them [82].

Finally, *socioeconomic factors* are derived from patients' inability (or difficulty) to afford their medication. They may include lack of adequate healthcare coverage, concerns about costs, unemployment, retirement, high medication costs, low health literacy, social deprivation, and poor social support. These factors are very important for the treatment of chronic cardiac conditions, for which multiple medications are required for life-long therapies. Cost-related non-adherence is an important problem in many healthcare systems, especially in elderly and people of low socioeconomic status [83,84].

Interventions to improve medication adherence

Interventions used to improve adherence can be grouped into two categories: unimodal and multimodal. In general, unimodal interventions have been found to be less successful than multimodal interventions [71]. Unimodal interventions that have demonstrated some success include counselling, reducing the number of daily single doses, and fixed combinations (polypills) to reduce the number of tablets and dose-dispensed medicine. Given that there are many factors resulting in non-adherence, a multifactorial approach is required. In order to be successful and sustainable, the interventions have to take into account the multiple barriers to adherence and to involve patients, healthcare provider, and healthcare system factors.

Although a variety of studies have highlighted some successful interventions to improve medication adherence, their implementation in everyday clinical practice is far from optimal. Several systematic reviews have shown that different types of interventions are effective in improving adherence for chronic medical conditions [85–87], ranging from single adjustments in the medication regimen to multimodal interventions addressing patients, healthcare providers, and the healthcare system (➲ Table 26.7). In general,

Table 26.7 Recommendations for promoting medication adherence

◆ Provide clear advice regarding the benefits and possible adverse effects of the medication, and the duration and timing of dosing
◆ Consider patients' habits and preferences
◆ Reduce dosage demands to the lowest feasible level
◆ Ask patients in a non-judgemental way how the medication works for them, and discuss possible reasons for non-adherence (e.g. side effects, worries)
◆ Implement repetitive monitoring and feedback
◆ In the case of lack of time, introduce physicians' assistants and/or trained nurses whenever it is necessary and feasible
◆ In the case of persistent non-adherence, offer multisession or combined behavioural interventions

From: European guidelines on cardiovascular disease prevention in clinical practice (version 2012). *EHJ* 2012 doi: 19.1093/eurheart/ehs092

evaluation of effective interventions was difficult because of the wide variations in study design, patient population, outcome measures, duration of follow-up, and the multifaceted nature of many of the interventions. Several types of interventions were found to be effective in improving medication adherence; however, effect sizes on adherence and clinical outcomes varied significantly between studies. Nonetheless, behavioural interventions, such as reducing dosage demands resulted in strong effects (effect size 0.89–1.20), but other interventions such as incorporating monitoring and feedback to patients and providers (effect size 0.27–0.81), multisession information (effect size 0.35–1.13), and combined behavioural interventions (effect size 0.43–1.20), demonstrated variable (small to large) effects. Several informational, behavioural, or combined studies showed improvement in at least one clinical outcome, but effects ranged from very small to large (effect size 0.17–3.41) [87].

In general, elements of successful interventions can be divided into patient, provider, and healthcare system factors [61]. One of the most effective patient-focused interventions is simplifying the treatment regimen [86]. Simpler and less frequent dosing regimens were associated with improved adherence across a variety of therapeutic classes [81]. Other studies found that minimizing the total number of daily doses was more effective at improving adherence than minimizing the total number of medications [88,89]. A reduction in the number of tablets is therefore important for the improvement of drug adherence.

Medication that is not effective (e.g. vitamins for the prevention of CVD) may be harmful by reducing adherence to effective medications. Furthermore, selection of 'more forgiving' medications with longer half-lives (drugs whose efficacy will not be affected by occasionally delayed or missed doses) may improve overall control of cardiac risk factors such as hypertension despite imperfect adherence. Fixed combinations (polypills) can contribute to a reduction in the number of single doses and to improving drug adherence, and has been proven to be cost-effective [90–93]. They could therefore be considered in patients with chronic conditions for the improvement of medication adherence, and subsequently the improvement of clinical outcomes.

Dose-dispensing of medicine such as the use of time-specific packs in the form of pre-packed medication dispensers containing each patient's medications is a relatively simple and efficacious method for improving drug adherence [90]. This was tested in a clinical trial of a pharmacy care programme on medication adherence and persistence in patients with hypertension and hyperlipidaemia taking a mean of nine chronic medications. Mean baseline medication adherence was 61% which increased to 97% after 6 months. The improved adherence was associated with improvements of systolic BP and LDL cholesterol [94]. It was demonstrated that a harmonized, structured pharmaceutical care programme improves the quality of life and the self-reported well-being, strongly suggesting that social and psychosocial aspects contribute to the effects of a pharmacy-based programme of weekly blisters [95].

In addition to simplifying the treatment regimens, motivational strategies such as monitoring and feedback, small group sessions, reminder calls, or patient education, although less effective, can still be valuable for improving adherence.

In contrast to patient-focused interventions, the evidence of the effect of provider-focused interventions is mixed and inconclusive [61]. Continuing medical education, audit, and feedback programmes have been least effective at improving medication adherence. Healthcare system interventions have been found to be successful in improving CV risk factor management, especially when team management approaches and nurse- or pharmacist-led intervention programmes were employed [96]. Furthermore, telephone counselling was found useful in a 2-year RCT in patients receiving five or more drugs for treatment of chronic disease [97].

Conclusions

Treatment adherence is essential for the optimal control of CV risk factors. Poor adherence is an increasingly recognized cause of adverse CV outcomes and increased healthcare costs. Non-adherence is not solely a patient problem but is influenced by providers and the healthcare system. Although a number of methods for measuring treatment adherence are available, each has its advantages and disadvantages and no particular method is considered the gold standard. Several types of intervention have been found to be effective in improving treatment adherence, but few were able to demonstrate an impact on clinical outcomes. Evidence suggests that simplifying dosage demands is the most effective single intervention for enhancing medication adherence. There is limited evidence about which interventions are the most effective in different patient groups. Interventions that involve monitoring and feedback, encouraging patients to participate in their care, and using information technologies to identify non-adherence and to start interventions are probably also effective. In clinical practice, physicians should always assess treatment adherence and identify reasons for possible non-adherence. Future research is needed to test the effects of interventions to improve adherence on clinical end-points.

Further reading

Measuring quality of care

Kotseva K, Wood D, De Backer G, et al.; on behalf of EUROASPIRE study Group. EUROASPIRE III: A survey on the lifestyle, risk factors and use of cardioprotective drug therapies in coronary patients from twenty two European countries. EUROASPIRE Study Group. *Eur J Cardiovasc Prev Rehabil* 2009; **16**: 121–37.

Kotseva K, Wood D, De Backer G, et al.; on behalf of EUROASPIRE study Group. Cardiovascular prevention guidelines—the clinical reality: a comparison of EUROASPIRE I, II and III surveys in 8 European countries. *Lancet* 2009; **372**: 929–40.

Kotseva K, Wood D, De Backer G, et al.; on behalf of EUROASPIRE study Group. EUROASPIRE III. Management of cardiovascular risk factors in asymptomatic high risk subjects in general practice: cross-sectional survey in 12 European countries. *Eur J Cardiovasc Prev Rehabil* 2010; **17**: 530–40.

Kotseva K, Wood D, De Bacquer D, et al. Use and effects of cardiac rehabilitation in patients with coronary heart disease: results from the EUROASPIRE III survey. *Eur J Prev Cardiol* 2013; **20**: 817–26.

Piepoli MF, Corrà U, Benzer W, et al.; Cardiac Rehabilitation Section of the European Association of Cardiovascular Prevention and Rehabilitation. Secondary prevention through cardiac rehabilitation: from knowledge to implementation. A position paper from the Cardiac Rehabilitation Section of the European Association of Cardiovascular Prevention and Rehabilitation. *Eur J Cardiovasc Prev Rehabil* 2010; **17**: 1–17.

Piepoli MF, Corrà U, Adamopoulos S, et al. Secondary prevention in the clinical management of patients with cardiovascular diseases. Core components, standards and outcome measures for referral and delivery. *Eur J Prev Cardiol* 2012; **21**: 664–81.

Redberg RF, Benjamin EJ, Bittner V, et al. AHA/ACCF 2009 performance measures for primary prevention in adults: a report of the American College of Cardiology Foundation/American Heart Association Task Force on performance measures (Writing Committee to develop performance measures for primary prevention of cardiovascular disease): Developed in collaboration with the American Academy of Family Physicians; American Association of Cardiovascular and Pulmonary Rehabilitation; and Preventive Cardiovascular Nurses Association. *Circulation* 2009; **120**: 1296–36.

Thomas RJ, King M, Lui K, et al. AACVPR/ACC/AHA 2007 performance measures on cardiac rehabilitation for referal to and delivery of cardiac rehabilitation/secondary prevention services. *Circulation* 2007; **116**: 1611–42.

Thomas RJ, King M, Lui K, et al. AACVPR/ACCF/AHA 2010 update: performance measures on cardiac rehabilitation for referral to cardiac rehabilitation/secondary prevention services: a report of the American Association of Cardiovascular and Pulmonary Rehabilitation and the American College of Cardiology Foundation/American Heart Association Task Force on Performance Measures. *Circulation* 2010; **122**: 1342–50.

Assessment of health-related quality of life

Committee for Medicinal Products for Human Use. *Reflection paper on the regulatory guidance for the use of health-related quality of life (HRQL) measures in the evaluation of medicinal products,* 2005. London: European Medicines Agency. URL: <http://www.ispor.org/workpaper/EMEA-HRQL-Guidance.pdf>

Drummond MF, Sculpher MJ, Torrance GW, et al. *Methods for the economic evaluation of healthcare programmes*, 3rd edn, 2005. Oxford: Oxford University Press.

Oldridge N, Guyatt G, Jones N, et al. Effects on quality of life with comprehensive rehabilitation after acute myocardial infarction. *Am J Cardiol* 1991; **67**: 1084–9.

Oldridge N, Höfer S, McGee H, et al. The HeartQoL: II. Validation of a new core health-related quality of life questionnaire for patients with ischemic heart disease. *Eur J Prev Cardiol* 2014; **21**: 98–106.

Rector TS, Kubo SH, Cohn JN. Patients' self-assessment of their congestive heart failure: Part 2. Content, reliability, and validity of a new measure, the Minnesota Living with Heart Failure questionnaire. *Heart Fail* 1987; **3**: 198–209.

Spertus JA, Winder JA, Dewhurst TA, et al. Development and evaluation of the Seattle Angina Questionnaire: a new functional status measure for coronary artery disease. *J Am Coll Cardiol* 1995; **25**: 1333–41.

Ware J, Kosinski M. *The SF-36 Physical and Mental Health Summary Scales: a manual for users of Version 1*, 2nd edn, 2005. Lincoln, RI: QualityMetric Incorporated.

Assessment and intervention to improve treatment adherence

Maddox TM, Ho PM. The role of treatment adherence in cardiac risk factor modification. In: Blumenthal R, Foody JM, Wong ND (eds), *Preventive cardiology. A companion to Brownwald's heart disease*, 2011, pp. 570–8. Amsterdam: Elsevier.

Perk J, De Backer G, Gohlke H, et al. European guidelines on cardiovascular disease prevention in clinical practice (version 2012) The Fifth Joint Task Force of the European Society of Cardiology and Other Societies on Cardiovascular Disease Prevention in Clinical Practice (constituted by representatives of nine societies and by invited experts). * Developed with the special contribution of the European Association for Cardiovascular Prevention and Rehabilitation (EACPR). *Eur Heart J* 2012; **33:** 1635–1701.

World Health Organization. *Adherence to long-term therapies: evidence for action*, 2003. Geneva: World Health Organization. URL: <http://apps.who.int/medicinedocs/en/d/Js4883e/1.html>

References

1 Berwick DM, Hackbarth AD. Eliminating waste in US healthcare. *J Am Med Assoc* 2012; **307**: 1513–16.

2 Lohr KN (ed.) *Medicare: a strategy for quality assurance*, Vol 1, p. 21. Washington, DC: National Academy Press.

3 Donabedian A. The quality of care. How can it be assessed? *J Am Med Assoc* 1988; **260**: 1743–8.

4 Pyörälä K, De Backer G, Graham I, et al. Prevention of coronary heart disease in clinical practice. Recommendations of the Task Force of the European Society of Cardiology, European Atherosclerotic Society and European Society of Hypertension. *Eur Heart J* 1994; **15**: 1300–31.

5 Wood D, De Backer G, Faergeman D, et al. Prevention of coronary heart disease in clinical practice. Recommendations of the Second Joint Task Force of European and other Societies on coronary prevention. *Eur Heart J* 1998; **19**: 1434–503.

6 De Backer G, Ambrosioni E, Borch-Johnsen K, et al. European guidelines on cardiovascular disease prevention in clinical practice. Third Joint Task Force of European and other Societies on Cardiovascular Disease Prevention in Clinical Practice (constituted by representatives of eight societies and by invited experts). *Eur J Cardiovasc Prev Rehabil* 2003; **10** (Suppl. 1): S1–S78.

7 Graham I, Atar D, Borch-Johnsen K, et al. European guidelines on cardiovascular disease prevention in clinical practice: Fourth Joint Task Force of the European Society of Cardiology and other Societies on Cardiovascular Disease Prevention in Clinical Practice (constituted by representatives of nine societies and by invited experts). *Eur J Cardiovasc Prev Rehabil* 2007; **14** (Suppl. 2): S1–113.

8 Perk J, De Backer G, Gohlke H, et al. European guidelines on cardiovascular disease prevention in clinical practice (version 2012): the Fifth Joint Task Force of the European Society of Cardiology and other Societies on Cardiovascular Disease Prevention in Clinical Practice (constituted by representatives of nine societies and by invited experts). *Eur Heart J* 2012; **33**: 1635–1701.

9 EUROASPIRE Study Group. EUROASPIRE. A European Society of Cardiology survey of secondary prevention of coronary heart disease: principal results. *Eur Heart J* 1997; **18**; 1569–82.

10 EUROASPIRE Study Group. Lifestyle and risk factor management and use of drug therapies in coronary patients from 15 countries. Principal results from EUROASPIRE II. Euro Heart Survey Programme. *Eur Heart J* 2001; **22**: 554–72.

11 EUROASPIRE Study Group. Clinical reality of coronary prevention guidelines: a comparison of EUROASPIRE I and II in nine countries. *Lancet* 2001; **357**: 995–1001.

12 Kotseva K, Wood D, De Backer G, et al., on behalf of EUROASPIRE study Group. EUROASPIRE III: a survey on the lifestyle, risk factors and use of cardioprotective drug therapies in coronary patients from twenty two European countries. EUROASPIRE Study Group. *Eur J Cardiovasc Prev Rehabil* 2009; **16**: 121–37.

13 Kotseva K, Wood D, De Backer G, et al., on behalf of EUROASPIRE study Group. Cardiovascular prevention guidelines—the clinical reality: a comparison of EUROASPIRE I, II and III surveys in 8 European countries. *Lancet* 2009; **372**: 929–40.

14 Kotseva K, Wood D, De Backer G, et al., on behalf of EUROASPIRE study Group. EUROASPIRE III. Management of cardiovascular risk factors in asymptomatic high risk subjects in general practice: cross-sectional survey in 12 European countries. *Eur J Cardiovasc Prev Rehabil* 2010; **17**: 530–40.

15 Kotseva K, Wood D, De Bacquer D, et al. Use and effects of cardiac rehabilitation in patients with coronary heart disease: results from the EUROASPIRE III survey. *Eur J Prev Cardiol* 2013; **20**: 817–26.

16 Banegas JR, López-García E, Dallongeville J, et al. Achievement of treatment goals for primary prevention of cardiovascular disease in clinical practice across Europe. The EURIKA study. *Eur Heart J* 2011; **32**: 2143–52.

17 Bhatt DL, Steg PG, Ohman EM, et al.; for the REACH Registry Investigators. International prevalence, recognition and treatment of cardiovascular risk factors in outpatients with atherothrombosis. *J Am Med Assoc* 2006; **295**: 180–9.

18 De Velasco JA, Cosin J, Lopez-Sendon JL, et al. Nuevos datos sobre la prevencion secundaria del infarto de miocardio en Espana. Resultados del estudio PREVESE II. [New data on secondary prevention of myocardial infarction in Spain. Results of the PREVESE II study.] *Rev Esp Cardiol* 2002; **55**: 801–9.

19 Muntner P, DeSalvo K, Wildman R, et al. Trends in the prevalence, awareness, treatment and control of cardiovascular risk factors among noninstitutionalized patients with a history of myocardial infarction and stroke. *Am J Epidemiol* 2006; **163**: 913–20.

20 Khot UN, Khot MB, Bajzer CT, et al. Prevalence of conventional risk factors in patients with coronary heart disease. *J Am Med Assoc* 2003; **290**: 898–904.

21 Ghandehary H, Kamal-Bahl S, Wong ND. Prevalence and extent of dyslipidaemia and recommended lipid levels in US adults with and without cardiovascular comorbidities: the National Health and Nutrition Examination Survey 2003–4. *Am Heart J* 2008; **156**: 112–19.

22 Van Ganse E, Laforest L, Alemao E, et al. Lipid-modifying therapy and attainment of cholesterol goals in Europe: the Return on Expenditure Achieved for Lipid Therapy (REALITY) study. *Curr Med Res Opinion* 2005; **21**: 1389–99.

23 Geller JC, Cassens S, Brosz M, et al. Achievement of guideline-defined treatment goals in primary care: the German Coronary Risk Management. (CoRiMa) study. *Eur Heart J* 2007; **28**: 3051–8.

24 Waters DD, Brotons C, Chiang CW, et al; Lipid Treatment Assessment Project 2 Investigators. Lipid treatment assessment project 2: a multinational survey to evaluate the proportion of patients achieving low-density lipoprotein cholesterol goals. *Circulation* 2009; **120**: 28–34.

25 Wang YR, Alexander GC, Stafford RS. Outpatient hypertension treatment, treatment intensification, and control in western Europe and the United States. *Arch Intern Med* 2007; **167**: 141–7.

26 Steinberg BA, Bhatt DL, Mehta S, et al. Nine-year trends in achievement of risk factor goals in the US and European outpatients with cardiovascular disease. *Am Heart J* 2008; **156**: 719–27.

27 Piepoli MF, Corrà U, Benzer W, et al.; Cardiac Rehabilitation Section of the European Association of Cardiovascular Prevention and Rehabilitation Secondary prevention through cardiac rehabilitation: from knowledge to implementation. A position paper from the Cardiac Rehabilitation Section of the European Association of Cardiovascular Prevention and Rehabilitation. *Eur J Cardiovasc Prev Rehabil* 2010; **17**: 1–17.

28 Piepoli MF, Corrà U, Adamopoulos S, et al. Secondary prevention in the clinical management of patients with cardiovascular diseases. Core components, standards and outcome measures for referral and delivery. *Eur J Prev Cardiol* 2012; **21**: 664–81.

29 Thomas RJ, King M, Lui K, et al. AACVPR/ACC/AHA 2007 performance measures on cardiac rehabilitation for referral to and delivery of cardiac rehabilitation/secondary prevention services. *Circulation* 2007; **116**: 1611–42.

30 Thomas RJ, King M, Lui K, et al. AACVPR/ACCF/AHA 2010 update: performance measures on cardiac rehabilitation for referral to cardiac rehabilitation/secondary prevention services: a report of the American Association of Cardiovascular and Pulmonary Rehabilitation and the American College of Cardiology Foundation/American Heart Association Task Force on Performance Measures. *Circulation* 2010; **122**: 1342–50.

31 Redberg RF, Benjamin EJ, Bittner V, et al. AHA/ACCF 2009 performance measures for primary prevention in adults: a report of the American College of Cardiology Foundation/American Heart Association Task Force on performance measures (Writing Committee to develop performance measures for primary prevention of cardiovascular disease): developed in collaboration with the American Academy of Family Physicians; American Association of cardiovascular and Pulmonary Rehabilitation; and Preventive Cardiovascular Nurses Association. *Circulation* 2009; **120**: 1296–336.

32 Committee for Medicinal Products for Human Use. *Reflection paper on the regulatory guidance for the use of health-related quality of life (HRQL) measures in the evaluation of medicinal products,* 2005. London: European Medicines Agency. URL: <http://www.ispor.org/workpaper/EMEA-HRQL-guidance.pdf>

33 US Department of Health and Human Services, Food and Drug Administration. *Guidance for industry. Patient-reported outcome measures: use in medical product development to support labeling claims*, 2009. Washington, DC: US Department of Health and Human Services. URL: <http://www.fda.gov/downloads/Drugs/Guidances/UCM193282.pdf>

34 Groene O, Klazinga N, Wagner C, et al. Investigating organizational quality improvement systems, patient empowerment, organizational culture, professional involvement and the quality of care in European hospitals: the 'Deepening our Understanding of Quality Improvement in Europe (DUQuE)' project. *BMC Health Serv Res* 2010; **10**: 281.

35 Groene O, Lombarts MJ, Klazinga N, et al. Is patient-centredness in European hospitals related to existing quality improvement strategies? Analysis of a cross-sectional survey (MARQuIS study). *Qual Saf Healthcare* 2009; **18** (Suppl. 1): i44–i50.

36 Rawlins M. In pursuit of quality: the National Institute for Clinical Excellence. *Lancet* 1999; **353**: 1079–82.

37 Roland M. Linking physicians' pay to the quality of care—a major experiment in the United Kingdom. *N Engl J Med* 2004; **351**: 1448–54.

38 Cella D, Yount S, Rothrock N, et al. The Patient-Reported Outcomes Measurement Information System (PROMIS): progress of an NIH roadmap cooperative group during its first two years. *Med Care* 2007; **45**: S3–S11.

39 Selby J, Beal A, Frank L. The Patient-Centered Outcomes Research Institute (PCORI) national priorities for research and initial research agenda. *J Am Med Assoc* 2012; **307**: 1583–4.
40 Rumsfeld JS, Alexander KP, Goff DC, Jr., et al. Cardiovascular health: the importance of measuring patient-reported health status: a scientific statement from the American Heart Association. *Circulation* 2013; **127**: 2233–49.
41 Anker SD, Agewall S, Borggrefe M, et al. The importance of patient-reported outcomes: a call for their comprehensive integration in cardiovascular clinical trials. *Eur Heart J* 2014;**35**:2001–9.
42 Campbell A. Subjective measures of well-being. *Am Psychol* 1976; **31**: 117–24.
43 Wilson IB, Cleary PD. Linking clinical variables with health-related quality of life. A conceptual model of patient outcomes. *J Am Med Assoc* 1995; **273**: 59–65.
44 Bottomley A, Jones D, Claassens L. Patient-reported outcomes: assessment and current perspectives of the guidelines of the Food and Drug Administration and the reflection paper of the European Medicines Agency. *Eur J Cancer* 2009; **45**: 347–53.
45 Snyder CF, Aaronson NK, Choucair AK, et al. Implementing patient-reported outcomes assessment in clinical practice: a review of the options and considerations. *Qual Life Res* 2012; **21**: 1305–14.
46 Dinan MA, Compton KL, Dhillon et al. Use of patient-reported outcomes in randomized, double-blind, placebo-controlled clinical trials. *Med Care* 2011; **49**: 415–19.
47 Drummond MF, Sculpher MJ, Torrance GW, et al. *Methods for the economic evaluation of healthcare programmes*, 3rd edn, 2005. Oxford: Oxford University Press.
48 Ware J, Kosinski M. *The SF-36 Physical and Mental Health Summary Scales: a manual for users of Version 1*, 2nd edn, 2005. Lincoln, RI: QualityMetric Incorporated.
49 Spertus JA, Winder JA, Dewhurst TA, et al. Development and evaluation of the Seattle Angina Questionnaire: a new functional status measure for coronary artery disease. *J Am Coll Cardiol* 1995; **25**: 333–41.
50 Rector TS, Kubo SH, Cohn JN. Patients' self-assessment of their congestive heart failure: Part 2. Content, reliability, and validity of a new measure, the Minnesota Living with Heart Failure questionnaire. *Heart Fail* 1987; **3**: 198–209.
51 Oldridge N, Guyatt G, Jones N, et al. Effects on quality of life with comprehensive rehabilitation after acute myocardial infarction. *Am J Cardiol* 1991; **67**: 1084–9.
52 Valenti L, Lim L, Heller RF, Knapp J. An improved questionnaire for assessing quality of life after myocardial infarction. *Qual Life Res* 1996; **5**: 151–61.
53 Oldridge N, Höfer S, McGee H, et al. The HeartQoL: I. Development of a new core health-related quality of life questionnaire for patients with ischemic heart disease. *Eur J Prev Cardiol* 2014; **21**: 90–7.
54 Oldridge N, Höfer S, McGee H, et al. The HeartQoL: II. Validation of a new core health-related quality of life questionnaire for patients with ischemic heart disease. *Eur J Prev Cardiol* 2014; **21**: 98–106.
55 Aaronson NK, Ahmedzai S, Bergman B, et al. The European Organization for Research and Treatment of Cancer QLQ-C30: a quality-of-life instrument for use in international clinical trials in oncology. *J Natl Cancer Inst* 1993; **85**: 365–76.
56 Cella DF, Tulsky DS, Gray G, et al. The Functional Assessment of Cancer Therapy scale: development and validation of the general measure. *J Clin Oncol* 1993; **11**: 570–9.
57 Valderas JM, Kotzeva A, Espallargues M, et al. The impact of measuring patient-reported outcomes in clinical practice: a systematic review of the literature. *Qual Life Res* 2008; **17**: 179–93.
58 Rahimi K, Malhotra A, Banning AP, Jenkinson C. Outcome selection and role of patient reported outcomes in contemporary cardiovascular trials: systematic review. *Br Med J* 2010; **341**: c5707.
59 World Health Organization. *Adherence to long-term therapies: evidence for action*, 2003. Geneva: World Health Organization. URL: <http://apps.who.int/medicinedocs/en/d/Js4883e/1.html>
60 Osterberg L, Blaschke T. Adherence to medication. *N Engl J Med* 2005; **353**: 487–97.
61 Maddox TM, Ho PM. The role of treatment adherence in cardiac risk factor modification. In: Blumenthal R, Foody JM, Wong ND (eds), *Preventive cardiology. A companion to Brownwald's heart disease*, 2011, pp. 570–8. Amsterdam: Elsevier.
62 Ho PM, Bryson CL, Rumsfeld JS. Medication adherence: its importance in cardiovascular outcomes. *Circulation* 2009; **119**: 3028–35.
63 Caetano PA, Lam JM, Morgan SG. Toward a standard definition and measurement of persistence with drug therapy: examples from research on statin and antihypertensive utilization. *Clin Ther* 2006; **28**: 1411–24.
64 Cramer JA, Roy A, Burell A, et al. Medication compliance and persistence: terminology and definitions. *Value Health* 2008; **11**: 44–7.
65 Cramer J, Rosenheck R, Kirk G, et al. Medication compliance feedback and monitoring in a clinical trial: predictors and outcomes. *Value Health* 2003; **6**: 566–73.
66 Haynes RB, McDonald HP, Garg AX. Helping patients follow prescribed treatment: clinical applications. *J Am Med Assoc* 2002; **288**: 2880–3.
67 Jackevicius CA, Mamdani M, Tu JV. Adherence with statin therapy in elderly patients with and without acute coronary syndromes. *J Am Med Assoc* 2002; **288**: 462–7.
68 Jackevicius CA, Li P, Tu JV. Prevalence, predictors, and outcomes of a primary nonadherence after acute myocardial infarction. *Circulation* 2008; **117**: 1028–36.
69 Ho PM, Spertus JA, Masoudi FA, et al. Impact of medication therapy discontinuation on mortality after myocardial infarction. *Arch Intern Med* 2006; **166**: 1842–7.
70 Vrijens B, Vincze G, Kristanto P, et al. Adherence to prescribed antihypertensive drug treatments: longitudinal study of electronically compiled dosing histories. *Br Med J* 2008; **336**: 1114–17.
71 Ho PM, Magid DJ, Shetterly SM, et al. Medication nonadherence is associated with a broad range of adverse outcomes in patients with coronary artery disease. *Am Heart J* 2008; **155**: 772–9.
72 DiMatteo MR, Giordani PJ, Lepper HS, et al. Patient adherence and medical treatment outcomes: a meta-analysis. *Med Care* 2002; **40**: 794–811.
73 Sokol MC, McGuigan KA, Verbrugge RR, et al. Impact of medication adherence on hospitalization risk and healthcare cost. *Med Care* 2005; **43**: 521–30.
74 Rasmussen JN, Chong A, Alter DA. Relationship between adherence to evidence-based pharmacotherapy and long-term mortality after acute myocardial infarction. *J Am Med Assoc* 2007; **297**: 177–86.
75 Simpson SH, Eurich DT, Majumdar SR, et al. A meta-analysis of the association between adherence to drug therapy and mortality. *Br Med J* 2006; **333**: 15.
76 Morisky DE, Green LW, Levine DM. Concurrent and predictive validity of a self-reported measure of medication adherence. *Med Care* 1986; **24**: 67–74.
77 Morisky DE, Ang A, Krousel-Wood M, et al. Predictive validity of a medication adherence measure in an outpatient setting. *J Clin Hypertens* 2008; **10**: 348–54.
78 Gehi AK, Ali S, Na B, et al. Self-reported medication adherence and cardiovascular events in patients with stable coronary heart disease. The Heart and Soul Study. *Arch Intern Med* 2007; **167**: 1798–803.
79 Lowry KP, Dudley TK, Oddone EZ, et al. Intentional and unintentional nonadherence to antihypertensive medication. *Ann Pharmacother* 2005; **39**: 1198–203.

80 Claxton AJ, Cramer J, Pierce C. A systematic review of the associations between dose regimens and medication compliance. *Clin Ther* 2001; **23**: 1296–310.

81 Naderi SH, Bestwick JP, Wald DS. Adherence to drugs that prevent cardiovascular disease: meta-analysis on 376,162 patients. *Am J Med* 2012; **125**: 882–7.

82 Schillinger D, Piette J, Grumbach K, et al. Closing the loop: physician communication with diabetic patients who have low health literacy. *Arch Intern Med* 2003; **163**: 83–90.

83 Doshi JA, Zhu J, Lee BY, et al. Impact of a prescription copayment increase on lipid-lowering medication adherence in veterans. *Circulation* 2009; **119**: 390–7.

84 Choudhry NK, Avorn JA, Glynn RJ, et al.; for the Post-Myocardial Infarction Free Rx Event and Economic Evaluation (MI-FREEE) Trial. Full coverage for preventive medications after myocardial infarction. *N Engl J Med* 2011; **365**: 2088–92.

85 Haynes RB, Yao X, Degani A, et al. Interventions to enhance medication adherence. *Cochrane Database Syst Rev* 2005; (4): CD000011.

86 Schroeder K, Fahey T, Ebrahim S. Interventions for improving adherence to treatment in patients with high blood pressure in ambulatory settings. *Cochrane Database Syst Rev* 2004; (2): CD004804.

87 Kripalani S, Yao X, Haynes RB. Interventions to enhance medication adherence in chronic medical conditions: a systematic review. *Arch Intern Med* 2007; **167**: 540–50.

88 Eisen SA, Miller DK, Woodward RS, et al. The effect of prescribed daily dose frequency on patient medication compliance. *Arch Intern Med* 1990; **150**: 1881.

89 Schroeder K, Fahey T, Ebrahim S. How can we improve adherence to blood pressure-lowering medication in ambulatory care? Systematic review of randomized controlled trials. *Arch Intern Med* 2004; **164**: 722–32.

90 Laufs U, Rettig-Ewen V, Böhm M. Strategies to improve drug adherence. *Eur Heart J* 2011; **32**: 264–8.

91 Bangalore S, Kamalakkannan G, Parkar S, et al. Fixed-dose combinations improve medication compliance: a meta-analysis. *Am J Med* 2007; **120**: 713–19.

92 Gaziano TA, Opie LH, Weinstein MC. Cardiovascular disease prevention with a multidrug regimen in the developing world: cost-effectiveness analysis. *Lancet* 2006; **368**: 679–86.

93 Yusuf S, Pais P, Afzal R, et al. Effects of a polypill (Polycap) on risk factors in middle-aged individuals without cardiovascular disease (TIPS): phase II, double-blind, randomised trial. *Lancet* 2009; **373**: 1341–51.

94 Lee JK, Grace KA, Taylor AJ. Effect of a pharmacy care program on medication adherence and persistence, blood pressure and low-density lipoprotein cholesterol: a randomised controlled trial. *J Am Med Assoc* 2006; **296**: 2563–71.

95 Bernsten C, Bjorkman I, Caramona M, et al. Improving the well-being of elderly patients via community based provision of pharmaceutical care: a multicentre study in seven European countries. *Drugs Aging* 2001; **18**: 63–7.

96 Fahey T, Schroeder K, Ebrahim S. Interventions used to improve control of blood pressure in patients with hypertension. *Cochrane Database Syst Rev* 2006; (4): CD005182.

97 Wu JY, Leung WY, Chang S, et al. Effectiveness of telephone counselling by a pharmacist in reducing mortality in patients receiving polypharmacy: randomised controlled trial. *Br Med J* 2006; **333**: 522.

Index